BASIC HUMAN NEUROPHYSIOLOGY

THIRD EDITION

ARTHUR C. GUYTON, M.D.

Chairman and Professor of the Department of Physiology and
Biophysics, University of Mississippi School of Medicine

1981

W. B. SAUNDERS COMPANY

Philadelphia London Toronto Mexico City Sydney Tokyo

W. B. Saunders Company: West Washington Square
Philadelphia, PA   19105

1 St. Anne's Road
Eastbourne, East Sussex BN21 3UN, England

1 Goldthorne Avenue
Toronto, Ontario M8Z 5T9, Canada

Apartado 26370 — Cedro 512
Mexico 4, D.F., Mexico

9 Waltham Street
Artarmon, N.S.W. 2064, Australia

Ichibancho, Central Bldg., 22-1 Ichibancho
Chiyoda-Ku, Tokyo 102, Japan

Listed here is the latest translated edition of this book together with
the language of the translation and the publisher.

Portuguese (*2nd Edition*) — Editora Interamericana Ltda. Rio de Janeiro, Brazil

Spanish (*2nd Edition*) — Nueva Editorial Interamericana S.A. Mexico 4 D.F., Mexico

Basic Human Neurophysiology   ISBN   0-7216-4367-1

Last digit is the print number: 9   8   7   6   5   4   3   2   1

PREFACE

In this third edition of this book, *Basic Human Neurophysiology,* several very important changes have been made. Foremost of these has been the addition of four new chapters on the somatic control functions of the nervous system, such as nervous control of the circulation, of the heart, of the gastrointestinal system, of the endocrine system, of body temperature, and even of sexual functions. These chapters should be especially valuable to students of physiological psychology, to help in understanding the way that the nervous system interfaces with the total body. To make it easier for the student to understand transmission at synapses, a new introductory chapter has also been added to the text, which discusses basic mechanisms of membrane transport, especially movement of ions through membranes.

Another new feature of this edition is the use of color in the figures and major headings of the text. This new format makes it possible to emphasize important essentials of the different structures and mechanisms. And, because major advances have been made in recent years, especially in the understanding of molecular and chemical bases for nervous function, much new information will be found in almost every chapter.

This text is intended for those persons — medical students, paramedical students, students of psychology, students of basic physiology, and others — who wish to study the general organization and function of the nervous system without the detail often associated with a research-oriented text. Also, neuroanatomy is presented only to the extent that it is important to understanding how the nervous system performs its many tasks; this means mainly emphasis on nerve tracts and on function of the nerve signals when they reach their destination.

I have tried above all to present the beauty and logic intrinsic in the design of the nervous system — the automaticity of such feats as walking, sleeping, waking, and even search for food; the inbred pace-setting effects of emotions; and the almost magic processes for channeling, storing, and deciphering information. The nervous system is an overall controller of our bodily function. It is a computer with capabilities that have never yet been duplicated by the most massive electronic computer. And it is that quality of our being that makes life meaningful, thoughtful, exciting.

At many points in the text, one will find discussion of neurological illnesses as examples of abnormal function of the nervous system. These are presented not with the view that this book is dedicated only to medical students but, instead, because of the enlightening experience that a student can achieve when he correlates basic conceptual knowledge with happenings in the world about him. Indeed, understanding neurological abnormalities adds immeasurably to one's understanding of basic neurophysiological concepts. Therefore, even for the non–medically oriented student, the discussions of abnormal function in the nervous system are meant to give values that are difficult to establish in other ways.

PREFACE

I wish to thank many others who have made this text possible, particularly Mrs. Billie Howard, Mrs. Jane Strickland, Miss Gwendolyn Robbins, and Mrs. Laveda Morgan for their excellent secretarial services, Miss Tomiko Mita for her superb work on the new and colored illustrations, and the staff of the W. B. Saunders Company for its continued excellence in editing and preparing the text for publication.

ARTHUR C. GUYTON

CONTENTS

PART I
MEMBRANE BIOPHYSICS, NERVE, AND MUSCLE

PART II
THE CENTRAL NERVOUS SYSTEM

CHAPTER 13

CORTICAL AND CEREBELLAR CONTROL OF MOTOR FUNCTIONS 160

CHAPTER 14

ACTIVATION OF THE BRAIN—THE RETICULAR ACTIVATING SYSTEM; THE GENERALIZED THALAMOCORTICAL SYSTEM; BRAIN WAVES; EPILEPSY; WAKEFULNESS AND SLEEP 179

CHAPTER 15

THE CEREBRAL CORTEX AND INTELLECTUAL FUNCTIONS OF THE BRAIN.................................. 192

PART III
THE SPECIAL SENSES

CONTENTS

PART IV
NERVOUS CONTROL OF BODY FUNCTIONS

INTRODUCTION

The nervous system is the major controller of man's activities. It is composed principally of *nerve cells,* also called *neurons.* The nerve cell, in turn, has two major parts, the *nerve cell body* itself and long extensions called *nerve fibers.*

In the central nervous system, the neurons form a complex network that functions as a central computer for storing information and for controlling the different functional units of the body.

Leading from the central nervous system to the periphery is a vast array of peripheral nerves containing millions of nerve fibers which are the filamentous extensions of the neurons mentioned above. These provide two-way communication between the brain and the periphery, carrying sensory signals from all parts of the body to the brain and in turn carrying motor control signals back to the separate organs and tissues.

Basically, nerve signals are transmitted by the nerve cell membranes. To achieve this, each membrane has an electrical charge across it between the inside and the outside of the membrane. When this charge is sufficiently disturbed in any part of the neuron, for instance in a peripheral nerve ending or in the central nervous system, electrical currents suddenly begin to flow through the membrane. These currents in turn induce similar discharges in rapid succession all the way along the neuronal membrane, creating a ripple current that spreads over the entire nerve fiber and even over the neuronal cell body itself. This is called the *nerve impulse*; it is by means of many such impulses that signals are transmitted in the nervous system.

Within the central nervous system, and also in a few areas in the periphery, nerve signals are relayed from one neuron to another. This is achieved through special contact points between the successive neurons called *neuronal synapses.* It is mainly the synapses that determine where in the nervous system the signals will be transmitted. Later in this text we shall discuss in detail the mechanisms of nerve signal control, for they are the bases of the different nerve reflexes, of the processes of memory and thinking and generally of all other intellectual processes.

The nerve fibers that provide the communicating linkages between the body periphery and the central nervous system are of two types: *sensory nerve fibers* and *motor nerve fibers.* The sensory fibers all originate at special nerve endings called *nerve receptors.* Examples of these are pain receptors, touch receptors, vision receptors, hearing receptors, and so forth. Each one of these receptors is specifically organized so that it can elicit the needed electrical disturbance in the nerve fiber to generate nerve impulses. The motor nerve fibers, on the other hand, carry nerve signals outward from the central nervous system to the functioning elements of the body, especially to the muscles, the visceral organs, and the glands.

The first requirement in understanding the function of the nervous system is to study the basic means by which the nerve impulses themselves are transmitted along the nerve cell membranes. But, to understand this, it is also necessary to become familiar with the mechanisms for movement of the different ions through the cell membrane. Therefore, in Chapter 1 we will begin not with a discussion of the neuronal network of the nervous system but instead with the much more fundamental mechanisms that underlie ion transport through the cell membrane. The membrane transport processes are essentially the same for all types of cells whether they be nerve cells or other cells; these processes have special significance for nerve signal transmission, as will become evident as we proceed to the discussion of membrane potentials and nerve impulse transmission in Chapter 2.

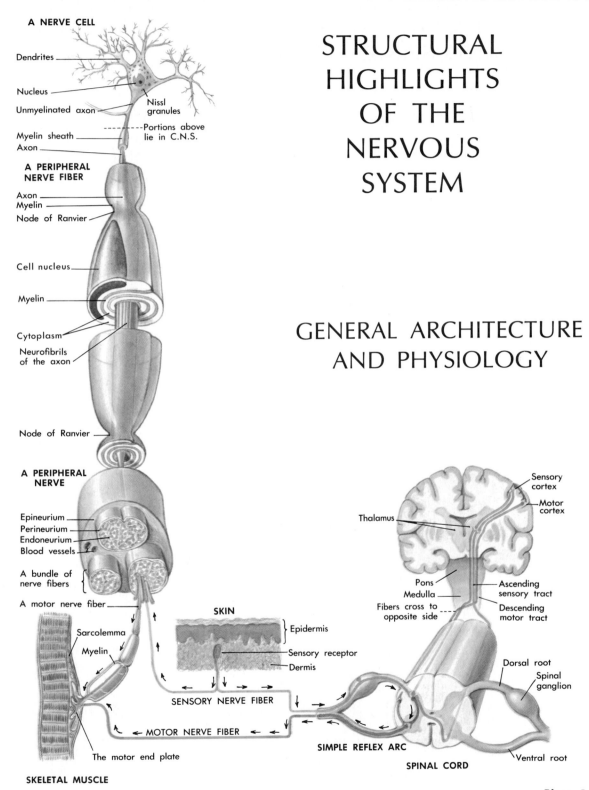

STRUCTURAL HIGHLIGHTS OF THE NERVOUS SYSTEM

GENERAL ARCHITECTURE AND PHYSIOLOGY

A NERVE CELL

Dendrites

Nucleus

Unmyelinated axon

Nissl granules

Myelin sheath

Axon

Portions above lie in C.N.S.

A PERIPHERAL NERVE FIBER

Axon

Myelin

Node of Ranvier

Cell nucleus

Myelin

Cytoplasm

Neurofibrils of the axon

Node of Ranvier

A PERIPHERAL NERVE

Epineurium

Perineurium

Endoneurium

Blood vessels

A bundle of nerve fibers

A motor nerve fiber

Sarcolemma

Myelin

The motor end plate

SKELETAL MUSCLE

SKIN

Epidermis

Sensory receptor

Dermis

SENSORY NERVE FIBER

← MOTOR NERVE FIBER ←

SIMPLE REFLEX ARC

Sensory cortex

Motor cortex

Thalamus

Pons

Medulla

Fibers cross to opposite side

Ascending sensory tract

Descending motor tract

Dorsal root

Spinal ganglion

Ventral root

SPINAL CORD

Plate 1

BRAIN AND SPINAL NERVES

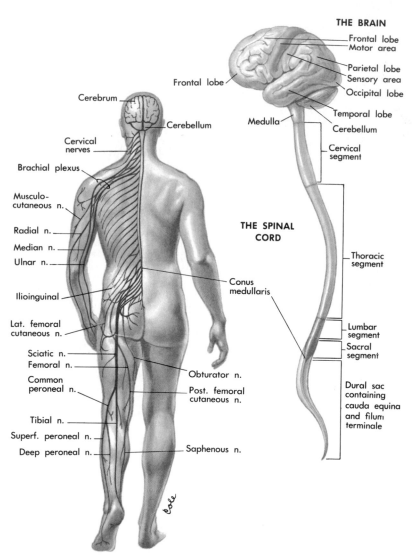

THE BRAIN

Frontal lobe
Motor area
Parietal lobe
Sensory area
Occipital lobe
Temporal lobe
Cerebellum

Frontal lobe

Medulla

Cerebrum

Cerebellum

Cervical
nerves

Cervical
segment

Brachial plexus

Musculo-
cutaneous n.

**THE SPINAL
CORD**

Radial n.

Thoracic
segment

Median n.

Ulnar n.

Conus
medullaris

Ilioinguinal

Lat. femoral
cutaneous n.

Lumbar
segment

Sacral
segment

Sciatic n.
Femoral n.

Obturator n.

Common
peroneal n.

Post. femoral
cutaneous n.

Dural sac
containing
cauda equina
and filum
terminale

Tibial n.

Superf. peroneal n.

Deep peroneal n.

Saphenous n.

THE MAJOR SPINAL NERVES

Plate 2

AUTONOMIC NERVES

Brain

Ciliary ganglion

Lacrimal gland

Oculomotor nerve III

Eye

Sphenopalatine ganglion

Facial nerve VII

Sup. cervical ganglion

Parotid gland

Glossopharyngeal nerve IX

Otic ganglion

Sublingual and submandibular glands

Submandibular ganglion

Vagus nerve X

Trachea

T1
2
3
4
5
6
7
8
9
10
11
12
L1
2
3

Lung

Heart

Greater splanchnic nerve

Lesser splanchnic nerve

Liver
Gallbladder

Least splanchnic nerve

Suprarenal gland

Renal plexus

Kidney

Stomach

Celiac plexus

Aortic plexus

Colon

Sup. mesenteric plexus

Small intestine

Inf. mesenteric plexus

Hypogastric plexus

S2
S3
S4

Pelvic nerves

Spinal cord

Vertebral ganglia (sympathetic trunk)

Ovary

Bladder

Pelvic plexus

Uterus

Testis

Urethra

SYMPATHETIC
Thoracolumbar outflow

Preganglionic sympathetic fibers
Postganglionic sympathetic fibers
Preganglionic parasympathetic fibers
Postganglionic parasympathetic fibers

PARASYMPATHETIC
Craniosacral outflow

Plate 3

ORGANS OF SPECIAL SENSE

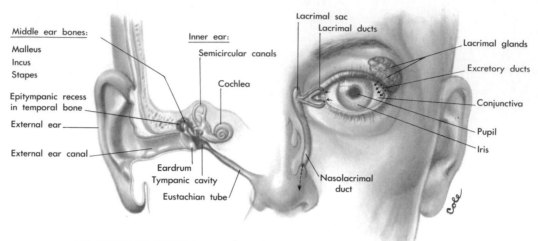

Middle ear bones:

Malleus
Incus
Stapes

Epitympanic recess in temporal bone

External ear

External ear canal

Inner ear:
Semicircular canals

Cochlea

Eardrum
Tympanic cavity

Eustachian tube

THE ORGAN OF HEARING

Lacrimal sac
Lacrimal ducts

Lacrimal glands

Excretory ducts

Conjunctiva

Pupil

Iris

Nasolacrimal duct

THE LACRIMAL APPARATUS AND THE EYE

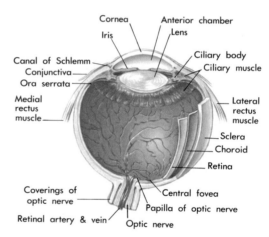

Cornea
Iris

Anterior chamber
Lens

Canal of Schlemm
Conjunctiva
Ora serrata
Medial rectus muscle

Ciliary body
Ciliary muscle

Lateral rectus muscle

Sclera
Choroid
Retina

HORIZONTAL SECTION OF THE EYE

Coverings of optic nerve

Retinal artery & vein

Optic nerve

Central fovea
Papilla of optic nerve

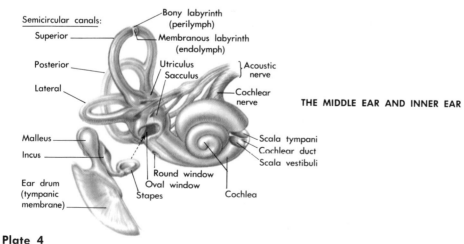

Semicircular canals:

Superior

Posterior

Lateral

Malleus

Incus

Ear drum (tympanic membrane)

Bony labyrinth (perilymph)

Membranous labyrinth (endolymph)

Utriculus
Sacculus

Acoustic nerve

Cochlear nerve

Scala tympani
Cochlear duct
Scala vestibuli

Round window
Oval window
Stapes

Cochlea

THE MIDDLE EAR AND INNER EAR

Plate 4

Part I
MEMBRANE BIOPHYSICS, NERVE, AND MUSCLE

1

Transport of Ions Through Cell Membranes

The fluid inside the cells of the body, called *intracellular fluid,* is very different from that outside the cells, called *extracellular fluid.* The extracellular fluid includes both the *interstitial fluid* that circulates in the spaces between the cells and also fluid of the *blood plasma* that mixes freely with the interstitial fluid through the capillary walls. It is the extracellular fluid that supplies the cells with nutrients and other substances needed for cellular function. But before the cell can utilize these substances, they must also be transported through the cell membrane.

Figure 1–1 gives the compositions of both the extracellular and intracellular fluids. Note that the extracellular fluid contains large quantities of *sodium* but only small quantities of *potassium.* Exactly the opposite is true of the intracellular fluid. Also, the extracellular fluid contains large quanti-

ties of chloride, while the intracellular fluid contains very little. But the concentrations of phosphates, essentially all of which are organic metabolic intermediates, and proteins in the intracellular fluid are considerably greater than in the extracellular fluid. These differences between the components of the intracellular and extracellular fluids are extremely important to the life of the cell. It is the purpose of this chapter to explain how these differences are brought about by the transport mechanisms in the cell membrane.

Substances are transported through the cell membrane by two major processes, *diffusion* and *active transport.* Though there are many different variations of these two basic mechanisms, as we shall see later in this chapter, basically, diffusion means free movement of substances in a random fashion caused by the normal kinetic motion of matter, whereas active transport means movement of substances in chemical combination with *carrier substances* in the membrane and also against an energy gradient, such as from a low concentration state to a high concentration state, a process that requires chemical energy to cause the movement.

DIFFUSION

All molecules and ions in the body fluids, including both water molecules and dissolved substances, are in constant motion, each particle moving its own separate way. Motion of these particles is what physicists call heat — the greater the motion, the higher is the temperature — and motion never ceases under any conditions except absolute zero temperature. When a moving molecule, A, approaches a stationary molecule, B, the electrostatic and internuclear forces of molecule A repel molecule B, adding some of the energy of motion to molecule B. Consequently, molecule B

	EXTRACELLULAR FLUID	INTRACELLULAR FLUID
Na⁺	142 mEq/l.	10 mEq/l.
K⁺	4 mEq/l.	140 mEq/l.
Ca⁺⁺	5 mEq/l.	<1 mEq/L
Mg⁺⁺	3 mEq/l.	58 mEq/l.
Cl⁻	103 mEq/l.	4 mEq/l.
HCO₃⁻	28 mEq/l.	10 mEq/l.
Phosphates	4 mEq/l.	75 mEq/l.
SO₄⁻⁻	1 mEq/l.	2 mEq/l.
Glucose	90 mgm.%	0 to 20 mgm.%
Amino acids	30 mgm.%	200 mgm.%?
Cholesterol Phospholipids Neutral fat	0.5 gm.%	2 to 95 gm.%
Po₂	35 mm.Hg	20 mm.Hg ?
Pco₂	46 mm.Hg	50 mm.Hg ?
pH	7.4	7.0
Proteins	2 gm.% (5 mEq./l.)	16 gm.% (40 mEq/l)

Figure 1–1. Chemical compositions of extracellular and intracellular fluids.

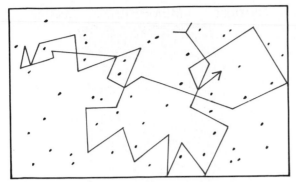

Figure 1–2. Diffusion of a fluid molecule during a fraction of a second.

gains kinetic energy of motion while molecule A slows down, losing some of its kinetic energy. Thus, as shown in Figure 1–2, a single molecule in solution bounces among the other molecules first in one direction, then another, then another, and so forth, bouncing randomly hundreds to millions of times each second. At times it travels a far distance before striking the next molecule, but at other times only a short distance.

This continual movement of molecules among each other in liquids, or in gases, is called *diffusion.* Ions diffuse in exactly the same manner as whole molecules, and even suspended colloid particles diffuse in a similar manner, except that because of their very large sizes they diffuse far less rapidly than molecular substances.

KINETICS OF DIFFUSION — THE CONCENTRATION DIFFERENCE

When a large amount of dissolved substance is placed in a solvent at one end of a chamber, it immediately begins to diffuse toward the opposite end of the chamber. If the same amount of substance is placed in the opposite end of the chamber, it begins to diffuse toward the first end, the same amount diffusing in each direction. As a result, the *net rate of diffusion* from one end to the other is zero. If, however, the concentration of the substance is greater at one end of the chamber than at the other end, the net rate of diffusion from the area of high concentration to low concentration is directly proportional to the larger concentration minus the lower concentration. The total concentration change along the axis of the chamber is called a *concentration difference,* and the concentration difference divided by the dis-

tance is called the *concentration* or *diffusion gradient.*

The rapidity with which a molecule diffuses from one point to another is less the greater the molecular size, because large particles are not impelled so intensely by collisions with other molecules. The rate of diffusion is approximately inversely proportional to the square root of the molecular weight but it is affected by the shape of the molecule as well.

If we consider all the different factors that affect the rate of diffusion of a substance from one area to another, they are the following:

(1) The greater the concentration difference, the greater is the rate of diffusion.

(2) The less the square root of the molecular weight, the greater is the rate of diffusion.

(3) The shorter the distance, the greater is the rate.

(4) The greater the cross-section of the chamber in which diffusion is taking place, the greater is the rate of diffusion.

(5) The greater the temperature, the greater is the molecular motion and also the greater is the rate of diffusion. All these can be expressed in an approximate formula, found at the bottom of this page, for diffusion in solutions.

DIFFUSION THROUGH THE CELL MEMBRANE

The cell membrane is essentially a sheet of lipid material, called the *lipid matrix,* with interspersed islands of globular protein molecules in the matrix. Some of these protein molecules penetrate all the way through the membrane. Water molecules and small dissolved molecules on each side of the membrane are believed to penetrate the protein portions of the membrane with ease, but the lipid portion of the membrane is an entirely different type of medium, acting as a limiting boundary between the extracellular and intracellular fluids.

Therefore, two different methods by which substances can diffuse through the membrane are (1) by becoming dissolved in the lipid matrix and diffusing through it in the same way that diffusion occurs in water, or (2) by diffusing through minute pores that pass directly through the membrane at wide intervals over its surface; these "pores" are probably intramolecular spaces within the structures of the protein molecules that penetrate all the way through the membrane.

$$\text{Diffusion rate} \propto \frac{\text{Concentration difference} \times \text{Cross-sectional area} \times \text{Temperature}}{\sqrt{\text{Molecular weight}} \times \text{Distance}}$$

Diffusion in the Dissolved State Through the Lipid Portion of the Membrane

A few substances are soluble in the lipid of the cell membrane as well as in water. These include oxygen, carbon dioxide, alcohol, fatty acids, and other less important substances. When one of these comes in contact with the membrane it immediately becomes dissolved in the lipid and continues to diffuse in exactly the same manner that it diffuses within the watery medium on either side of the membrane. In other words, the molecule continues its random motion within the substance of the membrane in exactly the same way that it undergoes random motion in the surrounding fluids. However, the viscosity of the lipid matrix is about 300 times that of water, and this slows the diffusion by this amount despite the lipid solubility.

Effect of Lipid Solubility on Diffusion Through the Lipid Matrix. The primary factor that determines how rapidly a substance can diffuse through the lipid matrix of a cell membrane is its solubility in lipids. If it is very soluble, it becomes dissolved in the membrane very easily and therefore passes on through. Indeed, if it is more than 300 times as soluble in lipid than in water, it actually diffuses even more rapidly through the membrane than in the water of the surrounding fluids. On the other hand, almost no substances that dissolve very poorly in lipids, such as water, glucose, and the electrolytes, pass through the lipid matrix.

Facilitated Diffusion Through the Lipid Matrix

Some substances are very insoluble in lipids and yet can still pass through the lipid matrix by a process called *carrier-mediated* or *facilitated diffusion*. This is the means by which some sugar and amino acids in particular cross the membrane. The most important of the sugars is glucose, the membrane transport of which is illustrated in Figure 1–3. This shows that glucose (G1) combines with a *carrier* substance (C) at point 1 to form the compound CG1. This combination is soluble in the lipid so that it can diffuse (or simply move by rotation of the large carrier molecule) to the other side of the membrane, where the glucose breaks away from the carrier (point 2) and passes to the inside of the cell, while the carrier moves back to the outside surface of the membrane to pick up still more glucose and transport it also to the inside. Thus, the effect of the carrier is to make the glucose soluble in the membrane; without it, glucose cannot pass through the membrane.

The rate at which a substance passes through a membrane by facilitated diffusion depends on the difference in concentration of the substance on the two sides of the membrane, the amount of carrier

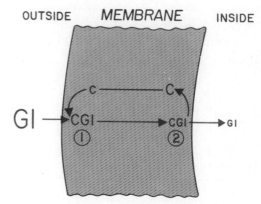

Figure 1–3. Facilitated diffusion of glucose through the cell membrane.

available, and the rapidity with which the chemical (or physical) reactions can take place. In the case of glucose transport and also transport of some of the amino acids, the overall rate is greatly increased by insulin, which is the primary hormone secreted by the pancreas. Large quantities of insulin can increase the rate of glucose transport about seven- to ten-fold, though it is not known whether this is caused by an effect of insulin to increase the quantity of carrier in the membrane or to increase the rate at which the chemical reactions take place between glucose and the carrier.

Very little is known about the carrier substance for transport of glucose through the membrane. It binds specifically with certain types of monosaccharides — glucose, mannose, galactose, xylose, and arabinose — but other monosaccharides are not transported at all or only slightly. A protein having a molecular weight of approximately 45,000 and also having the property of combining specifically and reversibly with the same types of monosaccharides that are transported has been discovered in the cell membrane. It is likely that this protein is the carrier substance for transport of glucose.

Many of the dynamics of facilitated diffusion are similar to those of active transport, which is discussed in detail later in the chapter. The primary difference between the two is that active transport can move substances through a membrane from a low concentration on one side to a high concentration on the other side, whereas in facilitated diffusion, the substance can move only from a high concentration toward a low concentration.

An important difference between facilitated diffusion and simple diffusion of free particles through a membrane is that the net diffusion rate of free particles is almost exactly proportional to the difference between the concentrations of the particles on the two sides of the membrane. However, for a carrier-transported substance, only when the concentrations of the substance are very small will this relationship hold. When the concentrations become great, the system becomes *saturated*, which means that then the rate at which facilitated diffusion will occur is determined by the quantity of available carrier or by the rates at which the chemical reactions between the mediated substance and the carrier can take place.

Diffusion Through the Membrane Pores

Some substances, such as water and many of the dissolved ions, seem to go through holes in the cell membrane called *membrane pores*. The nature of these pores is unknown. However, they are believed to be large protein molecules penetrating all the way through the cell membrane and providing pathways for movement of water-soluble substances within the intermolecular spaces of the protein. At any rate, these so-called "pores" in the cell membrane behave as if they were minute round holes approximately 0.8 nanometer (8 Angstroms) in diameter and as if the total area of the pores should equal approximately 1/5000 of the total surface area of the cell. Despite this very minute total area of the pores, water molecules diffuse so rapidly that the entire volume of fluid in some types of cells — the red blood cell for instance — can easily pass through the pores within one hundredth of a second.

Figure 1–4 illustrates a schematized structure of a pore, indicating that its surface is probably lined with negative charges, probably carboxyl or phosphate groups within the structure of the protein pore molecule. This figure shows several small particles passing through the pore and also shows that the maximum diameter of the particle that can pass through is approximately equal to the diameter of the pore itself, about 0.8 nanometer.

Effect of Pore Size on Diffusion Through the Pore — Permeability. Table 1–1 gives the effective diameters of various substances in comparison with the diameter of the pore, and it also gives the relative permeability of the pores for the different substances. *The permeability can be defined as the rate of transport through the membrane for a given concentration difference.* Note that some substances, such as the water molecule, urea molecule, and chloride ion, are considerably smaller in size than the pore. All these pass through most pores, particularly those of red cells, with great ease. For instance, the rate per second of diffusion of water in each direction through the pores of a red cell is about 100 times as great as the volume of the cell itself. It is fortunate that an identical amount of water normally diffuses in each direction, which keeps the cell from either swelling or shrinking despite the rapid rate of diffusion. The rates of diffusion of urea and chloride ions through the membrane are somewhat less than that of water, which is in keeping with the fact that their effective diameters are slightly greater than that of water.

Table 1–1 also shows that most of the sugars, including glucose, have effective diameters that are slightly greater than that of the pores. Obviously, not even a single molecule as large as these could go through a pore that is smaller than its size. For this reason essentially none of the

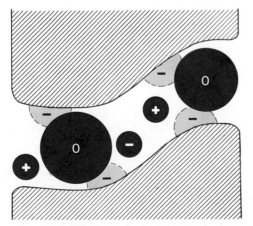

Figure 1–4. Postulated structure of the pore in the mammalian red cell membrane, showing the sphere of influence exerted by charges along the surface of the pore. (Modified from Solomon: *Sci. Am. 203*:146, 1960. ©1960 by Scientific American, Inc.)

TABLE 1–1 RELATIONSHIP OF EFFECTIVE DIAMETERS OF DIFFERENT SUBSTANCES TO PORE DIAMETER AND RELATIVE PERMEABILITIES

Substance	Diameter Å	Ratio to Pore Diameter	Approximate Relative Permeability
Water molecule	3	0.38	50,000,000
Urea molecule	3.6	0.45	1,500,000
Hydrated chloride ion			
(red cell)	3.86	0.48	500,000
(nerve membrane)	—	—	0.04
Hydrated potassium ion			
(red cell)	3.96	0.49	1.1
(nerve membrane)	—	—	0.02
Hydrated sodium ion			
(red cell)	5.12	0.64	1
(nerve membrane)	—	—	0.0003
Lactate ion	5.2	0.65	?
Glycerol molecule	6.2	0.77	?
Ribose molecule	7.4	0.93	?
Pore size	8 (Ave.)	1.00	—
Galactose	8.4	1.03	?
Glucose	8.6	1.04	0.4
Mannitol	8.6	1.04	?
Sucrase	10.4	1.30	?
Lactose	10.8	1.35	?

*These data have been gathered from different sources but relate primarily to the red cell membrane. Other cell membranes have different characteristics.

sugars can pass through the pores; instead, those that do enter the cell pass through the lipid matrix by the process of facilitated diffusion.

Effect of the Electrical Charge of Ions on Their Ability to Diffuse Through Membrane Pores. The electrical charges of ions often markedly affect their ability to diffuse through pores, sometimes impeding and sometimes enhancing their diffusion. Three major types of electrical forces affect ion diffusivity: (1) the intensity of electrical charges lining the pores, (2) the hydration energy of the ions, and (3) the potential difference across the membrane. Let us explain these.

First, there is reason to believe that different membrane pores are lined with either negative or positive charges. For instance, one set of pores, called *sodium channels,* seem especially to allow easy diffusion of sodium ions. It is believed that these pores are lined with strongly *negative* charges that attract sodium ions into the pores and then shuttle the sodium ions from one negative charge to the next, thus allowing rapid movement through the pores. On the other hand, larger-sized positive ions, such as potassium ions, have considerable difficulty passing through these channels, mainly because of their diameter.

Another instance in which the electrical charge of the pore probably affects ion diffusion is the following: It is believed that one end of the sodium channel sometimes becomes blocked by the presence of a *positive* charge appearing at the opening of the pore. This charge is called a *gate* because it repels the sodium ions and impedes their passage through the channel. We will discuss this gating theory for control of sodium transport through sodium channels in Chapter 2, in relation to transmission of the nerve impulse. Thus, ionic attraction in the pore can cause enhanced ion diffusion, while ionic repulsion can diminish ion diffusion.

The second factor that affects ion diffusion through pores, the hydration energy of the ion, mainly retards movement through pores. Most ions are loosely bound with water, and most or all of the water molecules bound with the ions must be removed before the particle size is small enough to allow passage through the pores. On the other hand, the smaller the ion, the greater is the hydration energy. For instance, the hydration energy for sodium is much greater than for potassium. Consequently, this factor impedes sodium transport through some pores far more than it does potassium transport because the water molecules can be broken away from potassium much more easily than from sodium. If the pores are very strongly negatively charged, as occurs in the sodium channels, this hydration energy can be overcome easily. However, in most cell membranes there seems to be a large population of either

uncharged pores or poorly charged pores that are relatively impermeable to sodium ions because of the high hydration energy of these ions but are relatively permeable to potassium ions because of their lower hydration energy. These pores are called *potassium channels.*

Third, many membranes have an electrical potential level in the fluid on one side of the membrane different from that on the other side; that is, the potential is more positive on one side and more negative on the other. Negative ions are attracted through the pores toward the positive fluid and positive ions toward the negative fluid. This is such an important effect that it will be discussed again later in this chapter and especially in Chapter 2.

Thus, several different factors determine the diffusivity of ions through cell membranes. In Chapter 2, we shall see that the permeability of the nerve membrane to sodium and potassium changes extremely rapidly, as much as 50- to 5000-fold, during the course of nerve impulse transmission. These changes presumably result from rapid alterations in the electrical charges lining the pores or guarding their entrances.

Effect of Different Factors on Pore Permeability. Pore permeability does not always remain exactly the same under different conditions. For instance, excess *calcium* in the extracellular fluid causes the permeability to decrease, and diminished calcium causes considerably increased permeability. This is extremely important in the function of nerves, for the enhanced permeability in extracellular fluid calcium deficiency causes excessive diffusion of ions, which results in spurious nerve discharge throughout the body.

Another factor that has an important effect on pore permeability of some cells is *antidiuretic hormone,* which is formed in the hypothalamus and secreted through the posterior pituitary gland. This hormone has an especially important effect on the membranes of the cells lining the collecting ducts of the kidney. Increased quantities of the hormone seem to increase the pore diameter, which allows water and other substances to diffuse from the tubules back into the blood with ease.

Net Diffusion Through the Cell Membrane and Factors That Affect It

From the preceding discussion, it is evident that many different substances can diffuse either through the lipid matrix of the cell membrane or through the pores. It should be noted, however, that substances that diffuse in one direction can also diffuse in the opposite direction. Usually it is not the total quantity of substances diffusing in both directions that is important to the cell but

7

instead the *net quantity* diffusing either into or out of the cell.

In addition to the permeability of the membrane, which has already been discussed, three other factors determine the rate of net diffusion of a substance: the concentration difference of the substance across the membrane, the electrical potential difference across the membrane, and the pressure difference across the membrane.

Effect of a Concentration Difference. Figure 1–5A illustrates a membrane with a substance in high concentration on the outside and low concentration on the inside. The rate at which the substance diffuses *inward* is proportional to the concentration of molecules on the outside, for this concentration determines how many of the molecules strike the outside of the pore each second. On the other hand, the rate at which the molecules diffuse *outward* is proportional to their concentration inside the membrane. Obviously, therefore, the rate of net diffusion into the cell is proportional to the concentration on the outside *minus* the concentration on the inside, or

$$\text{Net diffusion} \propto P(C_o - C_i)$$

in which C_o is the concentration on the outside, C_i is the concentration on the inside, and P is the permeability of the membrane for the substance.

Effect of an Electrical Potential Difference. If an electrical potential is applied across the membrane as shown in Figure 1–5B, ions, because of their electrical charges, will move through the membrane even though no concentration difference exists to cause their movement. Thus, to the left in Figure 1–5B, the concentrations of negative ions are exactly the same on both sides of the membrane, but a positive charge has been applied to the right side and a negative charge to the left, creating an electrical gradient across the membrane. The positive charge attracts the negative ions while the negative charge repels them. Therefore, net diffusion occurs from left to right. After much time large quantities of negative ions will have moved to the right (if we neglect, for the time being, the disturbing effects of the positive ions of the solution), creating the condition illustrated on the right in Figure 1–5B, in which a concentration difference of the same ions has developed in the direction opposite to the electrical potential difference. Obviously, the concentration difference is tending to move the ions to the left, while the electrical difference is tending to move them to the right. When the concentration difference rises high enough, the two effects exactly balance each other. At normal body temperature (38° C.), the electrical difference that will exactly balance a given concentration difference of univalent ions can be determined from the following formula called the *Nernst equation:*

$$\text{EMF (in millivolts)} = \pm 61 \log \frac{C_1}{C_2}$$

in which EMF is the electromotive force (voltage) between side 1 and side 2 of the membrane, C_1 is the concentration on side 1, and C_2 is the concentration on side 2. The polarity of the voltage on side 1 in the above equation is + for negative ions and − for positive ions. This relationship is extremely important in understanding the transmission of nerve impulses, for which reason it is discussed in even greater detail in Chapter 2.

Effect of a Pressure Difference. At times considerable pressure difference develops between the two sides of a membrane. This occurs, for instance, at the capillary membrane, which has a pressure approximately 23 mm. Hg greater inside the capillary than outside. Pressure actually means the sum of all the forces of the different molecules striking a unit surface area at a given instant. Therefore, when the pressure is increased on one side of a membrane, this means that the sum of all the forces of the molecules striking the pores on that side of the membrane is greater than

A

OUTSIDE *Membrane* INSIDE

B

C

Figure 1–5. Effect of (A) concentration difference, (B) electrical difference, and (C) pressure difference on diffusion of molecules and ions through a cell membrane.

on the other side. This can result either from greater numbers of molecules striking the membrane per second or from greater kinetic energy of the average molecule striking the membrane. In either event, increased amounts of energy are available to cause net movement of molecules from the high pressure side toward the low pressure side. This effect is illustrated in Figure 1–5C, which shows a piston developing high pressure on one side of a cell membrane, thereby causing net diffusion through the membrane to the other side.

For the usual red cell membrane, 1 mm. Hg pressure difference causes approximately 10^{-4} cubic micron of net diffusion of water through each square micron of membrane each second. This appears to be only a very minute rate of fluid movement through the membrane, but in relation to the normal cell size and the very large diffusion pressures that can develop at the cell membrane because of osmotic forces, as discussed later in the chapter, this rate can represent tremendous transport of fluid in only a few seconds.

Net Movement of Water Across Cell Membranes — Osmosis Across Semipermeable Membranes

By far the most abundant substance to diffuse through the cell membrane is water. It should be recalled again that enough water ordinarily diffuses in each direction through the red cell membrane per second to equal about *100 times the volume of the cell itself.* Yet, *normally,* the amount that diffuses in the two directions is so precisely balanced that not even the slightest *net* movement of water occurs. Therefore, the volume of the cell remains constant. However, under certain conditions, a *concentration difference for water* can develop across a membrane, just as concentration differences for other substances can also occur. When this happens, net movement of water does occur across the cell membrane, causing the cell either to swell or to shrink, depending on the direction of the net movement. This process of net movement of water caused by a concentration difference is called *osmosis.*

To give an example of osmosis, let us assume that we have the conditions shown in Figure 1–6, with pure water on one side of the cell membrane and a solution of sodium chloride on the other side. Referring back to Table 1–1, we see that water molecules pass through the cell membrane with extreme ease while sodium ions pass through only with extreme difficulty. And chloride ions cannot pass through the membrane because the positive charge of the sodium ions holds the negatively charged chloride ions back to maintain a balance between the negative and positive

charges in the solution, an effect called the *principle of electroneutrality.* Therefore, sodium chloride solution is actually a mixture of diffusible water molecules and non-diffusible sodium and chloride ions, and the membrane is said to be *semipermeable,* i.e., permeable to water but not to sodium and chloride ions. Yet, the presence of the sodium and chloride has reduced the concentration of water molecules to less than that of pure water. As a result, in the example of Figure 1–6, more water molecules strike the pores on the left side where there is pure water than on the right side where the water concentration has been reduced. Thus, net movement of water occurs from left to right — that is, osmosis occurs from left to right.

Osmotic Pressure

If in Figure 1–6 pressure were applied to the sodium chloride solution, osmosis of water into this solution could be slowed or even stopped. The amount of pressure required to stop osmosis completely is called the osmotic pressure of the sodium chloride solution.

The principle of a pressure difference opposing osmosis is illustrated in Figure 1–7, which shows a semipermeable membrane separating two separate columns of fluid, one containing water and the other containing a solution of water and some solute that will not penetrate the membrane. Osmosis of water from chamber B into chamber A causes the levels of the fluid columns to become farther and farther apart, until eventually a pressure difference is developed that is great enough to oppose the osmotic effect. The pressure difference

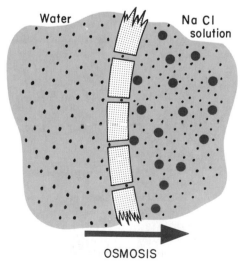

Figure 1–6. Osmosis at a cell membrane when a sodium chloride solution is placed on one side of the membrane and water on the other side.

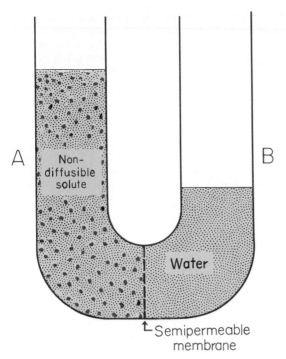

Figure 1–7. Demonstration of osmotic pressure on the two sides of a semipermeable membrane.

across the membrane at this time is the osmotic pressure of the solution containing the nondiffusible solute.

ACTIVE TRANSPORT

Often only a minute concentration of a substance is present in the extracellular fluid, and yet a large concentration of the substance is required in the intracellular fluid. For instance, this is true of potassium ions. Conversely, other substances frequently enter cells and must be removed even though their concentrations inside are far less than outside. This is true of sodium ions.

From the discussion thus far it is evident that *no substances can diffuse against a concentration gradient*, or, as is often said, "uphill." To cause movement of substances uphill, energy must be imparted to the substance. This is analogous to the compression of air by a pump. Compression causes the concentration of the air molecules to increase but to create this greater concentration, energy must be imparted to the air molecules by the piston of the pump as they are compressed. Likewise, as molecules are transported through a cell membrane from a dilute solution to a concentrated solution, energy must be imparted to the molecules. When a cell membrane moves molecules uphill against a concentration gradient (or uphill against an electrical or pressure gradient) the process is called *active transport.*

Among the different substances that are actively transported through cell membranes are sodium ions, potassium ions, calcium ions, iron ions, hydrogen ions, chloride ions, iodide ions, urate ions, several different sugars, and the amino acids.

BASIC MECHANISM OF ACTIVE TRANSPORT

The mechanism of active transport is believed to be similar for most substances and to depend on transport by *carriers.* Figure 1–8 illustrates the basic mechanism, showing a substance S entering the outside surface of the membrane where it combines with carrier C. At the inside surface of the membrane, S separates from the carrier and is released to the inside of the cell. C then moves back to the outside to pick up more S.

One will immediately recognize the similarity between this mechanism of active transport and that of facilitated diffusion discussed earlier in the chapter and illustrated in Figure 1–3. The difference, however, is that *energy is imparted to the system* in the course of active transport, so that transport can occur *against a concentration gradient* (or against an electrical or pressure gradient).

Though the mechanism by which energy is utilized to cause active transport is not entirely known, we do know some features of this process:

First, the energy is delivered to the inside surface of the membrane from high energy substances, principally adenosine triphosphate (ATP), inside the cytoplasm of the cell.

Second, active transport obeys the usual laws for chemical combination of one substance (the substance to be transported) with another substance (the carrier).

Third, a specific "carrier" molecule (or combination of molecules) is required to transport each type of substance or each class of similar substances.

Fourth, a specific enzyme (or enzymes) is required to promote active transport.

From this information, we can construct a theory for active transport, as follows: Referring again

Figure 1–8. Basic mechanism of active transport.

to Figure 1–8, we might suppose that the carrier has a natural affinity for the substance to be transported so that at the outer surface of the membrane the carrier and the substance readily combine. Then the combination of the two *diffuses* through the membrane to the inner surface. Here an enzyme-catalyzed reaction occurs, utilizing energy from ATP to split the substance away from the carrier. In other words, the enzyme-catalyzed reaction makes the affinity of the carrier for the transported substance very low and thereby displaces it from the combination. But the released substance, being insoluble in the membrane, cannot diffuse backward through the lipid matrix of the membrane. Therefore, it is released to the inside of the membrane while the carrier diffuses back to the outside surface to transport still another molecule of substance in the inward direction.

A special characteristic of active transport is that the mechanism *saturates* when the concentration of the substance to be transported is very high. This saturation results from limitation either of quantity of carrier available to transport the substance or of enzymes to promote the chemical reactions that release the substance from the carrier. Thus, the principle of saturation of active transport is almost identical with that of saturation of carrier-mediated facilitated diffusion, which was discussed earlier in the chapter.

Chemical Nature of Carrier Substances. Carrier substances are believed all to be proteins, conjugated proteins, or loose physical combinations of more than one protein molecule.

It has been suggested that the carrier might transport substances by a simple process of thermal motion, such as by rotating to expose its carrier site first to the outside surface of the cell membrane and then to the inside. But whether a "shuttling" of a "fixed" type of carrier exists, essentially the same principles of transport through the membrane would still apply.

Energetics of Active Transport. The amount of energy required to transport a substance actively through a membrane (aside from energy lost as heat in the chemical reactions) is determined by the degree that the substance is concentrated during transport. Compared to the energy required to concentrate a substance 10-fold, to concentrate it 100-fold requires twice as much energy, and to concentrate it 1000-fold requires three times as much. In other words, the energy required is proportional to the logarithm of the degree that the substance is concentrated as expressed by the following formula:

$$\text{Energy (in calories per osmole)} = 1400 \log \frac{C_1}{C_2}$$

Thus, in terms of calories, the amount of energy required to concentrate 1 osmole of substance 10-fold is about 1400 calories. One can see that the energy expenditure for concentrating substances in cells or for removing substances from cells against a concentration gradient can be tremendous. Some cells, such as those lining the renal tubules, expend almost 100 per cent of their energy for this purpose alone.

ACTIVE TRANSPORT OF SODIUM AND POTASSIUM

Referring back to Figure 1–1, one sees that the sodium concentration outside the cell is very high in comparison with its concentration inside, and the converse is true of potassium. Also, Table 1–1 shows that minute quantities of sodium and potassium can diffuse through the pores of the cell. If such diffusion should take place over a long period of time, the concentrations of the two ions would eventually become equal inside and outside the cell unless there were some means to remove the sodium from the inside and to transport potassium back in.

Fortunately, a mechanism for active transport of sodium and potassium ions is present in all cell membranes of the body. It is called the *sodium-potassium pump*. The basic principles of this pump are illustrated in Figure 1–9. The carrier for this mechanism transports sodium from inside the cell to the outside and potassium from the outside to the inside. And, because this carrier also has the capability of splitting ATP molecules and utilizing the energy from this source to promote the sodium and potassium transport, the carrier is called *sodium-potassium ATPase*. This ATPase is composed of two protein molecules, one a globulin with a molecular weight of 95,000 and the other a glycoprotein with a molecular weight of 55,000. The larger molecule actually binds with both the sodium and potassium ions and also with the ATP,

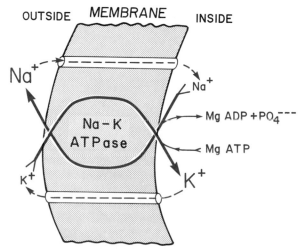

Figure 1–9. Postulated mechanism for active transport of sodium and potassium through the cell membrane, showing coupling of the two transport mechanisms and delivery of energy to the system at the inner surface of the membrane.

but the smaller molecule is also necessary to provide some facilitating function not yet understood.

Note in Figure 1–9 that *magnesium ATP* binds with the sodium-potassium ATPase at the inside surface of the membrane. The energy released from the ATP causes potassium ions to split away from the sodium-potassium ATPase carrier molecule and simultaneously causes sodium ions to bind. Then, at the outside surface of the membrane, the sodium ions split away from the carrier while potassium ions bind. But note that no energy source is required at the outside surface because the sodium release and potassium binding is an exothermic process that occurs without the need for additional energy. Thus, it is the intracellular ATP that provides the energy for transporting both the sodium and the potassium.

It should be noted especially that the sodium-potassium pump is powerful enough to transport sodium ions against concentration gradients as great as 20 to 1 and potassium gradients as great as 30 to 1.

One of the peculiarities of this sodium-potassium transport system is that it normally transports 3 sodium ions to the outside of the membrane for each 2 potassium ions transported to the inside. This gives a net transfer of 50 per cent more positive charges outward through the membrane than inward. Therefore, the sodium-potassium pump is called an *electrogenic pump* because it creates an electrical potential across the membrane whenever it pumps, creating negativity inside and positivity outside.

Another important feature of the pump is that it is strongly activated by an increase in sodium ion concentration inside the cell, the activity increasing in proportion to (sodium concentration)^3. This effect is extremely important because it allows even a slight excess buildup of sodium ions inside the cell to activate the pump very strongly and thereby return the intracellular sodium concentration back to its normal low level.

The sodium-potassium pump is so important to many different functioning systems of the body — such as to nerve and muscle fibers for transmission of impulses, various glands for the secretion of different substances, and all cells of the body to prevent cellular swelling — that we will discuss it at many different places in this text. In most instances it is the pumping of sodium rather than potassium that is especially important. Therefore, the sodium-potassium pump is called simply the *sodium pump*.

ACTIVE TRANSPORT OF OTHER IONS

Calcium and magnesium are transported by all cell membranes in much the same manner that sodium and potassium are transported, and certain cells of the body have the ability to transport still other ions. For instance, the glandular cell membranes of the thyroid gland can transport large quantities of iodide ion; the epithelial cells of the intestine can transport sodium, chloride, calcium, iron, hydrogen, and probably many other ions; and the epithelial cells of the renal tubules can transport calcium, magnesium, chloride, sodium, potassium, and a number of other ions.

REFERENCES

Andreoli, T. E., and Schaefer, J. A.: Mass transport across cell membranes: The effects of antidiuretic hormone on water and solute flows in epithelia. *Annu. Rev. Physiol.*, 38:451, 1976.

Andreoli, T. E., et al. (eds.): Membrane Physiology. New York, Plenum Press, 1980.

Avery, J. (ed.): Membrane Structure and Mechanisms of Biological Energy Transduction. New York, Plenum Press, 1974.

Bean, C. P.: The physics of porous membranes—neutral pores. *Membranes*, 1:1, 1972.

Ellory, C., and Lew, V. L. (eds.): Membrane Transport in Red Cells. New York, Academic Press, 1977.

Fettiplace, R., and Haydon, D. A.: Water permeability of lipid membranes. *Physiol. Rev.*, 60:510, 1980.

Finn, A. L.: Changing concepts of transepithelial sodium transport. *Physiol. Rev.*, 56:453, 1976.

Frizzell, R. A., and Heintze, K.: Transport functions of the gallbladder. *In* Javitt, N. B. (ed.): International Review of Physiology: Liver and Biliary Tract Physiology I. Vol. 21. Baltimore, University Park Press, 1980, p. 221.

Frizzell, R. A., and Schultz, S. G.: Models of electrolyte absorption and secretion by gastrointestinal epithelia. *In* Crane, R. K. (ed.): International Review of Physiology: Gastrointestinal Physiology III. Vol. 19. Baltimore, University Park Press, 1979, p. 205.

Gilles, R. (ed.): Mechanisms of Osmoregulation: Maintenance of Cell Volume. New York, John Wiley & Sons, 1979.

Glynn, I. M., and Karlish, S. J. D.: The sodium pump. *Annu. Rev. Physiol.*, 37:13, 1975.

Goresky, C. A.: Uptake in the liver: the nature of the process. *In* Javitt, N. B. (ed.): International Review of Physiology: Liver and Biliary Tract Physiology I. Vol. 21. Baltimore, University Park Press, 1980, p. 65.

Gregor, H. P., and Gregor, C. D.: Synthetic-membrane technology. *Sci. Am.*, 239(1):112, 1978.

Gupta, B. L., et al. (eds.): Transport of Ions and Water in Animals. New York, Academic Press, 1977.

Guyton, A. C., et al.: Dynamics and Control of the Body Fluids. Philadelphia, W. B. Saunders Co., 1975.

Hagiwara, S., and Jaffe, L. A.: Electrical properties of egg cell membranes. *Annu. Rev. Biophys. Bioeng.*, 8:385, 1979.

Hemmings, W. A. (ed.): Protein Transmission Through Living Membranes. New York, Elsevier/North-Holland, 1979.

Jacob, H. S. (ed.): Blood Cell Membranes. New York, Grune & Stratton, 1979.

Keynes, R. D.: Ion channels in the nerve-cell membrane. *Sci. Am.*, 240(3):126, 1979.

Korenbrot, J. I.: Ion transport in membranes: Incorporation of biological ion-translocating proteins in model membrane systems. *Annu. Rev. Physiol.*, 39:19, 1977.

Korn, E. D. (ed.): Methods in Membrane Biology. Vols. 1 and 2. New York, Plenum Press, 1974.

Korn, E. D.: Transport. New York, Plenum Publishing Corp., 1975.

Kotyk, A.: Mechanisms of nonelectrolyte transport. *Biochem. Biophys. Acta*, 300:183, 1973.

Lehninger, A. L.: The molecular organization of mitochondrial membranes. *Adv. Cytopharmacol.*, 1:199, 1971.

Lodish, H. F., and Rothman, J. E.: The assembly of cell membranes. *Sci. Am.*, 240(1):48, 1979.

Lux, S. E., et al. (eds.): Normal and Abnormal Red Cell Membranes. New York, A. R. Liss, 1979.

Macknight, A. D. C., and Leaf, A.: Regulation of cellular volume. *Physiol. Rev.*, 57:510, 1977.

Metcalfe, J. C. (ed.): Biochemistry of Cell Walls and Membranes II. Baltimore, University Park Press, 1978.

Packer, L.: Biomembranes: Architecture, Biogenesis, Bioenergetics, and Differentiation. New York, Academic Press, 1975.

Parsons, D. S. (ed.): Biological Membranes. New York, Oxford University Press, 1975.

Schultz, S. G.: Principles of electrophysiology and their application to epithelial tissues. *Int. Rev. Physiol., 4*:69, 1974.

Schultz, S. G., and Curran, P. F.: Role of sodium in non-electrolyte transport across animal cell membranes. *Physiologist, 12*:437, 1969.

Schultz, S. G., and Curran, P. F.: Coupled transport of sodium and organic solutes. *Physiol. Rev., 50*:637, 1970.

Sen, A. K., and Post, R. L.: Stoichiometry and localization of adenosine triphosphate-dependent sodium and potassium transport in the erythrocyte. *J. Biol. Chem., 239*:345, 1964.

Singer, S. J.: The molecular organization of membranes. *Annu. Rev. Physiol., 43*:805, 1974.

Solomon, A. K.: Properties of water in red cell and synthetic membranes. *Biomembranes, 3*:299, 1972.

Ullrich, K. L.: Sugar, amino acid, and Na^+ cotransport in the proximal tubule. *Annu. Rev. Physiol., 41*:181, 1979.

Van Winkle, W. B., and Schwartz, A.: Ions and inotrophy. *Annu. Rev. Physiol., 38*:247, 1976.

Wallick, E. T., *et al.*: Biochemical mechanism of the sodium pump. *Annu. Rev. Physiol., 41*:397, 1979.

Wright, E. M., and Diamond, J. M.: Anion selectivity in biological systems. *Physiol. Rev., 57*:109, 1977.

2

Membrane Potentials, Action Potentials, Excitation, and Rhythmicity

Electrical potentials exist across the membranes of essentially all cells of the body, and some cells, such as nerve and muscle cells, are "excitable" — that is, capable of self-generation of electrochemical impulses at their membranes and, in some instances, utilization of these impulses to transmit signals along the membranes. In still other types of cells, such as glandular cells, macrophages, and ciliated cells, changes in membrane potentials probably play significant roles in controlling many of the cell's functions. However, the present discussion is concerned with membrane potentials generated both at rest and during action by nerve and muscle cells.

BASIC PHYSICS OF MEMBRANE POTENTIALS

Before beginning this discussion, let us first recall that the fluids both inside and outside the cells are electrolytic solutions containing 150 to 160 mEq. per liter of positive ions and the same concentration of negative ions. Generally, a very minute excess of negative ions (anions) accumulates immediately inside the cell membrane along its inner surface, and an equal number of positive ions (cations) accumulates immediately outside the membrane. The effect of this is the establishment of a *membrane potential* between the inside and outside of the cell.

The two basic means by which membrane potentials can develop are: (1) active transport of ions through the membrane, thus creating an imbalance of negative and positive charges on the two sides of the membrane, and (2) diffusion of ions through the membrane as a result of ion concentration differences between the two sides of the membrane, thus also creating an imbalance of charges.

MEMBRANE POTENTIALS CAUSED BY ACTIVE TRANSPORT — THE "ELECTROGENIC PUMP"

Figure 2–1A illustrates how the process of active transport can create a membrane potential. In this figure equal concentrations of anions, which are *negatively charged,* are present both inside and outside the nerve fiber. However, the sodium "pump," which was discussed in Chapter 1, has transported some of the *positively charged* sodium ions to the exterior of the fiber. Thus, more negatively charged anions than positively charged sodium ions remain inside the nerve fiber, causing negativity on the inside. On the other hand, outside the fiber there are more positively charged sodium ions than negatively charged anions, thus causing positivity outside the fiber. A pump such as this, which causes the development of a membrane potential, is called an *electrogenic pump*.

In Chapter 1, it was pointed out that the sodium pump is also a potassium pump. That is, the same ATPase that acts as a carrier to transport sodium out of the cell also transports potassium inward at the same time. However, this pump normally transports three sodium ions outward for every two potassium ions inward. Thus, there is always more transfer of positively charged ions outward than inward. Because of this imbalance, the pump is still electrogenic. Therefore, as illustrated in Figure 2–1B, operation of this pump can still create electronegativity inside the nerve fiber membrane. We shall see in later sections of this chapter that this electrogenic pump is important in

ELECTROGENIC MEMBRANE POTENTIALS

DIFFUSION MEMBRANE POTENTIALS

Figure 2–1. A, Establishment of a membrane potential as a result of active transport of sodium ions out of the nerve fiber. B, Establishment of a membrane potential as a result of sodium and potassium pumping through the nerve membrane by the sodium-potassium electrogenic pump, three sodium ions passing out of the membrane for each two potassium ions entering the membrane. C, Establishment of a diffusion membrane potential caused by permeability of the membrane only to sodium ions while the membrane is impermeable to all other ions. D, Establishment of a diffusion membrane potential because of permeability of the membrane only to potassium ions while the membrane is impermeable to all other ions. Note that the internal membrane potential is positive in the case of sodium ion permeability and negative in the case of potassium ion permeability because of opposite concentration gradients.

establishing the membrane potential of probably all cells in the body.

MEMBRANE POTENTIALS CAUSED BY DIFFUSION

Figures 2–1C and D illustrate the nerve fiber when there is no active transport of either sodium or potassium. In Figure 2–1C the sodium concentration is very great outside the membrane while that inside is very low. Furthermore, the membrane is very permeable to the sodium ions but not to the anions. Because of the large sodium concentration gradient from the outside toward the inside, there is a strong tendency for sodium ions to diffuse inward. As they do so, they carry positive charges to the inside, thus creating a state of electropositivity inside the membrane, and electronegativity on the outside because of the negative anions that remain behind, that do not diffuse inward along with the sodium. This potential difference across the membrane tends to repel the sodium ions in the backward direction from inside

toward the outside. And within a millisecond or so the potential becomes great enough to block further diffusion of sodium ions to the interior. The potential at this point is called the Nernst potential, as we shall discuss below.

Figure 2–1D illustrates the same effect as that in Figure 2–1C but with a high concentration of potassium ions inside the membrane and a low potassium concentration outside. These ions are also positively charged. Also, the membrane is highly permeable to the potassium ions but impermeable to the anions. Diffusion of the potassium ions to the outside creates a membrane potential now of opposite polarity, with negativity inside and positivity outside, and, again, the membrane potential rises high enough within milliseconds to block further net diffusion of the potassium ions to the outside.

Thus, in both Figure 2–1C and D, we see that a concentration difference of ions across a semi-permeable membrane can, under appropriate conditions, cause the creation of a membrane potential. In later sections of this chapter, we shall also see that many of the membrane potential changes observed during the course of nerve and muscle impulse transmission result from the occurrence of rapidly changing diffusion membrane potentials.

Relationship of the Diffusion Potential to the Concentration Difference — The Nernst Equation. When a concentration difference of a single type of ions across a membrane causes diffusion of ions through the membrane, thus creating a membrane potential, the magnitude of the potential *inside* the membrane versus the outside is determined by the ratio of the tendency for the ions to diffuse in one direction versus the other direction, which is determined for positive ions by the following formula (*at body temperature, 38° C.*):

$$\text{EMF (millivolts)} = -61 \log \frac{\text{Conc. inside}}{\text{Conc. outside}}$$

Thus, when the concentration of positive ions on the inside of a membrane is 10 times that on the outside, the log of 10 is 1, and the potential difference calculates to be −61 millivolts. This equation is called the *Nernst equation*.

However, two conditions are necessary for this *Nernst potential* to develop as a result of diffusion: (1) The membrane must be semipermeable, allowing ions of one charge to diffuse through the pores while ions of the opposite charge do not diffuse. (2) The concentration of the diffusible ions must be greater on one side of the membrane than on the other side.

Using the above formula, let us now calculate the Nernst potential across the nerve membrane, first, when the membrane is permeable only to sodium ions, and, second, when the membrane is permeable only to potassium ions:

The normal concentration of sodium ions inside the nerve membrane is approximately 14 mEq. per liter and outside approximately 142 mEq. per liter. Thus, the ratio of these two is 0.10, and the logarithm of 0.10 is −1.00. Multiplying this by −61 millivolts gives a Nernst potential for sodium of +61 millivolts inside the nerve fiber membrane.

The normal concentration of potassium ions inside the nerve fiber is approximately 140 mEq. per liter and 4 mEq. per liter on the outside. The ratio of these two is 35. The logarithm of 35 is 1.54; this times −61 millivolts equals a Nernst potential for potassium of −94 millivolts inside the membrane.

Therefore, if there were no pumping of ions through the nerve membrane and if the membrane were permeable only to sodium but not at all to other ions, the potential inside the nerve fiber would be +61 millivolts. Conversely, if the membrane were permeable to potassium but not permeable to any other ions, the membrane potential would be −94 millivolts. We shall see later in this discussion that under resting conditions the membrane potential averages about −90 millivolts, which is very near to the −94 millivolts potassium Nernst potential. This is true because in the resting state the membrane is very permeable to potassium and only slightly permeable to sodium. On the other hand, when a nerve impulse is transmitted, the membrane, for a minute fraction of a second, becomes much more permeable to sodium than to potassium. Therefore, during this split second, the membrane potential rises to approximately +45 millivolts, which is much nearer the sodium Nernst potential than the potassium Nernst potential.

CALCULATION OF THE MEMBRANE POTENTIAL WHEN THE MEMBRANE IS PERMEABLE TO SEVERAL DIFFERENT IONS

When a membrane is permeable to several different ions, the diffusion potential that will develop depends on three factors: (1) the polarity of the electrical charge of each ion, (2) the permeability of the membrane (P) to each ion, and (3) the concentration of the respective ions on the two sides of the membrane. Thus, the following formula, called the *constant field equation* or the *Goldman equation*, gives the calculated membrane potential on the *inside* of the membrane when two univalent positive ions (cations, C) and

two univalent negative ions (anions, A) are involved.

$$\text{EMF (millivolts)} = -61 \log \frac{C_{1_i}^+ P_1 + C_{2_i}^+ P_2 + A_{3_o}^- P_3 + A_{4_o}^- P_4}{C_{1_o}^+ P_1 + C_{2_o}^+ P_2 + A_{3_i}^- P_3 + A_{4_i}^- P_4}$$

Note that a positive ion gradient from the inside (*i*) to the outside (*o*) of a membrane causes electronegativity inside the membrane, while a negative ion gradient in *exactly the opposite direction* also causes electronegativity on the inside.

The Cell Membrane as a Capacitor. Note in Figure 2–1A that the negative and positive ionic charges are shown lined up against the membrane. This occurs because the negative charges inside the membrane and the positive charges on the outside pull each other together at the membrane barrier, thus creating an abrupt change in electrical potential across the cell membrane.

This alignment of electrical charges on the two sides of the membrane is exactly the same process that takes place when an electrical capacitor becomes charged with electricity. In the cell membrane, the lipid matrix of the membrane is the *dielectric*, much as mica, paper, and mylar are frequently used as dielectrics in electrical capacitors. It will be recalled that a capacitor's capacity for holding electrical charges is inversely proportional to the thickness of the membrane. Because of the extreme thinness of the cell membrane (70 to 100 Angstroms), the capacitance of the cell membrane is tremendous for its area — about 1 microfarad per square centimeter (though only 1/1000 this much when insulated with a myelin sheath in the large nerve fibers).

Though the figures of this chapter will show large numbers of negative or positive ions (or charges) lined up against the nerve membrane, in actuality very few positive or negative ions need to line up on the two sides of the membrane to create the usual membrane potential of nerves. In the case of the usual large nerve fiber, only about 1/50,000 to 1/500,000 of the positive charges inside the nerve fiber need to be transferred to the outside of the fiber to create the normal nerve potential of −90 millivolts inside the fiber.

ORIGIN OF THE NERVE CELL MEMBRANE POTENTIAL

Distinction Between Original Development of a Membrane Potential and the Instantaneous Reestablishment of the Membrane Potential after Nerve Impulse Transmission. Let us assume that, in the beginning, the concentrations of all ions are the same inside and outside the nerve fiber. Under these conditions there will be no membrane potential. However, the normal cell will automatically develop a membrane potential. How does this come about? The answer to this lies in the function of the sodium-potassium pump and in the electrogenicity of this pump. That is, the continual pumping of more positive charges to the outside of the membrane than to the inside (three sodium ions pumped outward for every two potassium ions inward) eventually leads to the negative membrane potential inside the cell. Thus, the original development of the membrane potential results from this electrogenicity of the sodium-potassium pump.

But now let us write another scenario: First, assume that the sodium-potassium pump is nonfunctional but that there is already a high potassium concentration inside the cell and low potassium outside. Second, assume that the cell membrane is highly permeable to potassium while poorly permeable to sodium. Therefore, large numbers of potassium ions will diffuse to the outside while only a few sodium ions will diffuse to the inside. This results in far more transfer of positive ions to the outside than in the other direction. Consequently, once again a negative membrane potential develops inside the nerve membrane. It is in this manner that the negative membrane potential is re-established within less than a millisecond immediately following transmission of a nerve impulse along the nerve membrane.

Therefore, from the outset it is very important for the student to recognize the difference between the original development of the membrane potential, which is an electrogenic phenomenon, and the instantaneous re-establishment of the membrane potential following each nerve impulse (that is, following each action potential) which is a diffusion phenomenon. Now, let us discuss in detail the original development of the membrane potential.

Role of the Sodium-Potassium Pump and of Nondiffusible Anions in the Original Development of the Cell Membrane Potential. Before attempting to explain the original development of the cell membrane potential, several basic facts need to be understood:

1. The nerve membrane is endowed with a sodium-potassium pump, three sodium ions being pumped to the exterior for each two potassium ions pumped to the interior. This pump was discussed earlier in this chapter, and in even greater detail in Chapter 1.

2. The resting nerve membrane is normally 50 to 100 times as permeable to potassium as to sodium. Therefore, potassium diffuses with relative ease through the resting membrane, whereas sodium diffuses only with difficulty.

3. Inside the nerve fiber are large numbers of anions (negatively charged) that cannot diffuse through the nerve membrane at all or that diffuse

Figure 2–2. Establishment of a membrane potential of -90 millivolts in the normal resting nerve fiber and development of concentration differences of sodium and potassium ions between the two sides of the membrane. The dashed arrows represent diffusion and the solid arrows represent active transport (pumps).

very poorly. These anions include especially organic phosphate ions, sulfate ions, and protein ions.

Putting the above facts together, we can see how the resting nerve membrane potential comes about. First, sodium is pumped to the outside of the fiber, while potassium is pumped to the inside. However, because three sodium ions are pumped out of the fiber for every two potassium ions pumped in, more positive ions are continually being pumped out of the fiber than into it. Since most of the negatively charged anions inside the nerve fiber are nondiffusible, the negative charges remain inside the nerve fiber so that the inside of the fiber becomes electronegative, while the outside becomes electropositive, as illustrated in Figure 2–2.

Equilibration of Sodium Ion Transfer in the Two Directions Across the Membrane — Maximum Potential That Can Be Achieved by the Electrogenic Sodium-Potassium Pump. As progressively more sodium ions are pumped out of the nerve fiber, they begin to diffuse back into the nerve fiber for two reasons: (1) a sodium concentration gradient develops from the outside of the fiber toward the inside, and (2) a negative membrane potential develops inside the fiber and attracts the positively charged sodium ions inward. Eventually, there comes a point at which the inward diffusion equals the outward pumping by the sodium pump. When this occurs, the pump has reached its maximum capability to cause net transfer of sodium ions to the outside. This occurs when the sodium ion concentration inside the nerve fiber falls to about 14 mEq. per liter (in contrast to 142 mEq. per liter in the extracellular fluids) and when the membrane potential inside the fiber falls to −70 to −100 millivolts, averaging about −90 millivolts. Therefore, this −90 millivolts becomes the *resting potential* of the nerve membrane.

Equilibration of Potassium Ion Transfer Across the Membrane. At the same time that the sodium-potassium pump pumps sodium ions to the exterior, it pumps about two thirds as many potassium ions to the interior. However, the resting membrane is 50 to 100 times as permeable to potassium ions as to sodium ions, which means that each time potassium ions are pumped in they tend to diffuse back out of the fiber almost immediately. Therefore, the potassium pump by itself can build up only a slight excess of potassium ions inside the nerve fiber.

Yet, it is known that potassium ions do build up to a high concentration inside the nerve fiber. How could this be, if it is not caused by the potassium pump? The answer is the high degree of negativity created inside the fiber by the electrogenic sodium-potassium pump. The −90 millivolts inside the fiber attract the positive potassium ions from the exterior to the inside, and this attraction is essential for most of the buildup of potassium ions inside the fiber.

Thus, from a quantitative point of view, once the membrane has reached a steady state condition, three factors affect the equilibration of potassium ions on the two sides of the membrane: (1) the potassium pump pumping potassium ions *inward*, (2) the electrical gradient causing *inward* diffusion of potassium ions, and (3) the concentration gradient caused by the buildup of potassium ions inside the fiber causing diffusion of potassium ions *outward*. In the steady state condition, these three factors all come to exact quantitative equilibrium; that is, the two factors causing inward movement of potassium become exactly equal to the single factor causing outward movement.

Role of Chloride and Other Ions. Chloride ions are not pumped through the nerve membrane in either direction. However, they readily diffuse through the membrane. Because there is no pump to force buildup of a concentration difference of chloride ions across the membrane, the distribution of chloride ions on the two sides of the membrane is determined entirely by the degree and polarity of the membrane potential. That is,

the negativity that develops inside the membrane repels chloride ions from inside the fiber and causes the chloride concentration to fall to a very low value, about 4 mEq./liter in comparison with an extracellular fluid concentration of about 103 mEq./liter. Because there is no chloride pump, the Nernst equation can be used to calculate the exact concentration ratio of chloride ions on the two sides of the membrane when the membrane potential is known and when the membrane is in an equilibrium state. Thus, chloride ions play only a passive role. Later in the chapter we will discuss instantaneous changes in membrane potential caused by the so-called "action potential." Under these conditions, chloride ions move rapidly through the membrane and affect the duration and the magnitude of the action potential, but again their role is a passive one.

Essentially the same principles as those for sodium, potassium, and chloride distribution across the membrane also apply to other ions. Magnesium ions are affected in much the same way as potassium, and calcium ions in much the same manner as sodium ions. However, the concentrations and permeabilities of magnesium and calcium ions are small enough that the total number of electrical charges actually involved is also small. Yet both of these ions, especially calcium ions, affect membrane potentials in another way, by altering the permeability of the membrane to other ions, a subject that is discussed at greater length later in the chapter.

Membrane Potentials Measured in Nerve and Muscle Fibers. Figure 2–3 illustrates a method that has been used for measuring the resting membrane potential. A micropipet is made from a minute capillary glass tube so that the tip of the pipet has a diameter of only 0.25 to 2 microns. Inside the pipet is a solution of very concentrated potassium chloride, which acts as an electrical conductor. The fiber whose membrane is to be measured is pierced with the pipet and electrical connections are made from the pipet to an appropriate meter, as illustrated in the figure. The resting membrane potential measured in many different nerve and skeletal muscle fibers of mammals has usually ranged between −70 and −100 millivolts, with −90 millivolts as a reasonable average of the different measurements.

Figure 2–3. Measurement of the membrane potential of the nerve fiber using a micropipet.

THE ACTION POTENTIAL

In the above section we described the original development of the *resting membrane potential* and pointed out that it is normally about −90 mv. Now we will describe how membrane potentials are employed by nerve fibers to transmit nerve impulses, which is the means by which informational signals are transmitted from one part of the nervous system to another. This is achieved by means of *action potentials,* which are abrupt pulse-like changes in the membrane potential, lasting a few ten thousandths to a few thousandths of a second as illustrated in Figures 2–5, 2–6, 2–10, 2–11, and 2–12. And, for reasons that will be discussed below, the action potential moves along the length of the nerve, thus giving rise to the nerve signals.

An action potential can be elicited in a nerve fiber by almost any factor that suddenly increases the permeability of the membrane to sodium ions — such factors as electrical stimulation, mechanical compression of the fiber, application of chemicals to the membrane, or almost any other event that disturbs the normal resting state of the membrane. We shall see in Chapter 8 that the various nervous sensory receptors are also stimulated in one of these ways to initiate signals in the nervous system.

Role of Sodium and Potassium Membrane Diffusion Potentials in the Generation of the Action Potential. In the above discussion of the original development of the resting membrane potential, it became clear that the sodium-potassium pump is basically responsible for generating this resting potential. Furthermore, the sodium-potassium pump creates large sodium and potassium differences across the membranes, with very high sodium concentration outside the membrane and very high potassium concentration inside. But it is important to emphasize that once the sodium and potassium concentration differences have been created across the cell membrane, the occurrence of action potentials does not depend upon operation of the sodium-potassium pump. Indeed, many thousands of impulses can be transmitted even after the pump has been poisoned before the sodium and potassium concentration differences "run down." The action potential results from rapid changes in membrane permeability to sodium and potassium ions — the sodium permeability increasing about 5000-fold at the onset of the action potential, followed instantaneously by return of the sodium permeability to normal, and then the potassium permeability increases greatly. As a result, the membrane potential changes rapidly from its normal negative value to an instantaneous positive valve, then equally rapidly back to

its negative value. These changes will be discussed in the following sections.

Membrane Depolarization and Membrane Repolarization — the Two Stages of the Action Potential. The action potential occurs in two separate stages called *membrane depolarization* and *membrane repolarization,* each of which may be explained by referring to Figure 2–4. Figure 2–4A illustrates the resting state of the membrane, with negativity inside and positivity outside. When the permeability of the membrane to sodium ions suddenly increases, many of the sodium ions that are present in very high concentration outside the fiber rush to the inside, carrying enough positive charges to the inside to cause complete disappearance of the normal negative resting potential, and usually enough charges actually to develop a positive state inside the fiber. This sudden loss of normal negative potential inside the fiber is called *depolarization.* The positive potential that develops momentarily inside the fiber is called the *reversal potential.*

Almost immediately after depolarization takes place, the pores of the membrane again become almost impermeable to sodium ions, but at the same time considerably more permeable than normally to potassium ions. Therefore, sodium ions stop moving to the inside of the fiber, and, instead, potassium ions move to the outside because of the high potassium concentration on the inside. Thus, because the potassium ions are positively charged, the excess positive charges inside the fiber are transferred back out of the fiber, and the normal negative resting membrane potential returns. This effect, called *repolarization,* is illustrated in Fig-

Figure 2–4. Sequential events during the action potential, showing: A, the normal resting potential, B, development of a reversal potential during depolarization, and C, reestablishment of the normal resting potential during repolarization.

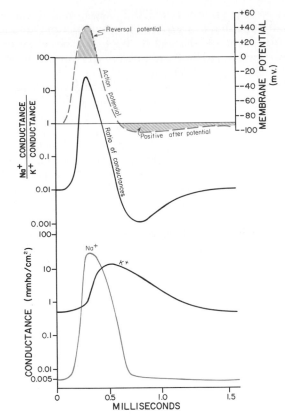

Figure 2–5. Changes in sodium and potassium conductances during the course of the action potential. Note that sodium conductance increases several thousand-fold during the early stages of the action potential, while potassium conductance increases only about 30-fold during the latter stages of the action potential and for a short period thereafter. (Curves constructed from data in Hodgkin and Huxley papers but transposed from squid axon to apply to the membrane potentials of large mammalian nerve fibers.)

ure 2–4C. The curve of Figure 2–5 shows the sequence of the recorded action potential inside the fiber membrane. Now let us explain in more detail *how* this sequence of events occurs.

Sodium "Channels" and Potassium "Channels." Most physiologists believe that the sodium and potassium ions diffuse mainly through separate types of pores. The pores through which the sodium ions diffuse are called *sodium channels* and those through which the potassium ions diffuse are called *potassium channels*. The actual anatomical structures of these channels are not known, but they have physiological properties *as if* the sodium channels were oval-shaped pores with dimensions of about 0.3 by 0.5 nanometer, and the potassium channels were round pores with dimensions of about 0.3 by 0.3 nanometer.

Each channel is believed to be guarded by an electrically charged "gate" that can open and close the channel. Under resting conditions, the gates of the sodium channels are almost completely closed, while those of the potassium channels are only partially closed; therefore, the potassium channels are some 50 to 100 times as permeable as the sodium channels. This difference allows far more potassium diffusion than sodium diffusion in the resting state, as has been explained. Yet, when the gates are widely opened, the permeability of the sodium channels can increase as much as 5000-fold, and the permeability of the potassium channels, which are already partially opened, can increase an additional 50-fold. It is this opening and closing of the gates to the sodium and potassium channels that is responsible for the depolarization and repolarization processes.

A Positive Feedback Regenerative Process that Opens the Sodium Gates to Cause Depolarization. The initial event in the causation of an action potential is a slight increase in the permeability of the membrane to sodium ions — that is, a slight opening of the sodium gates. When these gates open even a slight amount, a positive feedback effect immediately begins and initiates a regenerative cycle to open the gates still wider and wider until the sodium channel permeability increases within a few ten thousandths of a second about 5000-fold. This effect is illustrated by the abrupt rise in the sodium conductance curve (conductance = permeability × ion concentration) in Figure 2–5. At this instant the membrane is approximately 20 to 30 times as permeable to sodium as to potassium, because only the sodium channels open widely during the depolarization process. The result is that far more sodium ions now diffuse to the interior of the fiber than potassium ions to the exterior, carrying positive charges to the inside and leaving negative anions on the outside.

Mechanism of the Positive Feedback – The Gating Potential. Unfortunately, we do not know the exact means by which the gates of the sodium and potassium channels open and close. However, it is believed that the so-called gates are positive electrical charges which in turn are controlled by *gating potentials* that occur in the lipid matrix surrounding the sodium and potassium channels. When the gating potential is strong, the electrical charges are believed to repel the sodium or potassium ions and thereby close the gates. When weak, the channels open.

At the onset of the action potential, the first partial opening of the sodium channels allows enough sodium ions to flow to the interior of the fiber to cause partial depolarization. That is, the membrane potential changes from −90 mv. to approximately −60 mv. This change of potential inside the fiber is *in the positive direction* and it causes a *capacitative* change in the electrical field at the lining surfaces of the sodium channels to reduce the gating potentials of these channels. Consequently, the gates open more widely, still more sodium ions flow to the interior, the potential inside the fiber becomes still more positive, the gating potential becomes still weaker, the pores open even more widely, and still more sodium ions diffuse to the interior. Thus, the positive feedback regenerative cycle continues over and over again until the channels become fully opened. And the electrical potential inside the fiber becomes positive, about +45 mv., which is the *reversal potential,* as illustrated at the top of the action potential in Figure 2–5 (the upper curve).

Mechanism of Repolarization — Closure of the Sodium Channels and Opening of the Potassium Channels. Once the sodium channels become widely opened and the positive reversal potential appears inside the fiber, the sodium and potassium channel permeabilities make an about-face. The exact cause of this is not known, but it is known that the positive interior potential now causes electrical repulsion of the incoming sodium ions until their incoming movement slows or stops. This slowing of the sodium ion movement, for reasons not yet understood but it is possibly also an electrical field effect, causes the gating potential of the sodium channels to become strong once again. Consequently, at this point the sodium channels begin to close, but, just as rapidly, the potassium channels begin to open. This presumably results from the fact that the positive potential inside the membrane is now pushing potassium ions to the exterior at an extremely rapid rate. Loss of the potassium ions to the exterior carries positive charges to the exterior, and the potential on the interior of the fiber now returns toward the normal resting negative state. As the membrane becomes more negative, capacitative radiation of this negative field through the lipid matrix to the potassium channel gates opens the potassium channels.

Thus, during the repolarization process, a positive feedback regenerative cycle develops for opening the potassium channels, as illustrated by the increasing potassium conductance in Figure 2–5, in exactly the same way that a similar cycle had occurred during depolarization to open the sodium channels. More and more potassium ions pass to the exterior, and the electrical potential inside the fiber returns to the normal resting level of approximately −90 mv.

Once the membrane potential returns back to its negative resting level, it then remains at this level until the membrane is disturbed once again. The reason is that the potassium channels never close completely but only partially. Therefore, potassium ions continue to diffuse through the membrane with relative ease during the resting state, even though the permeability of the membrane to sodi-

um ions is greatly restricted. Thus, in the resting state, positive charges (the potassium ions) tend to diffuse out of the nerve fiber to the exterior, creating and maintaining negativity on the inside until the next action potential.

Role of Calcium Ions in Closing the Sodium Gates. When calcium ions are deficient in the extracellular fluid, the sodium gates will not close fully between action potentials, and the membrane remains very leaky to sodium ions — sometimes so much so that the membrane remains depolarized continuously or fires repetitively. Though the cause of this effect is not fully understood, a possible answer is the following: Since calcium ions tend to bind relatively strongly with proteins, it is possible that binding with the protein linings of the sodium channels creates an electrical field in or near the channels that blocks entry of sodium ions.

Quantity of Ions Lost from the Nerve Fiber During the Action Potential. The actual quantity of ions that must pass through the nerve membrane to cause the action potential — that is, to cause a 135 millivolt increase in the membrane potential and then to return this potential back to its normal resting level — is extremely slight. For large myelinated nerve fibers only about 1/100,000 to 1/500,000 of the ions normally inside the fiber are exchanged during this process. Nevertheless, this does cause a very slight increase of sodium ions inside the fiber and a corresponding very slight decrease in potassium ions. As we shall see later in the chapter, the active transport processes restore these ions within a few milliseconds or seconds.

RELATIONSHIP OF THE ACTION POTENTIAL TO THE POTASSIUM AND SODIUM NERNST POTENTIALS

Now that we have explained the events that transpire during the course of the action potential, let us review for a moment the relationship of this action potential to the potassium and sodium Nernst potentials. It was pointed out earlier in the chapter that under resting conditions the nerve membrane is highly permeable to potassium but only slightly permeable to sodium. Also, a calculation of the potassium Nernst potential earlier in the chapter showed this potential to be only a few millivolts more negative than the resting membrane potential. This is illustrated again in Figure 2–6, showing the potassium Nernst potential to be −94 mv. and a resting potential, −90 mv. Then, during the course of the action potential the membrane potential reverses and becomes approximately +45 mv, thus approaching the sodium Nernst potential of +61 mv., as also illustrated in the figure. However, the reversal potential is not as near to the sodium Nernst potential as the

Figure 2–6. Relationship of the action potential to the potassium and sodium Nernst potentials.

resting potential is to the potassium Nernst potential. The reason for this is that the ratio of sodium permeability to potassium permeability even at the peak of the action potential, about 20 to 1, never rises as high as the ratio of potassium permeability to sodium permeability during the resting state of the nerve fiber, about 75 to 1.

The reversal potential lasts for only a few fractions of a millisecond in a large myelinated nerve fiber, because the state of high permeability to sodium ions is a short-lived event. And when the permeability of the membrane to sodium decreases back to the normal level, the permeability to potassium ions now becomes highly dominant once again, which causes the resting potential to return to a level very near the potassium Nernst potential.

Thus, it can be seen that the potassium and sodium Nernst potentials represent the lower and upper limits of the membrane potential and that the action potential is displayed between these limits.

SOME EXPERIMENTAL METHODS THAT HAVE BEEN USED TO STUDY THE ACTION POTENTIAL

The events of the action potential, as discussed in the preceding few pages, have been studied most widely in the *squid axon*, a nerve fiber that is sometimes as large as 1 mm. in diameter. This fiber is large enough that potentials are easily measured on its inside, and it is even possible to remove the axoplasm from inside the fiber and to replace this with artificial solution. Also, electrodes can be placed inside the fiber to excite it or to "clamp" the voltage across the membrane — that is, to fix the voltage across the membrane at a constant level

by electronically controlling the current flow through the electrodes. Use of this clamping process has made it possible to study the effect of voltage changes on sodium and potassium permeabilities.

Two drugs have proved to be invaluable in the study of the sodium and potassium channels. One drug, *tetrodotoxin*, will block the sodium channels. However, it will block these channels only when applied to the outside of the nerve fiber. Nevertheless, when the sodium channels are blocked it is then possible to study the permeability of the potassium channels independently of the sodium channels. In a similar manner, application of *tetraethylammonium ion* to the inside of the fiber membrane blocks the potassium channels. In this state, the sodium channels can be studied independently of the potassium channels. Thus, by a painstaking process of elimination, the separate effects on the two types of channels are gradually being elucidated.

PROPAGATION OF THE ACTION POTENTIAL

In the preceding paragraphs we have discussed the action potential as it occurs at one spot on the membrane. However, an action potential elicited at any one point on an excitable membrane usually excites adjacent portions of the membrane, resulting in propagation of the action potential. The mechanism of this is illustrated in Figure 2–7. Figure 2–7A shows a normal resting nerve fiber, and Figure 2–7B shows a nerve fiber that has been excited in its midportion — that is, the midportion has suddenly developed increased permeability to sodium. The arrows illustrate a local circuit of current flow between the depolarized and the resting membrane areas; positive current flows inward through the depolarized membrane and outward through the resting membrane, thus completing a circuit. In some way not understood, *the outward current flow through the resting mem-*

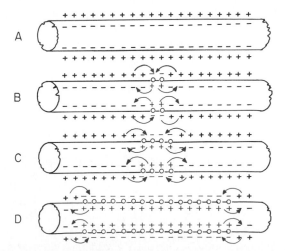

Figure 2–7. Propagation of action potentials in both directions along a conductive fiber.

brane *now increases the membrane's permeability to sodium,* which immediately allows sodium ions to diffuse inward through the membrane, thus setting up the vicious cycle of increasing sodium permeability discussed earlier in the chapter. As a result, depolarization occurs at this area of the membrane as well. Therefore, as illustrated in Figures 2–7C and D, successive portions of the membrane become depolarized. And these newly depolarized areas cause local circuits of current flow still farther along the membrane, causing progressively more and more depolarization. Thus, the depolarization process travels in both directions along the entire extent of the fiber. The transmission of the depolarization process along a nerve or muscle fiber is called a *nerve* or *muscle impulse.*

Direction of Propagation. It is now obvious that an excitable membrane has no single direction of propagation, but that the impulse can travel in both directions away from the stimulus — and even along all branches of a nerve fiber — until the entire membrane has become depolarized.

The All-or-Nothing Principle. It is equally obvious that, once an action potential has been elicited at any point on the membrane of a normal fiber, the depolarization process will travel over the entire membrane. This is called the all-or-nothing principle, and it applies to all normal excitable tissues. Occasionally, though, when the fiber is in an abnormal state the impulse will reach a point on the membrane at which the action potential does not generate sufficient voltage to stimulate the adjacent area of the membrane. When this occurs the spread of depolarization will stop. Therefore, for normal propagation of an impulse to occur, the ratio of action potential to threshold for excitation, called the *safety factor,* must at all times be greater than unity.

Propagation of Repolarization. The action potential normally lasts almost the same length of time at each point along a fiber. Therefore, repolarization normally occurs first at the point of original stimulus and then spreads progressively along the membrane, moving in the same direction that depolarization had previously spread. Figure 2–8 illustrates the same nerve fiber as that in Figure 2–7, showing that the polarization process

is propagated in the same direction as the depolarization process but a few ten thousandths of a second later.

"RECHARGING" THE FIBER MEMBRANE – IMPORTANCE OF ENERGY METABOLISM

Transmission of each impulse along the nerve fiber reduces the concentration differences of sodium and potassium between the inside and outside of the membrane. For a single action potential, this effect is so minute that it cannot even be measured. Indeed, 100,000 to 500,000 impulses can be transmitted by a large nerve fiber before the concentration differences have run down to the point that action potential conduction ceases. Yet, even so, with time it becomes necessary to re-establish these sodium and potassium membrane concentration differences. This is achieved by the action of the sodium and potassium pump in exactly the same way as that described in the first part of the chapter for establishment of the original resting potential. That is, the sodium ions that, during the action potentials, have diffused to the interior of the cell and the potassium ions that have diffused to the exterior are returned to their original state by the sodium and potassium pump. Since this pump requires energy for operation, this process of "recharging" the nerve fiber is an active metabolic one, utilizing energy derived from the adenosine triphosphate energy "currency" system of the cell.

A special feature of the sodium-potassium ATPase membrane pumping system is that its degree of activity is very strongly stimulated by excess sodium ions inside the cell membrane. In fact, the pumping activity increases approximately in proportion to the third power of the sodium concentration. That is, if the internal sodium concentration rises from 10 to 20 mEq. per liter, the activity of the pump does not merely double but instead

REPOLARIZATION

Figure 2–8. Propagation of repolarization in both directions along a conductive fiber.

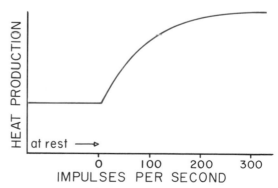

Figure 2–9. Heat production in a nerve fiber at rest and at progressively increasing rates of stimulation.

increases approximately 8-fold. Therefore, it can easily be understood how the recharging process of the nerve fiber can rapidly be set into motion whenever the concentration differences of sodium and potassium across the membrane begin to "run down."

Heat Production by the Nerve Fiber. Figure 2–9 illustrates the relationship of heat production in a nerve fiber to the number of impulses transmitted by the fiber each second. The rate of heat production is a measure of the rate of metabolism in the nerve, because heat is always liberated as a product of the chemical reactions of energy metabolism. Note that the heat production increases markedly as the number of impulses per second increases. It is this increased energy that causes the "recharging" process.

THE SPIKE POTENTIAL AND THE AFTER-POTENTIALS

Figure 2–10 illustrates an action potential recorded with a much slower time scale than that illustrated in Figure 2–5; many milliseconds of recording are shown in comparison with only the first 1.5 milliseconds of the action potential in Figure 2–5.

The Spike Potential. The initial, very large change in membrane potential shown in Figure 2–10 is called the spike potential. In large, type A myelinated nerve fibers it lasts for about 0.4 millisecond. The spike potential is the same as the first part of the action potential that has been discussed in the preceding paragraphs and is also called the *nerve impulse*.

The Negative After-Potential. At the termination of the spike potential, the membrane potential sometimes fails to return all the way to its resting level for another few milliseconds, as shown in Figure 2–10. This is particularly likely to occur after a series of rapidly repeated action potentials. This is called the *negative after-potential*. It is believed to result from a buildup of potassium ions immediately outside the membrane; this causes the concentration ratio of potassium across the membrane to be temporarily less than normal and therefore prevents full return of the normal resting membrane potential for a few additional milliseconds.

The Positive After-Potential. Once the membrane potential has returned to its resting value, it then becomes a little more negative than its normal resting value; this excess negativity is called the *positive after-potential*. It is a fraction of a millivolt to a few millivolts more negative than the normal resting membrane potential, but it lasts from 50 milliseconds to as long as many seconds.

The first part of this positive after-potential is caused by the excess permeability of the nerve membrane to potassium ions at the end of the spike potential, which drives the membrane potential nearer to the potassium Nernst potential, as was illustrated in Figure 2–6. However, the prolonged continuance of this potential is caused principally by the electrogenic pumping of excess sodium outward through the nerve fiber membrane, which is the recharging process that was discussed previously. If the active transport processes are poisoned, most of the positive after-potential is lost, though both the action potential and the negative after-potential continue to occur.

(The student might wonder why greater negativity in the resting membrane potential is called a positive rather than a negative after-potential, and, likewise, why the so-called negative after-potential is not named positive. The reason is that these potentials were first measured *outside* the nerve fibers rather than inside, and all potential changes on the outside are of exactly opposite polarity, whereas modern terminology expresses membrane potentials in terms of the inside potential rather than the outside potential.)

PLATEAU IN THE ACTION POTENTIAL

In some instances the excitable membrane does not repolarize immediately after depolarization, but, instead, the potential remains on a plateau near the peak of the spike sometimes for many milliseconds before repolarization begins. Such a plateau is illustrated in Figure 2–11, from which one can readily see that the plateau greatly prolongs the period of depolarization. It is this type of action potential that occurs in the heart, where the plateau lasts for as long as two- to three-tenths second and causes contraction of the heart muscle during this entire period of time.

The cause of the action potential plateau is probably a combination of several different factors. First, there is delay in closure of the sodium channels, which allows extra sodium ions to continue flowing into the fiber. Second, there is a small amount of calcium current flowing into the fiber at the same time, and these two currents together maintain the positive state inside the membrane that causes the plateau. However, third, probably equally as important is the fact that the permeability of the potassium channels decreases about five-fold at the onset of the action potential in excitable membranes that exhibit pla-

Figure 2–10. An idealized action potential, showing the initial spike followed by a negative after-potential and a positive after-potential.

Figure 2–11.   An action potential from a Purkinje fiber of the heart, showing a "plateau."

teaus, and this prevents rapid outflow of potassium ions to the outside of the fiber and, therefore, delays the repolarization process.

Yet, when closure of the sodium channels does begin, the process proceeds unabated; simultaneously, the potassium permeability of the membrane increases a hundred-fold or more. Therefore, sodium and calcium ions stop diffusing to the interior of the fiber, while potassium ions diffuse outward extremely rapidly. Consequently, the membrane potential returns quickly to its normal negative level, as illustrated in Figure 2–11, by the rapid decline of the potential at the end of the plateau.

RHYTHMICITY OF CERTAIN EXCITABLE TISSUES – REPETITIVE DISCHARGE

All excitable tissues can discharge repetitively if the threshold for stimulation is reduced low enough. For instance, even nerve fibers and skeletal muscle fibers, which normally are highly stable, discharge repetitively when they are placed in a solution containing the drug veratrine or when the calcium ion concentration falls below a critical value. Repetitive discharges, or rhythmicity, occur normally in the heart, in most smooth muscle, and also in many of the neurons of the central nervous system. It is these rhythmical discharges that cause the heart beat, that cause peristalsis, and that cause such neronal events as the rhythmical control of breathing.

The Re-Excitation Process Necessary for Rhythmicity.   For rhythmicity to occur, the membrane, even in its natural state, must be already permeable enough to sodium ions to allow automatic membrane depolarization. Thus, Figure 2–12 shows that the "resting" membrane potential is only −60 to −70 millivolts. This is not enough

negative voltage to keep the sodium channels closed. That is, (a) sodium ions flow inward, (b) this further increases the membrane permeability, (c) still more sodium ions flow inward, (d) the permeability increases more, and so forth, thus eliciting the regenerative process of sodium channel opening until an action potential is generated. Then, at the end of the action potential the membrane repolarizes. But shortly thereafter, the depolarization process begins again and a new action potential occurs spontaneously — this cycle continuing again and again and causing self-induced rhythmical excitation of the excitable tissue.

Yet why does the membrane not remain depolarized all the time instead of repolarizing, only to become depolarized again shortly thereafter? The answer to this can be found by referring back to Figure 2–5, which shows that toward the end of all action potentials, and continuing for a short period thereafter, the membrane becomes excessively permeable to potassium. The excessive outflow of potassium ions carries tremendous numbers of positive charges to the outside of the membrane, creating inside the fiber considerably more negativity than would otherwise occur for a short period after the preceding action potential is over. That is, the excessive potassium permeability counterbalances the naturally high sodium permeability, thus drawing the membrane potential nearer to the potassium Nernst potential. This is a state called *hyperpolarization*, which is illustrated in Figure 2–12. As long as this state exists, re-excitation will not occur; but gradually the excess potassium conductance (and the state of hyperpolarization) disappears, thereby allowing the onset of a new action potential.

Figure 2–12 illustrates this relationship between repetitive action potentials and potassium conductance. The state of hyperpolarization is established immediately after each preceding action potential; but it gradually recedes, and the membrane potential correspondingly increases until it reaches the *threshold* for excitation; then

Figure 2–12.   Rhythmic action potentials, and their relationship to potassium conductance and to the state of hyperpolarization.

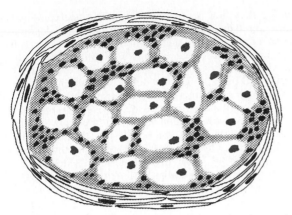

Figure 2–13. Cross-section of a small nerve trunk containing myelinated and unmyelinated fibers.

suddenly a new action potential results, the process occurring again and again.

SPECIAL ASPECTS OF IMPULSE TRANSMISSION IN NERVES

Myelinated and Unmyelinated Nerve Fibers. Figure 2–13 illustrates a cross-section of a typical small nerve trunk, showing a few very large nerve fibers that compose most of the cross-sectional area and many more small fibers lying between the large ones. The large fibers are *myelinated* and the small ones are *unmyelinated*. The average nerve trunk contains about twice as many unmyelinated fibers as myelinated fibers.

Figure 2–14 illustrates a typical myelinated fiber. The central core of the fiber is the *axon,* and the membrane of the axon is the actual *conductive membrane.* The axon is filled in its center with *axoplasm,* which is a viscid intracellular fluid. Surrounding the axon is a *myelin sheath* that is approximately as thick as the axon itself, and about once every millimeter along the extent of the axon the myelin sheath is interrupted by a *node of Ranvier.*

The myelin sheath is deposited around the axon by Schwann cells in the following manner: The membrane of a Schwann cell first envelops the axon. Then the cell rotates around the axon several times, laying down multiple layers of cellular membrane containing the lipid substance *sphingomyelin.* This substance is an excellent insulator that prevents almost all flow of ions. In fact, it increases the resistance to ion flow through the membrane approximately 5000-fold and also decreases the membrane capacitance as much as 1000-fold. However, at the juncture between each two successive Schwann cells along the axon, a small uninsulated area remains where ions can flow with ease between the extracellular fluid and the axon. This area is the node of Ranvier.

Saltatory Conduction in Myelinated Fibers from Node to Node. Even though ions cannot flow to a significant extent through the thick myelin sheaths of myelinated nerves, they can flow with considerable ease through the nodes of Ranvier. Indeed, the membrane at this point is 500 times as permeable as the membranes of some unmyelinated fibers.

Action potentials are conducted from node to node by the myelinated nerve rather than continuously along the entire fiber as occurs in the unmyelinated fiber. This process, illustrated in Figure 2–15, is called *saltatory conduction.* That is, electrical current flows through the surrounding extracellular fluids and also through the axoplasm from node to node, exciting successive nodes one after another. Thus, the impulse jumps down the fiber, which is the origin of the term "saltatory."

Figure 2–14. The myelin sheath and its formation by Schwann cells. (Modified from Elias and Pauley: Human Microanatomy. Philadelphia, F. A. Davis Company, 1966.)

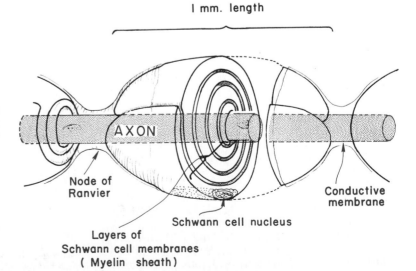

I mm. length

AXON

Node of
Ranvier

Schwann cell nucleus

Conductive
membrane

Layers of
Schwann cell membranes
(Myelin sheath)

Figure 2–15. Saltatory conduction along a myelinated axon.

Saltatory conduction is of value for two reasons: First, by causing the depolarization process to jump long intervals along the axis of the nerve fiber, this mechanism greatly increases the velocity of nerve transmission in myelinated fibers. Second, saltatory conduction conserves energy for the axon, for only the nodes depolarize, allowing several hundred times less loss of ions than would otherwise be necessary and therefore requiring little extra metabolism for re-establishing the sodium and potassium concentration differences across the membrane after a series of nerve impulses.

VELOCITY OF CONDUCTION IN NERVE FIBERS

The velocity of conduction in nerve fibers varies from as little as 0.5 meter per second in very small unmyelinated fibers up to as high as 130 meters per second (the length of a football field) in very large myelinated fibers. The velocity increases approximately with the fiber diameter in myelinated nerve fibers and approximately with the square root of fiber diameter in unmyelinated fibers.

EXCITATION — THE PROCESS OF ELICITING THE ACTION POTENTIAL

Chemical Stimulation. Basically, any factor that causes sodium ions to begin to diffuse inward through the membrane in sufficient numbers will set off the automatic, regenerative opening of the sodium channels, as noted earlier in the chapter, that eventuates in the action potential. Thus, certain chemicals can stimulate a nerve fiber by increasing the membrane permeability. Such chemicals include acids, bases, almost any salt solution of very strong concentration, and, most importantly, the substance *acetylcholine*. Many nerve fibers, when stimulated, secrete acetylcholine at their endings where they synapse with other neurons or

where they end on muscle fibers. The acetylcholine in turn stimulates the successive neuron or muscle fiber by opening pores in the membrane with diameters of 0.6 to 0.7 nanometer, large enough for sodium (as well as most other ions) to go through with ease. This is discussed in much greater detail in Chapter 4, and it is one of the most important means by which nerve and muscle fibers are stimulated. Likewise, *norepinephrine* secreted by sympathetic nerve endings can stimulate cardiac muscle fibers and some smooth muscle fibers, and still other hormonal substances can stimulate successive neurons in the central nervous system.

Mechanical Stimulation. Crushing, pinching, or pricking a nerve fiber can cause a sudden surge of sodium influx and, for obvious reasons, can elicit an action potential. Even slight pressure on some specialized nerve endings can stimulate these; this will be discussed in Chapter 8 in relation to sensory perception.

Electrical Stimulation. Electrical stimulation also can initiate an action potential. An electrical charge artificially induced across the membrane causes excess flow of ions through the membrane; this in turn can initiate an action potential. However, not all methods of applying electrical stimuli result in excitation, and, since this is the usual means by which nerve fibers are excited when they are studied in the laboratory, the process of electrical excitation deserves more detailed comment.

Cathodal Versus Anodal Currents. Figure 2–16 illustrates a battery connected to two electrodes on the surface of a nerve fiber. At the cathode, or negative electrode, the potential outside the membrane is negative with respect to that on the inside, and the positive current that flows outward through the membrane at this point is called *cathodal current*. At the anode, the electrode is positive with respect to the potential immediately inside the membrane, and the inward positive current flow at this point is called *anodal current*.

A cathodal current excites the fiber whereas an anodal current actually makes the fiber more resistant to excitation than normal. Though the cause of this difference between the two types of current cannot be explained completely, it is known that the normal impermeability of the membrane to sodium results partially from the high resting membrane potential across the membrane, and any condition that lessens this potential causes the membrane to become progressively more permeable to sodium. Obviously, at the cathode the applied voltage is opposite to the resting potential of the membrane, and this reduces the net potential. As a

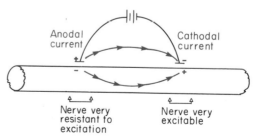

Figure 2–16. Effects of anodal and cathodal currents on excitability of the nerve membrane.

result, the membrane becomes far more permeable than usual to sodium followed by subsequent development of an action potential.

On the other hand, at the anode, the applied potential actually enhances the membrane potential. This makes the membrane less permeable to sodium than ever, resulting in increased resistance of the membrane to stimulation by other means.

Threshold for Excitation and "Acute Subthreshold Potential."   A very weak cathodal potential cannot excite the fiber. But, when this potential is progressively increased, there comes a point at which excitation takes place. Figure 2–17 illustrates the effects of successively applied cathodal stimuli of progressing strength. A very weak stimulus at point A causes the membrane potential to change from −90 to −85 millivolts, but this is not a sufficient change for the automatic regenerative processes of the action potential to develop. At point B the stimulus is greater, but, here again, the intensity still is not enough to set off the automatic action potential. Nevertheless, the membrane voltage is disturbed for as long as a millisecond or more after both of the weak stimuli; the potential changes during these short intervals of time are called *acute subthreshold potentials,* as illustrated in the figure.

At point C in Figure 2–17 the stimulus elicits an acute membrane potential that is not subthreshold but slightly more than the threshold value, and, after a short "latent period," it initiates an action potential. At point D the stimulus is still stronger, and the acute membrane potential initiates the action potential even sooner. Thus, this figure shows that even a very weak stimulus always causes a local potential change at the membrane, but that the intensity of the *local potential* must rise to a *threshold value* before the automatic action potential will be set off.

"Accommodation" to Stimuli.   When a cathodal potential applied to a nerve fiber is made to increase very slowly, rather than rapidly, the threshold voltage required to cause firing is considerably increased. This phenomenon is called *accommodation;* in other words, the excitable membrane is said to "accommodate" itself to slowly increasing potentials rather than firing. It is probable that a slowly increasing stimulatory current allows time for ions to build up (or become depleted) in the areas immediately adjacent to the fibers, these

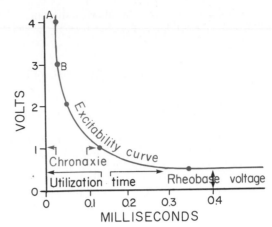

Figure 2–18.   Excitability of a large myelinated nerve fiber.

changes in ion concentrations partially opposing the stimulus.

Excitability Curve of Nerve Fibers.   A so-called "excitability curve" of a nerve fiber is shown in Figure 2–18. To obtain this curve a high voltage stimulus (4 volts, in this instance) is first applied to the fiber, and the minimum duration of stimulus required to excite the fiber is found. The voltage and minimal time are plotted as point A. Then a stimulus voltage of 3 volts is applied, and the minimal time required is again determined; the results are plotted as point B. The same is repeated at 2 volts, 1 volt, 0.5 volt, and so forth, until the least voltage possible at which the membrane is stimulated has been reached. On connection of these points, the excitability curve is generated.

The excitability curve of Figure 2–18 is that of a large myelinated nerve fiber. The least possible voltage at which it will fire is called the *rheobase,* and the time required for this least voltage to stimulate the fiber is called the *utilization time.* Then, if the voltage is increased to twice the rheobase voltage, the time required to stimulate the fiber is called the *chronaxie;* the chronaxie is often used as a means of expressing relative excitabilities of different excitable tissues. For instance, the chronaxie of a large type A fiber is about 0.0001 to 0.0002 second; of smaller myelinated nerve fibers, approximately 0.0003 second; of unmyelinated fibers, 0.0005 second; of skeletal muscle fibers, 0.00025 to 0.001 second; and of heart muscle, 0.001 to 0.003 second.

The Refractory Period.   A second action potential cannot occur in an excitable fiber as long as the membrane is still depolarized from the preceding action potential. Therefore, even an electrical stimulus of maximum strength applied before the first spike potential is almost over will not elicit a second one. This interval of inexcitability is called the *absolute refractory period.* The absolute refractory period of large myelinated nerve fibers is about 1/2500 second. Therefore, one can readily calculate that such a fiber can carry a maximum of about 2500 impulses per second. Following the absolute refractory period is a *relative refractory period* lasting about one quarter as long. During this period, stronger than normal stimuli are required to

Figure 2–17.   Effect of stimuli on the potential of the excitable membrane, showing the development of "acute subthreshold potentials" when the stimuli are below the threshold value required for eliciting an action potential.

excite the fiber. In some types of fibers, a short period of supernormal excitability follows the relative refractory period.

FACTORS THAT INCREASE MEMBRANE EXCITABILITY

Any condition that increases the natural permeability of the membrane usually causes it to become more excitable than usual. For instance, the drug *veratrine* has a direct action on the membrane to increase its permeability to sodium, and, as a consequence, the strength of stimulus needed to elicit an impulse is greatly reduced; or, on occasion, the fiber becomes so excitable that spontaneous impulses are generated without any extraneous excitation.

Low Calcium Tetany. An extremely important potentiator of excitability is low concentration of calcium ions in the extracellular fluids. Calcium ions normally decrease the permeability of the membrane to sodium. If sufficient calcium ions are not available, however, the permeability becomes increased, and, as a result, the membrane excitability greatly increases — sometimes so greatly that many spontaneous impulses result and cause muscular spasm. This condition is known as low calcium tetany. It often occurs in patients who have lost their parathyroid glands and who therefore cannot maintain normal calcium ion concentrations. This condition often causes respiratory muscle spasm and death.

INHIBITION OF EXCITABILITY — "STABILIZERS" AND LOCAL ANESTHETICS

Contrary to the factors that increase excitability, still others called *membrane stabilizing factors* can decrease excitability. For instance, a *high calcium ion concentration* decreases the membrane permeability and simultaneously reduces its excitability. Therefore, calcium ions are said to be a "stabilizer." Also, *low potassium ion concentration* in the extracellular fluids, because it increases the negativity of the resting membrane poten-

tial (a process called "hyperpolarization"), likewise acts as a stabilizer and reduces membrane excitability. Indeed, in a hereditary disease known as *familial periodic paralysis*, the extracellular potassium ion concentration is often so greatly reduced that the person actually becomes paralyzed but reverts to normal instantly after intravenous administration of potassium.

Local Anesthetics and the "Safety Factor." Among the most important stabilizers are the many substances used clinically as local anesthetics, including *cocaine, procaine, tetracaine,* and many other drugs. These act directly on the membrane, decreasing its permeability to sodium and, therefore, also reducing membrane excitability. When the excitability has been reduced so low that the ratio of *action potential strength to excitability threshold* (called the "safety factor") is reduced below unity, a nerve impulse fails to pass through the anesthetized area.

RECORDING MEMBRANE POTENTIALS AND ACTION POTENTIALS

The Cathode Ray Oscilloscope. Earlier in this chapter we noted that the membrane potential changes very rapidly throughout the course of an action potential. Indeed, most of the action potential complex of large nerve fibers takes place in less than $1/1000$ second. In some figures of this chapter a meter has been shown recording these potential changes. However, it must be understood that any meter capable of recording them must be capable of responding extremely rapidly. For practical purposes the only type of meter that is capable of responding accurately to the very rapid membrane potential changes of most excitable fibers is the cathode ray oscilloscope.

Figure 2–19 illustrates the basic components of a cathode ray oscilloscope. The cathode ray tube itself is composed basically of an *electron gun* and a *fluorescent surface* against which electrons are fired. Where the electrons hit the surface, the fluorescent material glows.

Figure 2–19. The cathode ray oscilloscope for recording transient action potentials.

If the electron beam is moved across the surface, the spot of glowing light also moves and draws a fluorescent line on the screen.

In addition to the electron gun and fluorescent surface, the cathode ray tube is provided with two sets of plates: one set, called the *horizontal deflection plates,* positioned on either side of the electron beam, and the other set, called the *vertical deflection plates,* positioned above and below the beam. If a negative charge is applied to the left-hand plate and a positive charge to the right-hand plate, the electron beam will be repelled away from the left plate and attracted toward the right plate, thus bending the beam toward the right, and this will cause the spot of light on the fluorescent surface of the cathode ray screen to move to the right. Likewise, positive and negative charges can be applied to the vertical deflection plates to move the beam up or down.

Since electrons travel at extremely rapid velocity and since the plates of the cathode ray tube can be alternately charged positively or negatively within less than a millionth of a second, it is obvious that the spot of light on the face of the tube can also be moved to almost any position in less than a millionth of a second. For this reason, the cathode ray tube oscilloscope can be considered to be an inertialess meter capable of recording with extreme fidelity almost any change in membrane potential.

To use the cathode ray tube for recording action potentials, two electrical circuits must be employed. These are (1) an *electronic sweep circuit* that controls the voltages on the horizontal deflection plates and (2) an *electronic amplifier* that controls the voltages on the vertical deflection plates. The sweep circuit automatically causes the spot of light to begin at the left-hand side and move slowly toward the right. When the spot reaches the right side it jumps back immediately to the left-hand side and starts a new trace.

The electronic amplifier amplifies signals that come from the nerve. If a change in membrane potential occurs while the spot of light is moving across the screen, this change in potential will be amplified and will cause the spot to rise above or fall below the mean level of the trace, as illustrated in the figure. In other words, the sweep circuit provides the lateral movement of the electron beam while the amplifier provides the vertical movement in direct proportion to the changes in membrane potentials picked up by appropriate electrodes.

Figure 2–19 also shows an electric stimulator used to stimulate the nerve. When the nerve is stimulated, a small *stimulus artifact* usually appears on the oscilloscope screen prior to the action potential.

Recording the Monophasic Action Potential. Throughout this chapter "monophasic" action potentials have been shown in the different diagrams. To record these, an electrode such as that illustrated earlier in the chapter, in Figure 2–3, must be inserted into the interior of the fiber. Then, as the action potential spreads down the fiber, the changes in the potential inside the fiber are recorded as illustrated earlier in the chapter, in Figures 2–5, 2–6, and 2–11.

Recording a Biphasic Action Potential. When one wishes to record impulses from a whole nerve trunk, it is not feasible to place electrodes inside the nerve fibers. Therefore, the usual method of recording is to place two

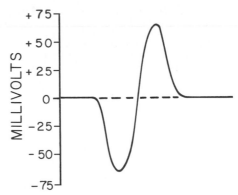

Figure 2–20. Recording of a biphasic action potential.

electrodes on the outside of fibers. However, the record that is obtained is then biphasic for the following reasons: When an action potential moving down the nerve fiber reaches the first electrode, it becomes charged negatively while the second electrode is still unaffected. This causes the oscilloscope to record in the negative direction. Then as the action potential is proceeding down the nerve, there comes a point when the membrane beneath the first electrode becomes repolarized while the second electrode is still negative, and the oscilloscope records in the opposite direction. When these changes are recorded by the oscilloscope, a graphic record such as that illustrated in Figure 2–20 is recorded, showing a potential change first in one direction and then in the opposite direction.

REFERENCES

Adrian, R. H.: Charge movement in the membrane of striated muscle. *Annu. Rev. Biophys. Bioeng.,* 7:85, 1978.

Agin, D.: Negative conductance and electrodiffusion in excitable membrane systems. *Membranes,* 1:249, 1972.

Aguayo, A. J., and Karpati, G. (eds.): Current Topics in Nerve and Muscle Research. New York, Elsevier/North-Holland, 1979.

Almers, W.: Gating currents and charge movements in excitable membranes. *In* Adrian, R. H., *et al.* (eds.): Reviews of Physiology, Biochemistry, and Pharmacology. New York, Springer-Verlag, 1978, p. 96.

Asbury, A. K., and Johnson, P. C.: Pathology of Peripheral Nerve. Philadelphia, W. B. Saunders Co., 1978.

Baker, P. F., and Reuter, H.: Calcium Movement in Excitable Cells. New York, Pergamon Press, 1975.

Baker, P. F., *et al.*: Replacement of the axoplasm of giant nerve fibers with artificial solutions. *J. Physiol. (Lond.),* 164:330, 1962.

Baker, P. F., *et al.*: The effects of changes in internal ionic concentrations on the electrical properties of perfused giant axons. *J. Physiol. (Lond.),* 164:355, 1962.

Brinley, F. J., Jr.: Calcium buffering in squid axons. *Annu. Rev. Biophys. Bioeng.,* 7:363, 1978.

Caldwell, P. C.: Factors governing movement and distribution of inorganic ions in nerve and muscle. *Physiol. Rev.,* 48:1, 1968.

Carmeliet, E., and Vereecke, J.: Electrogenesis of the action potential and automaticity. *In* Berne, R. M., *et al.* (eds.): Handbook of Physiology. Sec. 2, Vol. 1. Baltimore, Williams & Wilkins, 1979, p. 269.

Ceccarelli, B., and Clementi, F. (eds.): Neurotoxins, Tools in Neurobiology. New York, Raven Press, 1979.

Cohen, L. B.: Changes in neuron structure during action potential propagation and synaptic transmission. *Physiol. Rev.,* 53:373, 1973.

Cohen, L. B., and De Weer, P.: Structural and metabolic processes directly related to action potential propagation. *In* Brookhart, J. M., and Mountcastle, V. B. (eds.): Handbook of Physiology. Sec. 1, Vol. 1. Baltimore, Williams & Wilkins, 1977, p. 137.

Cole, K. S.: Electrodiffusion models for the membrane of squid giant axon. *Physiol. Rev., 45*:340, 1965.

Cuénod, M., *et al.* (eds.): Development and Chemical Specificity of Neurons. New York, Elsevier/North-Holland, 1979.

De Weer, P.: Aspects of the recovery process in nerve. *In* MTP International Review of Science: Physiology. Baltimore, University Park Press, 1975, Vol. 3, p. 231.

Ehrenstein, G., and Lecar, H.: The mechanism of signal transmission in nerve axons. *Annu. Rev. Biophys. Bioeng., 1*:347, 1972.

Finkelstein, A., and Mauro, A.: Physical principles and formalisms of electrical excitability. *In* Brookhart, J. M., and Mountcastle, V. B. (eds.): Handbook of Physiology. Sec. 1, Vol. 1. Baltimore, Williams & Wilkins, 1977, p. 161.

Fozzard, H. A.: Conduction of the action potential. *In* Berne, R. M., *et al.* (eds.): Handbook of Physiology. Sec. 2, Vol. 1., Baltimore, Williams & Wilkins, 1979, p. 335.

Glynn, I. M., and Karlish, S. J. D.: The sodium pump. *Annu. Rev. Physiol., 37*:13, 1975.

Greene, L. A., and Shooter, E. M.: The nerve growth factor: Biochemistry, synthesis, and mechanism of action. *Annu. Rev. Neurosci., 3*:353, 1980.

Guroff, G.: Molecular Neurobiology. New York, Marcel Dekker, 1979.

Hille, B.: Gating in sodium channels of nerve. *Annu. Rev. Physiol., 38*:139, 1976.

Hille, B.: Ionic basis of resting and action potentials. *In* Brookhart, J. M., and Mountcastle, V. B. (eds.): Handbook of Physiology. Sec. 1, Vol. 1. Baltimore, Williams & Wilkins, 1977, p. 99.

Hodgkin, A. L.: The Conduction of the Nervous Impulse. Springfield, Ill., Charles C Thomas, 1963.

Hodgkin, A. L., and Horowicz, P.: The effect of sudden changes in ionic concentrations on the membrane potential of single muscle fibres. *J. Physiol. (Lond.), 153*:370, 1960.

Hodgkin, A. L., and Huxley, A. F.: Movement of sodium and potassium ions during nervous activity. *Cold Spr. Harb. Symp. Quant. Biol., 17*:43, 1952.

Hodgkin, A. L., and Huxley, A. F.: Quantitative description of membrane current and its application to conduction and excitation in nerve. *J. Physiol. (Lond.), 117*:500, 1952.

Jack, J. J. B., *et al.*: Electric Current Flow in Excitable Cells. New York, Oxford University Press, 1975.

Jewett, D. L., and McCarroll, H. R., (eds.): Nerve Repair and Regeneration: Its Clinical and Experimental Basis. St. Louis, C. V. Mosby, 1979.

Jones, A. W.: Content and fluxes of electrolytes. *In* Bohr, D. F., *et al.* (eds.): Handbook of Physiology. Sec. 2, Vol. II. Baltimore, Williams and Wilkins, 1980, p. 253.

Katz, B.: Nerve, Muscle, and Synapse. New York, McGraw-Hill, 1968.

Keynes, R. D.: Ion channels in the nerve-cell membrane. *Sci. Am. 240*(3):126, 1979.

Kristensson, K.: Retrograde transport of macromolecules in axons. *Annu. Rev. Pharmacol. Toxicol., 18*:97, 1978.

Landowne, D., *et al.*: Structure-function relationships in excitable membranes. *Annu. Rev. Physiol., 37*:485, 1975.

Menaker, M., *et al.*: The physiology of circadian pacemakers. *Annu. Rev. Physiol., 40*:501, 1978.

Montal, M.: Experimental membranes and mechanisms of bioenergy transductions. *Annu. Rev. Biophys. Bioeng., 5*:119, 1976.

Mystrom, R. A.: Membrane Physiology. Englewood Cliffs, N.J., Prentice-Hall, 1973.

Narahashi, T.: Chemicals as tools in the study of excitable membranes. *Physiol. Rev., 54*:813, 1974.

Neher, E., and Stevens, C. F.: Conductance fluctuations and ionic pores in membranes. *Annu. Rev. Biophys. Bioeng., 6*:345, 1977.

Nelson, P. G.: Nerve and muscle cells in culture. *Physiol. Rev., 55*:1, 1975.

Noble, D.: Applications of Hodgkin-Huxley equations to excitable tissues. *Physiol. Rev., 46*:1, 1966.

Palay, S. L., and Chan-Palay, V.: General morphology of neurons and neuroglia. *In* Brookhart, J. M., and Mountcastle, V. B. (eds.): Handbook of Physiology. Sec. 1, Vol. 1. Baltimore, Williams & Wilkins, 1977, p. 5.

Patrick, J., *et al.*: Biology of cultured nerve and muscle. *Annu. Rev. Neurosci., 1*:417, 1978.

Pfenninger, K. H.: Organization of neuronal membrane. *Annu. Rev. Neurosci., 1*:445, 1978.

Rall, W.: Core conductor theory and cable properties of neurons. *In* Brookhart, J. M., and Mountcastle, V. B. (eds.): Handbook of Physiology. Sec. 1, Vol. 1. Baltimore, Williams & Wilkins, 1977, p. 39.

Ritchie, J. M.: A pharmacological approach to the structure of sodium channels in myelinated axons. *Annu. Rev. Neurosci., 2*:341, 1979.

Schultz, S. G.: Principles of electrophysiology and their application to epithelial tissues. *In* MTP International Review of Science: Physiology. Baltimore, University Park Press, 1974, Vol. 4, p. 69.

Schwartz, J. H.: Axonal transport: components, mechanisms, and specificity. *Annu. Rev. Neurosci., 2*:476, 1979.

Shanes, A. M.: Electrochemical aspects of physiological and pharmacological action in excitable cells. *Pharmacol. Rev., 10*:59, 165, 1958.

Somjem, G. G.: Electrogenesis of sustained potentials. *Prog. Neurobiol., 1*:201, 1973.

Spitzer, N. C.: Ion channels in development. *Annu. Rev. Neurosci., 2*:363, 1979.

Stevens, C. F.: The neuron. *Sci. Am., 241*(3):54, 1979.

Tasaki, I., and Hallett, M.: Bioenergetics of nerve excitation. *J. Bioenerg., 3*:65, 1972.

Trautwein, W.: Membrane currents in cardiac muscle fibers. *Physiol. Rev., 53*:793, 1973.

Ulbricht, W.: Ionic channels and gating currents in excitable membranes. *Annu. Rev. Biophys. Bioeng., 6*:7, 1977.

Varon, S. S., and Bunge, R. P.: Trophic mechanisms in the peripheral nervous system. *Annu. Rev. Neurosci., 1*:327, 1978.

Waggoner, A. S.: Dye indicators of membrane potential. *Annu. Rev. Biophys. Bioeng., 8*:47, 1979.

Walker, J. L., and Brown, H. M.: Intracellular ionic activity measurements in nerve and muscle. *Physiol. Rev., 57*:729, 1977.

Wallick, E. T., *et al.*: Biochemical mechanism of the sodium pump. *Annu. Rev. Physiol., 41*:397, 1979.

Waxman, S. G., (ed.): Physiology and Pathobiology of Axons. New York, Raven Press, 1978.

Zachar, J.: Electrogenesis and Contractility in Skeletal Muscle Cells. Baltimore, University Park Press, 1973.

3

Contraction of Skeletal Muscle

Approximately 40 per cent of the body is skeletal muscle and another 5 to 10 per cent is smooth and cardiac muscle. Many of the same principles of contraction apply to all these different types of muscle, but in the present chapter the function of skeletal muscle is considered mainly, while the specialized functions of smooth muscle will be discussed in the following chapter, and cardiac muscle in Chapter 5.

PHYSIOLOGIC ANATOMY OF SKELETAL MUSCLE

THE SKELETAL MUSCLE FIBER

Figure 3–1 illustrates the organization of skeletal muscle, showing that all skeletal muscles are made of numerous fibers ranging between 10 and 80 microns in diameter. Each of these fibers in

Figure 3–1. Organization of skeletal muscle, from the gross to the molecular level. F, G, H, and I are cross-sections at the levels indicated. (Drawing by Sylvia Colard Keene. From Bloom and Fawcett: A Textbook of Histology. Philadelphia, W. B. Saunders Company, 1975.)

Figure 3–2. Electron micrograph of muscle myofibrils, showing the detailed organization of actin and myosin filaments. Note the mitochondria lying between the myofibrils. (From Fawcett: The Cell. Philadelphia, W. B. Saunders Company, 1966.)

turn is made up of successively smaller subunits, also illustrated in Figure 3–1, that will be described in subsequent paragraphs.

In most muscles the fibers extend the entire length of the muscle, and, except for about 2 per cent of the fibers, each is innervated by only one nerve ending, located near the middle of the fiber.

The Sarcolemma. The sarcolemma is the cell membrane of the muscle fiber. However, the sarcolemma consists of a true cell membrane, called the *plasma membrane,* and a thin layer of polysaccharide material similar to that of the basement membrane surrounding blood capillaries; thin collagen fibrillae are also present in the outer layer of the sarcolemma. At the ends of the muscle fibers, these surface layers of the sarcolemma fuse with tendon fibers, which in turn collect into bundles to form the muscle tendons, and thence insert into the bones.

Myofibrils; Actin and Myosin Filaments. Each muscle fiber contains several hundred to several thousand *myofibrils,* which are illustrated by the many small open dots in the cross-sectional view of Figure 3–1C. Each myofibril (Figure 3–1D) in turn has, lying side-by-side, about 1500 *myosin filaments* and 3000 *actin filaments,* which are large polymerized protein molecules that are respons-

ible for muscle contraction. These can be seen in longitudinal view in the electron micrograph of Figure 3–2, and are represented diagrammatically in Figure 3–1E. The thick filaments are *myosin* and the thin filaments are *actin.* Note that the myosin and actin filaments partially interdigitate and thus cause the myofibrils to have alternate light and dark bands. The light bands, which contain only actin filaments, are called *I bands* because they are mainly *isotropic* to polarized light. The dark bands, which contain the myosin filaments as well as the ends of the actin filaments where they overlap the myosin, are called *A bands* because they are *anisotropic* to polarized light. Note also the small projections from the sides of the myosin filaments. These are called *crossbridges.* They protrude from the surfaces of the myosin filaments along the entire extent of the filament, except in the very center. It is interaction between these cross-bridges and the actin filaments that causes contraction.

Figure 3–1E also shows that the actin filaments are attached to the so-called *Z membrane* or *Z disc,* and the filaments extend on either side of the Z membrane to interdigitate with the myosin filaments. The Z membrane also passes from myofibril to myofibril, attaching the myofibrils to each other all the way across the muscle fiber. Therefore, the entire muscle fiber has light and dark bands, as is also true of the individual myofibrils. It is these bands that give skeletal and cardiac muscle their striated appearance.

The portion of a myofibril (or of the whole muscle fiber) that lies between two successive Z membranes is called a *sarcomere*. When the muscle fiber is at its normal fully stretched resting length, the length of the sarcomere is about 2.0 microns. At this length, the actin filaments completely overlap the myosin filaments and are just beginning to overlap each other. We shall see later that it is at this length that the sarcomere also is capable of generating its greatest force of contraction.

When a muscle fiber is stretched beyond its resting length, as it is in Figure 3–1, the ends of the actin filaments pull apart, leaving a light area in the center of the A band. This light area, called the *H zone*, is illustrated in Figure 3–2. Such an H zone rarely occurs in the normally functioning muscle because normal sarcomere contraction occurs when the length of the sarcomere is between 2.0 microns and 1.6 microns. In this range the ends of the actin filaments not only overlap the myosin filaments but also overlap each other.

The Sarcoplasm.   The myofibrils are suspended inside the muscle fiber in a matrix called *sarcoplasm*, which is composed of usual intracellular constituents. The fluid of the sarcoplasm contains large quantities of potassium, magnesium, phosphate, and protein enzymes. Also present are tremendous numbers of *mitochondria* that lie between and parallel to the myofibrils, a condition which is indicative of the great need of the contracting myofibrils for large amounts of ATP formed by the mitochondria.

The Sarcoplasmic Reticulum.   Also in the sarcoplasm is an extensive endoplasmic reticulum, which in the muscle fiber is called the *sarcoplasmic reticulum*. This reticulum has a special organization that is extremely important in the control of muscle contraction, which will be discussed later in the chapter. The electron micrograph of Figure 3–3 illustrates the arrangement of this sarcoplasmic reticulum and shows how extensive it can be. The more rapidly contracting types of muscle have especially extensive sarcoplasmic reticulums, indicating that this structure is important in causing rapid muscle contraction, as will also be discussed later.

MOLECULAR MECHANISM OF MUSCLE CONTRACTION

Sliding Mechanism of Contraction.   Figure 3–4 illustrates the basic mechanism of muscle contraction. It shows the relaxed state of a sarcomere (above) and the contracted state (below). In the relaxed state, the ends of the actin filaments derived from two successive Z membranes barely overlap each other while at the same time completely overlapping the myosin filaments. On the other hand, in the contracted state these actin filaments have been pulled inward among the myosin filaments so that they now overlap each other to a major extent. Also, the Z membranes have been pulled by the actin filaments up to the ends of the myosin filaments. Indeed, the actin filaments can be pulled together so tightly that the ends of the myosin filaments actually buckle during very intense contraction. Thus, muscle contraction occurs by a *sliding filament mechanism*.

But what causes the actin filaments to slide inward among the myosin filaments? Unfortunate-

Figure 3–3. Sarcoplasmic reticulum surrounding the myofibril, showing the longitudinal system paralleling the myofibrils. Also shown in cross-section are the T tubules that lead to the exterior of the fiber membrane and that contain extracellular fluid (arrows). (From Fawcett: The Cell. Philadelphia, W. B. Saunders Company, 1966.)

Figure 3–4. The relaxed and contracted states of a myofibril, showing sliding of the actin filaments into the channels between the myosin filaments.

ly, we do not completely know the answer to this question. Yet we do know that it is caused by attractive forces that develop between the actin and myosin filaments. Almost certainly, these attractive forces are the result of mechanical, chemical, or electrostatic forces generated by the interaction of the cross-bridges of the myosin filaments with the actin filaments.

Under resting conditions, the attractive forces between the actin and myosin filaments are inhibited, but when an action potential travels over the muscle fiber membrane, this causes the release of large quantities of calcium ions into the sarcoplasm surrounding the myofibrils. These calcium ions activate the attractive forces between the filaments and contraction begins. But energy is also needed for the contractile process to proceed. This energy is derived from the high energy bonds of adenosine triphosphate (ATP), which is degraded to adenosine diphosphate (ADP) to give the energy required.

In the next few sections we will describe what is known about the details of the molecular processes of contraction. To begin this discussion, however, we must first characterize in detail the myosin and actin filaments.

MOLECULAR CHARACTERISTICS OF THE CONTRACTILE FILAMENTS

The Myosin Filament. The myosin filament is composed of approximately 200 myosin molecules, each having a molecular weight of 490,000. Figure 3–5, section A illustrates an individual molecule; section B illustrates the organization of the molecules to form a myosin filament as well as its interaction with the ends of two actin filaments.

The myosin molecule is composed of two parts; *light meromyosin* and *heavy meromyosin*. The light meromyosin consists of two peptide strands

wound around each other in a helix. The heavy meromyosin in turn consists of two parts: first, a double helix similar to that of the light meromyosin; second, a *head* attached to the end of the double helix. The head itself is a composite of two globular protein masses.

It is believed that the myosin molecule is especially flexible at two points — the juncture between the light meromyosin and the heavy meromyosin and between the body of the heavy meromyosin and the head. These two areas are called *hinges*.

In section B of Figure 3–5 the central portion of a myosin filament is illustrated. The body of this filament is composed of parallel strands of light meromyosin from multiple myosin molecules. In fact, whenever myosin molecules are precipitated from solution, it is found that the light meromyosin portions of the myosin molecules have a natural tendency to aggregate together to form filaments almost precisely like those of the myosin filaments found in muscle. On the other hand, the heavy meromyosin portions of myosin molecules protrude from all sides of the myosin filament, as illustrated in the figure. These protrusions constitute the *cross-bridges*. The heads of the cross-bridges lie in apposition to the actin filaments, whereas the helix portions of the cross-bridges act as hinged arms that allow the heads either to extend far outward from the body of the myosin filament or to lie close to the body.

Note also that the arms of the cross-bridges extend in both directions away from the center-

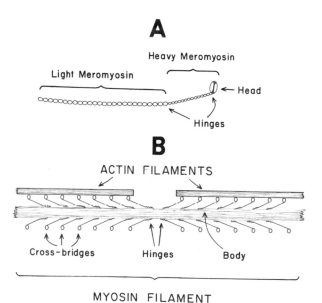

Figure 3–5. A, The myosin molecule. B, Combination of many myosin molecules to form a myosin filament. Also shown are the cross-bridges and the interaction between the heads of the cross-bridges and adjacent actin filaments.

most part of the filament. Therefore, in the very center of the myosin filament, for a length of about 0.2 micron, there are no cross-bridge heads.

The total length of the myosin filament is 1.6 microns, and the 200 myosin molecules allow the formation of 100 pairs of cross-bridges — 50 pairs on each end of the myosin filament.

Now, to complete the picture, the myosin filament is twisted so that it makes one complete revolution for each three pairs of cross-bridges. Each twist has a length of 42.9 nanometers with each pair of cross-bridges axially displaced from the previous pair by 120 degrees.

The Actin Filament. The actin filament is also complex. It is composed of three different components; *actin, tropomyosin,* and *troponin.*

The backbone of the actin filament is a double-stranded F-actin protein molecule, illustrated in Figure 3–6. The two strands are wound in a helix in the same manner as the myosin molecule, but with a complete revolution every 70 nanometers.

Each strand of the double F-actin helix is composed of polymerized G-actin molecules, each having a molecular weight of 47,000. There are approximately 13 of these molecules in each revolution of each strand of helix. Attached to each one of the G-actin molecules is one molecule of ADP. It is believed that these ADP molecules are the active sites on the actin filaments with which the cross-bridges of the myosin filaments interact to cause muscle contraction. The active sites on the two F-actin strands of the double helix are staggered, giving one active site on the overall actin filament approximately every 2.7 nanometers.

The Tropomyosin Strands. The actin filament also contains two additional protein strands that are polymers of *tropomyosin* molecules, each molecule having a molecular weight of 70,000 and extending a length of 40 nanometers. It is believed that each tropomyosin strand is loosely attached to an F-actin strand and that in the resting state it physically covers the active sites of the actin strands so that interaction cannot occur between the actin and myosin to cause contraction.

Troponin and Its Role in Muscle Contraction. Attached approximately two-thirds the distance along each tropomyosin molecule is a complex of three globular protein molecules called *troponin.* One of the globular proteins has a strong affinity for actin, another for tropomyosin, and a third for calcium ions. This complex is believed to attach the tropomyosin to the actin. The strong affinity of the troponin for calcium ions is believed to initiate the contraction process, as will be explained in the following section.

Interaction of Myosin and Actin Filaments to Cause Contraction

Inhibition of the Actin Filament by the Troponin-Tropomyosin Complex; Activation by Calcium Ions. A pure actin filament without the presence of the troponin-tropomyosin complex binds strongly with myosin molecules in the presence of magnesium ions and ATP, both of which are normally abundant in the myofibril. But, if the troponin-tropomyosin complex is added to the actin filament, this binding does not take place. Therefore, it is believed that the normal active sites on the normal actin filament of the relaxed muscle are inhibited (or perhaps physically covered) by the troponin-tropomyosin complex. Consequently, they cannot interact with the myosin filaments to cause contraction. Before contraction can take place the inhibitory effect of the troponin-tropomyosin complex must itself be inhibited.

Now, let us discuss the role of the calcium ions. In the presence of large amounts of calcium ions the inhibitory effect of the troponin-tropomyosin on the actin filaments is itself inhibited. The mechanism of this is not known, but one suggestion is the following: When calcium ions combine with the calcium binding subunit of troponin, which has an extremely high affinity for calcium ions even when they are present in minute quantities, the troponin complex supposedly undergoes a conformational change that in some way tugs on the tropomyosin protein strand. At the same time, the bonds between the troponin and the actin become loosened. This combination of effects supposedly moves the tropomyosin strand deeper into the groove between the two actin strands and thereby "uncovers" the active sites of the actin, thus allowing contraction to proceed. Though this is a hypothetical mechanism, nevertheless it does emphasize that the normal relationship between the tropomyosin-troponin complex and actin is altered by calcium ions — a condition which leads to contraction.

Interaction Between the "Activated" Actin Filament and the Myosin Molecule — The Ratchet Theory of Contraction. As soon as the actin filament becomes activated by the calcium ions, it is believed that the heads of the cross-bridges from the myosin filaments immediately become attracted to the active sites of the actin filament, and this in

Figure 3–6. The actin filament, composed of two helical strands of F-actin and two tropomyosin strands that lie in the grooves between the actin strands. Attaching the tropomyosin to the actin are several troponin complexes.

Figure 3–7. The ratchet mechanism for contraction of the muscle.

some way causes contraction to occur. Though the precise manner by which this interaction between the cross-bridges and the actin causes contraction is still unknown, a suggested hypothesis for which considerable circumstantial evidence exists is the so-called *ratchet theory of contraction.*

Figure 3–7 illustrates the postulated ratchet mechanism for contraction. This figure shows the heads of two cross-bridges attaching to and disengaging from the active sites of an actin filament. It is postulated that when the head attaches to an active site this attachment simultaneously causes profound changes in the intramolecular forces in the head and arm of the cross-bridge. The new alignment of forces causes the head to tilt toward the arm, and to drag the actin filament along with it. This tilt of the head of the cross-bridge is called the *power stroke.* Then, immediately after tilting, the head automatically splits away from the active site and returns to its normal perpendicular direction. In this position it combines with an active site further down along the actin filament; then, a similar tilt takes place again to cause a new power stroke, and the actin filament moves another step. Thus, the heads of the cross-bridges bend back and forth and step by step pull the actin filament toward the center of the myosin filament. Thus, the movements of the cross-bridges use the active sites of the actin filaments as cogs of a *ratchet.*

Each one of the cross-bridges is believed to operate independently of all others, each attaching and pulling in a continuous, alternating ratchet cycle. Therefore, the greater the number of cross-bridges in contact with the actin filament at any given time, the greater, theoretically, is the force of contraction.

ATP as the Source of Energy for Contraction — Chemical Events in the Ratchet Cycle. When a muscle contracts against a load, work is performed, and energy is required. It is found that large amounts of ATP are cleaved to form ADP during the contraction process. Furthermore, the greater the amount of work performed by the muscle, the greater is the amount of ATP that is cleaved, which is called the *Fenn effect.* However, unfortunately, it is still not known exactly how

ATP is used to provide the energy for contraction. Yet, the following is a sequence of events that has been suggested as the means by which this occurs:

1. When the inhibitory effect of the troponin-tropomyosin complex has itself been inhibited by calcium ions, the heads of the cross-bridges bind with uncovered sites on the actin filament, as illustrated in Figure 3–7.

2. It is assumed that the bond between the head of the cross-bridge and the active site of the actin filament causes a conformational change in the head, thus causing the head to tilt and to provide the power stroke for pulling the actin filament. This power stroke is believed to result from energy that has already been stored in the heavy meromyosin molecule and not from energy derived from ATP.

3. Once the head of the cross-bridge is tilted, the conformational change in the head exposes a site in the head where ATP can bind. Therefore, one molecule of ATP binds with the head, and this binding in turn causes detachment of the head from the active site.

4. Once the head bound with ATP splits away from the active site, the ATP is itself cleaved by a very potent ATPase activity of the heavy meromyosin. The energy released supposedly tilts the head back to its normal perpendicular condition and theoretically "cocks" the head in this position.

5. Then, when the "cocked" head, with its stored energy derived from the cleaved ATP, binds with a new active site on the actin filament, it becomes uncocked and once again provides the power stroke.

6. Thus, the process proceeds again and again until the actin filament pulls the Z membrane up against the ends of the myosin filaments or until the load on the muscle becomes too great for further pulling to occur.

RELATIONSHIP BETWEEN ACTIN AND MYOSIN FILAMENT OVERLAP AND TENSION DEVELOPED BY THE CONTRACTING MUSCLE

Figure 3–8 illustrates the relationship between the length of sarcomere and the tension developed by a single, contracting, *isolated* muscle fiber. To the right are illustrated different degrees of overlap of the myosin and actin filaments at different sarcomere lengths. At point D on the diagram, the actin filament has pulled all the way out to the end of the myosin filament with no overlap at all. At this point, the tension developed by the activated muscle is zero. Then, as the sarcomere shortens and the actin filament overlaps the myosin filament progressively more and more, the tension

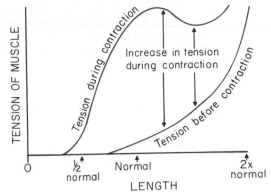

Figure 3–8. Length-tension diagram for a single sarcomere, illustrating maximum strength of contraction when the sarcomere is 2.0 to 2.2 microns in length. At the upper right are shown the relative positions of the actin and myosin filaments at different sarcomere lengths from point A to point D. (Modified from Gordon, Huxley, and Julian: *J. Physiol., 171:*28P, 1964.)

Figure 3–9. Relation of muscle length to force of contraction.

increases progressively until the sarcomere length decreases to about 2.2 microns. At this point the actin filament has already overlapped all the cross-bridges of the myosin filament but has not yet reached the center of the myosin filament. Upon further shortening, the sarcomere maintains full tension until point B at a sarcomere length of approximately 2.0 microns. It is at this point that the ends of the two actin filaments begin to overlap. As the sarcomere length falls from 2 microns down to about 1.65 microns, at point A, the strength of contraction decreases. It is at this point that the two Z membranes of the sarcomere abut the ends of the myosin filaments. Then, as contraction proceeds to still shorter sarcomere lengths, the ends of the myosin filaments are actually crumpled, and as illustrated in Figure 3–8, the strength of contraction also decreases precipitously.

This diagram illustrates that maximum contraction occurs when there is maximum overlap between the actin filaments and the cross-bridges of the myosin filaments, and it supports the idea that the greater the number of cross-bridges pulling the actin filaments, the greater is the strength of contraction.

Relation of Force of Contraction of the Intact Muscle to Muscle Length. The upper curve of Figure 3–9 is similar to that in Figure 3–8, but this illustrates the intact whole muscle rather than the isolated muscle fiber. The whole muscle has a large amount of connective tissue in it; also, the sarcomeres in different parts of the muscle do not necessarily contract exactly in unison. Therefore, the curve has somewhat different dimensions from those illustrated for the individual muscle fiber, but it nevertheless exhibits the same form.

Note in Figure 3–9 that when the muscle is at its normal resting length and is then activated, it contracts with maximum force of contraction. If the muscle is stretched to much greater than normal length prior to contraction, a large amount of *resting tension* develops in the muscle even before contraction takes place; this tension results from the elastic forces of the connective tissue, of the sarcolemma, the blood vessels, the nerves, and so forth. However, the *increase* in tension during contraction, called *active tension*, decreases as the muscle is stretched beyond its normal length.

Note also in Figure 3–9 that when the resting muscle is shortened to less than its normal length, the maximum tension of contraction decreases progressively and reaches zero when the muscle has shortened to approximately half its normal resting length.

RELATION OF VELOCITY OF CONTRACTION TO LOAD

A muscle contracts extremely rapidly when it contracts against no load — to a state of full

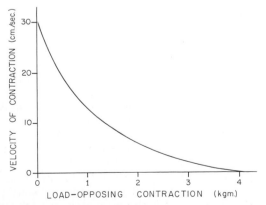

Figure 3–10. Relation of load to velocity of contraction in a skeletal muscle 8 cm. long.

contraction in approximately $1/20$ second for the average muscle. However, when loads are applied, the velocity of contraction becomes progressively less as the load increases, as illustrated in Figure 3–10. When the load increases to equal the maximum force that the muscle can exert, then the velocity of contraction becomes zero, and no contraction at all results, despite activation of the muscle fiber.

This decreasing velocity with load seems to be caused mainly by the fact that a load on a contracting muscle is a reverse force that opposes the contractile force caused by muscle contraction. Therefore, the net force that is available to cause velocity of shortening is correspondingly reduced.

INITIATION OF MUSCLE CONTRACTION: EXCITATION-CONTRACTION COUPLING

THE MUSCLE ACTION POTENTIAL

Initiation of contraction in skeletal muscle begins with action potentials in the muscle fibers. These elicit electrical currents that spread to the interior of the fiber where they cause release of calcium ions from the sarcoplasmic reticulum. It is the calcium ions that in turn initiate the chemical events of the contractile process.

Almost everything discussed in Chapter 2 regarding initiation and conduction of action potentials in nerve fibers applies equally well to skeletal muscle fibers, except for quantitative differences. Some of the quantitative aspects of muscle potentials are the following:

1. Resting membrane potential: Approximately -90 millivolts in skeletal fibers — the same as in large myelinated nerve fibers.

2. Duration of action potential: 1 to 5 milliseconds in skeletal muscle — about five times as long as large myelinated nerves.

3. Velocity of conduction: 3 to 5 meters per second — about $1/18$ the velocity of conduction in the large myelinated nerve fibers that excite skeletal muscle.

Excitation of Skeletal Muscle Fibers by Nerves. In normal function of the body, skeletal muscle fibers are excited by large myelinated nerve fibers. These attach to the skeletal muscle fibers at the neuromuscular junction, which will be discussed in detail in the following chapter. Except for 2 per cent of the muscle fibers, there is only one neuromuscular junction to each muscle fiber; this junction is located near the middle of the fiber. Therefore, the action potential spreads from the middle of the fiber towards its two ends. This

spreading is important because it allows nearly coincident contraction of all sarcomeres of the muscles so that they can all contract together rather than separately.

SPREAD OF THE ACTION POTENTIAL TO THE INTERIOR OF THE MUSCLE FIBER BY WAY OF THE TRANSVERSE TUBULE SYSTEM

The skeletal muscle fiber is so large that action potentials spreading along the membrane cause almost no current flow deep within the fiber. Yet, to cause contraction, these electrical currents must penetrate to the vicinity of all the separate myofibrils. This is achieved by transmission of the action potentials along *transverse tubules* (T tubules) that penetrate all the way through the muscle fiber from one side to the other. The T tubule action potentials in turn cause the sarcoplasmic reticulum to release calcium ions in the immediate vicinity of all the myofibrils, and it is these calcium ions that in turn cause contraction. Now, let us describe this system in much greater detail.

The Transverse Tubule–Sarcoplasmic Reticulum System. Figure 3–11 illustrates a group of myofibrils surrounded by the transverse tubule–sarcoplasmic reticulum system. The transverse tubules penetrate all the way from one side of the muscle fiber to the opposite side. Not shown in the figure is the fact that these tubules branch among themselves so that they form entire *planes* of T tubules interlacing among all the separate myofibrils. Also, it should be noted that where the T tubules originate from the cell membrane they are open to the exterior. Therefore, they communicate with the fluid surrounding the muscle fiber and contain extracellular fluid in their lumens. In other words, the T tubules are internal extensions of the cell membrane. Therefore, when an action potential spreads over a muscle fiber membrane, it spreads along the T tubules to the deep interior of the muscle fiber as well. The action potential currents surrounding these transverse tubules then elicit the muscle contraction.

Figure 3–11 shows the extensiveness of the *sarcoplasmic reticulum* as well. This is composed of two major parts: (1) long *longitudinal tubules* that terminate in (2) large chambers called *terminal cisternae*. The cisternae in turn abut the transverse tubules. When the muscle fiber is sectioned longitudinally and electron micrographs are made, one sees this abutting of the cisternae against the transverse tubule, which gives the appearance of a *triad* with a small central tubule and a large cisterna on either side. This is illustrated in Figure 3–11 and is also seen in the electron micrograph of Figure 3–3.

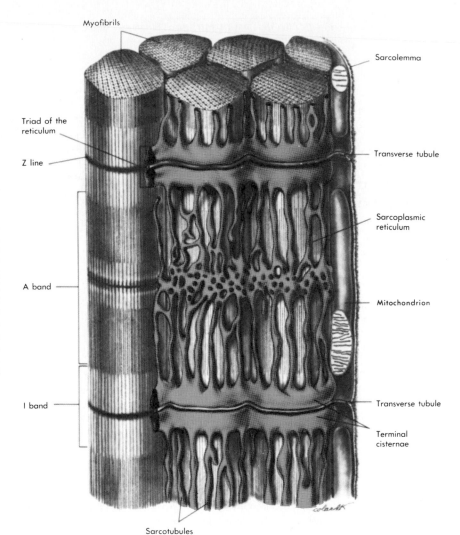

Myofibrils

Triad of the reticulum

Z line

A band

I band

Sarcolemma

Transverse tubule

Sarcoplasmic reticulum

Mitochondrion

Transverse tubule

Terminal cisternae

Sarcotubules

Figure 3–11. The transverse tubule–sarcoplasmic reticulum system. Note the *longitudinal tubules* that terminate in large *cisternae*. The cisternae in turn abut the transverse tubules. Note also that the transverse tubules communicate with the outside of the cell membrane. This illustration was drawn from frog muscle, which has one transverse tubule per sarcomere, located at the Z line. A similar arrangement is found in mammalian heart muscle, but mammalian skeletal muscle has two transverse tubules per sarcomere, located at the A-I junctions. (From Bloom and Fawcett: A Textbook of Histology. Philadelphia, W. B. Saunders Company, 1975. Modified after Peachey: *J. Cell Biol. 25*:209, 1965. Drawn by Sylvia Colard Keene.)

In the muscle of lower animals such as the frog, there is a single T tubule network for each sarcomere, located at the level of the Z membrane as illustrated in Figure 3–11. Cardiac muscle also has this type of T tubule system. However, in mammalian skeletal muscle there are two T tubule networks for each sarcomere located near the two ends of the myosin filaments, which are the points where the actual mechanical forces of muscle contraction are created. Thus, mammalian skeletal muscle is optimally organized for rapid excitation of muscle contraction.

RELEASE OF CALCIUM IONS BY THE CISTERNAE OF THE SARCOPLASMIC RETICULUM

One of the special features of the sarcoplasmic reticulum is that it contains calcium ions in very high concentration, and many of these ions are released when the adjacent T tubule is excited.

Figure 3–12 shows that the action potential of the T tubule causes current flow through the cisternae where they abut the T tubule. The cisternae project *junctional feet* that surround the T tubule, presumably facilitating passage of electrical current from the T tubule into the cisternae. It is possible that the current entering the cisternae elicits action potentials along the membranes of the sarcoplasmic reticulum in the same manner that action potentials spread along the T tubules. Indeed, such action potentials have been demonstrated under special conditions, but it is not known whether they occur normally. At any rate, current flow into the cisternae from the T tubules does cause rapid release of calcium ions from the cisternae. Presumably this results from the opening of calcium pores similar to the opening of sodium pores at the onset of the action potential, though the actual mechanism is still unknown.

The calcium ions that are thus released from the cisternae diffuse to the adjacent myofibrils where

Figure 3-12. Excitation-contraction coupling in the muscle, showing an action potential that causes release of calcium ions from the sarcoplasmic reticulum and then re-uptake of the calcium ions by a calcium pump.

they bind strongly with troponin, as discussed in an earlier section, and this in turn elicits the muscle contraction, as has also been discussed. However, the calcium ions also bind less strongly with the myosin filaments, which could theoretically be another factor in initiating contraction.

The Calcium Pump for Removing Calcium Ions from the Sarcoplasmic Fluid. Once the calcium ions have been released from the cisternae and have diffused to the myofibrils, muscle contraction will then continue as long as the calcium ions are still present in high concentration in the sarcoplasmic fluid. However, a continually active calcium pump located in the walls of the sarcoplasmic reticulum pumps calcium ions out of the sarcoplasmic fluid back into the vesicular cavities of the reticulum. This pump can concentrate the calcium ions about 2000-fold inside the reticulum, a condition which allows massive buildup of calcium in the sarcoplasmic reticulum and also causes almost total depletion of calcium ions in the fluid of the myofibrils. Therefore, except immediately after an action potential, the calcium ion concentration in the myofibrils is kept at an extremely low level.

The Excitatory "Pulse" of Calcium Ions. The normal concentration (about 10^{-7} molar) of calcium ions in the sarcoplasm that bathes the myofibrils is too little to elicit contraction. Therefore, in the resting state, the troponin-tropomyosin complex keeps the actin filaments inhibited and maintains a relaxed state of the muscle.

On the other hand, full excitation of the T tubule–sarcoplasmic reticulum system causes enough release of calcium ions to increase the concentration in the myofibrillar fluid to as high as 2×10^{-4} molar concentration, which causes maximum muscle contraction. Immediately thereafter, the calcium pump depletes the calcium ions again. The total duration of this calcium "pulse" in the usual skeletal muscle fiber lasts about $1/30$ of a second, though it may last several times as long as this in some skeletal muscle fibers and be several times shorter in others (in heart muscle the pulse lasts for as long as 0.3 second). It is during this calcium pulse that muscle contraction occurs. If the contraction is to continue without interruption for longer intervals, a series of such pulses must be initiated by a continuous series of repetitive action potentials, as will be discussed in more detail later in the chapter.

THE SOURCE OF ENERGY FOR MUSCLE CONTRACTION

We have already seen that muscle contraction depends upon energy supplied by ATP. Most of this energy is required to actuate the ratchet mechanism by which the cross-bridges pull the actin filaments, but small amounts are required for (1) pumping calcium from the sarcoplasm into the sarcoplasmic reticulum, and (2) pumping sodium and potassium ions through the muscle fiber membrane to maintain an appropriate ionic environment for the propagation of action potentials.

However, the amount of ATP that is present in the muscle fiber is sufficient to maintain full contraction for less than 1 second. Fortunately, after the ATP is broken into ADP to release its energy, the ADP is rephosphorylated to form new ATP within a fraction of a second. There are several sources of the energy required for this rephosphorylation:

The first source of energy that is used to reconstitute the ATP is the substance *creatine phosphate*, which carries a high-energy phosphate bond similar to those of ATP. The high-energy phosphate bond of the creatine phosphate is cleaved and the released energy causes bonding of a new phosphate ion to ADP to reconstitute the ATP. However, the total amount of creatine phosphate is also very little — only about five times as great as the ATP. Therefore, the combined energy of both the stored ATP and the creatine phosphate in the muscle is still capable of causing maximal muscle contraction for no longer than a few seconds.

The next source of energy used to reconstitute both the creatine phosphate and the ATP is energy released from the foodstuffs — from carbohydrates, fats, and proteins. Most of this energy is released in the course of oxidation of these foodstuffs. This oxidative release of energy takes place almost entirely in the mitochondria, which utilize the released energy to form new ATP. Thus, the ultimate source of energy for muscle contraction is the basic food substances and oxygen. The energy is especially derived from the metabolism of carbohydrates and fats.

Efficiency of Muscle Contraction. The "efficiency" of an engine or a motor is calculated as the percentage of energy input that is converted into work instead of heat. The percentage of the input energy to a muscle (the chemical energy in the nutrients) that can be converted into work is less than 20 to 25 per cent, the remainder becoming heat. Maximum efficiency can be realized only when the muscle contracts at a moderate velocity. If the muscle contracts very slowly, large amounts of *maintenance heat* are released during the process of contraction, thereby decreasing the efficiency. On the other hand, if contraction is too rapid, large proportions of the energy are used to overcome the viscous friction within the muscle itself, and this, too, reduces the efficiency of contraction. Ordinarily, maximum efficiency is developed when the velocity of contraction is about 30 per cent of maximum.

CHARACTERISTICS OF A SINGLE MUSCLE TWITCH

Many features of muscle contraction can be especially well demonstrated by eliciting single *muscle twitches*. This can be accomplished by instantaneously exciting the nerve to a muscle or by passing a short electrical stimulus through the muscle itself, giving rise to a single, sudden contraction lasting for a fraction of a second.

Isometric Versus Isotonic Contraction. Muscle contraction is said to be *isometric* when the muscle does not shorten during contraction and *isotonic* when it shortens but the tension on the muscle remains constant. Systems for recording the two types of muscle contraction are illustrated in Figure 3–13.

To the right is the isometric system in which the muscle is suspended between a solid rod and a lever of an electronic force transducer. This transducer records force with almost zero movement of the lever; therefore, in effect, the muscle is bound between fixed points so that it cannot contract significantly. To the left is shown an isotonic recording system: the muscle simply

Figure 3–13. Isotonic and isometric recording systems.

lifts a pan of weights so that the force against which the muscle contracts remains constant, though the length of the muscle changes considerably.

There are several basic differences between isometric and isotonic contractions. First, isometric contraction does not require much sliding of myofibrils among each other. Second, in isotonic contraction a load is moved, which involves the phenomena of inertia. That is, the weight or other type of object being moved must first be accelerated, and once a velocity has been attained the load has momentum that causes it to continue moving even after the contraction is over. Therefore an isotonic contraction is likely to last considerably longer than an isometric contraction of the same muscle. Third, isotonic contraction entails the performance of external work. Therefore, in accordance with the Fenn effect discussed previously, a greater amount of energy is used by the muscle.

In comparing the rapidity of contraction of different types of muscle, isometric recordings such as those illustrated in Figure 3–14 are usually used instead of isotonic recordings because the duration of an isotonic recording is almost as dependent on the inertia of the recording system as on the contraction itself, and this makes it difficult to compare time relationships of contractions from one muscle to another.

Muscles can contract both isometrically and isotonically in the body, but most contractions are actually a mixture of the two. When standing, a person tenses the quadriceps muscles to tighten the knee joints and to

Figure 3–14. Duration of isometric contractions of different types of mammalian muscles, showing also a latent period between the action potential and muscle contraction.

keep the legs stiff. This is isometric contraction. On the other hand, when a person lifts a weight using the biceps, this is mainly an isotonic contraction. Finally, contractions of leg muscles during running are a mixture of isometric and isotonic contractions —isometric mainly to keep the limbs stiff when the legs hit the ground and isotonic mainly to move the limbs.

The Series Elastic Component of Muscle Contraction. When muscle fibers contract against a load, those portions of the muscle that do not contract — the tendons, the sarcolemmal ends of the muscle fibers where they attach to the tendons, and perhaps even the hinged arms of the cross-bridges — will stretch slightly as the tension increases. Consequently, the muscle must shorten an extra 3 to 5 per cent to make up for the stretch of these elements. The elements of the muscle that stretch during contraction are called the *series elastic component* of the muscle.

Characteristics of Isometric Twitches Recorded from Different Muscles. The body has many different sizes of skeletal muscles — from the very small stapedius muscle of only a few millimeters length and a millimeter or so in diameter up to the very large quadriceps muscle. Furthermore, the fibers may be as small as 10 microns in diameter or as large as 80 microns. And, finally, the energetics of muscle contraction vary considerably from one muscle to another. These different physical and chemical characteristics often manifest themselves in the form of different characteristics of contraction, some muscles contracting rapidly while others contract slowly.

Fast Versus Slow Muscle. Figure 3–14 illustrates isometric contractions of three different types of skeletal muscles: an ocular muscle, which has a duration of contraction of less than $1/100$ second; the gastrocnemius muscle, which has a duration of contraction of about $1/30$ second; and the soleus muscle, which has a duration of contraction of about $1/10$ second. It is interesting that these durations of contractions are adapted to the function of each of the respective muscles, for ocular movements must be extremely rapid to maintain fixation of the eyes upon specific objects, the gastrocnemius muscle must contract moderately rapidly to provide sufficient velocity of limb movement for running and jumping, while the soleus muscle is concerned principally with slow reactions for continual support of the body against gravity.

Thus, there is a wide range of gradations from *fast* to *slow* muscles. In general, the slow muscles are used more for prolonged performance of work. Their muscle fibers generally are smaller, are surrounded by more blood capillaries, and have far more mitochondria than the fast muscles. They also have a large amount of *myoglobin* in the sarcoplasm (myoglobin is a substance similar to the hemoglobin in red blood cells and can combine with oxygen and store this oxygen inside the muscle cell until it is needed by the mitochondria). On the other hand, the fast muscles generally have a much more extensive sarcoplasmic reticulum, which allows very rapid release of calcium ions and then rapid re-uptake of the calcium ions so that the contraction can be rapid. The slow muscle is frequently called *red muscle* because of the reddish tint caused by the myoglobin as well as by the large amount of red blood cells in the capillaries; the fast muscle is called *white muscle*

because of a whitish appearance caused by a paucity of these elements.

MECHANICS OF SKELETAL MUSCLE CONTRACTION

THE MOTOR UNIT

Each motor neuron that leaves the spinal cord usually innervates many different muscle fibers, the number depending on the type of muscle. All the muscle fibers innervated by a single motor nerve fiber are called a *motor unit.* In general, small muscles that react rapidly and whose control is exact have few muscle fibers (as few as 2 to 3 in some of the laryngeal muscles) in each motor unit and have a large number of nerve fibers going to each muscle. On the other hand, the large muscles which do not require very fine degree of control, such as the gastrocnemius muscle, may have several hundred muscle fibers in a motor unit. An average figure for all the muscles of the body can be considered to be about 150 muscle fibers to the motor unit.

Usually muscle fibers of adjacent motor units overlap, with small bundles of 10 to 15 fibers from one motor unit lying among similar bundles of the second motor unit. This interdigitation allows the separate motor units to contract in support of each other rather than entirely as individual segments.

Macromotor Units. Loss of some of the nerve fibers to a muscle causes the remaining nerve fibers to sprout forth and innervate many of the paralyzed muscle fibers. When this occurs, such as following poliomyelitis, one occasionally develops *macromotor units,* which can contain as many as 5 times the normal number of muscle fibers. This obviously decreases the degree of control that one has over the muscles, but, nevertheless, allows the muscles to regain function.

SUMMATION OF MUSCLE CONTRACTION

Summation means the adding together of individual muscle twitches to make strong and concerted muscle movements. In general, summation occurs in two different ways: (1) by increasing the number of motor units contracting simultaneously and (2) by increasing the rapidity of contraction of individual motor units. These are called, respectively, *multiple motor unit summation* and *wave summation* (or spatial summation and temporal summation).

Multiple Motor Unit Summation. Even within a single muscle, the numbers of muscle fibers and their sizes in the different motor units vary tremendously, so that one motor unit may be as much as 50 times as strong as another. The smaller motor units are far more easily excited than are the larger ones because they are innervated by smaller nerve fibers whose cell bodies in the spinal cord have a naturally high level of excitability. This effect causes the gradations of muscle strength during weak muscle contraction to occur in very small steps, while the steps become progressively greater as the intensity of contraction increases because the larger motor units then begin to contract.

Figure 3–15. Wave summation and tetanization.

Wave Summation. Figure 3–15 illustrates the principles of wave summation, showing in the lower left-hand corner several single muscle twitches followed by successive muscle twitches at various frequencies. When the frequency of twitches rises above 10 per second, the first muscle twitch is not completely over by the time the second one begins. Therefore, since the muscle is already in a partially contracted state when the second twitch begins, the degree of muscle shortening this time is slightly greater than that which occurs with the single muscle twitch. At more rapid rates of contraction, the degree of summation of successive contractions becomes greater and greater, because the successive contractions appear at earlier times following the preceding contraction.

Tetanization. When a muscle is stimulated at progressively greater frequencies, a frequency is finally reached at which the successive contractions fuse together and cannot be distinguished one from the other. This state is called *tetanization,* and the lowest frequency at which it occurs is called the *critical frequency.*

Tetanization results partly from the viscous properties of the muscle and partly from the nature of the contractile process itself. The muscle fibers are filled with sarcoplasm, which is a viscous fluid, and the fibers are encased in fasciae and muscle sheaths that have a viscous resistance to change in length. Therefore, undoubtedly these viscous factors play a role in causing the successive contractions to fuse with each other.

But in addition to the viscous property of muscle, the activation process itself lasts for a definite period of time, and successive pulsatile states of activation of the muscle fiber can occur so rapidly that they fuse into a long continual state of activation; that is, free calcium ions persist continuously in the myofibrils and provide an uninterrupted stimulus for maintenance of contraction. Once the critical frequency for tetanization is reached, further increase in rate of stimulation increases the force of contraction only a few more per cent, as shown in Figure 3–15.

Asynchronous Summation of Motor Units. Actually it is rare for either multiple motor unit summation or wave summation to occur separately from each other in normal muscle function. Instead, special neurogenic mechanisms in the spinal cord normally increase both the impulse rate and the number of motor units firing at the same time. If a motor unit fires at all, it usually fires at least 5 times per second, but this can increase to as

high as 50 per second for most muscles or much more than this for the very fast muscles — to frequencies sufficient to cause complete tetanization.

Yet, even when tetanization of individual motor units of a muscle is not occurring, the tension exerted by the whole muscle is still continuous and nonjerky because *the different motor units fire asynchronously;* that is, while one is contracting another is relaxing; then another fires, followed by still another, and so forth. Consequently, even when motor units fire as infrequently as 5 times per second, the muscle contraction, though weak, is nevertheless very smooth.

Maximum Strength of Contraction. The maximum strength of tetanic contraction of a muscle operating at a normal muscle length is about 3.5 kilograms per square centimeter of muscle, or 50 pounds per square inch. Since a quadriceps muscle can at times have as much as 16 square inches of muscle belly, as much as 800 pounds of tension may at times be applied to the patellar tendon. One can readily understand, therefore, how it is possible for muscles sometimes to pull their tendons out of the insertions in bones. This often occurs where the patellar tendon inserts in the tibia, and it occurs even more frequently where the Achilles tendon of the gastrocnemius muscle inserts at the heel.

Changes in Muscle Strength at the Onset of Contraction — The Staircase Effect (Treppe). When a muscle begins to contract after a long period of rest, its initial strength of contraction may be as little as one-half its strength 30 to 50 muscle twitches later. That is, the strength of contraction increases to a plateau, a phenomenon called the *staircase effect* or *treppe.* This phenomenon has interested physiologists greatly because it gives possible insights into the mechanism of muscle contraction.

Though all the possible causes of the staircase effect are not yet known, it is believed to be caused primarily by electrolyte changes that occur when a series of contractions begins. For instance, there is a net increase in calcium ions inside the muscle fiber because of movement of calcium ions inward through the membrane with each action potential. There is probably also further increase of calcium ions in the sarcoplasm because of release of these ions from the sarcoplasmic reticulum and failure to recapture the ions immediately. In addition, there is decreased potassium inside the cell as well as increased sodium; it has been suggested that the changes in these two ions increase the rate of liberation of calcium ions from the sarcoplasmic reticulum. Recalling the earlier discussion of the relationship of calcium ions to the contractile process, one can readily understand that progressive increase in calcium ion concentration in the sarcoplasm, caused either directly or as a consequence of sodium and potassium movement, could progressively increase the strength of muscle contraction, giving rise to the staircase effect.

SKELETAL MUSCLE TONE

Even when muscles are at rest, a certain amount of tautness usually remains. This residual degree of contraction in skeletal muscle is called *muscle tone.* Since skeletal muscle fibers do not contract without an actual action potential to stimulate the fibers except in certain pathological conditions, it is believed that skeletal muscle tone results entirely from nerve impulses coming from the spinal cord. These in turn are controlled partly by impulses transmitted from the brain to the appropriate anterior motor neurons and partly by impulses that originate in *muscle spindles* located in the muscle itself.

Muscle spindles are sensory receptors that exist throughout essentially all skeletal muscles to detect the degree of muscle contraction. These will be discussed in detail in Chapter 11, but, briefly, they transmit impulses almost continually through the posterior roots into the spinal cord, where they excite the anterior motor neurons, which in turn provide the necessary nerve stimuli for muscle tone. Simply cutting the posterior roots, thereby blocking the muscle spindle impulses, usually reduces muscle tone to such a low level that the muscle becomes almost completely flaccid.

Many other neurogenic factors, originating especially in the brain, enter into the control of muscle tone. These will be discussed in detail in relation to muscle spindle and spinal cord function in Chapter 11.

MUSCLE FATIGUE

Prolonged and strong contraction of a muscle leads to the well-known state of muscle fatigue. This results simply from inability of the contractile and metabolic processes of the muscle fibers to continue supplying the same work output. The nerve continues to function properly, the nerve impulses pass normally through the neuromuscular junction into the muscle fiber, and even normal action potentials spread over the muscle fibers, but the contraction becomes weaker and weaker because of reduction of ATP formation in the muscle fibers themselves.

Interruption of blood flow through a contracting muscle leads to almost complete muscle fatigue in a minute or more because of the obvious loss of nutrient supply.

THE LEVER SYSTEMS OF THE BODY

Muscles obviously operate by applying tension to their points of insertion into bones, and the bones in turn form various types of lever systems. Figure 3–16

Figure 3–16. The lever system activated by the biceps muscle.

illustrates the lever system activated by the biceps muscle to lift the forearm. If we assume that a large biceps muscle has a cross-sectional area of 6 square inches, then the maximum force of contraction would be about 300 pounds. When the forearm is exactly at right angles with the upper arm, the tendon attachment of the biceps is about 2 inches anterior to the fulcrum at the elbow, and the total length of the forearm lever is about 14 inches. Therefore, the amount of lifting power that the biceps would have at the hand would be only one seventh of the 300 pounds force, or about 43 pounds. When the arm is in the fully extended position the attachment of the biceps is much less than 2 inches anterior to the fulcrum, and the force with which the forearm can be brought forward is much less than 43 pounds.

In short, an analysis of the lever systems of the body depends on (a) a discrete knowledge of the point of muscle insertion and (b) its distance from the fulcrum of the lever, as well as (c) the length of the lever arm and (d) the position of the lever. Obviously, many different types of movement are required in the body, some of which need great strength and others large distances of movement. For this reason there are all varieties of muscles; some are long and contract a long distance and some are short but have large cross-sectional areas and therefore can provide extreme strengths of contraction over short distances. The study of different types of muscles, lever systems, and their movements is called *kinesiology* and is a very important phase of human physioanatomy.

Accommodation of Muscle Length to the Length of the Lever System.   If a bone is broken and then heals in a shortened state, the force of contraction of the muscles lying along this broken bone would obviously become decreased because of the shortened lengths of muscles. However, muscles shortened in this manner undergo *physical shortening* during the next few weeks. That is, the muscle fibers actually shorten and re-establish new muscle lengths approximately equal to the maximum length of the lever system itself, thus re-establishing optimum force of contraction by the muscles.

The same shortening process also occurs in muscles of limbs immobilized for several weeks in casts if the muscles during this time are in a shortened position. When the cast is removed, the muscles must often be restretched over a period of weeks before full mobility is restored.

SPECIAL FEATURES AND ABNORMALITIES OF SKELETAL MUSCLE FUNCTION

MUSCLE HYPERTROPHY

Forceful muscular activity causes the muscle size to increase, a phenomenon called hypertrophy. The diameters of the individual muscle fibers increase, the sarcoplasm increases, and the fibers gain in various nutrient and intermediary metabolic substances, such as adenosine triphosphate, creatine phosphate, glycogen, intracellular lipids, and even many additional mitochondria. It is likely that the myofibrils also increase in size and perhaps in numbers as well, but this has not been proved. Briefly, muscular hypertrophy increases both the motive power of the muscle and the nutrient mechanisms for maintaining increased motive power.

Weak muscular activity, even when sustained over long periods of time, does not result in significant hypertrophy. Instead, hypertrophy results mainly from *very* forceful muscle activity, though the activity might occur for only a few minutes each day. For this reason, strength can be developed in muscles much more rapidly when "resistive" or "isometric" exercise is used rather than simply prolonged mild exercise. Indeed, essentially no enlargement of the muscle fibers occurs unless the muscle contracts to at least 75 per cent of its maximum tension.

On the other hand, prolonged muscle activity does increase muscle endurance, causing increases in the oxidative enzymes, myoglobin, and even blood capillaries — all of which are essential to increased muscle metabolism.

MUSCLE ATROPHY

Muscle atrophy is the reverse of muscle hypertrophy; it results any time a muscle is not used or even when a muscle is used only for very weak contractions. Atrophy is particularly likely to occur when limbs are placed in casts, thereby preventing muscular contraction. As little as one month of disuse can sometimes decrease the muscle size to one-half normal.

Atrophy Caused by Muscle Denervation. When a muscle is denervated it immediately begins to atrophy, and the muscle continues to decrease in size for several years. If the muscle becomes reinnervated during the first three to four months, full function of the muscle usually returns, but after four months of denervation some of the muscle fibers usually will have degenerated. Re-innervation after two years rarely results in return of any function at all. Pathological studies show that the muscle fibers have by that time been replaced by fat and fibrous tissue.

Prevention of Muscle Atrophy by Electrical Stimulation. Strong electrical stimulation of denervated muscles, particularly when the resulting contractions occur against loads, will delay and in some instances prevent muscle atrophy despite denervation. This procedure is used to keep muscles alive until reinnervation can take place.

Physical Contracture of Muscle Following Denervation. When a muscle is denervated, its fibers tend to shorten if the muscle is kept in a shortened position, and even the associated nerves and fasciae shorten. All this is a natural characteristic of protein fibers called "creep." That is, unless continual movement keeps stretching the muscle and other structures, they will creep toward a shortened length. This is one of the most difficult problems in the treatment of patients with denervated muscles, such as occur in poliomyelitis or nerve trauma. Unless passive stretching is applied daily to the muscles, they may become so shortened that even when re-innervated they will be of little value. But, more important, the shortening can often result in extremely contorted positions of different parts of the body.

RIGOR MORTIS

Several hours after death all the muscles of the body go into a state of *contracture* called rigor mortis; that is, the muscle contracts and becomes rigid even without action potentials. It is believed that this rigidity is caused by loss of all the ATP, which is required to cause separation of the cross-bridges from the actin filaments during the relaxation process. The muscles remain in rigor until the muscle proteins are destroyed, which usually results from autolysis caused by enzymes released from the lysosomes some 15 to 25 hours later.

FAMILIAL PERIODIC PARALYSIS

Occasionally, a hereditary disease called familial periodic paralysis occurs. In persons so afflicted, the extracellular fluid potassium concentration periodically falls to very low levels, causing various degrees of paralysis. The paralysis is caused in the following manner: A great decrease in extracellular fluid potassium increases the muscle fiber membrane potential to a very high value. This results in strong *hyperpolarization* of the membrane (a membrane potential more negative than the normal −90 millivolts) making the fiber almost totally inexcitable; that is, the membrane potential is so high that the normal stimulus at the neuromuscular junction is incapable of exciting the fiber.

THE ELECTROMYOGRAM

Each time an action potential passes along a muscle fiber a small portion of the electrical current spreads away from the muscle as far as the skin. If many muscle fibers contract simultaneously, the summated electrical potentials at the skin may be very great. By placing two electrodes on the skin or inserting needle electrodes into the muscle, an electrical recording called the electromyogram can be made when the muscle is stimulated. Figure 3–17 illustrates a typical electromyographic recording from the gastrocnemius muscle during a moderate contraction. Electromyograms are frequently used clinically to discern abnormalities of muscle excitation. Two such abnormalities are muscle *fasciculation* and *fibrillation*.

Muscle Fasciculation. When an abnormal impulse occurs in a motor nerve fiber its whole motor unit contracts. This often causes sufficient contraction in the muscle that one can see a slight ripple in the skin over the muscle. This process is called fasciculation.

Fasciculation occurs especially following destruction of anterior motor neurons in poliomyelitis or following

Figure 3–17. Electromyogram recorded during contraction of the gastrocnemius muscle.

traumatic interruption of a nerve. As the peripheral nerve fibers die, spontaneous impulses are generated during the first few days, and fasciculatory muscle movements result in the muscle. Typical electromyographic records of weak periodic potentials can be obtained from the skin overlying the muscle.

Muscle Fibrillation. After all nerves to a muscle have been destroyed and the nerve fibers themselves have become nonfunctional, which requires three to five days, spontaneous impulses begin to appear in the denervated muscle fibers. At first, these occur at a rate of once every few seconds, but, after a few more days or a few weeks, the impulses become as rapid as 3 to 10 times per second. Thus, skeletal muscle fibers, when released from innervation, develop an intrinsic rhythmicity. After several more weeks the muscle fibers atrophy to such an extent that the fibrillatory impulses finally cease. To record an electromyogram of fibrillation, minute bipolar needle electrodes must be inserted into the muscle belly itself because adjacent muscle fibers do not fire simultaneously and, therefore, do not summate. As a result, the potentials are not strong enough to record from the surface of the skin.

REFERENCES

Aguayo, A. J., and Karpati, G. (eds.): Current Topics in Nerve and Muscle Research. New York, Elsevier/North-Holland, 1979.

Baker, P. F., and Reuter, H.: Calcium Movement in Excitable Cells. New York, Pergamon Press, 1975.

Basmajian, J. V.: Muscles Alive; Their Functions Revealed by Electromyography. Baltimore, Williams & Wilkins, 1978.

Becker, P. E.: Myotonia Congenita and Syndromes Associated with Myotonia: Clinical-Genetic Studies of the Nondystrophic Myotonias. Stuttgart, Thieme, 1977.

Bourne, G. H. (ed.): The Structure and Function of Muscle, 2nd Ed. New York, Academic Press, 1973.

Buchthal, F., and Schmalbruch, H.: Motor unit of mammalian muscle. Physiol. Rev., 60:90, 1980.

Buller, A. J.: The physiology of skeletal muscle. In MTP International Review of Science: Physiology. Baltimore, University Park Press, 1975, Vol. 3, p. 279.

Caputo, C.: Excitation and contraction processes in muscle. Annu. Rev. Biophys. Bioeng., 7:63, 1978.

Clausen, J. P.: Effect of physical training on cardiovascular adjustments to exercise in man. Physiol. Rev., 57:779, 1977.

Cohen, C.: The protein switch of muscle contraction. Sci. Am., 233(5): 36, 1975.

Cosgrove, M.: Your Muscles and Ways to Exercise Them. New York, Dodd, Mead, 1980.

Costantin, L. L.: Activation in striated muscle. In Brookhart, J. M., and Mountcastle, V. B. (eds.): Handbook of Physiology. Sec. 1, Vol. 1. Baltimore, Williams & Wilkins, 1977, p. 215.

Curtin, N. A., and Woledge, R. C.: Energy changes in muscular contraction. Physiol. Rev., 58:690, 1978.

Ebashi, S.: Regulatory mechanism of muscle contraction with special reference to the Ca-troponin-tropomyosin system. Essays Biochem., 10:1, 1974.

Ebashi, S.: Excitation-contraction coupling. Annu. Rev. Physiol., 38:293, 1976.

Endo, M.: Calcium release from the sarcoplasmic reticulum. Physiol. Rev., 57:71, 1977.

Fabiato, A., and Fabiato, F.: Calcium and cardiac excitation-contraction coupling. Annu. Rev. Physiol., 41:473, 1979.

Feldman, S. A.: Muscle Relaxants, 2nd Ed. Philadelphia, W. B. Saunders Co., 1979.

Fozzard, H. A.: Heart: Excitation-contraction coupling. Annu. Rev. Physiol., 39:201, 1977.

Fuchs, F.: Striated muscle. Annu. Rev. Physiol., 36:461, 1974.

Grimby, G., and Saltin, B.: Physiological effects of physical training. Scand. J. Rehabil. Med., 3:6, 1971.

Harper, P. S.: Myotonic Dystrophy. Philadelphia, W. B. Saunders Co., 1979.

Hess, A.: Vertebrate slow muscle fibers. Physiol. Rev., 50:40, 1970.

Hill, A. L., et al.: Physiology of voluntary muscle. Br. Med. Bull., 12(Sept.): 1956.

Holloszy, J. O., and Booth, F. W.: Biochemical adaptations to endurance exercise in muscle. Annu. Rev. Physiol., 38:273, 1976.

Holman, M. E., and Hirst, G. D. S.: Junctional transmission in smooth muscle and the autonomic nervous system. In Brookhart, J. M., and Mountcastle, V. B. (eds.): Handbook of Physiology. Sec. 1, Vol. 1. Baltimore, Williams & Wilkins, 1977, p. 417.

Homsher, E., and Kean, C. J.: Skeletal muscle energetics and metabolism. Annu. Rev. Physiol., 40:93, 1978.

Hughes, J. T.: Pathology of Muscle. Philadelphia, W. B. Saunders Co., 1975.

Huxley, A. F., and Gordon, A. M.: Striation patterns in active and passive shortening of muscle. Nature (Lond.), 193:280, 1962.

Huxley, H. E.: Muscular contraction and cell motility. Nature, 243: 445, 1973.

Ingels, N. B., Jr., (ed.): The Molecular Basis of Force Development in Muscle. Palo Alto, Cal., Palo Alto Medical Research Foundation, 1979.

Johnson, E. W., (ed.): Practical Electromyography. Baltimore, Williams & Wilkins, 1979.

Kaldor, G., and DiBattista, W. J. (eds.): Aging in Muscle. New York, Raven Press, 1978.

Lyman, R. W.: Kinetic analysis of myosin and actinomysin ATPase. Annu. Rev. Biophys. Bioeng., 8:145, 1979.

Mauro, A., and Bischoff, R., (eds.): Muscle Regeneration. New York, Raven Press, 1979.

Nakano, K. K.: Neurology of Musculoskeletal and Pneumatic Disorders. Boston, Houghton Mifflin, 1978.

Nelson, P. G.: Nerve and muscle cells in culture. Physiol. Rev., 55:1, 1975.

Northrip, J. W., et al.: Introduction to Biomechanic Analysis of Sport. Dubuque, Iowa, W. C. Brown Co., 1979.

Rasch, P. J., and Burke, R. K.: Kinesiology and Applied Anatomy: The Science of Human Movement. Philadelphia, Lea & Febiger, 1978.

Sahlin, K.: Intracellular pH and Energy Metabolism in Skeletal Muscle of Man: with Special Reference to Exercise. Stockholm, Acta Physiologica Scandinavica, 1978.

Schneck, A. G., and Vandecasserie, C., (eds.): Myoglobin. Brussels, l'Université de Bruxelles, Faculté des Sciences, 1977.

Sugi, H., and Pollack, G. H., (eds.): Cross-Bridge Mechanism in Muscle Contraction. Baltimore, University Park Press, 1979.

Tada, M., et al.: Molecular mechanism of active calcium transport by sarcoplasmic reticulum. Physiol. Rev., 58:1, 1978.

Taylor, C. R.: Exercise and environmental heat loads: different mechanisms for solving different problems: Int. Rev. Physiol., 15:119, 1977.

Toida, N., et al.: Obliquely striated muscle. Physiol. Rev., 55:700, 1975.

Tregear, R. T., and Marston, S. B.: The crossbridge theory. Annu. Rev. Physiol., 41:723, 1979.

Walton, J. N. (ed.): Disorders of Voluntary Muscle. New York, Churchill Livingstone, 1974.

Weber, A., and Murray, J. M.: Molecular control mechanisms in muscle contraction. Physiol. Rev., 53:612, 1973.

Winter, D. A.: Biomechanics of Human Movement. New York, John Wiley & Sons, 1979.

Zak, R., and Rabinowitz, M.: Molecular aspects of cardiac hypertrophy. Annu. Rev. Physiol., 41:539, 1979.

4

Neuromuscular Transmission; Function of Smooth Muscle

TRANSMISSION OF IMPULSES FROM NERVES TO SKELETAL MUSCLE FIBERS: THE NEUROMUSCULAR JUNCTION

The skeletal muscles are innervated by large myelinated nerve fibers that originate in the large motoneurons of the anterior horns of the spinal cord. It was pointed out in the previous chapter that each nerve fiber normally branches many times and stimulates from 3 to several hundred skeletal muscle fibers. The nerve ending makes a junction, called the *neuromuscular junction* or the *myoneural junction*, with the muscle fiber approximately at the fiber's midpoint so that the action potential in the fiber travels in both directions. With the exception of about 2 per cent of the muscle fibers there is only one such junction per muscle fiber.

Physiologic Anatomy of the Neuromuscular Junction. Figure 4–1, Parts A and B, illustrates the neuromuscular junction between a large myelinated nerve fiber and a skeletal muscle fiber. The nerve fiber branches at its end to form a complex of branching nerve *terminals* called the *end-plate*, which invaginates into the muscle fiber but lies entirely outside the muscle fiber plasma membrane. The entire structure is covered by one or more Schwann cells that insulate the end-plate from the surrounding fluids.

Figure 4–1C shows an electronmicrographic sketch of the juncture between a single-branch axon terminal and the muscle fiber membrane. The invagination of the membrane is called the *synaptic gutter* or *synaptic trough*, and the space

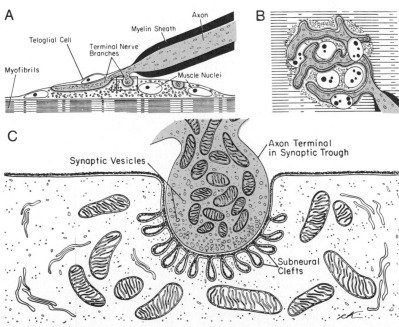

Figure 4–1. Different views of the motor end-plate. A, Longitudinal section through the end-plate. B, Surface view of the end-plate. C, Electronmicrographic appearance of the contact point between one of the axon terminals and the muscle fiber membrane, representing the rectangular area shown in A. (From Bloom and Fawcett, as modified from R. Couteaux: A Textbook of Histology. Philadelphia, W. B. Saunders Company, 1975.)

A

Teloglial Cell
Terminal Nerve Branches
Myelin Sheath
Axon
Myofibrils
Muscle Nuclei

B

C

Synaptic Vesicles
Axon Terminal in Synaptic Trough
Subneural Clefts

47

between the terminal and the fiber membrane is called the *synaptic cleft*. The synaptic cleft is 20 to 30 nanometers wide and is filled with a gelatinous "ground" substance through which diffuses extracellular fluid. At the bottom of the gutter are numerous *folds* of the muscle membrane which form *subneural clefts* that greatly increase the surface area at which the synaptic transmitter can act. In the axon terminal are many mitochondria that supply energy mainly for synthesis of the excitatory transmitter *acetylcholine* that, in turn, excites the muscle fiber. The acetylcholine is synthesized in the cytoplasm of the terminal but is rapidly absorbed into many small synaptic vesicles, approximately 300,000 of which are normally in all the terminals of a single end-plate. In the matrix of the subneural clefts are large quantities of the enzyme *cholinesterase*, which is capable of destroying acetylcholine, as is explained in further detail below.

Secretion of Acetylcholine by the Axon Terminals. When a nerve impulse reaches the neuromuscular junction, about 300 vesicles of acetylcholine are released by the terminals into the synaptic clefts between the terminals and the muscle fiber membrane. This results from movement of calcium ions from the extracellular fluid into the membranes of the terminals when the action potential depolarizes their membranes. The calcium ions cause the vesicles of acetylcholine to rupture through the membrane. In the absence of calcium or in the presence of excess magnesium, the release of acetylcholine is greatly depressed.

Destruction of the Released Acetylcholine by Cholinesterase. Within approximately 1 millisecond after acetylcholine is released by the axon terminal, a small portion of it diffuses out of the synaptic gutter and no longer acts on the muscle fiber membrane, but the greater bulk of it is destroyed by the cholinesterase in the subneural clefts. The very short period of time that the acetylcholine remains in contact with the muscle fiber membrane — about 1 millisecond — is almost always sufficient to excite the muscle fiber, and yet the rapid removal of the acetylcholine prevents re-excitation after the muscle fiber has recovered from the first action potential.

The "End-Plate Potential" and Excitation of the Skeletal Muscle Fiber. Even though the acetylcholine released into the space between the end-plate and the muscle membrane lasts for only a minute fraction of a second, during this period of time it can affect the muscle membrane sufficiently to open large pores with diameters of 0.6 to 0.7 nanometers (6 to 7 Angstroms) in the membrane. This makes the membrane very permeable to sodium ions (as well as to most other ions), allowing rapid influx of sodium into the muscle fiber. As a result, the membrane potential rises *in*

the local area of the end-plate as much as 50 to 75 millivolts, creating a *local potential* called the *end-plate potential*.

The mechanism by which acetylcholine increases the permeability of the muscle membrane is probably the following: It is believed that the muscle membrane contains special protein molecules called *acetylcholine receptors* to which the acetylcholine binds. Under the influence of the acetylcholine this receptor supposedly undergoes a conformational change that increases the permeability of the membrane to ions. Rapid influx of sodium ions ensues, and this elicits the end-plate potential that is responsible for initiation of the action potential at the muscle fiber membrane.

An end-plate potential is illustrated at point A in Figure 4–2. This potential was recorded after the muscle had been poisoned with curare, which made the end-plate potential too weak to excite an action potential in the muscle fiber. However, in the normal muscle fiber, the effect shown at point B occurs: The end-plate potential begins, but before it can complete its course the intense local current flow created by this potential initiates an action potential; this in turn spreads in both directions along the muscle fiber. The threshold voltage at which the skeletal muscle fiber is stimulated is approximately −50 millivolts. Thus, if the resting membrane potential of the muscle is at the normal level of about −90 millivolts, then an end-plate potential of +40 millivolts is required to elicit an action potential in the muscle fiber.

At point C, another situation is illustrated in which only a small quantity of acetylcholine is released at the end-plate. This also causes an end-plate potential that is less than the threshold value required to cause an action potential. Note that the potential dies in a few milliseconds. Thus,

Figure 4–2. End-plate potentials: A, weakened end-plate potential recorded in a curarized muscle, too weak to elicit an action potential; B, normal end-plate potential eliciting a muscle action potential; and C, weakened end-plate potential caused by botulinum toxin that decreases end-plate release of acetylcholine, again too weak to elicit a muscle action potential.

failure to transmit a signal to the muscle fiber can result from either diminished receptivity of the muscle membrane, as occurs when the muscle has been poisoned with curare, or decreased release of acetylcholine, as occurs when the end-plates have been poisoned with botulinum toxin.

"Safety Factor" for Transmission at the Neuromuscular Junction; Fatigue of the Junction. Ordinarily, each impulse that arrives at the neuromuscular junction creates an end-plate current flow about three to four times that required to stimulate the muscle fiber. Therefore, the normal neuromuscular junction is said to have a very high *safety factor*. However, artificial stimulation of the nerve fiber at rates greater than 100 times per second for several minutes often diminishes the number of vesicles of acetylcholine released with each impulse so much that impulses then often fail to pass into the muscle fiber. This is called *fatigue* of the neuromuscular junction, and it is analogous to fatigue of the synapse in the central nervous system. However, under normal functioning conditions, fatigue of the neuromuscular junction rarely occurs, because almost never do the spinal nerves stimulate even the most active neuromuscular junctions more than 100 times per second.

Drugs that Affect Transmission at the Neuromuscular Junction. *Drugs that Stimulate the Muscle Fiber by Acetylcholine-Like Action.* Many different compounds, including *methacholine, carbachol,* and *nicotine,* have the same effect on the muscle fiber as does acetylcholine. The difference between these drugs and acetylcholine is that they are not destroyed by cholinesterase or are destroyed very slowly, so that when once applied to the muscle fiber the action persists for many minutes to several hours. Moderate quantities of the above three drugs applied to a muscle fiber cause localized areas of depolarization, and every time the muscle fiber becomes repolarized elsewhere, these depolarized areas, by virtue of their leaking ions, cause new action potentials, thereby causing a state of spasm. On the other hand, when extreme doses of these drugs are used, so much of the membranes becomes depolarized that the fibers can no longer pass impulses at all, and a state of flaccid paralysis exists instead of the spasm that occurs with moderate dosages.

Drugs that Block Transmission at the Neuromuscular Junction. A group of drugs, known as the *curariform drugs,* can prevent passage of impulses from the end-plate into the muscle. Thus, D-tubocurarine affects the membrane, probably by competing with acetylcholine for the receptor sites of the membrane, so that the acetylcholine cannot increase the permeability of the membrane sufficiently to initiate a depolarization wave.

Drugs that Stimulate the Neuromuscular Junction by Inactivating Cholinesterase. Three particularly well-known drugs, *neostigmine, physostigmine,* and *diisopropyl fluorophosphate,* inactivate cholinesterase so that the cholinesterase normally in the synapses will not hydrolyze acetylcholine released at the end-plate. As a result, acetylcholine increases in quantity with successive nerve impulses so that extreme amounts of ace-

tylcholine can accumulate and repetitively stimulate the muscle fiber. This causes *muscular spasm* when even a few nerve impulses reach the muscle; this can cause death due to laryngeal spasm, which smothers the person.

Neostigmine and physostigmine combine with cholinesterase to inactivate it for several hours, after which they are displaced from the cholinesterase so that it once again becomes active. On the other hand, diisopropyl fluorophosphate, which has military potential as a very powerful "nerve" gas, actually inactivates cholinesterase for several weeks, which makes this a particularly lethal drug.

MYASTHENIA GRAVIS

The disease *myasthenia gravis,* which occurs in rare instances in human beings, causes the person to become paralyzed because of inability of the neuromuscular junctions to transmit signals from the nerve fibers to the muscle fibers. Pathologically, the number of subneural clefts in the synaptic gutter is reduced and the synaptic cleft itself is widened as much as 50 per cent. Also, antibodies that attack the muscle fibers have been demonstrated in the bloods of many of these patients. Therefore, it has been postulated that myasthenia gravis is an autoimmune disease in which patients have developed antibodies against their own muscles. And the antibodies in turn have damaged the muscle fibers — one of the effects being partial destruction of the receptor membrane of the neuromuscular junction.

Though it has not been possible to make precise neurophysiological measurements at the neuromuscular junctions in these patients, circumstantial evidence suggests that the end-plate potentials in these patients are greatly reduced, perhaps or probably because of the damaged receptor membrane of the junction.

Regardless of the cause, the end-plate potentials developed in the muscle fibers are too weak to stimulate the muscle fibers adequately. If the disease is intense enough, the patient dies of paralysis — in particular, of paralysis of the respiratory muscles. However, the disease can usually be ameliorated with several different drugs, as follows:

Treatment with Drugs. When a patient with myasthenia gravis is treated with a drug, such as neostigmine, that is capable of inactivating or destroying cholinesterase, the acetylcholine secreted by the end-plate is not destroyed immediately. If a sequence of nerve impulses arrives at the end-plate, the quantity of acetylcholine present at the membrane increases progressively until finally the end-plate potential caused by the acetylcholine rises above threshold value for stimulating the muscle fiber. Thus, it is possible by diminishing the quantity of cholinesterase in the muscles of a patient with myasthenia gravis to allow even the inadequate quantities of acetylcholine secreted at the end-plates to effect almost normal muscular activity.

CONTRACTION OF SMOOTH MUSCLE

In the previous chapter and thus far in the present chapter, the discussion has been concerned with skeletal muscle. We now turn to smooth muscle, which is composed of far smaller fibers — usually 2 to 5 microns in diameter and only 50 to 200 microns in length — in contrast to the skeletal muscle fibers that are as much as 20 times as large (in diameter) and thousands of times as long. Nevertheless, many of the same principles of contraction apply to both smooth muscle and skeletal muscle. Most important, essentially the same chemical substances cause contraction in smooth muscle as in skeletal muscle, but the physical arrangement of smooth muscle fibers is entirely different, as we shall see.

TYPES OF SMOOTH MUSCLE

The smooth muscle of each organ is distinctive from that of most other organs in several different ways: physical dimensions, organization into bundles or sheets, response to different types of stimuli, characteristics of its innervation, and function. Yet, for the sake of simplicity, smooth muscle can generally be divided into two major types, which are illustrated in Figure 4–3: *multiunit smooth muscle* and *visceral smooth muscle*.

Multiunit Smooth Muscle.   This type of smooth muscle is composed of discrete smooth muscle fibers. Each fiber operates entirely independently of the others and is often innervated by a single nerve ending, as occurs for skeletal muscle fibers. Furthermore, the outer surfaces of these fibers, like those of skeletal muscle fibers, are covered by a thin layer of "basement membrane-like" substance, a glycoprotein that helps to insulate the separate fibers from each other.

The most important characteristic of multiunit smooth muscle fibers is that their control is exerted almost entirely by nerve signals and very little by other stimuli such as local tissue factors. This is in contrast to a major share of the control of visceral smooth muscle by non-nervous stimuli. An additional characteristic is that they rarely exhibit spontaneous contractions.

Some examples of multiunit smooth muscle found in the body are the smooth muscle fibers of the ciliary muscle of the eye, the iris of the eye, the nictitating membrane that covers the eyes in some lower animals, the piloerector muscles that cause erection of the hairs when stimulated by the sympathetic nervous system, and the smooth muscle of many of the larger blood vessels.

Visceral Smooth Muscle.   Visceral smooth muscle fibers are similar to multiunit fibers except that they are usually arranged in sheets or bundles and the cell membranes contact each other at multiple points to form many *gap junctions,* or *nexi.* Thus the fibers form a *functional syncytium* that usually contracts in large areas at once. For this reason, this type of smooth muscle is also known as *single-unit* or *unitary smooth muscle.* This type of muscle is found in most of the organs of the body, especially in the walls of the gut, the bile ducts, the ureters, the uterus, and so forth.

When one portion of a visceral muscle tissue is stimulated, the action potential is conducted to the surrounding fibers by *ephaptic conduction.* This means that the action potential generated in one area of the muscle electrically excites the adjacent fibers without secretion of any excitatory substance. Visceral smooth muscle fibers can transmit action potentials one to another in this manner because the gap junctions between adjacent fibers exhibit greatly enhanced permeability so that the electrical resistance between the inside of one fiber and the next is only a fraction of the normal membrane resistance. This obviously allows easy flow of current from the interior of one cell to the next and therefore allows ease of transmission of action potentials over the surface membranes of the muscle mass.

THE CONTRACTILE PROCESS IN SMOOTH MUSCLE

The Chemical Basis for Contraction.   Smooth muscle contains both *actin* and *myosin filaments,* having chemical characteristics similar to but not exactly the same as those of the actin and myosin filaments in skeletal muscle. Smooth muscle also contains *tropomyosin,* but it is doubtful whether troponin or a troponin-like substance exists in smooth muscle. This raises a question about the mechanism for control of smooth muscle contraction, which will be discussed in more detail in a subsequent section of this chapter.

Chemical studies have shown that actin and myosin derived from smooth muscle interact with each other in the same way that this occurs for actin and myosin derived from skeletal muscle. Furthermore, the contractile process is activated by calcium ions, and ATP is degraded to ADP to provide the energy for contraction.

On the other hand, there are major differences

VISCERAL   MULTIUNIT

Figure 4–3. Visceral smooth muscle fibers and multiunit smooth muscle fibers.

in the physical organization of smooth muscle and skeletal muscle, as well as differences in other aspects of smooth muscle function such as excitation-contraction coupling, control of the contractile process by calcium ions, duration of contraction, and amount of energy required for the contractile process.

The Physical Basis for Smooth Muscle Contraction. Smooth muscle does not have the same striated arrangement of the actin and myosin filaments as that found in skeletal muscle. And, for a long time, it was impossible to discern even in electronmicrographs any specific organization in the smooth muscle cell that could account for contraction. However, recent special staining techniques suggest the physical organization illustrated in Figure 4-4. This shows large numbers of actin filaments attached to so-called *dense bodies*. Some of these bodies in turn are attached to the cell membrane while others are dispersed throughout the sarcoplasm. There also appear to be enough cross-attachments from one dense body to another to hold these in relatively fixed positions within the cell. Interspersed among the actin filaments are a few thick filaments about 2.5 times the diameter of the thin actin filaments. These are assumed to be myosin filaments. However, there are only one twelfth to one fifteenth as many of these "myosin filaments" as actin filaments.

Despite the relative paucity of myosin filaments, it is assumed that they have sufficient

Figure 4-4. Arrangement of actin and myosin filaments in the smooth muscle cell. Note the attachment of the actin filaments to "dense bodies," some of which are themselves attached to the cell membrane.

cross-bridges to attract the many actin filaments and cause contraction by the sliding filament mechanism in essentially the same way that this occurs in skeletal muscle. And it is especially interesting to note that the maximum strength of contraction of smooth muscle is approximately equal to that of skeletal muscle, about 2 to 3 kg. per square centimeter of cross-sectional area of the muscle.

Slowness of Contraction and Relaxation of Smooth Muscle. Though each smooth muscle tissue in the body has its own characteristics quite distinctive from the others, a typical smooth muscle tissue will begin to contract 50 to 100 milliseconds after it is excited, and will reach full contraction about half a second later. Then the contraction declines in another 1 to 2 seconds, giving a total contraction time of 1 to 3 seconds, which is about 30 times as long as the single-twitch contraction of skeletal muscle. However, smooth muscle contractions as short as 0.2 second and as long as 30 seconds have been recorded.

A major share of the prolonged contractile state of smooth muscle seems to be caused by slowness of the chemical reactions that cause the contraction. For instance, assuming that smooth muscle contraction occurs by the same ratchet mechanism as that proposed for skeletal muscle, it has been calculated that the frequency of power strokes by the heads of the cross-bridges is only one fiftieth to one hundredth as rapid as in skeletal muscle. This apparently results from the fact that the cross-bridge heads have far less ATPase activity than that exhibited by the cross-bridge heads in skeletal muscle.

Energy Required to Sustain Smooth Muscle Contraction. Measurements have shown that as little as one five-hundredth as much energy is required to sustain the same tension of contraction in smooth muscle as in skeletal muscle. This presumably results from the very slow activity of the myosin ATPase and also from the fact that there are far fewer myosin filaments in smooth muscle than in skeletal muscle.

This economy of energy utilization by smooth muscle is exceedingly important to overall function of the body, because organs such as the intestines, the urinary bladder, the gallbladder, and other viscera must maintain moderate degrees of muscle contractile tone day in and day out.

MEMBRANE POTENTIALS AND ACTION POTENTIALS IN SMOOTH MUSCLE

Smooth muscle exhibits membrane potentials and action potentials similar to those that occur in skeletal muscle fibers. Furthermore, smooth muscle contraction can be elicited by depolarization of the membrane in the same way that contraction is initiated by depolarization of skeletal muscle fibers. However, there are both quantitative and qualitative differences in the membrane potentials and action potentials of smooth muscle that require special attention.

Membrane Potentials in Smooth Muscle. The

quantitative value of the membrane potential of smooth muscle is variable from one type of smooth muscle to another, and it also depends on the momentary condition of the muscle. However, in the normal resting state, the membrane potential is usually about −50 to −60 millivolts, or about 30 millivolts less negative than in skeletal muscle.

Action Potentials in Visceral Smooth Muscle. Action potentials occur in visceral smooth muscle in the same way that they occur in skeletal muscle. However, action potentials probably do not normally occur in multiunit types of smooth muscle, as will be discussed in a subsequent section.

The action potentials of visceral smooth muscle occur in two different forms: (1) spike potentials and (2) action potentials with plateaus.

Spike Potentials. Typical spike action potentials, such as those seen in skeletal muscle, occur in most types of visceral smooth muscle. The duration of this type of action potential is 10 to 50 milliseconds, as illustrated in Figure 4–5A. Such action potentials can be elicited in many ways, such as by electrical stimulation, by the action of hormones on the smooth muscle, by the action of transmitter substances from nerve fibers, or as a result of spontaneous generation in the muscle fiber itself, as discussed below.

Action Potentials with Plateaus. Figure 4–6 illustrates an action potential with a plateau. The onset of this action potential is similar to that of the typical spike potential. However, instead of rapid repolarization of the muscle fiber membrane, the repolarization is delayed for several hundred

Figure 4–6. Monophasic action potential from a smooth muscle fiber of the rat uterus.

to several thousand milliseconds. Plateaus as long as 30 seconds have been recorded. The importance of the plateau is that it can account for the prolonged periods of contraction that occur in at least some types of smooth muscle. This type of action potential often occurs in the ureter, in the uterus under some conditions, and in some types of vascular smooth muscle. (Also, this is the type of action potential seen in cardiac muscle fibers that have a prolonged period of contraction, as we shall discuss in the next two chapters.)

Slow Wave Potentials in Visceral Smooth Muscle and Spontaneous Generation of Action Potentials. Some smooth muscle is self-excitatory. That is, action potentials arise within the smooth muscle itself without an extrinsic stimulus. This is usually associated with a basic *slow wave rhythm* of the membrane potential. A typical slow wave of this type is illustrated in Figure 4–5B. The slow wave itself is not an action potential. It is not a self-regenerative process that spreads progressively over the membranes of the muscle fibers. Instead, it is a local property of the smooth muscle fibers that make up the muscle mass.

The cause of the slow wave rhythm is as yet unknown; one suggestion, for which there is circumstantial evidence, is that the slow waves are caused by waxing and waning of the pumping of sodium outward through the muscle fiber membrane; the membrane potential becomes more negative when sodium is pumped rapidly and less negative when the sodium pump becomes less active.

The importance of the slow waves lies in the fact that they can initiate action potentials. The slow waves themselves cannot cause muscle contraction, but when the potential of the slow wave rises above the level of approximately −35 millivolts (the approximate threshold for eliciting action potentials in most visceral smooth muscle), an action potential develops and spreads over the visceral smooth muscle mass, and then contraction does occur. Figure 4–5B illustrates this effect, showing that at each peak of the slow wave, one or more action potentials occur. This effect can obviously promote a series of rhythmical contractions of the smooth muscle mass. There-

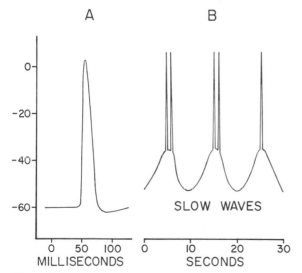

Figure 4–5. *A,* A typical smooth muscle action potential (spike potential) elicited by an external stimulus. *B,* A series of spike action potentials elicited by rhythmical slow electrical waves occurring spontaneously in the smooth muscle wall of the intestine.

fore, the slow waves are frequently called *pacemaker waves*. This type of activity is especially prominent in tubular types of smooth muscle masses, such as in the gut, the ureter, and so forth. In fact, this type of activity controls the rhythmical contractions of the gut.

Spread of Action Potentials Through Visceral Smooth Muscle. Because of the *gap junctions* that allow easy spread of electrical current from one smooth muscle fiber to the next in visceral smooth muscle, once an action potential begins, it spreads slowly through the muscle mass. For instance, if it begins at the upper end of the gastrointestinal tract, it can spread variable distances downward along the intestinal wall, creating a constrictive ring that moves forward. The constrictive ring propels the intestinal contents forward. This process is called *peristalsis*, an important end result of smooth muscle function.

Excitation of Visceral Smooth Muscle by Stretch. When visceral smooth muscle is stretched sufficiently, spontaneous action potentials are usually generated. These result from a combination of the normal slow wave potentials plus a decrease in the membrane potential caused by the stretch itself. This response to stretch is an especially important function of visceral smooth muscle because it allows a hollow organ that is excessively stretched to contract automatically and therefore to resist the stretch. For instance, when the gut is overstretched by intestinal contents, a local automatic contraction sets up a peristaltic wave that moves the contents away from the super-stretched intestine.

Depolarization of Multiunit Smooth Muscle Without Action Potentials. The smooth muscle fibers of multiunit smooth muscle normally contract only in response to nerve stimuli. The nerve endings secrete acetylcholine in the case of some multiunit smooth muscles and norepinephrine in the case of others. In both instances, these transmitter substances cause depolarization of the smooth muscle membrane, and this response in turn elicits the contraction. However, action potentials most often do not develop. The presumed reason for this is that the fibers are too small to generate an action potential. In fact, when action potentials are elicited in visceral smooth muscle, as many as 30 to 40 smooth muscle fibers must depolarize simultaneously before a self-propagating action potential ensues. Yet, even without an action potential in the multiunit smooth muscle fibers, the local depolarization caused by the nerve transmitter substance itself spreads "electrotonically" over the entire fiber and is all that is needed to cause the muscle contraction.

Role of Calcium Ions in Causing Smooth Muscle Action Potentials. It will be recalled from the discussion in Chapter 2 that the depolarization process during the action potential of nerve fibers (and also of skeletal muscle fibers) is caused almost entirely by rapid influx of sodium ions to the interior of the cell membrane. In the action potential of smooth muscle fibers, the rapid influx of ions includes not only sodium ions but also a large quantity of calcium ions. Indeed, it is believed that for many types of smooth muscle, the onset of depolarization is caused mainly by influx of calcium ions rather than of sodium ions. This is particularly important in view of the fact that influx of calcium ions seems also to be the major means by which muscle contraction itself is elicited, as will be discussed in the following section.

EXCITATION-CONTRACTION COUPLING – ROLE OF CALCIUM IONS

In the previous chapter it was pointed out that the actual contractile process in skeletal muscle is activated by calcium ions. This is also true in smooth muscle. However, the source of the calcium ions differs in smooth muscle because the sarcoplasmic reticulum of smooth muscle is poorly developed, in contrast to the sarcoplasmic reticulum of skeletal muscle which is very extensive and is the source of very nearly 100 per cent of the contraction-inducing calcium ions.

In some types of smooth muscle, most of the calcium ions that cause contraction enter the muscle fiber from the extracellular fluid at the time of the action potential. There is a reasonably high concentration of calcium ions in the extracellular fluid, and as was pointed out in the previous section, the action potential is caused at least partly by influx of calcium ions into the muscle fiber. Because the smooth muscle fibers are extremely small (in contrast to the sizes of the skeletal muscle fibers), these calcium ions can diffuse to all parts of the smooth muscle and elicit the contractile process. The time required for this diffusion to occur is usually 200 to 300 milliseconds and is called the *latent period* before the contraction begins; this latent period is some 50 times as great as that for skeletal muscle contraction.

Yet, in some smooth muscle there is a moderately developed sarcoplasmic reticulum. However, there are no T tubules. Instead, the cisternae of the reticulum abut the cell membrane. Therefore, it is believed that the membrane action potentials in these smooth muscle fibers cause release of calcium ions from these cisternae, thereby providing a greater degree of contraction than would occur on the basis of calcium ions entering through the cell membrane alone.

The Calcium Pump. To cause relaxation of the smooth muscle contractile elements, it is necessary to remove the calcium ions. This removal is achieved by a calcium pump that pumps the calcium ions out of the smooth muscle fiber and back into the extracellular fluid, or pumps the calcium ions into the sarcoplasmic reticulum. However, this pump is very slow-acting in comparison with the fast-acting sarcoplasmic reticulum pump in skeletal muscle. Therefore, the duration of smooth muscle contraction is often in the order of seconds rather than in tens of milliseconds, as occurs for skeletal muscle.

Mechanism by Which Calcium Ions Excite Contraction in Smooth Muscle. In skeletal muscle, calcium ions activate contraction by binding with troponin. This in turn causes conformational changes in the tropomyosin, then activation of the actin filament, and finally the contractile process itself. However, troponin has not been proved to be present in smooth muscle cells. Therefore, it is doubtful that calcium ions initiate smooth muscle contraction in the same way that they initiate skeletal muscle contraction. Instead, in smooth muscle, calcium ions strongly excite the ATPase activity of the heads of the myosin cross-bridges. In skeletal muscle this activation by calcium ions is weak, but in smooth muscle it occurs at very low calcium ion concentrations. In contrast to skeletal muscle, therefore, this activation of the myosin ATPase system is believed to initiate smooth muscle contraction. That is, the ATPase begins to split ATP; in turn, the released energy sets into motion the contractile process. It is possible that the troponin-tropomyosin system is not involved.

NEUROMUSCULAR JUNCTIONS OF SMOOTH MUSCLE

Physiologic Anatomy of Smooth Muscle Neuromuscular Junctions. Neuromuscular junctions of the type found on skeletal muscle fibers do not occur in smooth muscle. Instead, the nerve fibers generally branch diffusely on top of a sheet of muscle fibers, as was illustrated in Figure 4–3. In most instances these fibers do not make direct contact with the smooth muscle fibers at all but instead form so-called *diffuse junctions* that secrete their transmitter substance into the interstitial fluid a few microns away from the muscle cells; the transmitter substance then diffuses to the cells. Furthermore, where there are many layers of muscle cells, the nerve fibers often innervate only the outer layer, and the muscle excitation then travels from this outer layer to the inner layers by direct action potential conduction or by subsequent diffusion of the transmitter substance. But, less often, terminal branches of the axons do penetrate into the muscle mass.

The axons innervating smooth muscle fibers also do not have typical end-feet as observed in the end-plate on skeletal muscle fibers. Instead, the fine terminal axons have multiple varicosities spread along their axes. At these points the Schwann cells are interrupted so that transmitter substance can be secreted through the walls of the

varicosities. In the varicosities are vesicles similar to those present in the skeletal muscle end-plate containing transmitter substance. However, in contrast to the vesicles of skeletal muscle junctions that contain only acetylcholine, the vesicles of the autonomic nerve fiber varicosities contain acetylcholine in some fibers and norepinephrine in others.

In a few instances, particularly in the multiunit type of smooth muscle, the varicosities lie directly on the muscle fiber membrane with a separation from this membrane of only 20 nanometers — the same width as the synaptic cleft that occurs in the skeletal muscle junction. These *contact junctions* function in much the same way as the skeletal muscle neuromuscular junction, and the latent period of contraction of these smooth muscle fibers is considerably shorter than of fibers stimulated by the diffuse junctions.

Excitatory and Inhibitory Transmitter Substances at the Smooth Muscle Neuromuscular Junction. Two different transmitter substances known to be secreted by the autonomic nerves innervating smooth muscle are *acetylcholine* and *norepinephrine*. Acetylcholine is an excitatory substance for smooth muscle fibers in some organs but an inhibitory substance for smooth muscle in other organs. And when acetylcholine excites a muscle fiber, norepinephrine ordinarily inhibits it, or when acetylcholine inhibits a fiber norepinephrine excites it.

It is believed that *receptor substances* in the membranes of the different smooth muscle fibers determine which will excite them, acetylcholine or norepinephrine. Thus, there are *excitatory receptors* and *inhibitory receptors*. These receptor substances will be discussed in more detail in Chapter 17 in relation to function of the autonomic nervous system.

Excitation of Action Potentials in Smooth Muscle Fibers — The Junctional Potential. Transmission of impulses from terminal nerve fibers to smooth muscle fibers occurs in very much the same manner as transmission at the neuromuscular junction of skeletal muscle fibers except for temporal differences. When an action potential reaches the terminal of an excitatory nerve fibril, there is a typical latent period of 50 milliseconds before any change in the membrane potential of the smooth muscle fiber can be detected. Then the potential rises to a maximal level in approximately 100 milliseconds. If an action potential does not occur, this potential gradually disappears at a rate of approximately one-half every 200 to 500 milliseconds. This complete sequence of potential changes is called the *junctional potential;* it is analogous to the end-plate potential of the skeletal muscle fibers except that its duration is 20 to 100 times as long.

If the junctional potential rises to the threshold

level for discharge of the smooth muscle membrane, an action potential will occur in the smooth muscle fiber in exactly the same way that an action potential occurs in a skeletal muscle fiber. A typical smooth muscle fiber has a normal resting membrane potential of −50 to −60 millivolts, and the threshold potential at which the action potential occurs is about −30 to −35 millivolts.

Inhibition at the Smooth Muscle Neuromuscular Junction. When a transmitter substance at the nerve ending interacts with an inhibitory receptor instead of an excitatory receptor, the membrane potential of the muscle fiber becomes more negative than ever, for instance −70 millivolts; that is, it becomes *hyperpolarized* and therefore becomes much more difficult to excite than is usually the case.

SMOOTH MUSCLE CONTRACTION WITHOUT ACTION POTENTIALS — EFFECT OF LOCAL TISSUE FACTORS AND HORMONES

Though we have thus far discussed smooth muscle contraction elicited only by nervous signals and smooth muscle membrane action potentials, we must quickly disavow the fact that all smooth muscle contraction occurs in this way. In fact, probably half or more of all smooth muscle contraction is initiated not by action potentials but by stimulatory factors acting directly on the smooth muscle contractile machinery. The two types of non-nervous and nonaction potential stimulating factors most often involved are (1) local tissue factors, and (2) various hormones.

Smooth Muscle Contraction in Response to Local Tissue Factors. In later chapters we shall discuss the control of contraction of the arterioles, meta-arterioles, and precapillary sphincters. The smaller of these vessels have little or no nervous supply. Yet, the smooth muscle is highly contractile, responding rapidly to changes in local conditions in the surrounding interstitial fluid. In this way a powerful local feedback control system exists to maintain appropriate local fluid environmental conditions. Some of the specific control factors are:

(1) Lack of oxygen in the local tissues causes smooth muscle relaxation and therefore vasodilatation.
(2) Excess carbon dioxide causes vasodilatation.
(3) Increased hydrogen ion concentration also causes increased vasodilatation.

And such factors as lactic acid, increased potassium ions, diminished calcium ion concentration, and decreased body temperature will also cause local vasodilatation.

Effects of Hormones on Smooth Muscle Contraction. Most of the circulating hormones in the body affect smooth muscle contraction at least to some degree, and some often have very profound effects. Some of the more important hormones are norepinephrine, epinephrine, acetylcholine, angiotensin, vasopressin, oxytocin, serotonin, and histamine.

A hormone will cause contraction of smooth muscle when the smooth muscle cells contain an *excitatory receptor* for the respective hormone. However, the hormone will cause inhibition instead of contraction if the cells contain an *inhibitory receptor* rather than an excitatory receptor. Thus, most of the hormones will cause excitation of some smooth muscle but inhibition of other muscle.

Some of the hormones — especially norepinephrine, vasopressin, and angiotensin — have such a powerful excitatory effect that they can cause smooth muscle spasm for hours.

Mechanism of Muscle Excitation by Local Tissue Factors and Hormones. It is believed that the local tissue factors and hormones that cause smooth muscle contraction do so by activating the calcium mechanism for control of the contractile process. Some of these factors change the membrane potential a moderate amount but without necessarily causing an action potential, and this increases the flow of calcium ions to the interior of the cell. However, most of them can activate contraction even when the membrane potential is not altered and even when calcium ions are not available to enter the cell. In these circumstances calcium ions probably are released from the sarcoplasmic reticulum. In some instances, possibly the affinity of the contractile mechanism for calcium ions is increased by the local factor or the hormone.

MECHANICAL CHARACTERISTICS OF SMOOTH MUSCLE CONTRACTION

From the foregoing discussion of the many different types of smooth muscle and the different ways in which contraction can be elicited, one can readily understand why smooth muscle in different parts of the body has many different characteristics of contraction. For instance, the multiunit smooth muscle of the large blood vessels contracts mainly in response to nerve impulses, whereas in many types of visceral smooth muscle — the smaller blood vessels, the ureter, the bile ducts, and other glandular ducts — a self-excitatory process controlled mainly by local factors and by hormones causes continuous rhythmic contraction.

Tone of Smooth Muscle. Smooth muscle can maintain a state of long-term, steady contraction that has been called either *tonus* contraction of smooth muscle or simply *smooth muscle tone*. This is an important feature of smooth muscle contraction because it allows prolonged or even indefinite continuance of the smooth muscle function. For instance, the arterioles are maintained in a state of tonic contraction almost throughout the entire life of the person. Likewise, tonic contraction in the gut wall maintains steady pressure on the contents of the gut, and tonic contraction of the urinary bladder wall maintains a moderate amount of pressure on the urine in the bladder.

Tonic contractions of smooth muscle can be caused in either of two ways:

(1) They are sometimes caused by *summation of individual contractile pulses;* each contractile pulse is initiated by a separate action potential in the same way that tetanic contractions are produced in skeletal muscle.

(2) However, most smooth muscle tonic contractions probably result from *prolonged direct smooth muscle excitation* without action potentials, usually caused by local tissue factors or circulating hormones. For instance, prolonged tonic contractions of the blood vessels without the mediation of action potentials are regularly caused by angiotensin, vasopressin, or norepinephrine, and these play important roles in the long-term regulation of arterial pressure as well as in the control of other bodily functions.

A typical example of a tonic contraction (also frequently called simply *tonus*) is illustrated in Figure 4–7. This figure also shows that rhythmic contractions can be superimposed onto the tonic contraction because of simultaneous (a) rhythmical nerve discharges or (b) rhythmical pacemaker slow waves that periodically excite the smooth muscle.

Degree of Shortening of Smooth Muscle During Contraction. A special characteristic of smooth muscle — one that is also different from skeletal muscle —is its ability to shorten a far greater percentage of its length than can skeletal muscle. Skeletal muscle has a useful distance of contraction equal to only 25 to 35 per cent of its length, while smooth muscle can often contract quite effectively from a length two times its normal length to as short as one-half its normal length, giving as much as a four-fold distance of contraction. This allows smooth muscle to perform important functions in the hollow viscera — for instance, allowing the gut, the bladder, blood vessels, and other internal structures of the body to change their lumen diameters from almost zero up to very large values.

Stress-Relaxation of Smooth Muscle. A very important characteristic of smooth muscle is its ability to change length greatly without marked changes in tension. This results from a phenomenon called *stress-relaxation*, which may be explained as follows:

If a segment of smooth muscle 1 inch long is suddenly stretched to 2 inches, the tension between the two ends increases tremendously at first, but the extra tension also begins to disappear immediately, and within a few minutes it has returned almost to its level prior to the stretch, even though the muscle is now twice as long. This possibly results from the loose arrangement of the actin and myosin filaments in smooth muscle. Over a period of time, the filaments of the stretched muscle presumably rearrange their bonds and gradually allow the sliding process to take place, thus allowing the tension to return almost to its original amount.

Exactly the converse effect occurs when smooth muscle is shortened. Thus, if the 2 inch segment of smooth muscle is shortened back to 1 inch, essentially all tension will be lost from the muscle immediately. Gradually, over a period of 1 minute or more, much of the tension returns, this again presumably resulting from slow sliding of the filaments. This is called *reverse stress-relaxation*.

REFERENCES

Baker, P. F., and Reuter, H.: Calcium Movement in Excitable Cells. New York, Pergamon Press, 1975.

Bolton, T. B.: Mechanisms of action of transmitters and other substances on smooth muscle. *Physiol. Rev.,* 59:606, 1979.

Bulbring, E., *et al.* (eds.): Physiology of Smooth Muscles; Twenty-sixth International Congress of Physiological Sciences. New York, Raven Press, 1975.

Ceccarelli, B., and Hurlbut, W. P.: Vesicle hypothesis of the release of quanta of acetylcholine. *Physiol. Rev.,* 60:396, 1980.

Chamley-Campbell, J., *et al.*: Smooth muscle cell in culture. *Physiol. Rev.,* 59:1, 1979.

Daniel, E. E., and Sarna, S.: The generation and conduction of activity in smooth muscle. *Annu. Rev. Pharmacol. Toxicol.,* 18:145, 1978.

Dau, P. C. (ed.): Plasmapheresis and the Immunobiology of Myasthenia Gravis. Boston, Houghton Mifflin, 1979.

De Robertis, E., and Schacht, J. (eds.): Neurochemistry of Cholinergic Receptors. New York, American Elsevier Publishing Co., 1974.

Devine, C. E.: Morphology and ultrastructure. *In* Kaley, G., and Altura, B. M. (eds.): Microcirculation. Vol. II. Baltimore, University Park Press, 1977.

Fambrough, D. M.: Control of acetylcholine receptors in skeletal muscle. *Physiol. Rev.,* 59:165, 1979.

Gage, P. W.: Generation of end-plate potentials. *Physiol. Rev.,* 56:177, 1976.

Guyton, A. C., and MacDonald, M. A.: Physiology of botulinus toxin. *Arch. Neurol. Psychiat.,* 57:578, 1947.

Guyton, A. C., and Reeder, R. C.: The dynamics of curarization. *J. Pharmacol. Exp. Ther.,* 97:322, 1949.

Hall, Z. W., *et al.*: Chemistry of Synaptic Transmission. Newton, Mass., Chiron Press, 1974.

Hartshorne, D. J., and Gorecka, A.: Biochemistry of the contractile proteins of smooth muscle. *In* Bohr, D. F., *et al.* (eds.): Handbook of Physiology. Sec. 2, Vol. II. Baltimore, Williams & Wilkins, 1980, p. 93.

Heuser, J. E., and Reese, T. S.: Structure of the synapse. *In* Brookhart, J. M., and Mountcastle, V. B. (eds.): Handbook of Physiology. Sec. 1, Vol. 1. Baltimore, Williams & Wilkins, 1977, p. 261.

Johansson, B.: Vascular smooth muscle biophysics. *In* Kaley, G., and Altura, B. M. (eds.): Microcirculation. Vol. II. Baltimore, University Park Press, 1977.

Johansson, B., and Somlyo, A. P.: Electrophysiology and excitation-contraction coupling. *In* Bohr, D. F., *et al.* (eds.): Handbook of Physiology. Sec. 2, Vol. II. Baltimore, Williams & Wilkins, 1980, p. 301.

Landmesser, L. T.: The generation of neuromuscular specificity. *Annu. Rev. Neurosci.,* 3:279, 1980.

Figure 4–7. Record of rhythmic and tonic smooth muscle contraction.

Lester, H. A.: The response to acetylcholine. *Sci. Am., 236*(2):106, 1977.

Lunt, G. G., and Marchbanks, R. M.: The Biochemistry of Myasthenia Gravis and Muscular Dystrophy. New York, Academic Press, 1978.

Mark, R. F.: Synaptic repression at neuromuscular junctions. *Physiol. Rev., 60*:355, 1980.

Martin, A. R.: Junctional transmission. II. Presynaptic mechanisms. *In* Brookhart, J. M., and Mountcastle, V. B. (eds.): Handbook of Physiology. Sec. 1, Vol. I. Baltimore, Williams & Wilkins, 1977, p. 329.

McGeachie, J. K.: Smooth Muscle Regeneration; A Review and Experimental Study. Basel, S. Karger, 1975.

Minton, S. A., Jr.: Venom Diseases. Springfield, Ill., Charles C Thomas, 1974.

Murphy, R. A.: Filament organization and contractile function in vertebrate smooth muscle. *Annu. Rev. Physiol., 41*:737, 1979.

Paul, R. J.: Chemical energetics of vascular smooth muscle. *In* Bohr, D. F., *et al.* (eds.): Handbook of Physiology. Sec. 2, Vol. II. Baltimore, Williams & Wilkins, 1980, p. 201.

Paul, R. J., and Rüegg, J. C.: Biochemistry of vascular smooth muscle: Energy metabolism and proteins. *In* Kaley, G., and Altura, B. M. (eds.): Microcirculation. Vol. II. Baltimore, University Park Press, 1977.

Pepeu, G., *et al.* (eds.): Receptors for Neurotransmitters and Peptide Hormones. New York, Raven Press, 1980.

Prosser, C. L.: Smooth muscle. *Annu. Rev. Physiol., 36*:503, 1974.

Prosser, C. L.: Evolution and diversity of nonstriated muscles. *In* Bohr, D. F., *et al.* (eds.): Handbook of Physiology. Sec. 2, Vol. II. Baltimore, Williams & Wilkins, 1980, p. 635.

Rémond, A., and Izard, C. (eds.): Electrophysiological Effects of Nicotine. New York, Elsevier/North-Holland, 1979.

Somlyo, A. P.: Excitation-contraction coupling in vertebrate smooth muscle: Correlation of ultrastructure with function. *Physiologist, 15*: 338, 1972.

Somlyo, A. P.: Ultrastructure of vascular smooth muscle. *In* Bohr, D. F., *et al.* (eds.): Handbook of Physiology. Sec. 2, Vol. II. Baltimore, Williams & Wilkins, 1980, p. 33.

Takeuchi, A.: Junctional transmission. I. Postsynaptic mechanisms. *In* Brookhart, J. M., and Mountcastle, V. B. (eds.): Handbook of Physiology. Sec. 1, Vol. I. Baltimore, Williams & Wilkins, 1977, p. 295.

5

The Heart: Its Rhythmical Excitation and Nervous Control

The heart is a muscular organ. Like other muscles of the body, it is, in a sense, an extension of the nervous system, for its pumping function is at least partly controlled by nerves.

To perform its pumping function, the heart is divided into four separate chambers. The right and left atria pump blood respectively into the right and left ventricles. The right ventricle then pumps blood through the lungs, and the left ventricle pumps blood through the remainder of the body.

The atria actually function as "primer" pumps for the ventricles. Normally, they contract about one-eighth of a second ahead of the ventricles, thus allowing time for extra blood to enter the ventricles prior to their contraction; this greatly increases the effectiveness of ventricular pumping.

The complexity of the heart's pumping cycle requires both rhythmical control of the heart beat and special timing mechanisms for sequential control of the atria and the ventricles. Furthermore, the rate of rhythmicity, as well as the strength of heart beat, can be increased or decreased by signals from the central nervous system. These control mechanisms will be explained later in the chapter. However, first, let us discuss the basic physiology of cardiac muscle itself, especially how it differs from skeletal muscle, which was discussed in Chapter 3.

PHYSIOLOGY OF CARDIAC MUSCLE

The heart is composed of three major types of cardiac muscle: atrial muscle, ventricular muscle, and specialized excitatory and conductive muscle fibers. The atrial and ventricular types of muscle contract in much the same way as the skeletal muscle fibers. On the other hand, the specialized excitatory and conductive fibers contract only feebly because they contain few contractile fibrils; instead, because of their rhythmical properties

and their rapidity of conduction, they provide an excitatory system for the heart and a transmission system for rapid conduction of impulses throughout the heart.

PHYSIOLOGIC ANATOMY OF CARDIAC MUSCLE

Figure 5–1 illustrates a typical histologic picture of cardiac muscle, showing the cardiac muscle fibers arranged in a latticework, the fibers dividing, then recombining, and then spreading again. One notes immediately from this figure that cardiac muscle is *striated* in the same manner as typical skeletal muscle. Furthermore, cardiac muscle has typical myofibrils that contain *actin* and *myosin filaments* almost identical to those found in skeletal muscle, and these filaments interdigitate the slide along one another during the process of contraction in the same manner as occurs in skeletal muscle. (See Chapter 3.)

Cardiac Muscle as Syncytium. The angulated dark areas crossing the cardiac muscle fibers in Figure 5–1 are called *intercalated discs;* however, they are actually cell membranes that separate individual cardiac muscle cells from each other. That is, cardiac muscle fibers are made up of many

Intercalated discs

Figure 5–1. The "syncytial" nature of cardiac muscle.

cardiac muscle cells connected in series with each other. Yet electrical resistance through the intercalated disc is only one four-hundredth the resistance through the outside membrane of the cardiac muscle fiber, because the cell membranes fuse with each other to form "tight junctions" that allow almost completely free diffusion of ions. Therefore, from a functional point of view, ions move with ease along the axes of the cardiac muscle fibers so that action potentials travel from one cardiac muscle cell to another, past the intercalated discs, without significant hindrance. Therefore, cardiac muscle is a *syncytium*, in which the cardiac muscle cells are so tightly bound that when one of these cells becomes excited, the action potential spreads to all of them, spreading from cell to cell and spreading throughout the latticework interconnections.

The heart is composed of two separate syncytiums, the *atrial syncytium* and the *ventricular syncytium*. These are separated from each other by the fibrous tissue surrounding the valvular rings, but an action potential can be conducted from the atrial syncytium into the ventricular syncytium by way of a specialized conductive system, the *A-V bundle*, which will be discussed in detail later in this chapter.

All-or-Nothing Principle as Applied to the Heart. Because of the syncytial nature of cardiac muscle, stimulation of any single atrial muscle fiber causes the action potential to travel over the entire atrial muscle mass, and, similarly, stimulation of any single ventricular fiber causes excitation of the entire ventricular muscle mass. If the A-V bundle is intact, the action potential passes also from the atria to the ventricles. This is called the all-or-nothing principle; and it is precisely the same as that discussed in Chapter 2 for nerve fibers. However, because the cardiac muscle fibers interconnect with each other, the all-or-nothing principle applies to the entire functional syncytium of the heart rather than to single muscle fibers as in the case of skeletal muscle fibers.

ACTION POTENTIALS IN CARDIAC MUSCLE

The *resting membrane potential* of normal cardiac muscle is approximately −85 to −95 millivolt (mv.) and approximately −90 to −100 mv. in the specialized conductive fibers, the Purkinje fibers, which are discussed later in this chapter.

The *action potential* recorded in ventricular muscle, shown at the bottom of Figure 5–2, is 105 mv., which means that the membrane potential rises from its normally very negative value to a slightly positive value of about +20 mv. Because of this change of potential from negative to positive, the positive portion is called the *reversal potential*. The basic principles of the genesis of resting, action, and reversal potentials were discussed in Chapter 2.

Cardiac muscle has a peculiar type of action potential. After the initial *spike* the membrane remains depolarized for 0.15 for atrial muscle to 0.3 second for ventricular muscle, exhibiting a *plateau* as illustrated in Figure 5–2, followed at the end of the plateau by abrupt repolarization. The presence of this plateau in the action potential causes the action potential to last 20 to 50 times as long in cardiac muscle as in skeletal muscle and causes a correspondingly increased period of contraction.

At this point we must ask the question: Why does the action potential of cardiac muscle have a plateau while that of skeletal muscle does not? There are at least two major differences between the membrane properties of these two types of muscle that presumably account for the plateau in cardiac muscle. First, a moderate quantity of calcium ions diffuses to the inside of the cardiac muscle fiber during the action potential, while only a very small quantity diffuses into skeletal muscle. Furthermore, the calcium ion influx does not occur only at the onset of the action potential, as is true for sodium ions, but instead continues for 0.2 to 0.3 second. The plateau occurs during this prolonged influx of calcium ions.

The second major functional difference between cardiac muscle and skeletal muscle that helps to account for the plateau is this: immediately after the onset of the action potential the permeability of the cardiac muscle membrane for potassium *decreases* about five-fold, an effect that does not occur in skeletal muscle. It is believed that this decreased potassium permeability is caused by the excess calcium influx noted above. The decreased potassium permeability greatly decreases the out-

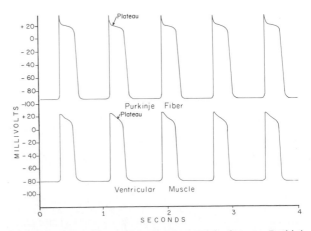

Figure 5–2. Rhythmic action potentials from a Purkinje fiber and from a ventricular muscle fiber, recorded by means of microelectrodes.

flux of potassium ions for the next 0.2 to 0.3 second, which prevents rapid repolarization of the membrane and thus gives rise to the plateau. Then, at the end of this time, the membrane permeability for potassium begins to increase so that more and more potassium leaves the fiber. This becomes a self-regenerative process; that is, the greater the rate of potassium outflux, the greater becomes the permeability of the membrane for potassium so that the potassium outflux becomes still greater. This regenerative cycle causes an almost explosive increase in potassium permeability, and the rapid loss of potassium from the fiber returns the membrane potential to its resting level, thus ending the action potential.

Velocity of Conduction in Cardiac Muscle. The velocity of conduction of the action potential in both atrial and ventricular muscle fibers is about 0.3 to 0.5 meter per second, or about 1/250 the velocity in very large nerve fibers and about one tenth the velocity in skeletal muscle fibers. The velocity of conduction in the specialized conductive system varies from 0.02 to 4 meters per second in different parts of the system, as is explained later in the chapter.

Refractory Period of Cardiac Muscle. Cardiac muscle, like an excitable tissue, is refractory to restimulation during the action potential. An extremely strong electrical stimulus can sometimes initiate a new spike at the very end of the action potential plateau, but this is a very abnormal situation and the spike is not propagated along the muscle. Therefore, the refractory period of the heart is usually stated to be the interval of time, as shown to the left in Figure 5–3, during which a normal cardiac impulse cannot re-excite an already excited area of cardiac muscle. The normal refractory period of the ventricle is 0.25 to 0.3 second, which is approximately the duration of the action potential. There is an additional *relative refractory period* of about 0.05 second during

which the muscle is more difficult than normal to excite but nevertheless can be excited, as illustrated by the early premature contraction in Figure 5–3.

The refractory period of atrial muscle is much shorter than that for the ventricles (about 0.15 second), and the relative refractory period is another 0.03 second. Therefore, the rhythmical rate of contraction of the atria can be much faster than that of the ventricles.

CONTRACTION OF CARDIAC MUSCLE

Excitation-Contraction Coupling — Function of Calcium Ions and of the T Tubules. The term excitation-contraction coupling means the mechanism by which the action potential causes the myofibrils of muscle to contract. This was discussed in detail for skeletal muscle in Chapter 3. However, once again there are differences in this mechanism in cardiac muscle that have important effects on the characteristics of cardiac muscle contraction.

As is true for skeletal muscle, when an action potential passes over the cardiac muscle membrane, the action potential also spreads to the interior of the cardiac muscle fiber along the membranes of the T tubules. The T tubule action potentials in turn cause instantaneous release of calcium ions into the muscle sarcoplasm from the cisternae of the sarcoplasmic reticulum. Then the calcium ions diffuse in another few thousandths of a second into the myofibrils where they catalyze the chemical reactions that promote sliding of the actin and myosin filaments along each other; this in turn produces the muscle contraction. Thus far, this mechanism of excitation-contraction coupling is the same as that for skeletal muscle, but at this point a major difference begins to appear. In addition to the calcium ions that are released into the sarcoplasm from the cisternae of the sarcoplasmic reticulum, large quantities of calcium ions also diffuse during the action potential from the T tubules into the sarcoplasm. Indeed, without this extra calcium from the T tubules, it is probable that the strength of cardiac muscle contraction would be considerably reduced, because the cisternae of cardiac muscle are less well developed than those of skeletal muscle and do not store enough calcium. On the other hand, the T tubules of cardiac muscle have a diameter 5 times as great as that of the skeletal muscle tubules; inside the T tubules is a large quantity of mucopolysaccharides that are electronegatively charged and bind an abundant storehouse of calcium ions, keeping this always available for diffusion to the interior of the cardiac muscle fiber when the T tubule action potential occurs. This extra supply of calcium from the T tubules is at least one of the factors that

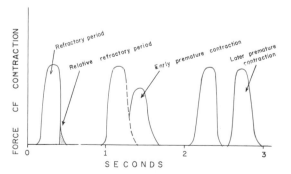

Figure 5–3. Contraction of the heart, showing the durations of the refractory period and the relative refractory period, the effect of an early premature contraction, and the effect of a later premature contraction. Note that the premature contractions do not cause wave summation as occurs in skeletal muscle.

prolongs the cardiac muscle action potential and maintains cardiac muscle contraction for as long as a third of a second rather than one-tenth that time as occurs in skeletal muscle.

At the end of the plateau of the action potential the supply of new calcium ions to the interior of the muscle fiber is suddenly cut off, and the calcium ions in the sarcoplasm are rapidly pumped back into the sarcoplasmic reticulum and T tubules — thus, the end of contraction until a new action potential occurs.

It is especially interesting that the strength of contraction of cardiac muscle depends partly upon the concentration of calcium ions in the extracellular fluids, which normally is not the case for skeletal muscle. The probable reason for this is that the quantity of calcium ions in the T tubules is directly proportional to the extracellular fluid calcium concentration, because the T tubules themselves are actually filled with extracellular fluid. Consequently, the availability of calcium ions to cause cardiac muscle contraction directly depends upon the extracellular fluid calcium.

Another difference between the tubules of cardiac muscle and those of skeletal muscle is that the T tubules in the skeletal muscle are located adjacent to actin and myosin filaments where they overlap each other so that there are two T tubule systems to each sarcomere. On the other hand, in cardiac muscle there is only one T tubule system per sarcomere located at the Z line but composed of much larger T tubules. This difference in structure is compatible with the fact that cardiac muscle contracts much more slowly than skeletal muscle so that there is adequate time for calcium ions to diffuse from the Z line to the middle of the sarcomere where the contractile process occurs.

Duration of Contraction. Cardiac muscle begins to contract a few milliseconds after the action potential begins and continues to contract for a few milliseconds after the action potential ends. Therefore, the duration of contraction of cardiac muscle is mainly a function of the duration of the action potential —about 0.15 second in atrial muscle and 0.3 second in ventricular muscle.

Effect of Heart Rate on Duration of Contraction. When the heart rate increases, the duration of each total cycle of the heart, including both the contraction phase and the relaxation phase, obviously decreases. The duration of the action potential and the period of contraction (systole) also decrease but not as great a percentage as does the relaxation phase (diastole). At a normal heart rate of 72 beats per minute, the period of contraction is about 0.4 of the entire cycle. At 3 times normal heart rate, this period is about 0.65 of the entire cycle, which means that the heart under some conditions does not remain relaxed long enough to allow complete filling of the cardiac chambers prior to the next contraction.

THE SPECIAL EXCITATORY AND CONDUCTIVE SYSTEM OF THE HEART

The adult human heart normally contracts at a rhythmic rate of about 72 beats per minute. Figure 5–4 illustrates the special excitatory and conductive system of the heart that controls these cardiac contractions. The figure shows: (A) the *S-A node* in which the normal rhythmic self-excitatory impulse is generated, (B) the *internodal pathways* that conduct the impulse from the S-A node to the A-V node, (C) the *A-V node* in which the impulse from the atria is delayed before passing into the ventricles, (D) the *A-V bundle,* which conducts the impulse from the atria into the ventricles, and (E) the *left* and *right bundles of Purkinje fibers,* which conduct the cardiac impulse to all parts of the ventricles.

THE SINO-ATRIAL NODE

The sino-atrial (S-A) node is a small, crescent strip of specialized muscle approximately 3 mm. wide and 1 cm. long; it is located in the posterior wall of the right atrium immediately beneath and medial to the opening of the superior vena cava. The fibers of this node are each 3 to 5 microns in diameter, in contrast to a diameter of 15 to 20 microns for the surrounding atrial muscle fibers. However, the S-A fibers are continuous with the atrial fibers so that any action potential that begins in the S-A node spreads immediately into the atria.

Automatic Rhythmicity of the Sino-Atrial Fibers. Most cardiac fibers have the capability of *self-excitation,* a process which can cause automatic rhythmical contraction. This is especially true of the fibers of the heart's specialized conducting system; the portion of this system that displays self-excitation to the greatest extent is the fibers of the S-A node. For this reason, the sino-atrial (S-A) node ordinarily controls the rate of beat of the entire heart, as will be discussed in detail later in this chapter. First, however, let us describe this automatic rhythmicity.

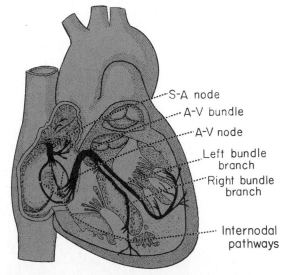

S-A node
A-V bundle
A-V node
Left bundle branch
Right bundle branch
Internodal pathways

Figure 5–4. The S-A node and the Purkinje system of the heart.

The sino-atrial fibers are somewhat different from most other cardiac muscle fibers, having a resting membrane potential of only −55 to −60 millivolts in comparison with −85 to −95 millivolts in most of the other fibers. This low resting potential is caused by a natural leakiness of the membranes to sodium ions. And it is also this leakage of sodium that causes the self-excitation of the S-A fibers. Figure 5–5 illustrates the rhythmical repetitiveness of the action potentials in the S-A node, which can be explained as follows:

Immediately after each action potential is over, the membrane is even more permeable to potassium ions than normally, as was discussed in Chapter 2, and this contrasts with a very low permeability at this instant for sodium ions. Recalling the Goldman equation from Chapter 2, one may note that when the ratio of potassium ion to sodium ion permeability is very high, the potential inside the membrane becomes very highly negative because potassium ions diffusing out of the cell carry positive charges away from the interior of the cell. Therefore, immediately after the action potential is over, the membrane potential reaches its greatest degree of negativity, a state called *hyperpolarization*. At this time the membrane potential is much too negative for the fiber to fire again. However, this does not last long because the high degree of negativity inside the membrane causes the membrane to become progressively less permeable to potassium during the next few tenths of a second, and the natural leakiness of the membrane to sodium returns and causes the membrane potential to "drift" slowly back toward a less negative value. This is illustrated after each one of the action potentials in Figure 5–5.

After a few tenths of a second, the so-called "resting" potential will have drifted enough for it finally to reach the threshold level for excitation of the fiber. When this occurs, the flux of sodium ions to the interior of the fiber accelerates, causing the fiber to become even more conductive to sodium. Thus a self-regeneration process begins that leads to extremely high sodium permeability and rapid total depolarization of the membrane, followed by overshoot of the membrane potential to a positive potential of approximately +20 millivolts, called a *reversal potential,* as pointed out in Chapter 2. For slightly over 0.10 second, the membrane remains depolarized; then the permeability of the membrane for potassium increases while that for sodium decreases to a low value.

After approximately 0.12 second the permeability for potassium is now great enough that a self-regenerative process begins in the opposite direction, with accelerating flux of potassium ions to the exterior; this recreates the negative potential inside the fiber. After the action potential is over, an especially high potassium permeability persists again for a few tenths of a second, thus maintaining a new state of hyperpolarization. Then the process begins again, with gradual decrease in permeability of the membrane to potassium, more and more leakage of sodium, and then a new regenerative cycle that causes depolarization. This process continues over and over throughout the life of the person, thereby providing rhythmical excitation of the S-A nodal fibers at a normal resting rate of about 72 times per minute.

INTERNODAL PATHWAYS AND TRANSMISSION OF THE CARDIAC IMPULSE THROUGH THE ATRIA

The ends of the S-A nodal fibers fuse with the surrounding atrial muscle fibers, and action potentials originating in the S-A node travel outward into these fibers. In this way, the action potential spreads through the entire atrial muscle mass and eventually also to the A-V node. The velocity of conduction in the atrial muscle is approximately 0.3 meter per second. However, conduction is somewhat more rapid in several small bundles of atrial muscle fibers, some of which pass directly from the S-A node to the A-V node and conduct the cardiac impulse at a velocity of 0.45 to 0.6 meter per second. Some physiologists claim that these bundles contain specialized conduction fibers similar to the Purkinje fibers of the ventricles, which will be discussed subsequently. However, other physiologists believe that this more rapid conduction is caused simply by the greater mass of muscle and the more direct orientation of the muscle fibers in the special bundles. Nevertheless, these pathways do conduct the impulse from the S-A node to the A-V node more rapidly than the conduction in the general mass of atrial muscle; these *internodal pathways* are illustrated in Figure 5–4.

THE ATRIOVENTRICULAR (A-V) NODE AND THE PURKINJE SYSTEM

Delay in Transmission at the A-V Node. Fortunately, the conductive system is organized so that

Figure 5–5. Rhythmic discharge of an S-A nodal fiber.

the cardiac impulse will not travel from the atria into the ventricles too rapidly; this allows time for the atria to empty their contents into the ventricles before ventricular contraction begins. It is primarily the A-V node and its associated conductive fibers that delays this transmission of the cardiac impulse from the atria into the ventricles.

Figure 5–6 shows diagrammatically the different parts of the A-V node and its connections with the atrial internodal pathway fibers and the A-V bundle. The figure also shows the approximate intervals of time in fractions of a second between the genesis of the cardiac impulse in the S-A node and its appearance at different points in the A-V nodal system. Note that the impulse, after traveling through the internodal pathway, reaches the A-V node approximately 0.04 second after its origin in the S-A node. However, between this time and the time that the impulse emerges in the A-V bundle, another 0.11 second elapses. About one half of this time lapse occurs in the *junctional fibers*, which are very small fibers that connect the normal atrial fibers with the fibers of the node itself (illustrated in Figures 5–6 and 5–7). The velocity of conduction in these fibers is about 0.02 meter per second (about one twenty-fifth that in normal cardiac muscle), which greatly delays entrance of the impulse into the A-V node. After entering the node proper, the velocity of conduction in the *nodal fibers* is still quite low, only 0.1 meter per second, about one-fourth the conduction velocity in normal cardiac muscle. Therefore, a further delay in transmission occurs as the impulse travels through the A-V node into the *transitional fibers* and finally into the *A-V bundle* (also called the *bundle of His*).

Figure 5–7 illustrates a functional diagram of the A-V nodal region showing the atrial fibers leading into the minute junctional fibers, then progressive enlargement of the fibers again as they

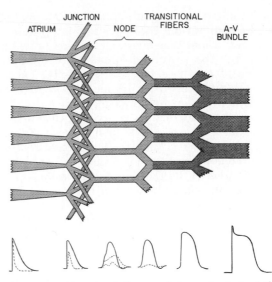

Figure 5–7. Functional diagram of the anatomical relationships in the region of the atrioventricular node. The action potentials at the bottom were recorded under normal conditions (solid lines) and under the influence of acetylcholine (dashed lines), showing blockage of conduction by this substance. (From Hoffman and Cranefield: Electrophysiology of the Heart. New York, McGraw-Hill Book Company, 1960.)

spread through the node, through the transitional region, and into the A-V bundle. The characteristics of the action potential in the different parts of the node are illustrated at the bottom.

The cause of the extremely slow conduction in the junctional and other A-V nodal fibers is probably three-fold: (1) The fibers are very small, a fact which in itself makes the conduction rate very slow. (2) The number of tight junctions at the intercalated discs from one cardiac cell to the next in these fibers is much less than in the usual cardiac muscle fibers — that is, the number of *nexi* (points of tight fusion between the cell membranes) is greatly reduced between these cardiac muscle cells, thereby reducing the rapidity of ionic transport along the axis of the fiber. (3) These fibers are made up of a much more embryonic type of cell with much less differentiation than in the usual cardiac muscle cell, this also presumably reducing the capability of the cell to transmit the cardiac impulse.

TRANSMISSION IN THE PURKINJE SYSTEM

The *Purkinje fibers* that lead from the A-V node through the A-V bundle and into the ventricles have functional characteristics quite the opposite of those of the A-V nodal fibers; they are very large fibers, even larger than the normal ventricular muscle fibers, and they transmit impulses at a velocity of 1.5 to 4.0 meters per second, a velocity about 6 times that in the usual cardiac muscle and 150 times that in the junctional fibers. This allows

Internodal pathway fibers (.04)
Junctional fibers (.06)
Node (.11)
Transitional fibers (.13)
A-V bundle (.15)

Figure 5–6. Organization of the A-V node. The numbers represent the interval of time from the origin of the impulse in the S-A node. The values have been extrapolated to the human being. (This figure is based on studies in lower animals discussed and illustrated in Hoffman and Cranefield: Electrophysiology of the Heart. New York, McGraw-Hill Book Company, 1960.)

almost immediate transmission of the cardiac impulse throughout the entire ventricular system.

The very rapid transmission of action potentials by Purkinje fibers is probably caused by increased numbers of nexi between the successive cardiac cells that make up the Purkinje fibers. At these nexi, ions are transmitted easily from one cell to the next, thus enhancing the velocity of transmission. The Purkinje fibers also have very few myofibrils, which means that they barely contract during the course of impulse transmission.

Distribution of the Purkinje Fibers in the Ventricles. The Purkinje fibers, after originating in the A-V node, form the A-V bundle, which then threads through the fibrous tissue between the valves of the heart and thence into the ventricular system, as shown in Figure 5–4. The A-V bundle divides almost immediately into the *left* and *right* *bundle branches* that lie beneath the endocardium of the respective sides of the septum. Each of these branches spreads downward toward the apex of the respective ventricle, but then divides into small branches and spreads around each ventricular chamber and finally back toward the base of the heart along the lateral wall. The terminal Purkinje fibers form swirls underneath the endocardium and penetrate about one-third of the way into the muscle mass to terminate on the muscle fibers.

From the time that the cardiac impulse first enters the A-V bundle until it reaches the terminations of the Purkinje fibers, the total time that lapses is only 0.03 second; therefore, once a cardiac impulse enters the Purkinje system, it spreads almost immediately to the entire endocardial surface of the ventricular muscle.

CONTROL OF EXCITATION AND CONDUCTION IN THE HEART

THE S-A NODE AS THE PACEMAKER OF THE HEART

In the above discussion of the genesis and transmission of the cardiac impulse through the heart, it was stated that the impulse normally arises in the S-A node. However, this need not be the case under abnormal conditions, for other parts of the heart can exhibit rhythmic contraction in the same way that the fibers of the S-A node can; this is particularly true of the A-V nodal and Purkinje fibers.

The A-V nodal fibers, when not stimulated from some outside source, discharge at an intrinsic rhythmic rate of 40 to 60 times per minute, and the Purkinje fibers discharge at a rate of somewhere between 15 and 40 times per minute. These rates are in contrast to the normal rate of the S-A node of 70 to 80 times per minute.

Therefore, the question that we must ask is: Why does the S-A node control the heart's rhythmicity rather than the A-V node or the Purkinje fibers? The answer to this is simply that the rate of the S-A node is considerably greater than that of either the A-V node or the Purkinje fibers. Each time the S-A node discharges, its impulse is conducted into both the A-V node and the Purkinje fibers, discharging their excitable membranes. Then these tissues, as well as the S-A node, recover from the action potential and become hyperpolarized. But the S-A node loses this hyperpolarization much more rapidly than does either of the other two and emits a new impulse before either one of them can reach its own threshold for self-excitation. The new impulse again discharges both the A-V node and Purkinje fibers. This process continues on and on, the S-A node always exciting these other potentially self-excitatory tissues before self-excitation can actually occur.

Thus, the S-A node controls the beat of the heart, because its rate of rhythmic discharge is greater than that of any other part of the heart. Therefore, it is said that the S-A node is the normal *pacemaker* of the heart.

Abnormal Pacemakers — The Ectopic Pacemaker. Occasionally some other part of the heart develops a rhythmic discharge rate that is more rapid than that of the S-A node. For instance, this frequently occurs in the A-V node or in the Purkinje fibers. In either of these cases, the pacemaker of the heart shifts from the S-A node to the A-V node or to the excitable Purkinje fibers. Under rare conditions a point in the atrial or ventricular muscle develops excessive excitability and becomes the pacemaker.

A pacemaker elsewhere than the S-A node is called an *ectopic pacemaker*. Obviously, an ectopic pacemaker causes an abnormal sequence of contraction of the different parts of the heart.

ROLE OF THE PURKINJE SYSTEM IN CAUSING SYNCHRONOUS CONTRACTION OF THE VENTRICULAR MUSCLE

It is clear from the above description of the Purkinje system that the cardiac impulse arrives at almost all portions of the ventricles within a very narrow span of time, exciting the first ventricular muscle fiber only 0.06 second ahead of excitation of the last ventricular muscle fiber. Since the ventricular muscle fibers remain contracted for a total period of 0.30 second, one can see that this rapid spread of excitation throughout the entire ventricular muscle mass causes all portions of the ventricular muscle in both ventricles to contract at almost exactly the same time. Effective pumping by the two ventricular chambers requires this synchronous type of contraction. If the cardiac impulse traveled through the ventricular muscle very slowly, then much of the ventricular mass would contract prior to contraction of the remainder, in which case the overall pumping effect would be greatly depressed. Indeed, in some types of cardiac debilities, such slow transmission does indeed occur, and the pumping effectiveness of the ventricles is decreased perhaps as much as 20 to 30 per cent.

CONTROL OF HEART RHYTHMICITY AND CONDUCTION BY THE AUTONOMIC NERVES

The heart is supplied with both sympathetic and parasympathetic nerves, as illustrated in Figure 5–8. The parasympathetic nerves are distributed mainly to the S-A and A-V nodes, to a lesser extent to the muscle of the two atria, and even less to the ventricular muscle. The sympathetic nerves are distributed to these same areas but with a strong representation to the ventricular muscle as well as to the other parts of the heart.

Effect of Parasympathetic (Vagal) Stimulation on Cardiac Rhythm and Conduction — Ventricular Escape. Stimulation of the parasympathetic nerves to the heart (the vagi) causes the hormone acetylcholine to be released at the vagal endings. This hormone has two major effects on the heart. First, it decreases the rate of rhythm of the S-A node, and, second, it decreases the excitability of the A-V junctional fibers between the atrial musculature and the A-V node, thereby slowing transmission of the cardiac impulse into the ventricles. Very strong stimulation of the vagi can completely stop the rhythmic contraction of the S-A node or completely block transmission of the cardiac impulse through the A-V junction. In either case, rhythmic impulses are no longer transmitted into the ventricles. The ventricles stop beating for 4 to 10 seconds, but then some point in the Purkinje fibers, usually in the A-V bundle, develops a rhythm of its own and causes ventricular contraction at a rate of 15 to 40 beats per minute. This phenomenon is called *ventricular escape*.

Mechanism of the Vagal Effects. The acetylcholine released at the vagal nerve endings greatly increases the permeability of the fiber membranes to potassium, which allows rapid leakage of potassium to the exterior. This causes increased negativity inside the fibers, an effect called *hyperpolarization*, which makes excitable tissue much less excitable, as was explained in Chapter 2.

In the A-V node, the state of hyperpolarization makes it difficult for the minute junctional fibers, which can generate only small quantities of current during the action potential, to excite the nodal fibers. Therefore, the *safety factor* for transmission of the cardiac impulse through the junctional fibers and into the nodal fibers decreases. A moderate decrease in this simply delays conduction of the impulse, but a decrease in safety factor below unity (which means so low that the action potential of one fiber cannot cause an action potential in the successive fiber) completely blocks conduction.

Effect of Sympathetic Stimulation on Cardiac Rhythm and Conduction. Sympathetic stimulation causes essentially the opposite effects on the heart to those caused by vagal stimulation as follows: First, it increases the rate of S-A nodal discharge. Second, it increases the rate of conduction and the excitability in all portions of the heart. Third, it increases greatly the force of contraction of all the cardiac musculature, both atrial and ventricular, as discussed in the previous chapter.

In short, sympathetic stimulation increases the overall activity of the heart. Maximal stimulation can almost triple the rate of heartbeat and can increase the strength of heart contraction as much as two-fold.

Mechanism of the Sympathetic Effect. Stimulation of the sympathetic nerves releases the hormone norepinephrine at the sympathetic nerve endings. The precise mechanism by which this hormone acts on cardiac muscle fibers is still somewhat doubtful, but the present belief is that it increases the permeability of the fiber membrane to sodium and calcium. In the S-A node, an increase of sodium permeability would cause increased tendency for the resting membrane potential to decay to the threshold level for self--excitation, which obviously would accelerate the onset of self-excitation after each successive heartbeat and therefore increase the heart rate.

In the A-V node, increased sodium permeability would make it easier for each fiber to excite the succeeding fiber, thereby decreasing the conduction time from the atria to the ventricles.

The increase in permeability to calcium ions is probably at least partially responsible for the increase in contractile strength of the cardiac muscle under the influence of sympathetic stimulation, because calcium ions play a powerful role in exciting the contractile process of the myofibrils.

CONTROL OF HEART PUMPING BY THE NERVES

The autonomic nerves affect cardiac pumping in two ways: (1) by changing the heart rate and (2) by changing the strength of contraction of the heart. As discussed previously, parasympathetic stimulation decreases heart rate, and sympathetic stimulation increases heart rate. The range of control is from as little as 20 to 30 heart beats per minute with maximum vagal stimulation up to as high as 250 or, rarely, 300 heart beats per minute with maximum sympathetic stimulation.

Effect of Heart Rate on Function of the Heart as a Pump. In general, the more times the heart beats per minute, the more blood it can pump, but there are important limitations to this effect. For instance, once the heart rate rises above a critical level, the heart strength itself decreases, presumably because of overutilization of metabolic substrates in the cardiac muscle. In addition, the period of diastole between the contractions becomes so reduced that blood does not have time to flow adequately from the atria into the ventricles. For these reasons, when the heart rate is increased artificially by electrical stimulation, the heart has its peak ability to pump large quantities of blood at a heart rate between 100 and 150 beats per minute. On the other hand, when its rate is increased by sympathetic stimulation, it reaches its peak ability to pump blood at a heart rate between 170 and 250 beats per minute. The reason for this difference is that sympathetic stimulation not only increases the heart rate but also increases heart strength as well.

When the atrial pressures are high, the higher heart rates are especially effective in increasing the output of the heart.

Nervous Regulation of Contractile Strength of the Heart. The two atria are especially well supplied with large numbers of both sympathetic and parasympathetic nerves, but the ventricles are supplied mainly by sympathetic nerves and far fewer parasympathetic fibers. In general, sympathetic stimulation increases the strength of heart muscle contraction, whereas parasympathetic stimulation decreases the strength of contraction.

Under normal conditions the sympathetic nerve fibers to the heart continually discharge at a slow rate that maintains a strength of ventricular contraction about 20 per cent above its strength with no sympathetic stimulation at all. Therefore, one method by which the nervous system can decrease the strength of ventricular contraction is simply to slow or stop the transmission of sympathetic impulses to the heart. On the other hand, maximal sympathetic stimulation can increase the strength of ventricular contraction to approximately 100 per cent greater than normal.

Maximal parasympathetic stimulation of the heart decreases ventricular contractile strength about 30 per cent. Thus, the parasympathetic effect is, by contrast with the sympathetic effect, relatively small.

REFERENCES

Brown, H., et al.: The initiation of the heartbeat and its control by autonomic transmitters. In Dickinson, C. J., and Marks, J. (eds.): Developments in Cardiovascular Medicine. Lancaster, England, MTP Press, 1978, p. 31.

Brutsaert, D. L., and Paulus, W. J.: Contraction and relaxation of the heart as muscle and pump. In Guyton, A. C., and Young, D. B. (eds.): International Review of Physiology: Cardiovascular Physiology III. Vol. 18. Baltimore, University Park Press, 1979, p. 1.

Chung, E. K. (ed.): Artificial Cardiac Pacing: Practical Approach. Baltimore, Williams & Wilkins, 1978.

Cobb, L. A., et al.: Community cardiopulmonary resuscitation. Annu. Rev. Med., 31:453, 1980.

Cranefield, P. F.: The Conduction of the Cardiac Impulse. New York, Futura Publishing Co., 1975.

Durrer, D., et al.: Human cardiac electrophysiology. In Dickinson, C. J., and Marks, J. (eds.): Developments in Cardiovascular Medicine. Lancaster, England, MTP Press, 1978, p. 53.

Fozzard, H. A.: Heart: Excitation-contraction coupling. Annu. Rev. Physiol., 39:201, 1977.

Guyton, A. C., and Satterfield, J.: Factors concerned in electrical defibrillation of the heart, particularly through the unopened chest. Am. J. Physiol., 167:81, 1951.

Irisawa, H.: Comparative physiology of the cardiac pacemaker mechanism. Physiol. Rev., 58:461, 1978.

Jones, P.: Cardiac Pacing. New York, Appleton-Century-Crofts, 1980.

Josephson, M. E., and Seides, S. F.: Clinical Cardiac Electrophysiology Techniques and Interpretations. Philadelphia, Lea & Febiger, 1979.

Levy, M. N., and Martin, P. J.: Cardiac excitation and contraction. In MTP International Review of Science: Physiology. Baltimore, University Park Press, 1974, Vol. 1, p. 49.

Levy, M. N., and Martin, P. J.: Neural control of the heart. In Berne, R. M., et al. (eds.): Handbook of Physiology. Sec. 2, Vol. I. Baltimore, Williams & Wilkins, 1979, p. 581.

Narula, O. S. (ed.): Cardiac Arrhythmias: Electrophysiology, Diagnosis, and Management. Baltimore, Williams & Wilkins, 1979.

Nobel, D.: The Initiation of the Heartbeat. New York, Oxford University Press, 1979.

Pick, A., and Langendorf, R.: Interpretation of Complex Arrhythmias. Philadelphia, Lea & Febiger, 1980.

Reuter, H., and Winegrad, S.: Excitation-contraction coupling of the heart: Neurohumoral effects. In Hayase, S., and Murao, S. (eds.): Cardiology: Proceedings of the VIII World Congress of Cardiology, Tokyo, 1978. New York, Elsevier/North-Holland, 1979, p. 800.

Sperelakis, N.: Origin of the cardiac resting potential. In Berne, R. M., et al. (eds.): Handbook of Physiology. Sec. 2, Vol. I. Baltimore, Williams & Wilkins, 1979, p. 187.

Sperelakis, N.: Propagation mechanisms in heart. Annu. Rev. Physiol., 41:441, 1979.

Stent, G. S., et al.: Neural control of heartbeat in the leech and in some other invertebrates. Physiol. Rev., 59:101, 1979.

Stull, J. T., and Mayer, S. E.: Biochemical mechanisms of adrenergic and cholinergic regulation of myocardial contractility. In Berne, R. M., et al. (eds.): Handbook of Physiology. Sec. 2, Vol. I. Baltimore, Williams & Wilkins, 1979, p. 741.

Vasselle, M.: Electrogenesis of the plateau and pacemaker potential. Annu. Rev. Physiol., 41:425, 1979.

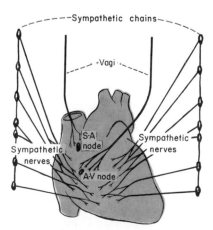

Figure 5–8. The cardiac nerves.

Part II

THE CENTRAL
NERVOUS SYSTEM

6

Organization of the Nervous System; Basic Functions of Synapses

The nervous system, along with the endocrine system, provides most of the control functions for the body. In general, the nervous system controls the rapid activities of the body, such as muscular contractions, rapidly changing visceral events, and even the rates of secretion of some endocrine glands. The endocrine system, by contrast, regulates principally the metabolic functions of the body.

The nervous system is unique in the vast complexity of the control actions that it can perform. It receives literally thousands of bits of information from the different sensory organs and then integrates all these to determine the response to be made by the body. The purpose of this chapter is to present, first, a general outline of the overall mechanisms by which the nervous system performs such functions. Then we will discuss the function of central nervous system synapses, the basic structures that control the passage of signals into, through, and then out of the nervous system. In succeeding chapters we will analyze in detail the functions of the individual parts of the nervous system. Before beginning this discussion, however, the reader should refer to Chapters 2 and 4, which present, respectively, the principles of membrane potentials and transmission of impulses through neuromuscular junctions.

GENERAL DESIGN OF THE NERVOUS SYSTEM

THE SENSORY DIVISION — SENSORY RECEPTORS

Most activities of the nervous system are initiated by sensory experience emanating from *sensory receptors,* whether these be visual receptors, auditory receptors, tactile receptors on the surface of the body, or other kinds of receptors. This sensory experience can cause an immediate reaction, or its memory can be stored in the brain for minutes, weeks, or years and then can help to determine the bodily reactions at some future date.

Figure 6–1 illustrates a portion of the sensory system, the *somatic* portion that transmits sensory information from the receptors of the entire surface of the body and deep structures. This information enters the nervous system through the spinal nerves and is conducted into (a) the spinal cord at all levels, (b) the reticular substance of the medulla, pons, and mesencephalon, (c) the cerebellum, (d) the thalamus, and (e) the somesthetic areas of the cerebral cortex. But in addition to these ''primary sensory'' areas, signals are then relayed to essentially all other segments of the nervous system.

THE MOTOR DIVISION — THE EFFECTORS

The most important ultimate role of the nervous system is control of bodily activities. This is achieved by controlling (a) contraction of skeletal muscles throughout the body, (b) contraction of smooth muscle in the internal organs, and (c) secretion by both exocrine and endocrine glands in many parts of the body. These activities are collectively called *motor functions* of the nervous system, and the muscles and glands are called *effectors* because they perform the functions dictated by the nerve signals. That portion of the nervous system directly concerned with transmitting signals to the muscles and glands is called the motor division of the nervous system.

Figure 6–2 illustrates the *motor axis* of the nervous system for controlling skeletal muscle contraction. Operating parallel to this axis is another similar system for control of the smooth

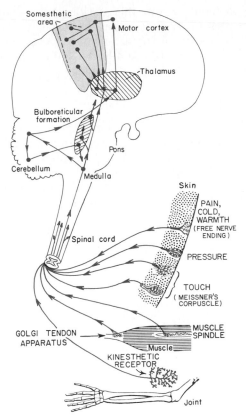

Figure 6–1. The somatic sensory axis of the nervous system.

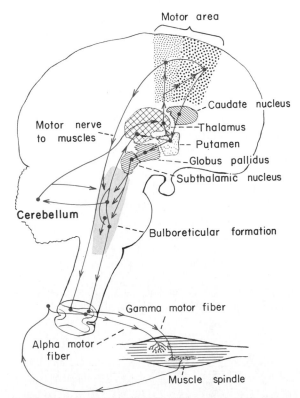

Figure 6–2. The motor axis of the nervous system.

muscles and glands; it is the *autonomic nervous system,* which will be presented in detail in Chapter 17. Note in Figure 6–2 that the skeletal muscles can be controlled from many different levels of the central nervous system, including (a) the spinal cord, (b) the reticular substance of the medulla, pons, and mesencephalon, (c) the basal ganglia, (d) the cerebellum, and (e) the motor cortex. Each of these different areas plays its own specific role in the control of body movements, the lower regions being concerned primarily with automatic, instantaneous responses of the body to sensory stimuli and the higher regions with deliberate movements controlled by the thought processes of the cerebrum.

PROCESSING OF INFORMATION

The nervous system would not be at all effective in controlling bodily functions if each bit of sensory information caused some motor reaction. Therefore, one of the major functions of the nervous system is to process incoming information in such a way that *appropriate* motor responses occur. Indeed, more than 99 per cent of all sensory information is discarded by the brain as irrelevant and unimportant. For instance, one is ordinarily totally unaware of the parts of the body that are in contact with clothing and is also unaware of the seat pressure when sitting. Likewise, attention is drawn only to an occasional object in one's field of vision, and even the perpetual noise of our surroundings is usually relegated to the background.

After the important sensory information has been selected, it is then channeled into proper motor regions of the brain to cause the desired responses. Thus, if a person places a hand on a hot stove, the desired response is to lift the hand, plus other associated responses such as moving the entire body away from the stove and perhaps even shouting with pain. Yet even these responses represent activity by only a small fraction of the total motor system of the body.

Role of Synapses in Processing Information. The synapse is the junction point from one neuron to the next and, therefore, is an advantageous site for control of signal transmission. Later in this chapter we will discuss the details of synaptic function. However, it is important to point out here that the synapses determine the directions that the nervous signals spread in the nervous system. Some synapses transmit signals from one neuron to the next with ease, while others transmit signals only with difficulty. Also, facilitatory and inhibitory signals from other areas in the nervous system can control synaptic activity, sometimes opening the synapses for transmission and at other times closing them. In addition, some post-synaptic neurons respond with large numbers of impulses, while others respond with only a few. Thus, the synapses perform a selective action, often blocking the weak signals while allowing the strong signals to pass, often selecting and amplifying certain weak signals, and often channeling the signal in many different directions rather than simply in one direction. The basic principles of this processing of information by the synapses are so important that they are discussed in detail in the latter part of this chapter and in the entire following chapter.

STORAGE OF INFORMATION — MEMORY

Only a small fraction of the important sensory information causes an immediate motor response. Much of the remainder is stored for future control of motor activities and for use in the thinking processes. Most of this storage occurs in the *cerebral cortex,* but not all, for even the basal regions of the brain and perhaps even the spinal cord can store small amounts of information.

The storage of information is the process we call *memory,* and this too is a function of the synapses. That is, each time a particular sensory signal passes through a sequence of synapses, these synapses become more capable of transmitting the same signal the next time, which process is called *facilitation.* After the sensory signal has passed through the synapses a large number of times, the synapses become so facilitated that signals generated within the brain itself can also cause transmission of impulses through the same sequence of synapses even though the sensory input has not been excited. This gives the person a perception of experiencing the original sensation, though in effect it is only a memory of the sensation.

Unfortunately, we do not know the precise mechanism by which facilitation of synapses occurs in the memory process, but what is known about this and other details of the memory process will be discussed in Chapter 15.

Once memories have been stored in the nervous system, they become part of the processing mechanism. The thought processes of the brain compare new sensory experiences with the stored memories; the memories help to select the important new sensory information and to channel this into appropriate storage areas for future use or into motor areas to cause bodily responses.

THE THREE MAJOR LEVELS OF NERVOUS SYSTEM FUNCTION

The human nervous system has inherited specific characteristics from each stage of evolutionary development. From this heritage, there remain three major levels of the nervous system that have special functional significance: (1) the spinal cord level, (2) the lower brain level, and (3) the higher brain or cortical level.

THE SPINAL CORD LEVEL

The spinal cord of the human being still retains many functions of the multisegmental animal. Sensory signals are transmitted through the spinal nerves into each *segment* of the spinal cord, and these signals can cause localized motor responses either in the segment of the body from which the sensory information is received or in adjacent segments. Essentially all the spinal cord motor responses are automatic and occur almost instantaneously in response to the sensory signal. In addition, they occur in specific patterns of response called *reflexes.*

Figure 6–3 illustrates two of the simpler cord reflexes. To the left is the neural control of the *muscle stretch reflex.* If a muscle suddenly becomes stretched, a sensory nerve receptor in the muscle called the *muscle spindle* becomes stimulated and transmits nerve impulses through a sensory nerve fiber into the spinal cord. This fiber synapses directly with a motoneuron in the anterior horn of the cord gray matter, and the motoneuron in turn transmits impulses back to the muscle to cause the muscle, the effector, to contract. The muscle contraction opposes the original muscle stretch. Thus, this reflex acts as a *feedback* mechanism, operating from a receptor to an effector, to prevent sudden change in the length of the muscle. This allows a person to maintain the limbs and other parts of the body in desired positions despite sudden outside forces that tend to move the parts out of position.

To the right in Figure 6–3 is illustrated the neural control of another reflex called the *with-*

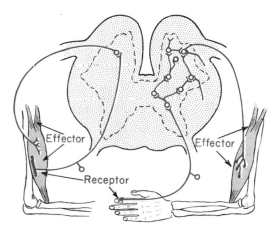

Figure 6–3. *Left*: The simple stretch reflex. *Right*: A withdrawal reflex.

drawal reflex. This is a protective reflex that causes withdrawal of any part of the body from an object that causes pain. For instance, let us assume that the hand is placed on a sharp object. Pain signals are transmitted into the gray matter of the spinal cord, and, after appropriate selection of information by the synapses, signals are channeled to the appropriate motoneurons to cause flexion of the biceps muscle. This obviously lifts the hand away from the sharp object.

We see, then, that the withdrawal reflex is much more complex than the stretch reflex, for it involves many neurons in the gray matter of the cord, and signals are transmitted to many adjacent segments of the cord to cause contraction of the appropriate muscles.

Cord Functions After the Brain is Removed. The many reflexes of the spinal cord will be discussed in Chapter 11; however, the following list of important cord reflex functions that occur even after the brain is removed illustrates the many capabilities of the spinal cord:

1. An animal can under certain conditions be made to stand up. This is caused primarily by reflexes initiated from the pads of the feet. Sensory signals from the pads cause the extensor muscles of the limbs to tighten, which in turn allows the limbs to support the animal's body.

2. An animal with its spinal cord transected, when held in a sling so that its feet hang downward, often begins walking or galloping movements involving one, two, or all of its legs. This illustrates that the basic patterns for causing the limb movements of locomotion are present in the spinal cord.

3. A flea crawling on the skin of a spinal animal causes reflex to-and-fro scratching by the paw, and the paw can actually localize the flea on the surface of the body.

4. Cord reflexes exist to cause emptying of the urinary bladder and of the rectum.

5. Segmental temperature reflexes are present throughout the body. Local cooling of the skin causes vasoconstriction, which helps to conserve heat in the body. Conversely, local heating in the skin causes vasodilatation, resulting in loss of heat from the body.

This list of some of the segmental and multisegmental reflexes of the spinal cord demonstrates that many of our day-by-day and moment-by-moment activities are controlled locally by the respective segmental levels of the spinal cord, and the brain plays only a modifying role in these local controls.

THE LOWER BRAIN LEVEL

Many if not most of what we call subconscious activities of the body are controlled in the lower areas of the brain — in the medulla, pons, mesen-cephalon, hypothalamus, thalamus, cerebellum, and basal ganglia. Subconscious control of arterial blood pressure and respiration is achieved primarily in the reticular substance of the medulla and pons. Control of equilibrium is a combined function of the older portions of the cerebellum and the reticular substance of the medulla, pons, and mesencephalon. The coordinated turning movements of the head, of the entire body, and of the eyes are controlled by specific centers located in the mesencephalon, paleocerebellum, and lower basal ganglia. Feeding reflexes, such as salivation in response to taste of food and licking of the lips, are controlled by areas in the medulla, pons, mesencephalon, amygdala, and hypothalamus. And many emotional patterns, such as anger, excitement, sexual activities, reactions to pain, or reactions of pleasure, can occur in animals without a cerebral cortex.

In short, the subconscious but coordinate functions of the body, as well as many of the life processes themselves — arterial pressure and respiration, for instance — are controlled by the lower regions of the brain, regions that usually, but not always, operate below the conscious level.

THE HIGHER BRAIN OR CORTICAL LEVEL

We have seen from the above discussion that many of the intrinsic life processes of the body are controlled by subcortical regions of the brain or by the spinal cord. What then is the function of the cerebral cortex? The cerebral cortex is primarily a vast information storage area. Approximately three quarters of all the neuronal cell bodies of the entire nervous system are located in the cerebral cortex. It is here that most of the memories of past experiences are stored, and it is here that many of the patterns of motor responses are stored, which information can be called forth at will to control motor functions of the body.

Relation of the Cortex to the Thalamus and Other Lower Centers. The cerebral cortex is actually an outgrowth of the lower regions of the brain, particularly of the thalamus. For each area of the cerebral cortex there is a corresponding and connecting area of the thalamus, and activation of a minute portion of the thalamus activates the corresponding and much larger portion of the cerebral cortex. It is presumed that in this way the thalamus can call forth cortical activities at will. Also, activation of regions in the mesencephalon transmits diffuse signals to the cerebral cortex, partially through the thalamus and partially through other pathways, to activate the entire cortex. This is the process that we call *wakefulness*. On the other hand, when these areas of the mesencephalon become inactive, the thalamic and cortical regions also become inactive, which is the process we call *sleep*.

Function of the Cerebral Cortex in Thought Processes.   Some areas of the cerebral cortex are not directly concerned with either sensory or motor functions of the nervous system — for example, the prefrontal lobes and large portions of the temporal and parietal lobes. These areas are set aside for the more abstract processes of thought, but even they also have direct nerve connections with the lower regions of the brain.

Large areas of the cerebral cortex can be destroyed without blocking the subconscious and even many involuntary conscious activities of the body. For instance, destruction of the somesthetic cortex does not destroy one's ability to feel objects touching the skin, but it does destroy the ability to distinguish the shapes of objects, their character, and the precise points on the skin where the objects are touching. Thus, the cortex is not required for perception of sensation, but it does add immeasurably to its depth of meaning. Likewise, destruction of the prefrontal lobe does not destroy one's ability to think, but it does destroy the ability to think in deeply abstract terms. In other words, each time a portion of the cerebral cortex is destroyed, a vast amount of information is lost to the thinking process and some of the mechanisms for processing this information are also lost. Therefore, total loss of the cerebral cortex causes a vegetative type of existence rather than a ''living'' existence.

Telencephalization.   In the process of evolution, the higher regions of the human nervous system have taken over many sensory and motor functions performed by the less developed brain of lower animals. For instance, if the spinal cord of an opossum is cut in the midthoracic region, the opossum can still walk perfectly well on both its forelimbs and hindlimbs, except that the hindlimbs are then unsynchronized with the forelimbs. A similar transection of the spinal cord in the human being causes complete loss of ability to use the legs for locomotion.

This process by which the progressively higher centers of the brain have taken over more and more of the function of the lower centers is called *telencephalization*. Yet, despite telencephalization, some of the very basic functions of the lower centers still remain active or at least partially active in the human being, such as many of the cord reflexes and the stereotyped control systems of the basal regions of the brain that were just discussed.

COMPARISON OF THE NERVOUS SYSTEM WITH AN ELECTRONIC COMPUTER

When electronic computers were first developed in many different laboratories of the world by as many

Figure 6–4.   Block diagram of a general-purpose electronic computer, showing the basic components and their interrelationships.

different scientists, it soon became apparent that all these machines have many features in common with the nervous system. First, they all have input circuits that are comparable to the sensory portion of the nervous system, and output circuits that are comparable to the motor portion of the nervous system. In the conducting pathway between the inputs and the outputs are the mechanisms for performing the different types of computations.

In simple computers, the output signals are controlled directly by the input signals, operating in a manner similar to that of the simple reflexes of the spinal cord. But, in the more complex computers, the output is determined both by the input signals and by information that has already been stored in memory in the computer, which is analogous to the more complex reflex and processing mechanisms of our higher nervous system. Furthermore, as the computers become even more complex it is necessary to add still another unit, called the *central programming unit,* which determines the sequence of all operations. This unit is analogous to the mechanism in our brain that allows us to direct our attention first to one thought or sensation or motor activity, then to another, and so forth, until complex sequences of thought or action take place.

Figure 6–4 illustrates a simple block diagram of a modern computer. Even a rapid study of this diagram will demonstrate its similarity to the nervous system. Furthermore, general purpose computers designed and built by many different scientific groups have ended up with almost completely the same basic components. The fact that these components are analogous to those of the human nervous system demonstrates that the brain is basically a computer that continuously collects sensory information and uses this along with stored information to compute the daily course of bodily activity.

FUNCTION OF CENTRAL NERVOUS SYSTEM SYNAPSES

Every medical student is aware that information is transmitted in the central nervous system mainly in the form of nerve impulses through a succession of neurons, one after another. However, it is not immediately apparent that each impulse may be (a) blocked in its transmission from one neuron to the next, (b) changed from a single impulse into repetitive impulses, or (c) integrated with impulses from other neurons to cause highly intricate patterns of impulses in successive neurons. All these functions can be classified as *synaptic functions of neurons*.

PHYSIOLOGIC ANATOMY OF THE SYNAPSE

The junction between one neuron and the next is called a *synapse*. Figure 6–5 illustrates a typical *motoneuron* in the anterior horn of the spinal cord. It is comprised of three major parts: the *soma*, which is the main body of the neuron; a single *axon*, which extends from the soma into the peripheral nerve; and the *dendrites*, which are thin projections of the soma that extend up to 1 mm. into the surrounding areas of the cord.

An average of about 6000 small knobs called *synaptic knobs* lie on the surfaces of the dendrites and soma of the motoneuron, approximately 80 to 90 per cent of them on the dendrites. These knobs are the terminal ends of nerve fibrils that originate in many other neurons, and usually not more than a few of the knobs are derived from any single previous neuron. Later it will become evident that many of these synaptic knobs are *excitatory* and

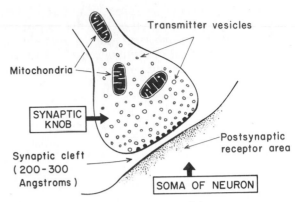

Figure 6–6. Physiologic anatomy of the synapse.

secrete a substance that excites the neuron, while others are *inhibitory* and secrete a substance that inhibits the neuron.

Neurons in other parts of the cord and brain differ markedly from the motoneuron in (1) the size of the cell body, (2) the length, size, and number of dendrites, ranging in length from almost none at all up to as long as one meter (the peripheral sensory nerve fiber), (3) the length and size of the axon, and (4) the number of synaptic knobs, which may range from only a few to more than a hundred thousand. These differences make neurons in different parts of the nervous system react differently to incoming signals and therefore perform different functions, as will be explained in subsequent chapters.

The Synaptic Knobs. Electron microscope studies of the synaptic knobs show that they have varied anatomical forms, but most resemble small round or oval knobs and therefore are frequently called *terminal knobs, boutons, end-feet,* or simply *presynaptic terminals*.

Figure 6–6 illustrates the basic structure of the synaptic knob (presynaptic terminal). It is separated from the neuronal soma by a *synaptic cleft* having a width usually of 200 to 300 Angstroms. The knob has two internal structures important to the excitatory or inhibitory functions of the synapse: the *synaptic vesicles* and the *mitochondria*. The synaptic vesicles contain a *transmitter substance* which, when released into the synaptic cleft, either *excites* or *inhibits* the neurons — excites if the neuronal membrane contains *excitatory receptors,* inhibits if it contains *inhibitory receptors*. The mitochondria provide ATP, which is required to synthesize new transmitter substance. The transmitter must be synthesized extremely rapidly because the amount stored in the vesicles is sufficient to last for only a few seconds to a few minutes of maximum activity.

When an action potential spreads over a presynaptic terminal, the membrane depolarization causes emptying of a small number of vesicles into

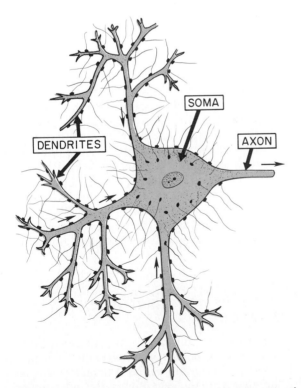

Figure 6–5. A typical motoneuron, showing synaptic knobs on the neuronal soma and dendrites. Note also the single axon.

the cleft; and the released transmitter in turn causes an immediate change in the permeability characteristics of the subsynaptic neuronal membrane, which leads to excitation or inhibition of the neuron, depending on the type of receptor substance.

Mechanism by Which the Synaptic Knob Action Potential Causes Release of Transmitter Vesicles. Unfortunately, we can only guess at the mechanism by which an action potential causes the vesicles to release transmitter substance into the synaptic cleft on reaching the synaptic knob. However, the number of vesicles released with each action potential is greatly reduced (a) when the quantity of calcium ions in the extracellular fluid is diminished, (b) when the quantity of sodium ions in the extracellular fluid is diminished, (c) when the quantity of magnesium ions in the extracellular fluids is increased, or (d) when the membrane of the synaptic knob has already been partially depolarized prior to transmission of the action potential so that the action potential is weaker than usual. On the basis of these characteristics, it has been suggested that the spread of the action potential over the membrane of the knob causes small amounts of calcium ions to leak into the knob. The calcium ions then are believed to cause several submembranal transmitter vesicles to fuse with the membrane and shortly thereafter to rupture, thus allowing spillage of their contents into the synaptic cleft.

At any rate, it is known that each time an action potential travels over the surface of the synaptic knob, a few vesicles of transmitter substance are emptied into the synaptic cleft, the number of vesicles depending upon the factors mentioned above. After emptying its contents, each vesicle then separates from the membrane and is used over and over again for transmitter storage and release.

One transmitter substance that occurs in certain parts of the nervous system is acetylcholine, as is discussed later. It has been calculated that about 3000 molecules of acetylcholine are present in each vesicle, and enough vesicles are present in the synaptic knob on a neuron to transmit a few thousand impulses.

Synthesis of New Transmitter Substance. Fortunately, the synaptic knobs have the capability of continually synthesizing new transmitter substance. Were it not for this ability, synaptic transmission would become completely ineffective within a few minutes. The synthesis usually occurs either partially or totally in the cytoplasm of the synaptic knobs, and then the newly synthesized or partially synthesized transmitter is immediately absorbed into the vesicles and stored or further processed until needed. Thus, each time a vesicle empties its contents into the synaptic cleft,

soon thereafter it becomes filled again with new transmitter.

Acetylcholine is synthesized from acetyl-CoA and choline in the presence of the enzyme *choline acetyltransferase,* an enzyme that is present in abundance in the cytoplasm of the cholinergic type of synaptic knob. When acetylcholine is released from the knob into the synaptic cleft, it is rapidly split again to acetate and choline by the enzyme cholinesterase that is adherent to the outer surface of the knob. Then the choline is actively transported back into the knob to be used once more for synthesis of new acetylcholine. Thus, the vesicles are used again and again. But even so, both the vesicles and the mitochondria that supply the energy for transmitter synthesis eventually disintegrate. Fortunately, new vesicles and mitochondria are continually transported from the cell soma down the axon to the synaptic knob, moving along the axon at a velocity of about 10 cm. per day, thus replenishing the supply in the knobs.

The formation, release, and re-uptake of norepinephrine by synaptic knobs of the sympathetic nervous system will be discussed in detail in Chapter 17 in relation to function of the autonomic nervous system.

Action of the Transmitter Substance on the Postsynaptic Neuron. The membrane of the postsynaptic neuron where a synaptic knob abuts is believed to contain specific receptor molecules that bind the transmitter substance. These receptors are probably proteins that, in response to the binding, change their shapes or activities in such a way that they increase the membrane permeability to most ions when the membrane receptor is excitatory and increase the permeability mainly to chloride ions when the receptor is inhibitory.

The ribosomes and the endoplasmic reticulum are both increased in the area immediately beneath the synapse, as illustrated by the density of the postsynaptic area in Figure 6–6. It is possible that the degree of development of this postsynaptic receptor area increases with the intensity of activity of the synapse; therefore, this is possibly a means by which the synapse can subserve the memory function, as will be discussed in detail in Chapter 15.

CHEMICAL AND PHYSIOLOGICAL NATURES OF THE TRANSMITTER SUBSTANCES

Excitation and Inhibition. Whether a transmitter will cause excitation or inhibition is determined not only by the nature of the transmitter but also by the nature of the receptor in the postsynaptic membrane. To give an example, the same neuron might be excited by a synapse that releases acetylcholine but inhibited by still another synapse that releases glycine. Thus, the neuronal membrane contains an *excitatory receptor* for acetylcholine and an *inhibitory receptor* for glycine. To give another example, norepinephrine released by some synapses in the central nervous system causes inhibition while at other synapses it causes excitation. In the first case, the neuronal membranes contain an inhibitory receptor for norepinephrine while the others contain an excitatory receptor for the same transmitter.

Differences in Function of Different Transmitters. Aside from the fact that transmitter substances sometimes cause excitation and sometimes inhibition, they also have other differences, the most important of which is duration of stimulation. For instance, the excitatory synapses on the anterior motoneurons of the spinal cord develop their excitatory stimulus in 1 to 2 milliseconds, and the excited state then lasts for another 10 to 20 milliseconds. On the other hand, some inhibitory synapses in the brain require as long as 10 to 15 milliseconds to develop full effect, and the effect often lasts for as long as 200 to 300 milliseconds. Still other substances have been isolated from the cerebrospinal fluid which, when infused into the aqueduct of Sylvius, cause brain stem inhibition and make an animal go to sleep for as long as several hours. This suggests that these substances might be synaptic transmitters the effects of which can last for hours.

Another difference among transmitters is that some cause an increase in the rate of firing of neurons while others have no effect at all on the firing rate but do change the neuron's sensitivity to still other transmitter substances. This type of transmitter is called a *modulator*.

One can readily see, therefore, that the brain can call on many different types of transmitters, each having its own special attributes. Obviously, these can be used in many different ways to achieve the varied functions of the nervous system. This is an area of neurophysiological research that is only now beginning to be understood.

Release of Only a Single Type of Transmitter Substance by Each Neuron. A single neuron releases only one type of transmitter, and it releases it at all its nerve terminals. Therefore, release of the different types of transmitters in the central nervous system requires different types of neurons.

In general, there are special neuronal *systems* for secreting the different transmitters. For example, most of the neurons located in the substantia nigra of the brain stem give rise to a system of nerve fibers that projects upward into the basal ganglia and into closely associated areas; all of these fibers release dopamine. The dopamine in turn has an inhibitory effect on that entire region of the brain. A similar system for release of norepinephrine originates in the reticular substance of the brain stem. And other similar systems exist for other transmitter substances elsewhere in the brain.

Some of the Important Transmitter Substances. There now exists very good evidence for about thirty different nervous system transmitters. Some types of evidence that have been used for discovering the different transmitters include the following: (1) the transmitter substance has been isolated from the neuronal tissue or shown to exist in specific neurons by chemical or immunological techniques; (2) the enzymes required for synthesis of the specific transmitter have been isolated from the nervous tissue or shown to exist specifically in the synaptic knobs; (3) injection of the transmitter substance into the local neuronal areas will cause excitation or inhibition; (4) substances that prevent destruction of the transmitter will potentiate its effect on the local neurons; and (5) specific mechanisms for removing a specific transmitter after it is released have been discovered in the local tissue area. Almost none of the presumed nervous system transmitter substances fulfill all these criteria, but some of the substances that fulfill many of them are the following:

Acetylcholine is secreted by neurons in many areas of the brain. Two places where this has been proved beyond doubt are in the striate region of the basal ganglia and at the endings of the recurrent nerve fibers from the anterior motoneurons where they terminate on the Renshaw cells in the anterior horns of the cord. In addition, histochemical studies suggest that acetylcholine is a widely used transmitter throughout the brain. It probably has an excitatory effect either everywhere or almost everywhere that it is released, even though it is known to have inhibitory effects in some portions of the peripheral parasympathetic nervous system, such as inhibition of the heart by the vagus nerves.

Norepinephrine is secreted by many neurons of which the cell bodies are located in the reticular formation of the brain stem and also in the hypothalamus. These neurons send nerve fibers to widespread areas of the brain. In most instances they probably cause inhibition, though it is probable that they cause excitation in some areas.

Epinephrine is secreted by a fewer number of neurons, but in general they parallel the norepinephrine system.

Dopamine is secreted by neurons that originate in the substantia nigra. The terminations of these neurons are mainly in the striatal region of the basal ganglia. The effect of dopamine is usually inhibition.

Glycine is secreted mainly at synapses in the

spinal cord. It probably always acts as an inhibitory transmitter.

Gamma amino butyric acid (GABA) is secreted by nerve terminals in the spinal cord, the cerebellum, the basal ganglia, and many other areas. It is believed always to cause inhibition.

Glutamic acid is probably secreted by the synaptic knobs in some or many of the sensory pathways. It probably always causes excitation.

Substance P is probably released by pain fiber terminals in the substantia gelatinosa of the spinal cord. In general, it causes excitation.

Enkephalins and endorphins are probably secreted by nerve terminals in the spinal cord, in the brain stem, in the thalamus, and in the hypothalamus. These probably act as excitatory transmitters to excite another system that inhibits the transmission of pain.

Serotonin is secreted by nuclei that originate in the median raphe of the brain stem and project to many brain areas, especially to the dorsal horns of the spinal cord and to the hypothalamus. Serotonin acts as an inhibitor of pain pathways in the cord, and it is also believed to help control the mood of the person, perhaps even to cause sleep.

Despite this long list of transmitter substances, it is only a partial list. Other substances that have been proved or suggested include various peptides, other amino acids, histamine, prostaglandins, cyclic AMP, and many others.

ELECTRICAL EVENTS DURING NEURONAL EXCITATION

The electrical events in neuronal excitation have been studied mainly in the large motoneuron of the anterior horn of the spinal cord. Therefore, the events to be described in the following few sections pertain essentially to these neurons. However, except for some quantitative differences, they apply to most other neurons of the nervous system as well.

The Resting Membrane Potential of the Neuronal

Soma. Figure 6–7 illustrates the soma of a motoneuron, showing the resting membrane potential to be about −70 millivolts. This is somewhat less than the −90 millivolts found in large peripheral nerve fibers and in skeletal muscle fibers; the lower voltage is important, however, because it allows both positive and negative control of the degree of excitability of the neuron. That is, decreasing the voltage to a less negative value makes the membrane of the neuron more excitable, while increasing this voltage to a more negative value makes the neuron less excitable. This is the basis of the two modes of function of the neuron — either excitation or inhibition — as we will explain in detail in the following sections.

Concentration Differences of Ions Across the Neuronal Somal Membrane. Figure 6–7 also illustrates the concentration differences across the neuronal somal membrane of the three ions that are most important for neuronal function: sodium ions, potassium ions, and chloride ions.

At the top, the sodium ion concentration is shown to be very great in the extracellular fluid but low inside the neuron. This sodium concentration gradient is caused by a strong sodium pump that continually pumps sodium out of the neuron.

The figure also shows that the potassium ion concentration is large inside the neuronal soma but very low in the extracellular fluid. It illustrates that there is a weak potassium pump that tends to pump potassium to the interior while there is a very high degree of permeability to potassium. The pump is relatively unimportant because potassium ions leak through the neuronal somal pores so readily that this nullifies most of the effectiveness of the pump. Therefore, for most purposes one can consider the membrane to be relatively permeable to potassium and the potassium pump to be of only slight importance.

Figure 6–7 shows the chloride ion to be of high concentration in the extracellular fluid but low concentration inside the neuron. It also shows that the membrane is highly permeable to chloride ions

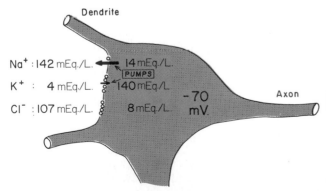

Figure 6–7. Distribution of sodium, potassium, and chloride ions across the neuronal somal membrane; origin of the intrasomal membrane potential.

and that there is no chloride pump. Therefore, the chloride ions become distributed across the membrane passively. The reason for the low concentration of chloride ions inside the neuron is the −70 millivolts in the neuron. That is, this negative voltage repels the negatively charged chloride ions, forcing them outward through the pores until the concentration difference is so great that its tendency to move chloride ions inward exactly balances the tendency of the electrical difference to move them outward. That is, the chloride ions become distributed across the membrane in accordance with the Nernst equation for equilibrium conditions. This equation was discussed in detail in Chapter 2.

Origin of the Resting Membrane Potential of the Neuronal Soma. The basic cause of the −70 millivolt resting membrane potential of the neuronal soma is the sodium-potassium pump. This pump causes the extrusion of more positively charged sodium ions to the exterior than potassium to the interior — 3 sodium ions for each 2 potassium ions. Since there are large numbers of negatively charged ions inside the soma that cannot diffuse through the membrane — protein ions, phosphate ions, and many others — extrusion of the positively charged sodium ions to the exterior leaves all these nondiffusible negative ions unbalanced by positive ions on the inside. Therefore, the interior of the neuron becomes negatively charged as the result of the sodium-potassium pump. This principle was discussed in more detail in Chapter 2 in relation to the resting membrane potential of nerves.

Uniform Distribution of the Potential Inside the Soma. The interior of the neuronal soma contains a very highly conductive electrolytic solution, the intracellular fluid of the neuron. Furthermore, the diameter of the neuronal soma is very large (from 10 to 80 microns in diameter) causing there to be almost no resistance to conduction of electrical current from one part of the somal interior to another part. Therefore, any change in potential in any part of the intrasomal fluid causes an almost exactly equal change in potential at all other points in the soma. This is an important principle because it plays a major role in the summation of signals entering the neuron from multiple sources, as we shall see in subsequent sections of this chapter.

Effect of Synaptic Excitation on the Postsynaptic Membrane — The Excitatory Postsynaptic Potential. Figure 6–8A illustrates the resting neuron with an unexcited synaptic knob resting upon its surface. The resting membrane potential everywhere in the soma is −70 millivolts.

Figure 6–8B illustrates a synaptic knob that has secreted a transmitter into the cleft between the knob and the neuronal somal membrane. This

Figure 6–8. Three states of a neuron. A, A resting neuron. B, A neuron in an excited state, with increased intraneuronal potential caused by sodium influx. C, A neuron in an inhibited state, with decreased intraneuronal membrane potential caused by potassium ion efflux.

transmitter acts on a membrane excitatory receptor *to increase the membrane's permeability to all ions.* However, because of the large electrochemical gradient that tends to move sodium inward and because both the potassium and chloride concentration gradients are almost in equilibrium with the electrical potential, this large opening of the membrane pores mainly allows sodium ions to rush to the inside of the membrane.

The rapid influx of the positively charged sodium ions to the interior of the neuron neutralizes part of the negativity of the resting membrane potential. Thus, in Figure 6–8B the resting membrane potential has been increased from −70 millivolts to −59 millivolts. This increase in voltage above the normal resting neuronal potential — that is, to a less negative value — is called the *excitatory postsynaptic potential* (or EPSP) because when this potential rises high enough it will elicit an action potential in the neuron, thus exciting it.

However, we must issue a word of warning at this point. Discharge of a single synaptic knob can never increase the neuronal potential from −70 millivolts up to −59 millivolts. Instead, an increase of this magnitude requires the simultaneous discharge of many knobs — ten or more usually — at the same time or in rapid succession. This occurs by a process called *summation*, which will be discussed in detail in the following sections.

Generation of Action Potentials at the Initial Segment of the Axon — Threshold for Excita-

tion. When the membrane potential inside the neuron rises high enough, there comes a point that this initiates an action potential in the neuron. However, the action potential does not begin on the somal membrane adjacent to the excitatory synapses. Instead, it begins in the initial segment of the axon (the "axon hillock"). This may be explained as follows: Any factor that increases the potential inside the soma at any single point also increases this potential everywhere in the soma at the same time because of the very low resistance inside the soma, as explained earlier. Yet, because of physical differences in the membrane and differences in geometrical arrangement of the membrane in different parts of the neuron, the most excitable part of the neuron by far is the initial segment of the axon — that is, the first 50 to 100 microns of the axon after it leaves the neuronal soma. The excitatory postsynaptic potential that will elicit an action potential at this point on the neuron is approximately 11 millivolts. This is in contrast to approximately 30 millivolts required on the soma itself. Therefore, the new action potential originates in the initial segment of the axon and not on the soma. Once the action potential begins, it travels peripherally along the axon and also travels backward over the soma of the neuron (however, it usually does not travel backward very far into the dendrites).

Thus, in Figure 6–8B, it is shown that under normal conditions the *threshold* for excitation of the neuron is −59 millivolts, which represents an excitatory postsynaptic potential of +11 millivolts — that is, 11 millivolts more positive than the normal resting neuronal potential of −70 millivolts.

ELECTRICAL EVENTS IN NEURONAL INHIBITION

Effect of Inhibitory Synapses on the Postsynaptic Membrane — The Inhibitory Postsynaptic Potential. It was pointed out above that excitatory synapses increase the permeability of the somal membrane to all ions — including sodium, potassium, and chloride. The inhibitory synapses, in contrast, increase the permeability of the postsynaptic membrane only to potassium and chloride ions. And the opened channels are too small to allow the large hydrated sodium ions to pass through. However, potassium efflux does occur, as illustrated in Figure 6–8C. The reason potassium flows outward through the membrane is the following: In the resting state, a weak potassium pump has been pumping a slight excess of potassium ions to the interior of the neuron. Therefore, there are too many potassium ions on the inside to be in an exact equilibrium state as described by the Nernst equation for equilibrium conditions.

Consequently, opening of the pores causes outward diffusion of some of the excess potassium ions, thereby decreasing the positive ions inside the neuron and leaving the nondiffusible negative ions of the neuron (protein ions, phosphate ions, and others). This concentration of negative ions makes the internal potential of the neuron more negative, as illustrated by the −75 millivolt potential inside the neuron in Figure 6–8C. This is called a *hyperpolarized state*. And the 5 millivolt decrease in intraneuronal voltage below the normal resting potential of −70 millivolts caused by the inhibitory transmitter is called the *inhibitory postsynaptic potential*.

Obviously, the increased negativity of the membrane potential (−75 millivolts) makes the neuron less excitable than it is normally. Since the potential must rise to −59 millivolts to excite the neuron, an excitatory postsynaptic potential must now be 16 millivolts instead of the normal 11 millivolts to cause excitation. Thus, in this way the inhibitory transmitter inhibits the neuron.

"Clamping" of the Resting Membrane Potential as a Means to Inhibit Neurons. Sometimes, excitation of the inhibitory synapses causes little or no inhibitory postsynaptic potential, but it still inhibits the neuron. The reason that the potential does not change is that in some neurons the summated concentration differences across the membrane for the potassium and chloride ions are only barely able to create a diffusion potential equal to the normal resting potential. Therefore, when the inhibitory pores open, there is no net flow of ions to cause an inhibitory postsynaptic potential. Yet, both the potassium and the chloride ions do diffuse bidirectionally through the wide-open pores many times as rapidly as normally, and this high flux of these two ions inhibits the neuron in the following way: When excitatory synapses fire and sodium ions flow into the neuron, this raises the intraneuronal voltage far less than usual because any tendency for the membrane potential to change away from the resting potential is immediately opposed by rapid flux of potassium and chloride ions through the inhibitory pores to bring the potential back to the resting value. Therefore, the amount of influx of sodium ions required to cause excitation may be increased to as much as 5 to 20 times normal.

This tendency for the potassium and chloride ions to maintain a membrane potential near the resting value when the inhibitory pores are wide open is called "clamping" of the potential.

To express the phenomenon for clamping more mathematically, one needs to recall the Goldman equation from Chapter 2. This equation indicates that the membrane potential is determined by summation of the tendencies for the different ions to carry electrical charges through the membrane in the two directions. The membrane potential will approach the Nernst equilibrium potential for those ions that permeate the membrane to the greatest extent. When the inhibitory channels are wide open, the chloride and potassium ions permeate the membrane very greatly. Therefore, when the excitatory channels open, it is difficult to raise the neuronal potential up to the threshold value for excitation.

It is also interesting that some recent studies suggest that inhibitory channels are considerably more permeable to chloride ions than to potassium ions. Since chloride permeability inhibits neurons only by the clamping mechanism, this emphasizes the importance of clamping in the inhibitory process.

Presynaptic Inhibition

In addition to the inhibition caused by inhibitory synapses operating at the neuronal membrane, called *postsynaptic inhibition,* another type of inhibition often occurs before the signal reaches the synapse. This type of inhibition, called *presynaptic inhibition,* is believed to occur in the following way:

In presynaptic inhibition, instead of the postsynaptic neuron being inhibited, the presynaptic terminal fibrils and synaptic knobs are inhibited. This inhibition is caused by "presynaptic" synapses that lie on the terminal fibrils and synaptic knobs before the knobs themselves terminate on the following neuron. It is believed that these presynaptic synapses secrete a transmitter substance that in some way not yet understood depresses the voltage of the action potential that occurs at the membrane of the knob and, as has already been pointed out, this greatly decreases the amount of transmitter released by the knob. Therefore, the degree of excitation of the neuron is also greatly suppressed, or inhibited.

The nature of the transmitter substance released at the presynaptic synapses is not known. However, presynaptic inhibition is blocked by *picrotoxin* and also by *bicuculline.* Since these two substances also block the action of the transmitter substance GABA, it has been suggested that the transmitter that causes presynaptic inhibition is GABA. On the other hand, the transmitter substance probably associated with most postsynaptic inhibition in the spinal cord is glycine. The reason for believing this is that strychnine inhibits this type of inhibition, and it also blocks the inhibitory action of glycine, but not of GABA, on neurons.

Presynaptic inhibition is different from postsynaptic inhibition in its time sequence. It requires many milliseconds to develop, but once it does occur, it can last for as long as a half second or perhaps even longer, while postsynaptic inhibition, at least of the anterior motoneurons, lasts for only 10 to 15 milliseconds.

Presynaptic inhibition occurs especially at the more peripheral synapses of the sensory pathways. Shortly after a strong sensory signal enters the sensory pathways, negative feedback automatically causes increasing presynaptic inhibition. This, in turn, reduces the degree of transmission of the sensory signals. Therefore, the greater the intensity of the input signal, the greater also becomes the negative feedback inhibition. In this way presynaptic inhibition acts as a sensitivity control on the sensory input. It also sharpens the boundaries between stimulated and nonstimulated areas of the sensory pathway because it prevents excessive spread of the sensory signals to the unexcited neurons. This process is called "contrast enhancement."

SUMMATION OF POSTSYNAPTIC POTENTIALS

Time Course of Postsynaptic Potentials. When a synapse excites the anterior motoneuron, the neuronal membrane becomes highly permeable for only 1 to 2 milliseconds. During this time sodium ions diffuse rapidly to the interior of the cell to increase the intraneuronal potential, thus creating the *excitatory postsynaptic potential.* This potential then persists for about 15 milliseconds because this is the time required for the sodium ions to be pumped out or for potassium ions to leak out or chloride ions to leak in to re-establish the normal resting membrane potential.

Precisely the same effect occurs for the inhibitory postsynaptic potential. That is, the inhibitory synapse increases the permeability of the membrane to potassium and chloride ions for 1 to 2 milliseconds, and this usually decreases the intraneuronal potential to a more negative value than normal, thereby creating the *inhibitory postsynaptic potential.* This potential also persists for about 15 milliseconds.

However, other types of transmitter substances acting on other neurons can perhaps excite or inhibit for hundreds of milliseconds or even for seconds, minutes, or hours.

Spatial Summation of the Postsynaptic Potentials. It has already been pointed out that excitation of a single synaptic knob on the surface of a neuron will almost never excite the neuron. The reason for this is that sufficient transmitter substance is released by a single knob to cause an excitatory postsynaptic potential usually no more than a millivolt at most, instead of the required 10 or more millivolts that is the usual threshold for excitation. However, during an excitatory state in a neuronal pool of the nervous system, many synaptic knobs are usually stimulated at the same time, and even though these knobs are spread over wide areas of the neuron, their effects can still summate. The reason for this summation is the following: It has already been pointed out that a change in the potential at any single point within the soma will cause the potential to change everywhere in the soma almost exactly equally. Therefore, for each excitatory synapse that discharges simultaneously, the intrasomal potential rises another quantal amount — up to about 1 millivolt. When the excitatory postsynaptic potential becomes great enough, the threshold for firing will be reached, and an action potential will generate at the initial segment of the axon. This effect is illustrated in Figure 6–9, which shows several excitatory postsynaptic potentials. The bottom postsynaptic potential in the figure was caused by stimulation of only four excitatory synapses; then the next higher potential was caused by stimulation of two times as many synapses; finally, a still higher excitatory postsynaptic potential was caused by stimulation of four times as many synapses. This time an action potential was generated at the axon hillock.

This effect of summing simultaneous postsynaptic potentials by excitation of multiple knobs on widely spaced areas of the membrane is called *spatial summation*.

Temporal Summation. Most synaptic knobs can fire repetitively in rapid succession only a few milliseconds apart. Each time a knob fires, the released transmitter substance opens the membrane pores for a millisecond or so. Since the postsynaptic potential lasts for up to 15 milliseconds, a second opening of the same pore can increase the postsynaptic potential to a still greater level so that the more rapid the rate of knob stimulation, the greater the effective postsynaptic potential. Thus, successive postsynaptic potentials of individual synaptic knobs, if they occur rapidly enough, can summate in the same way that postsynaptic potentials can summate

from widely distributed knobs over the surface of the neuron. This summation is called *temporal summation*.

Simultaneous Summation of Inhibitory and Excitatory Postsynaptic Potentials. Obviously, if an inhibitory postsynaptic potential is tending to decrease the membrane potential to a more negative value while an excitatory postsynaptic potential is tending to increase the potential at the same time, these two effects can either completely nullify each other or partially nullify each other. Also, inhibitory "clamping" of the membrane potential can nullify much of an excitatory potential. Thus, if a neuron is currently being excited by an excitatory postsynaptic potential, then an inhibitory signal from another source can easily reduce the postsynaptic potential below the threshold value for excitation, thus turning off the activity of the neuron.

Facilitation of Neurons. Often the summated postsynaptic potential is excitatory in nature but has not risen high enough to reach the threshold for excitation. When this happens the neuron is said to be *facilitated*. That is, its membrane potential is nearer the threshold for firing than normally, but it is not yet to the level of firing. Nevertheless, a signal entering the neuron from some other source can then excite the neuron very easily. Diffuse signals in the nervous system often facilitate large groups of neurons so that they can respond quickly and easily to signals arriving from secondary sources.

SPECIAL FUNCTIONS OF DENDRITES IN EXCITING NEURONS

The Large Spatial Field of Excitation of the Dendrites. The dendrites of the anterior motoneurons extend for 0.5 to 1 millimeter in all directions from the neuronal soma. Therefore, these dendrites can receive signals from a large spatial area around the motoneuron. This provides vast opportunity for summation of signals from many separate presynaptic neurons.

It is also important that between 80 and 90 per cent of all the synaptic knobs terminate on the dendrites of the anterior motoneuron in contrast to only 10 to 20 per cent terminating on the neuronal soma. Therefore, the preponderant share of the excitation of the neuron is provided by signals transmitted over the dendrites.

Failure of Many Dendrites to Transmit Action Potentials. Many dendrites fail to transmit action potentials because their thresholds for excitation are very high. Yet they do transmit *electrotonic current* down the dendrites to the soma. (Transmission of electrotonic current means the direct spread of current by electrical conduction in the

Figure 6–9. Excitatory postsynaptic potentials, showing that simultaneous firing of only a few synapses will not cause sufficient summated potential to elicit an action potential, but that simultaneous firing of many synapses will raise the summated potential to the threshold for excitation and cause a superimposed action potential.

Figure 6–10. Stimulation of a neuron by synaptic knobs located on dendrites, showing, especially, decremental conduction of electrotonic potentials in the two dendrites to the left and inhibition of dendritic excitation in the dendrite that is uppermost.

fluids in the dendrites with no generation of action potentials.) Stimulation of the neuron by this current has special characteristics, as follows:

Decrement of Electrotonic Conduction in the Dendrites — Greater Excitation by Synapses Near the Soma. In Figure 6–10 a number of excitatory and inhibitory synapses are shown stimulating the dendrites of a neuron. On the two dendrites to the left in the figure are shown excitatory effects near the ends of the dendrites; note the high levels of the excitatory postsynaptic potentials at these ends — that is, the less negative potentials. However, a large share of the excitatory postsynaptic potential is lost before it reaches the soma. The reason for this is that the dendrites are long and thin, and their membranes are also very leaky to electrical current. Therefore, before the excitatory potentials can reach the soma, a large share of the potential is lost by leakage through the membrane. This decrease in membrane potential as it spreads along dendrites toward the soma is called *decremental conduction.*

It is also obvious that the nearer the excitatory synapse is to the soma of the neuron, the less will be the decrement of conduction. Therefore, those synapses that lie near the soma have far more excitatory effect than those that lie far away from the soma.

Rapid Re-excitation of the Neuron by the Dendrites After the Neuron Fires. When an action potential is generated in a neuron, this action potential spreads back over the soma but not always over the dendrites. Furthermore, the postsynaptic potentials in the dendrites often remain relatively undisturbed by the action potential. Therefore, just as soon as the action potential is over, the potentials still existing in the dendrites are ready and waiting to re-excite the neuron. Thus, the

dendrites have a "holding capacity" for the excitatory signal from presynaptic sources.

Summation of Excitation and Inhibition in Dendrites. The uppermost dendrite of Figure 6–10 is shown to be stimulated by both excitatory and inhibitory synapses. At the tip of the dendrite is a strong excitatory postsynaptic potential, but much of this is lost by decremental conduction along the dendrite. Then near the soma two inhibitory synapses are stimulating the same dendrite. These inhibitory synapses provide a hyperpolarizing voltage in the dendrite that completely nullifies the excitatory effect and indeed transmits a small amount of inhibition by decremental electrotonic conduction toward the soma. Thus, dendrites can summate excitatory and inhibitory postsynaptic potentials in the same way that the soma can. In those instances when action potentials do develop in dendrites, inhibitory synapses located near the soma can completely block the action potentials and can prevent their ever entering the soma of the neuron. It is interesting that the inhibitory synapses are especially abundant on or near the soma.

RELATION OF STATE OF EXCITATION OF THE NEURON TO THE RATE OF FIRING

The "Central Excitatory State." The "central excitatory state" of a neuron is defined as the degree of excitatory drive to the neuron. If there is a higher degree of excitation than inhibition of the neuron at any given instant, then it is said that there is a *central excitatory state.* On the other hand, if there is more inhibition than excitation, then it is said that there is a *central inhibitory state.*

When the central excitatory state of a neuron rises above the threshold for excitation, then the neuron will fire repetitively as long as the excitatory state remains at this level. However, the rate at which it will fire is determined by how much above threshold it is. To explain this, we must first consider what happens to the neuronal somal potential during and following the action potential.

Changes in Neuronal Somal Potential During and Following the Action Potential. Figure 6–11 illustrates an action potential initiated by an excitatory postsynaptic potential. Following the spike portion of the action potential, there is a very long *positive after-potential* lasting for many milliseconds. During this interval the somal membrane potential falls below the normal resting membrane potential of -70 millivolts. This is probably caused by a very high degree of permeability of the neuronal membrane to potassium ions that persists for many milliseconds after the action potential is over. As a result, potassium ions diffuse from inside the neuron to the exterior carrying positive charges out of the neuron and, therefore, creating an excessively high degree of negativity inside the neuron. This is called *hyperpolarization*.

The importance of this state of hyperpolarization after the spike potential is that the neuron remains in an *inhibited state* during this period of time. Therefore, a far greater central excitatory state is required during this time than normally to cause re-excitation of the neuron.

Relationship of Central Excitatory State to Frequency of Firing. The curve shown at the top of Figure 6–11, labeled "central excitatory state required for re-excitation," depicts the relative level of the central excitatory state required at each instant after an action potential is over to re-excite the neuron. Note that very soon after an action potential is over a very high central excitatory state is required. That is, a very large number of excitatory synapses must be firing simultaneously. Then, after many milliseconds have passed and the state of hyperpolarization of the neuron has begun to disappear, the central excitatory state required becomes greatly reduced.

Therefore, it is immediately evident that when the central excitatory state is high a second action potential will appear very soon after the previous one. Then still a third action potential will appear soon after the second, and this process will continue indefinitely. Thus, at a very high central excitatory state the frequency of firing of the neuron is great.

On the other hand, when the central excitatory state is only barely above threshold, the neuron must recover almost completely from the hyperpolarization, which requires many milliseconds,

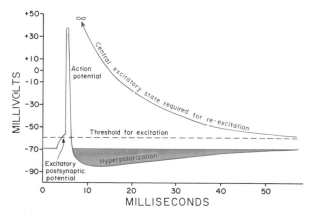

Figure 6–11. A neuronal potential followed by a prolonged period of neuronal hyperpolarization. Also shown is the central excitatory state required for re-excitation of the neuron at given intervals after the action potential is over.

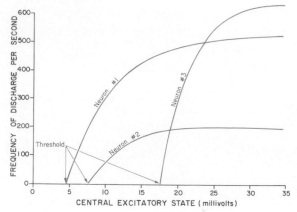

Figure 6–12. Response characteristics of different types of neurons to progressively increasing central excitatory states.

before it will fire again. Therefore, the frequency of neuronal firing is low.

(Note that the increase in the central excitatory state that is required for re-excitation is far greater than the decrease in the neuronal potential during the state of hyperpolarization. The reason for this is that at the same time that the neuron is hyperpolarized its voltage is also "clamped" to a great extent by the high permeability of the membrane to potassium and chloride ions. This clamping mechanism of neuronal inhibition was discussed earlier in the chapter.)

Response Characteristics of Different Neurons to Increasing Levels of Central Excitatory State. Histological study of the nervous system immediately convinces one of the widely varying types of neurons in different parts of the nervous system. And, physiologically, the different types of neurons perform different functions. Therefore, as would be expected, the ability to respond to stimulation by the synapses varies from one type of neuron to another.

Figure 6–12 illustrates theoretical responses of three different types of neurons to varying levels of central excitatory state. Note that neuron number 1 will not discharge at all until the excitatory state rises to 5 millivolts. Then, as the excitatory state rises progressively to 35 millivolts the frequency of discharge rises to slightly over 500 per second.

Neuron number 2 is quite a different type, having a threshold for excitation of 8 millivolts and a maximum rate of discharge of only 190 per second. Finally, neuron number 3 has a high threshold for excitation, about 18 millivolts, but its discharge rate rises rapidly to over 600 per second as the central excitatory state rises only slightly above threshold.

Thus, different neurons respond differently, have different thresholds for excitation, and have widely differing maximal frequencies of discharge. With a little imagination one can readily understand the importance of having neurons with many different types of response characteristics to perform the widely varying functions of the nervous system.

SOME SPECIAL CHARACTERISTICS OF SYNAPTIC TRANSMISSION

Forward Conduction Through Synapses. From the above discussion, it should be evident by now that impulses are conducted through synapses only from the synaptic knobs to the successive neurons and never in the reverse direction. This is called the *principle of forward conduction*.

Fatigue of Synaptic Transmission. When excitatory synapses are repetitively stimulated at a rapid rate, the number of discharges by the postsynaptic neuron is at first very great, but it becomes progressively less in succeeding milliseconds or seconds. This is called *fatigue* of synaptic transmission.

Fatigue is an exceedingly important characteristic of synaptic function, for when areas of the nervous system become overexcited, fatigue causes them to lose this excess excitability after a while. For example, fatigue is probably the most important means by which the excess excitability of the brain during an epileptic fit is finally subdued so that the fit ceases. Thus, the development of fatigue is a protective mechanism against excess neuronal activity. This will be discussed further in the description of reverberating neuronal circuits in the following chapter.

The mechanism of fatigue is mainly exhaustion of the stores of transmitter substance in the synaptic knobs, particularly since it has been calculated that the excitatory knobs can store enough excitatory transmitter for only 10,000 normal synaptic transmissions, an amount that can be exhausted in only a few seconds to a few minutes. However, part of the fatigue process might also result from progressive inactivation of the membrane receptors.

Post-Tetanic Facilitation. When a rapidly repetitive series of impulses stimulates an excitatory synapse for a period of time and then a rest period is allowed, the postsynaptic neuron will usually be even more responsive to subsequent stimulation than normally. This is called *post-tetanic facilitation*.

Experiments have shown that at least two factors help to cause post-tetanic facilitation. First, for reasons not yet fully understood, a rapidly stimulated synaptic knob develops a state of hyperpolarization (more negative membrane potential than normal), and this causes the action potentials of the synaptic knob to become considerably increased, an effect that also causes increased release of transmitter substance. Second, the transmitter vesicles in the synaptic knob seem to become more mobile, or at least to release their transmitter substances more easily than usual, and this also increases the amount of transmitter substance released. This probably results from enhanced permeability of the synaptic knobs to calcium, the calcium in turn increasing the vesicular release of transmitter. (It is possible that the postsynaptic receptor membrane also becomes more sensitive to the transmitter substance, but this has not yet been proved.) At any rate, post-tetanic facilitation causes the excitatory postsynaptic potential to increase to as much as 2 times normal.

The physiological significance of post-tetanic facilitation is still very doubtful, and it may have no real significance at all. However, since post-tetanic facilitation can last from a few seconds in some neurons to several hours in others, it is immediately apparent that neurons could possibly store information by this mechanism. Therefore post-tetanic facilitation might well be a mechanism of "short-term" memory in the central nervous system. This possibility will be discussed at length in Chapter 15 in relation to the memory function of the cerebral cortex.

Effect of Acidosis and Alkalosis on Synaptic Transmission. The neurons are highly responsive to changes in pH of the surrounding interstitial fluids. *Alkalosis greatly increases neuronal excitability.* For instance, a rise in arterial pH from the normal of 7.4 to about 7.8 often causes cerebral convulsions because of increased excitability of the neurons. This can be demonstrated especially well by having a person who is normally predisposed to epileptic fits overbreathe. The overbreathing elevates the pH of the blood only momentarily, but even this short interval can often precipitate an epileptic convulsive attack.

On the other hand, *acidosis greatly depresses neuronal activity;* a fall in pH from 7.4 to below 7.0 usually causes a comatose state. For instance, in very severe diabetic or uremic acidosis, coma always develops.

Effect of Hypoxia on Synaptic Transmission. Neuronal excitability is also highly dependent on an adequate supply of oxygen. Cessation of oxygen supply for only a few seconds can cause complete inexcitability of the neurons. This is often seen when the cerebral circulation is temporarily interrupted, for within 3 to 5 seconds the person becomes unconscious.

Effect of Drugs on Synaptic Transmission. Many different drugs are known to increase the excitability of neurons, and others are known to decrease the excitability. For instance, caffeine, theophylline, and theobromine, which are found in coffee, tea, and cocoa, respectively, all increase neuronal excitability, presumably by reducing the threshold for excitation of the neurons. However, strychnine, which is one of the best known of all the agents that increase the excitability of neurons, does not reduce the threshold for excitation of the neurons at all but, instead, *inhibits the action of at least some of the inhibitory transmitters* on the neurons, probably especially the inhibitory effect of glycine in the spinal cord. In consequence, the effects of the excitatory transmitters become overwhelming, and the neurons become so excited that they go into rapidly repetitive discharge, resulting in severe convulsions.

Most anesthetics have long been believed to increase membrane threshold for excitation and thereby to decrease neuronal activity throughout the body. This is based principally on the fact that most of the volatile anesthetics are chemically inert compounds but are lipid soluble. Therefore, it has been reasoned that these substances might change the physical characteristics of the neuronal membranes, making them less responsive to excitatory agents.

Synaptic Delay. In transmission of an impulse from a synaptic knob to a postsynaptic neuron, a certain amount of time is consumed in the process of (a) discharge of the transmitter substance by the knob, (b) diffusion of the transmitter to the subsynaptic neuronal membrane, (c) action of the transmitter on the membrane receptor, (d) action of the receptor to increase the membrane permeability, and (e) inward diffusion of sodium to raise the excitatory postsynaptic potential to a high enough value to elicit an action potential. The *minimal* period of time required for all these events to take place, even when large numbers of presynaptic terminals are stimulated simultaneously, is 0.3 to 0.5 millisecond. This is called the *synaptic delay*. It is important for the following reason: Neurophysiologists can measure the *minimal* delay time between an input volley of impulses and an output volley and from this can estimate the number of series neurons in the circuit.

REFERENCES

Adams, D. J., *et al.*: Ionic currents in molluscan soma. *Annu. Rev. Neurosci., 3*:141, 1980.

Baker, P. F., and Reuter, H.: Calcium Movement in Excitable Cells. New York, Pergamon Press, 1975.

Barker, J. L.: Peptides: Roles in neuronal excitability. *Physiol. Rev., 56*:435, 1976.

Bennett, M. V. L.: Electrical transmission: A functional analysis and comparison with chemical transmission. *In* Brookhart, J. M., and Mountcastle, V. B. (eds.): Handbook of Physiology. Sec. 1, Vol. 1. Baltimore, Williams & Wilkins, 1977, p. 357.

Bourne, G. II., *et al.* (eds.): Neuronal Cells and Hormones. New York, Academic Press, 1978.

Ceccarelli, B., and Clementi, F. (eds.): Neurotoxins, Tools in Neurobiology. New York, Raven Press, 1979.

Ceccarelli, B., and Hurlbut, W. P.: Vesicle hypothesis of the release of quanta of acetylcholine. *Physiol. Rev., 60*:396, 1980.

Cobb, W. A., and vanDuijn, H. (eds.): Contemporary Clinical Neurophysiology. New York, Elsevier Scientific Publishing Co., 1978.

Cooper, J. R. *et al.*: The Biochemical Basis of Neuropharmacology. New York, Oxford University Press, 1978.

Cuénod, M., *et al.* (eds.): Development and Chemical Specificity of Neurons. New York, Elsevier Scientific Publishing Co., 1979.

Duggan, A. W.: Pharmacology of mammalian central inhibition: *In* Porter, R. (ed.): International Review of Physiology: Neurophysiology III. Vol. 17. Baltimore, University Park Press, 1978, p. 119.

Eccles, J. C.: My scientific odyssey. *Annu. Rev. Physiol., 39*:1, 1977.

Fuxe, K. (ed.): Peptidergic Neuron. New York, Plenum Press, 1979.

Gotto, A. M., Jr., *et al.* (eds.): Brain Peptides: A New Endocrinology. New York, Elsevier/North-Holland, 1979.

Guroff, G.: Molecular Neurobiology. New York, Marcel Dekker, 1979.

Horn, A. S., *et al.* (eds.): The Neurology of Dopamine. New York, Academic Press, 1979.

Iversen, L. L.: The chemistry of the brain. *Sci. Am. 241*(3):134, 1979.

Johnston, G. A. R.: Neuropharmacology of amino acid inhibitory transmitters. *Annu. Rev. Pharmacol. Toxicol., 18*:269, 1978.

Kelly, R. B., *et al.*: Biochemistry of neurotransmitter release. *Annu. Rev. Neurosci., 2*:399, 1979.

Krogsgaard-Larsen, P., *et al.*: (eds.): GABA-Neuro-Transmitters. New York, Academic Press, 1979.

Kupfermann, I.: Modulatory actions of neurotransmitters. *Annu. Rev. Neurosci., 2*:447, 1979.

Langer, S. Z., *et al.* (eds.): Presynaptic Receptors. New York, Pergamon Press, 1979.

Lynch, G., and Schubert, P.: The use of in vitro brain slices for multidisciplinary studies of synaptic function. *Ann. Rev. Neurosci., 3*:1, 1980.

Maelicke, A., *et al.*: Biochemical aspects of neurotransmitter receptors. *In* Brookhart, J. M., and Mountcastle, V. B. (eds.): Handbook of Physiology. Sec. 1, Vol. 1. Baltimore, Williams & Wilkins, 1977, p. 493.

Mandel, P., and DeFeudis, F. V. (eds.): GABA — Biochemistry and CNS Functions. New York, Plenum Press, 1979.

McLachlan, E. M.: The statistics of transmitter release at chemical synapses. *In* Porter, R. (ed.): International Review of Physiology: Neurophysiology III. Vol. 17. Baltimore, University Park Press, 1978, p. 49.

Moore, R. Y., and Bloom, F. E.: Central catecholamine neuron systems: Anatomy and physiology of the dopamine systems. *Annu. Rev. Neurosci., 1*:129, 1978.

Nicoll, R. A., *et al.*: Substance P as a transmitter candidate. *Ann. Rev. Neurosci., 3*:227, 1980.

Oja, S. S., *et al.*: Amino Acids as Inhibitory Neurotransmitters. New York, Fischer, 1977.

Otsuka, M., and Hall, Z. W. (eds.): Neurobiology of Chemical Transmission. New York, John Wiley & Sons, 1978.

Passonneau, J. V., *et al.*: Cerebral Metabolism and Neural Function. Baltimore, Williams & Wilkins, 1980.

Pepeu, G., *et al.* (eds.): Receptors for Neurotransmitters and Peptide Hormones. New York, Raven Press, 1980.

Redman, S. J.: A quantitative approach to integrative function of dendrites. *Int. Rev. Physiol., 10*:1, 1976.

Rose, F. C. (ed.): Physiological Aspects of Clinical Neurology. Oxford, Blackwell Scientific Publications, 1977.

Schulster, D., and Levitzki, A. (eds.): Cellular Receptors for Hormones and Neurotransmitters. New York, John Wiley & Sons, 1980.

Simon, P. (ed.): Neurotransmitters. New York, Pergamon Press, 1979.

Snyder, S. H., and Bennett, J. P., Jr.: Neurotransmitter receptors in the brain: Biochemical identification. *Annu. Rev. Physiol., 38*:153, 1976.

Spencer, W. A.: The physiology of supraspinal neurons in mammals. *In* Brookhart, J. M., and Mountcastle, V. B. (eds.): Handbook of Physiology. Sec. 1, Vol. 1. Baltimore, Williams & Wilkins, 1977, p. 969.

Stephenson, W. K.: Concepts of Neurophysiology. New York, John Wiley & Sons, 1980.

Stevens, C. F.: The neuron. *Sci. Am. 241*(3):54, 1979.

Tipton, K. F. (ed.): Neurochemistry and Biochemical Pharmacology. Baltimore, University Park Press, 1978.

Vernadakis, A., *et al.* (eds.): Maturation of Neurotransmission: Biochemical Aspects. New York, S. Karger, 1977.

7

Neuronal Mechanisms and
Circuits for Processing
Information

The primary role of the nervous system is to control a major share of the body's functions. To do this, it gains information from the body's surroundings and from within the body itself and then transmits this information, stores it, changes it, and uses it in any other way that can be advantageous for bodily control. The entire section of this book on the nervous system addresses these many functions of the nervous system.

Throughout the nervous system, certain special neuronal mechanisms and neuronal circuits are used again and again. The purpose of this chapter is to characterize some of these and to preview some of their important uses.

INFORMATION, SIGNALS, AND IMPULSES

The term *information,* as it applies to the nervous system, means a variety of different things, such as knowledge, facts, quantitative values, intensity of pain, intensity of light, temperature, and any other aspect of the body or its immediate surroundings that has meaning. Thus, pain from a pin prick is information, pressure on the bottom of the feet is information, degree of angulation of the joints is information, and a stored memory in the brain is information.

However, information cannot be transmitted in its original form but only in the form of nerve impulses. Thus, a part of the body that is subjected to pain must first convert this information into *nerve impulses;* specific areas of the brain convert abstract thoughts also into nerve impulses that are then transmitted either elsewhere in the brain or into peripheral nerves to motor effectors throughout the body. The retina of the eye converts vision into nerve impulses, the nerve endings of the joints convert degree of angulation of the joints into nerve impulses, and so forth.

Signals. In the transmission of information, it is frequently not desirable to speak in terms of the individual impulses but instead of the overall pattern of impulses; this pattern is called a *signal.* As an example, when pressure is applied to a large area of skin, impulses are transmitted by large numbers of parallel nerve fibers, and the total pattern of impulses transmitted by all these fibers is called a signal. Thus, we can speak of visual signals, auditory signals, somesthetic sensory signals, motor signals, and so forth.

TRANSMISSION OF SIGNALS IN NERVE TRACTS

SIGNAL STRENGTH

Obviously, one of the characteristics of information that must be conveyed is the quantitative intensity of the information, for instance the intensity of pain. The different gradations of intensity can be transmitted either by utilizing increasing numbers of parallel fibers or by sending more impulses along a single fiber. These two mechanisms are called, respectively, spatial summation and temporal summation.

Spatial Summation (Multiple Fiber Summation). Figure 7–1 illustrates the phenomenon of spatial summation, whereby increasing signal strength is transmitted by using progressively greater numbers of fibers. This figure shows a section of skin innervated by a large number of parallel pain nerve fibers. Each of these arborizes into hundreds of minute *free nerve endings* that serve as pain receptors. The entire cluster of fibers from one pain fiber frequently covers an area of skin as large as 5 cm. in diameter, and this area is called the *receptive field*. The number of endings is large in the center of the field but becomes less and less toward the periphery. One can also see from the figure that the arborizing nerve fibrils overlap those from other pain fibers. Therefore, a pin prick of the skin usually stimulates endings from many different pain fibers simultaneously. But, if the pin prick is in the center of the receptive field of a particular pain fiber, the degree of stimulation is far greater than if it is in the periphery of the field. Thus, a mild pin prick might stimulate only the pain fiber receiving the signal from the center of its receptive field, but a strong pin prick would stimulate all the pain fibers whose receptive fields overlap at that point.

Thus, in the lower part of Figure 7–1 is shown three separate views of the cross-section of the nerve bundle leading from the skin area. To the left is shown the effect of a weak stimulus, with only a single nerve fiber in the middle of the bundle stimulated very strongly (represented by the solid fiber) while several adjacent fibers are stimulated weakly (half-solid fibers). The other two views of the nerve cross-section show the effect respectively of a moderate stimulus and a strong stimulus, with progressively more fibers being stimulated. Thus, the signal spreads to more and more fibers. This phenomenon is called *spatial summation,* which means simply that one of the means by which signals of increasing strength are transmitted in the nervous system is by utilizing progressively greater numbers of fibers. The increase in number of fibers as the strength of signal increases is called *recruitment* of the additional fibers.

Temporal Summation. A second means by which signals of increasing strength are transmitted is by increasing the *frequency* of nerve impulses in each fiber, which is called *temporal summation*. Figure 7–2 illustrates this type of summation, showing in the upper part a changing strength of signal and in the lower part the actual impulses transmitted by the nerve fiber.

Figure 7–2. Translation of signal strength into a frequency-modulated series of nerve impulses, showing *above* the strength of signal and *below* the separate nerve impulses.

SPATIAL ORIENTATION OF SIGNALS IN FIBER TRACTS

How does the brain detect the area on the body that is receiving a sensory stimulus, and how does the brain transmit impulses to individual skeletal muscles? It does this by transmitting their signals in spatial patterns through the nerve tracts. All the different nerve tracts, both in the peripheral nerves and in the fiber tracts of the central nervous system, are spatially organized. For instance, in the dorsal columns of the spinal cord the sensory fibers from the feet lie toward the midline, while those fibers entering the dorsal columns at higher levels of the body lie progressively more toward the lateral sides of the dorsal columns. This spatial organization is maintained with precision in this sensory pathway all the way to the somesthetic cortex. Likewise, the fiber tracts within the brain and those extending into motor nerves are spatially oriented in the same way.

As an example, Figure 7–3 illustrates, on the left, three separate pins stimulating the skin; on the

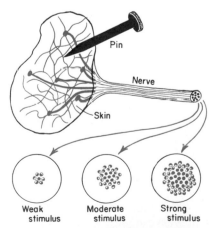

Figure 7–1. Pattern of stimulation of pain fibers in a nerve trunk leading from an area of skin pricked by a pin.

Figure 7–3. Spatial pattern of nerve fiber stimulation in a nerve trunk following stimulation of the skin by three separate but simultaneous pinpricks.

right, the spatial orientation of the stimulated fibers in the nerve is shown. Each pin in this example stimulates a single fiber strongly and adjacent fibers less strongly.

TRANSMISSION AND PROCESSING OF SIGNALS IN NEURONAL POOLS

The central nervous system is made up of literally hundreds or even thousands of separate neuronal pools, some of which contain very few neurons, while others hold vast numbers. For instance, the entire cerebral cortex could be considered to be a single large neuronal pool. If all the surface area of the cerebral cortex were flattened out, including the surfaces of the penetrating folds, the total area of this large flat pool would be several square feet. It has many separate fiber tracts coming to it (afferent fibers) and others leaving it (efferent fibers). Furthermore it maintains the same quality of spatial orientation as that found in the nerve bundles, individual points of the cortex connecting with specific points elsewhere in the nervous system or connecting through the peripheral nerves with specific points in the body. However, within this pool of neurons are large numbers of short nerve fibers whereby signals spread horizontally from neuron to neuron within the pool itself.

Other neuronal pools include the different basal ganglia and the specific nuclei in the thalamus, cerebellum, mesencephalon, pons, and medulla. Also, the entire dorsal gray matter of the spinal cord could be considered to be one long pool of neurons, and the entire anterior gray matter another long neuronal pool. Each pool has its own special characteristics of organization which cause it to process signals in its own special way. It is these special characteristics of the different pools that allow the multitude of functions of the nervous system. Yet, despite their differences in function, the pools also have many similarities which are described in the following pages.

RELAYING OF SIGNALS THROUGH NEURONAL POOLS

Organization of Neurons for Relaying Signals. Figure 7–4 is a schematic diagram of several neurons in a neuronal pool, showing "input" fibers to the left and "output" fibers to the right. Each input fiber divides hundreds to thousands of times, providing an average of a thousand or more terminal fibrils that spread over a large area in the pool to synapse with the dendrites or cell bodies of the neurons in the pool. The dendrites of some of

Figure 7–4. Basic organization of a neuronal pool.

the neurons also arborize and spread in the pool. The neuronal area stimulated by each incoming nerve fiber is called its *stimulatory field*. Note that each input fiber arborizes so that large numbers of its synaptic knobs lie on the centermost neurons in its "field," but progressively fewer knobs lie on the neurons farther from the center of the field.

Threshold and Subthreshold Stimuli — Facilitation. In the discussion of synaptic function in the previous chapter, it will be recalled that stimulation of a single excitatory synaptic knob almost never stimulates the postsynaptic neuron. Instead, large numbers of knobs must discharge on the same neuron either simultaneously or in rapid succession to cause excitation. For instance, let us assume that 6 separate knobs must discharge simultaneously or in rapid succession to excite any one of the neurons in Figure 7–4. Note that input fiber 1 contributes a total of 10 synaptic knobs to neuron *a*. Therefore, an incoming impulse in fiber 1 will cause neuron *a* to discharge. This same incoming fiber has two knobs on neuron *b* and three on neuron *c*. Neither of these two neurons will fire.

Incoming nerve fiber 2 has 12 synaptic knobs on neuron *d*, three on neuron *c*, and two on neuron *b*. In this case, an impulse in fiber 2 excites only neuron *d*.

Though fiber 1 fails to stimulate neurons *b* and *c*, discharge of the synaptic knobs changes the membrane potentials of these neurons so that they can be more easily excited by other incoming signals. Thus, a stimulus to a neuron can be either (1) an *excitatory stimulus*, also called a *threshold stimulus* because it is above the threshold required for excitation, or (2) a *subthreshold stimulus*. A subthreshold stimulus fails to excite the neuron but does make the neuron more excitable to impulses from other sources. The neuron that is made more excitable but does not discharge is said to be *facilitated*.

"Convergence" of Subthreshold Stimuli to Cause Excitation.   Let us now assume that both fibers 1 and 2 in Figure 7–4 transmit concurrent impulses into the neuronal pool. In this case, neuron *c* is stimulated by six synaptic knobs simultaneously, which is the required number to cause excitation. Thus, subthreshold stimuli can *converge* from several sources and *summate* at a neuron to cause an excitatory stimulus.

Summation of Facilitation.   Now, let us consider neuron *b* of Figure 7–4 when both input nerve fibers are stimulated. In this case each fiber excites two synaptic knobs on neuron *b*, but the total of four excited knobs still is not up to the threshold value required to excite the neuron. However, the degree of facilitation does become greatly increased so that now only two additional knobs excited from another source need fire to cause discharge.

The "Field" of Terminals.   It must be recognized that Figure 7–4 represents a highly condensed version of the neuronal pool, for each input nerve fiber gives off terminals that spread to as many as 100 or more separate neurons, and the surface of each neuron is covered by many hundred or many thousand synapses. In the centralmost portion of this *field* of terminals, almost all the neurons are stimulated by the incoming fiber; while farther toward the periphery of the field, the neurons are facilitated but do not discharge. Figure 7–5 illustrates this effect, showing the field of a single input nerve fiber. The area in the neuronal pool in which all the neurons discharge is called the *discharge* or *excited* or *liminal zone,* and the area to either side in which the neurons are facilitated but do not discharge is called the *facilitated* or *subthreshold* or *subliminal* zone.

Facilitation of the Neuronal Pool by Signals from Accessory Sources.   A neuronal pool frequently receives input nerve fibers from many different sources. Thus, in Figure 7–6 a neuron in a given pool receives impulses from a *primary source* and

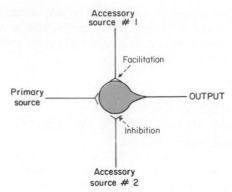

Figure 7–6.   Basic neuronal circuit for facilitation or inhibition.

from two *accessory sources*. The nerve fiber from accessory source #1 is an excitatory fiber that stimulates excitatory synapses. If enough synapses from this source are stimulated, the postsynaptic neuron discharges. However, in many parts of the nervous system the accessory sources supply only a few nerve fibers to the pool, not enough usually to cause excitation but yet enough to *facilitate* the neurons. Thus, in Figure 7–6, if a facilitatory signal is entering the pool from accessory source #1, a much weaker than usual signal from the primary source is then able to excite the postsynaptic neuron. In this way the signal from accessory source #1 controls the ease with which signals pass from the primary source to the output, which explains one of the means by which different parts of the nervous system control the degree of activity of other parts.

Inhibition of a Neuronal Pool by Signals from an Accessory Source.   It will be recalled from the previous chapter that many synapses in the central nervous system are inhibitory instead of excitatory. Thus, in Figure 7–6, stimulation of the inhibitory fibers from accessory source #2 strongly inhibits the neuronal pool so that a much stronger than usual signal from the primary source is now required to cause even normal output.

Mechanism By Which a Single Input Signal Can Cause Both Excitation and Inhibition — The Inhibitory Circuit.   Figure 7–7 illustrates the so-called inhibitory circuit which can change an excitatory signal into an inhibitory signal. In this figure the

Figure 7–5.   "Discharge" and "facilitated" zones of a neuronal pool.

Figure 7–7.   Inhibitory circuit. Neuron 2 is an inhibitory neuron.

input fiber divides and provides excitatory synapses at both its endings. This causes excitation of both neurons 1 and 2. However, the synapse between neurons 2 and 3 is inhibitory. Excitation of this neuron therefore inhibits neuron 3.

In short, the usual means to cause inhibition is for a signal *to be transmitted through a neuron that terminates at an inhibitory synapse*.

Convergence. The term *convergence* means control of a single neuron by converging signals from two or more separate input nerve fibers. One type of convergence was illustrated in Figure 7–4, in which two excitatory input nerve fibers from the same source converged upon several separate neurons to stimulate them. This type of convergence from a single source is illustrated again in Figure 7–8A.

However, convergence can also result from input signals (excitatory or inhibitory) from several different sources, which is illustrated in Figure 7–8B. For instance, the interneurons of the spinal cord receive converging signals from (a) peripheral nerve fibers entering the cord, (b) propriospinal fibers passing from one segment of the cord to another, (c) corticospinal fibers from the cerebral cortex, and (d) several other long pathways descending from the brain into the spinal cord. Then the signals from the interneurons converge on the motoneurons to control muscle function.

Such convergence allows summation of information from different sources, and the resulting response is a summated effect of all the different types of information. Obviously, therefore, convergence is one of the important means by which the central nervous system correlates, summates, and sorts different types of information.

Divergence. Divergence means that excitation of a single input nerve fiber stimulates multiple output fibers from the neuronal pool. The two major types of divergence are illustrated in Figure 7–9 and may be described as follows:

An *amplifying* type of divergence often occurs, illustrated in Figure 7–9A. This means simply

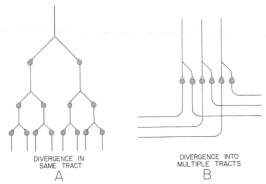

Figure 7–9. "Divergence" in neuronal pathways. A, Divergence within a pathway to cause "amplification" of the signal. B, Divergence into multiple tracts to transmit the signal to separate areas.

that an input signal spreads to an increasing number of neurons as it passes through successive pools of a nervous pathway. This type of divergence is characteristic of the corticospinal pathway in its control of skeletal muscles as follows: Stimulation of a single large pyramidal cell in the motor cortex transmits a single impulse into the spinal cord. Yet, under appropriate conditions of very strong cord facilitation, this impulse can stimulate perhaps several hundred interneurons and anterior motoneurons. Each of the motoneurons then stimulates as many as 100 to 1000 muscle fibers. Thus, there is a total divergence, or amplification, of as much as 10,000-fold.

The second type of divergence, illustrated in Figure 7–9B, is *divergence into multiple tracts*. In this case, the signal is transmitted in two separate directions from the pool, to different parts of the nervous system where it is needed. For instance, information transmitted in the dorsal columns of the spinal cord takes two courses in the lower part of the brain, (1) into the cerebellum and (2) on through the lower regions of the brain to the thalamus and cerebral cortex. Likewise, in the thalamus almost all sensory information is relayed both into deep structures of the thalamus and to discrete regions of the cerebral cortex.

TRANSMISSION OF SPATIAL PATTERNS THROUGH SUCCESSIVE NEURONAL POOLS

Most information is transmitted from one part of the nervous system to another through several successive neuronal pools. For instance, sensory information from the skin passes first through the peripheral nerve fibers, then through second order neurons that originate either in the spinal cord or in the cuneate and gracile nuclei of the medulla, and finally through third order neurons originating in the thalamus to the cerebral cortex. Such a

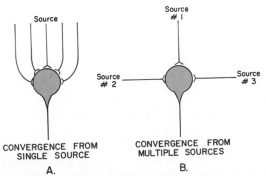

Figure 7–8. "Convergence" of multiple input fibers on a single neuron. A, Input fibers from a single source. B, Input fibers from multiple sources.

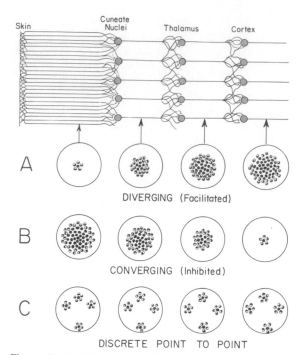

Figure 7–10. *Above,* Typical organization of a sensory pathway from the skin to the cerebral cortex. *Below,* The patterns of fiber stimulation at different points in the pathway following stimulation by a pinprick when the pathway is (A) facilitated, (B) inhibited, and (C) normally excitable.

Yet, it is true that a signal passing through *highly facilitated neuronal pools* could diverge so much that the spatial pattern at the terminus of the pathway would be completely obscured. This effect is illustrated in Figure 7–10A, which shows successively expanding spatial patterns of neuron stimulation in such a facilitated, diverging pathway.

However, the degree of facilitation of the different neuronal pools varies from time to time. Under some conditions the degree of facilitation is so low that the pathway becomes converging, as illustrated in Figure 7–10B. In this case, a broad area of the skin is stimulated, but the signal loses part of its fringe stimuli as it passes through each successive pool until the breadth of the stimulus becomes contracted at the opposite end. One can achieve this type of stimulation by pressing ever so lightly with a flat object on the skin. The signal converges to give the person a sensation of almost a point contact.

In Figure 7–10C, four separate points are simultaneously stimulated on the skin, and the degree of excitability in each neuronal pool is exactly that amount required to prevent either divergence or convergence. Therefore, a reasonably true spatial pattern of each of the four points of stimulation is transmitted through the entire pathway.

Centrifugal Control of Neuronal Facilitation in the Sensory Pathways. It is obvious from the above discussion that the degree of facilitation of each neuronal pool must be maintained at exactly the proper level if faithful transmission of the spatial pattern is to occur. Recent discoveries have demonstrated that the degrees of inhibition or facilitation of most — indeed, probably all — neuronal pools in the different sensory pathways are controlled by *centrifugal nerve fibers* that pass from the respective sensory areas of the cortex downward to the separate sensory relay neuronal pools. Thus, these nerve fibers undoubtedly help to control the faithfulness of signal transmission.

Lateral Inhibition to Provide Contrast in the Spatial Pattern. When a single point of the skin or other sensory area is stimulated, not only is a single fiber excited but a number of "fringe" fibers are excited less strongly at the same time, as already explained above. Therefore, the spatial pattern is blurred even before the signal begins to be transmitted through the pathway. However, in many pathways — if not all — such as in the visual pathway and in the somesthetic pathway, lateral *inhibitory circuits* inhibit the fringe neurons and re-establish a truer spatial pattern.

Figure 7–11A illustrates one of the postulated types of lateral inhibitory circuits, showing that the nerve fibers of a pathway give off collateral fibers that excite inhibitory neurons. These inhib-

pathway is illustrated at the top of Figure 7–10. Note that the sensory nerve endings in the skin overlap each other tremendously; and the terminal fibrils of each nerve fiber, on entering each neuronal pool, spread to many adjacent neurons, innervating perhaps 100 or more separate neurons. On first thought, one would expect signals from the skin to become completely mixed up by this haphazard arrangement of terminal fibrils in each neuronal pool. For statistical reasons, however, this does not occur, which can be explained as follows:

First, if a single point is stimulated in the skin, the nerve fiber with the most nerve endings in that particular spot becomes stimulated to the strongest extent, while the immediately adjacent nerve fibers become stimulated less strongly, and the nerve fibers still farther away become stimulated only weakly. When this signal arrives at the first neuronal pool, the stimulus spreads in many directions in the terminal fibrils of the neuronal pool. Yet the *greatest number* of *excited presynaptic terminals* lies very near the point of entry of the most excited input nerve fiber. Therefore, the neuron closest to this central point is the one that becomes stimulated to the greatest extent. Exactly the same effect occurs in the second neuronal pool in the thalamus and again when the signal reaches the cerebral cortex.

Figure 7–11. A, One type of lateral inhibitory circuit by which an excited fiber of a neuronal pool can cause inhibition of adjacent fibers. B, Increase in contrast of the stimulus pattern caused by the inhibitory circuit.

itory neurons in turn inhibit the less excited fringe neurons in the signal pathway. The effect of this on transmission of the spatial pattern is illustrated in Figure 7–11B, which shows the same point-to-point transmission pattern that was illustrated in Figure 7–10C. The left-hand pattern illustrates four strongly excited fibers (the solid fibers) with penumbras of fringe excitation surrounding each of these. In the illustration to the right, the penumbras have been removed by the lateral inhibitory circuits; obviously, this increases the contrast in the signal and helps in the faithfulness of transmission of the spatial pattern. Unfortunately, we still know too little about the mechanism or mechanisms of this lateral inhibition, but the more we learn the more it becomes clear that this is one of the most useful of all the neuronal circuits of the nervous system to differentiate and analyze sensory signals. We shall discuss this much more fully in the following chapters.

PROLONGATION OF A SIGNAL BY A NEURONAL POOL— "AFTER-DISCHARGE"

Thus far, we have considered signals that are merely relayed through neuronal pools. However, in many instances, a signal entering a pool causes a prolonged output discharge, called *after-discharge,* even after the incoming signal is over and lasting from a few milliseconds to as long as many minutes. The three basic mechanisms by which after-discharge occurs are the following:

Synaptic After-Discharge. When excitatory synapses discharge on the surfaces of dendrites or the soma of a neuron, a postsynaptic potential develops in the neuron and lasts for many milliseconds — in the anterior motoneuron for about 15 milliseconds, though perhaps much longer in other neurons — especially so when some of the long-acting synaptic transmitter substances are in-

volved. As long as this potential lasts it can continue to excite the neuron, causing it to transmit a continuous train of output impulses, as was explained in the previous chapter. Thus, as a result of this synaptic after-discharge mechanism alone, it is possible for a single instantaneous input to cause a sustained signal output (a series of repetitive discharges) lasting as long as 15 or more milliseconds.

The Parallel Circuit Type of After-Discharge. Figure 7–12 illustrates a second type of neuronal circuit that can cause short periods of after-discharge. In this case, the input signal spreads through a series of neurons in the neuronal pool, and from many of these neurons impulses keep converging on an output neuron. It will be recalled that a signal is delayed at each synapse for about 0.5 millisecond, which is called the *synaptic delay.* Therefore, signals that pass through a succession of intermediate neurons reach the output neuron one by one after varying periods of delay. Therefore, the output neuron continues to be stimulated for many milliseconds.

It is doubtful that more than a few dozen successive neurons ordinarily enter into a parallel after-discharge circuit. Therefore, one would suspect that this type of after-discharge circuit could cause after-discharges that last for no more than perhaps 25 to 50 milliseconds. Yet, this circuit does represent a means by which a single input signal, lasting less than 1 millisecond, can be converted into a sustained output signal lasting many milliseconds.

The Reverberatory (Oscillatory) Circuit as a Cause of After-Discharge. Many neurophysiologists believe that one of the most important of all circuits in the entire nervous system is the *reverberatory,* or *oscillatory, circuit.* Such circuits are caused by positive feedback within the neuronal pool. That is, the output of a neuronal circuit feeds back to re-excite the same circuit. Consequently, once stimulated, the circuit discharges repetitively for a long time.

Several different postulated varieties of reverberatory circuits are illustrated in Figure 7–13, the simplest — in Figure 7–13A — involving only a single neuron. In this case, the output

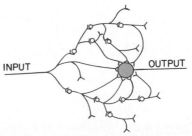

Figure 7–12. The parallel after-discharge circuit.

neuron simply sends a collateral nerve fiber back to its own dendrites or soma to restimulate itself; therefore, once the neuron should discharge, the feedback stimuli could theoretically keep the neuron discharging for a long time thereafter.

Figure 7–13B illustrates a few additional neurons in the feedback circuit, which would give a longer period of time between the initial discharge and the feedback signal. Figure 7–13C illustrates a still more complex system in which both facilitatory and inhibitory fibers impinge on the reverberating pool. A facilitatory signal increases the ease with which reverberation takes place, while an inhibitory signal decreases the ease of reverberation.

Figure 7–13D illustrates that most reverberating pathways are constituted of many parallel fibers, and at each cell station the terminal fibrils diffuse widely. In such a system the total reverberating signal can be either weak or strong, depending on how many parallel nerve fibers are momentarily involved in the reverberation.

Finally, reverberation need not occur only in a single neuronal pool, for it can occur through a circuit involving two or more successive pools in the positive feedback pathway.

Characteristics of After-Discharge from a Rever-

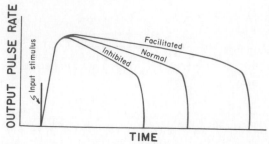

Figure 7–14. Typical pattern of the output signal from a reverberatory circuit following a single input stimulus, showing the effects of facilitation and inhibition.

beratory Circuit. Figure 7–14 illustrates postulated output signals from a reverberatory after-discharge circuit. The input stimulus need last only 1 millisecond or so, and yet the output can last for many milliseconds or even minutes. The figure demonstrates that the intensity of the output signal increases to a reasonably high value early in the reverberation, then decreases to a critical point, and suddenly ceases entirely. Furthermore, the duration of the after-discharge is determined by the degree of inhibition or facilitation of the neuronal pool. In this way, signals from other parts of the brain can control the reaction of the pool to the input stimulus.

Almost these exact patterns of output signals can be recorded from the motor nerves exciting a muscle involved in the flexor reflex (discussed in Chapter 11), which is believed to be caused by a reverberating type of after-discharge following stimulation of pain fibers.

Importance of Synaptic Fatigue in Determining the Duration of Reverberation. It was pointed out in the previous chapter that synapses fatigue if stimulated for prolonged periods of time. Therefore, one of the most important factors that determines the duration of the reverberatory type of after-discharge is probably the rapidity with which the involved synapses fatigue. Rapid fatigue would obviously tend to shorten the period of after-discharge.

Furthermore, the greater the number of neurons in the reverberatory pathway and the greater the number of collateral feedback fibrils, the easier would it be to keep the reverberation going. Therefore, it is to be expected that longer reverberating pathways would in general sustain after-discharges for longer periods of time.

Duration of Reverberation. Even though neurophysiologists are not certain which functions of the nervous system can rightfully be ascribed to reverberatory circuits, some of those that have been postulated have reverberatory durations as short as 10 milliseconds or as long as several minutes, or perhaps even hours. Some examples

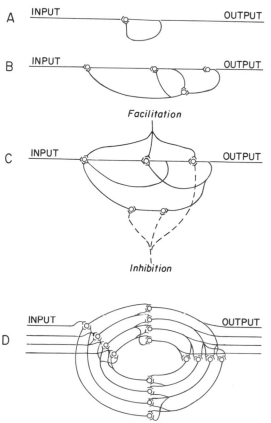

Figure 7–13. Reverberatory circuits of increasing complexity.

include: (1) In an animal whose spinal cord is transected in the neck, a sudden painful stimulus to the animal's paw will cause the flexor muscles to contract and remain contracted a fraction of a second to more than a second after the stimulus ends. It is believed that this is caused by an after-discharge of the reverberatory type. (2) During respiration the inspiratory neuronal pool in the medulla becomes excited for about 2 seconds during each respiratory cycle. One theory suggests that this is caused by reverberation within the inspiratory neuronal pool. And (3) a theory of wakefulness is that continual reverberation occurs somewhere within the brain stem to keep a wakefulness area excited during the waking hours. If this be true, then this would represent a 14 to 18 hour period of reverberation.

CONTINUOUS SIGNAL OUTPUT FROM NEURONAL POOLS

Some neuronal pools emit output signals continuously even without excitatory input signals. At least two different mechanisms theoretically can cause this effect: (1) intrinsic neuronal discharge and (2) reverberatory signals.

Continuous Discharge Caused by Intrinsic Neuronal Excitability. Neurons, like other excitable tissues, discharge repetitively if their membrane potentials rise above certain threshold levels. The membrane potentials of many neurons even normally are high enough to cause them to emit impulses continually. This occurs especially in large numbers of the neurons of the cerebellum as well as in most of the interneurons of the spinal cord. The rates at which these cells emit impulses can be increased by facilitatory signals or decreased by inhibitory signals; the latter can sometimes decrease the rate to extinction.

Continuous Signals Emitted from Reverberating Circuits. Obviously, a reverberating circuit that never fatigues to extinction could also be a source of continual impulses. Facilitatory impulses entering the reverberating pool, as illustrated in Figure 7–13C, could increase the output signal, and inhibition could decrease or even extinguish the output signal.

Figure 7–15 illustrates a continual output signal from a pool of neurons, whether it be a pool emitting impulses because of intrinsic neuronal excitability or as a result of reverberation. Note that an excitatory (or facilitatory) input signal greatly increases the output signal, whereas an inhibitory input signal greatly decreases the output. Those students who are familiar with radio transmitters will recognize this to be a *carrier wave* type of information transmission. That is,

Figure 7–15. Continuous output either from a reverberating circuit or from a pool of intrinsically discharging neurons. This figure also shows the effect of excitatory or inhibitory input signals.

the excitatory and inhibitory control signals are not the *cause* of the output signal, but they do *control* it. Note that this carrier wave system allows decrease in signal intensity as well as increase, whereas, up to this point, the types of information transmission that we have discussed have been only positive information rather than negative information. This type of information transmission is used by the autonomic nervous system to control such functions as vascular tone, gut tone, degree of constriction of the iris, heart rate, and others.

RHYTHMIC SIGNAL OUTPUT

Many neuronal circuits emit rhythmic output signals — for instance, the rhythmic respiratory signal originating in the reticular substance of the medulla and pons. This repetitive rhythmic signal continues throughout life, while other rhythmic signals, such as those that cause scratching movements by the hind leg of a dog or the walking movements in an animal, require input stimuli into the respective circuits to initiate the signals.

Many rhythmic signals are postulated to result from reverberating pathways. One can readily understand that each time a signal passes around a reverberatory loop, collateral impulses could be transmitted into the output pathway. Thus, the rhythmic respiratory signals could result from such a reverberatory mechanism.

Obviously, facilitatory or inhibitory signals can affect rhythmic signal output in the same way that they can affect continual signal outputs. Figure 7–16, for instance, illustrates the rhythmic respiratory signal in the phrenic nerve. However, when the carotid body is stimulated by arterial oxygen deficiency, the frequency and amplitude of the rhythmic signal pattern increase progressively.

Figure 7–16. The rhythmical output from the respiratory center, showing that progressively increasing stimulation of the carotid body increases both the intensity and frequency of oscillation.

INSTABILITY AND STABILITY OF NEURONAL CIRCUITS

Almost every part of the brain connects either directly or indirectly with every other part, and this creates a serious problem. If the first part excites the second, the second the third, the third the fourth, and so on until finally the signal re-excites the first part, it is clear that an excitatory signal entering any part of the brain would set off a continuous cycle of re-excitation of all parts. If this should occur, the brain would be inundated by a mass of uncontrolled reverberating signals —signals that would be transmitting no information but, nevertheless, would be consuming the circuits of the brain so that none of the informational signals could be transmitted. Such an effect actually occurs in widespread areas of the brain during *epileptic fits*.

How does the central nervous system prevent this from happening all the time? The answer seems to lie in two basic mechanisms that function throughout the central nervous system: (1) inhibitory circuits, and (2) fatigue of synapses.

INHIBITORY CIRCUITS AS A MECHANISM FOR STABILIZING NERVOUS SYSTEM FUNCTION

The phenomenon of lateral inhibition that was discussed earlier in the chapter prevents signals in an informational pathway from spreading diffusely everywhere. In addition, two other types of inhibitory circuits in widespread areas of the brain help to prevent excessive spread of unwanted signals: (a) inhibitory feedback circuits that return from the termini of pathways back to the initial excitatory neurons of the same pathways — these inhib-

it the input neurons when the termini become overly excited, and (b) some neuronal pools that exert gross inhibitory control over widespread areas of the brain — for instance, many of the basal ganglia exert inhibitory influences throughout the motor control system.

SYNAPTIC FATIGUE AS A MEANS FOR STABILIZING THE NERVOUS SYSTEM (DECREMENTAL CONDUCTION)

Synaptic fatigue means simply that the signal becomes progressively weaker the more prolonged the period of excitation. This phenomenon is also frequently called *decremental conduction* because the output signal from a strongly excited pathway *decrements* with time.

Figure 7–17 illustrates typical synaptic fatigue, showing a muscle response during the flexor reflex. That is, stimulation of the pain sensory endings in a limb causes reflex contraction of the flexor muscles of the limb, leading to withdrawal of the limb from the painful stimulus. However, if this stimulus is repeated at close intervals, as was done in Figure 7–17, the response progressively decreases. But how does this fatigue, as illustrated by the decreasing response of the flexor reflex, play a role in stabilizing nervous system function? To answer this, let us assume that a large series of interconnecting neurons in a single pool becomes excessively excitable. As soon as this occurs, positive feedback and reverberation will begin. But so also will fatigue begin, and after a period of time the level of excitability of the entire neuronal pool will automatically return below the threshold level for continued reverberation.

Neuronal Circuits That Exhibit Fatigue; Those That Do Not. Fortunately, some synaptic pathways exhibit very little fatigue, while others exhibit extreme degrees. One type of pathway that exhibits almost no fatigue is the fast-conducting sensory pathways from the peripheral parts of the

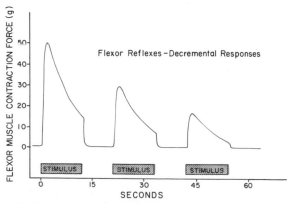

Figure 7–17. Successive flexor reflexes illustrating fatigue of conduction through the reflex pathway.

body to the brain, such as the pathways through the dorsal columns to the thalamus and thence to the somesthetic cortex. This seems to be of purposeful benefit to nervous function because it allows faithful transmission of sensory information into the brain.

On the other hand, the interconnecting links through the short interneurons between the sensory system and the motor system frequently exhibit extreme degrees of fatigue. This was illustrated in Figure 7–17 for the flexor reflex pathway, because it is the interneurons between the sensory input and the motor output of the spinal cord that fatigue. At least in certain parts of the nervous system, this fatigue has been shown to result from exhaustion of transmitter substance in the synaptic knobs.

Recovery From Fatigue.   After a major degree of fatigue has occurred in the conduction of a synapse, the conduction recovers if an adequate period of rest between stimuli is allowed. Thus, when a pathway is not used often, it becomes progressively more excitable until full conduction returns.

Automatic Adjustment of Sensitivity of Pathways by the Fatigue Mechanism.   It is clear by now that if the excitability of a pathway in the nervous system is too great, then too many impulses will be transmitted and the fatigue mechanism will automatically adjust the sensitivity of the pathway to a lower level. Conversely, if the sensitivity is too low, then too few impulses will be transmitted, and the sensitivity of the system will automatically adjust to a higher level. Therefore, this fatigue mechanism, and its recovery during rest, is probably an extremely important mechanism for maintaining a proper balance among the conductivities of the respective pathways throughout the brain.

REFERENCES

An der Heiden, U.: Analysis of Neural Networks. New York, Springer-Verlag, 1980.

Andreassen, S.: Interval Pattern of Single Motor Units. Aalborg, Denmark, Institute of Electronic Systems, Aalborg University Centre, 1978.

Anderson, H., *et al.*: Developmental neurobiology of invertebrates. *Annu. Rev. Neurosci., 3*:97, 1980.

Asanuma, H., and Wilson V. J. (eds.): Integration in the Nervous System. New York, Igaku-Shoin, 1979.

Bennett, M. V. L. (ed.): Synaptic Transmission and Neuronal Interaction. New York, Raven Press, 1975.

Björklund, A., and Stenevi, U.: Regeneration of monoaminergic and cholinergic neurons in the mammalian central nervous system. *Physiol. Rev., 59*:62, 1979.

Blumenthal, R., *et al.* (eds.): Dynamic Patterns of Brain Cell Assemblies. Neurosciences Research Program Bulletin. Vol. 12, No. 1. Cambridge, Mass., Massachusetts Institute of Technology, 1974.

Cowan, W. M.: The development of the brain. *Sci. Am. 241*(3):112, 1979.

Freides, D.: Human information processing and sensory modality: Cross-modal functions, information complexity, memory, and deficit. *Psychol. Bull., 81*:284, 1974.

Friesen, W. O., and Stent, G. S.: Neural circuits for generating rhythmic movements. *Annu. Rev. Biophys. Bioeng., 7*:37, 1978.

Grinnell, A. D.: Specificity of neurons and their interconnections. *In* Brookhart, J. M., and Mountcastle, V. B. (eds.): Handbook of Physiology. Sec. 1, Vol. 1. Baltimore, Williams & Wilkins, 1977, p. 803.

Kandel, E. R.: Small systems of neurons. *Sci. Am. 241*(3):66, 1979.

Karlin, A., *et al.* (eds.): Neuronal Information Transfer. New York, Academic Press, 1978.

Kater, S. B., *et al.*: Identifiable neurons and invertebrate behavior. *In* MTP International Review of Science: Physiology. Vol. 3. Baltimore, University Park Press, 1974, p. 1.

Kennedy, D., and Davis, W. J.: Organization of invertebrate motor systems. *In* Brookhart, J. M., and Mountcastle, V. B. (eds.): Handbook of Physiology. Sec. 1, Vol. 1. Baltimore, Williams & Wilkins, 1977, p. 1023.

Levi-Montalcini, R., and Calissano, P.: The nerve-growth factor. *Sci. Am. 240*(6):68, 1979.

Macagno, E. R., *et al.*: Three-dimensional computer reconstruction of neurons and neuronal assemblies. *Ann. Rev. Biophys. Bioeng. 8*:323, 1979.

Martin, A. R.: Synaptic transmission. *In* MTP International Review of Science: Physiology. Vol. 3. Baltimore, University Park Press, 1974, p. 53.

Nicholls, J. C., and Van Essen, D.: The nervous system of the leech. *Sci. Am., 230*:38, 1974.

Patterson, P. H., *et al.*: The chemical differentiation of nerve cells. *Sci. Am., 239*(1):50, 1978.

Pinsker, H. M., and Willis, W. D., Jr. (eds.): Information Processing in the Nervous System. New York, Raven Press, 1980.

Purves, D., and Lichtman, J. W.: Formation and maintenance of synaptic connections in autonomic ganglia. *Physiol. Rev., 58*:821, 1978.

Rovainen, C. M.: Neurobiology of lampreys. *Physiol. Rev., 59*:1007, 1979.

Schmidt, R. F. (ed.): Fundamentals of Neurophysiology. New York, Springer-Verlag, 1978.

Schmidt, R. F. (ed.): Fundamentals of Sensory Physiology. New York, Springer-Verlag, 1978.

Shepherd, B. M.: The Synaptic Organization of the Brain: an Introduction. New York, Oxford University Press, 1974.

Shepherd, G. M.: Microcircuits in the nervous system. *Sci. Am., 238*(2):92, 1978.

Szentagothai, J., *et al.* (eds.): Conceptual Models of Neural Organization. Neurosciences Research Program. Cambridge, Mass., Massachusetts Institute of Technology, 1974.

Uttley, A. M.: Information Transmission in the Nervous System. New York, Academic Press, 1979.

Wooldridge, D. E.: Sensory Processing in the Brain: An Exercise in Neuroconnective Modeling. New York, John Wiley & Sons, 1979.

8

Sensory Receptors and Their Basic Mechanisms of Action

Input to the nervous system is provided by the sensory receptors that detect such sensory stimuli as touch, sound, light, pain, cold, warmth, and so forth. The purpose of this chapter is to discuss the basic mechanisms by which these receptors change sensory stimuli into nerve signals and, also, how both the type of sensory stimulus and its strength are detected by the brain.

TYPES OF SENSORY RECEPTORS AND THE SENSORY STIMULI THEY DETECT

The student of medical physiology will have already studied many different anatomical types of nerve endings, and Table 8–1 gives a list and classification of most of the body's sensory receptors. This table shows that there are basically five different types of sensory receptors: (1) *mechanoreceptors,* which detect mechanical deformation of the receptor or of cells adjacent to the receptor; (2) *thermoreceptors,* which detect changes in temperature, some receptors detecting cold and others warmth; (3) *nociceptors,* which detect damage in the tissues, whether it be physical damage or chemical damage; (4) *electromagnetic receptors,* which detect light on the retina of the eye; and (5) *chemoreceptors,* which detect taste in the mouth, smell in the nose, oxygen level in the arterial blood, osmolality of the body fluids, carbon dioxide concentration, and perhaps other factors that make up the chemistry of the body.

This chapter will discuss the function of a few specific types of receptors, primarily the peripheral mechanoreceptors, to illustrate some of the basic principles by which receptors in general operate. Other receptors will be discussed in rela-

tion to the sensory systems that they subserve, mainly in the next few chapters. Figure 8–1 illustrates some of the different types of mechanoreceptors found in the skin or in the deep structures of the body, and Table 8–1 gives their respective sensory functions. All these receptors will be discussed in the following chapters in relation to the respective sensory systems. However, the functions of some of these are described here briefly as follows:

Free nerve endings are found in all parts of the body. A large proportion of these detect pain. However, other free nerve endings detect crude touch, pressure, and tickle sensations and possibly warmth and cold.

Several of the more complex receptors listed in Figure 8–1 detect tissue deformation. These include the *Merkel's discs,* the *tactile hairs, pacinian corpuscles, Meissner's corpuscles, Krause's corpuscles,* and *Ruffini's end-organs.* In the skin, these receptors detect the tactile sensations of touch, pressure, and vibration. In the deep tissues, they detect stretch, deep pressure, or any other type of tissue deformation — even the stretch of joint capsules and ligaments to determine the angulation of a joint.

The *Golgi tendon apparatus* detects degree of tension in tendons, and the *muscle spindle* detects relative changes in muscle length. These receptors will be discussed in Chapter 11 in relation to the muscle and tendon reflexes.

DIFFERENTIAL SENSITIVITY OF RECEPTORS

The first question that must be answered is, how do two types of sensory receptors detect different types of sensory stimuli? The answer is by virtue of differential sensitivities. That is, each type of receptor is very highly sensitive to one type of

TABLE 8–1 CLASSIFICATION OF SENSORY RECEPTORS

Mechanoreceptors

Skin tactile sensibilities (epidermis and dermis)
  Free nerve endings
  Expanded tip endings
    Merkel's discs
    Plus several other variants
  Spray endings
    Ruffini's endings
  Encapsulated endings
    Meissner's corpuscles
    Krause's corpuscles
  Hair end-organs
Deep tissue sensibilities
  Free nerve endings
  Expanded tip endings
    Plus a few other variants
  Spray endings
    Ruffini's endings
  Encapsulated endings
    Pacinian corpuscles
    Plus a few other variants
  Muscle endings
    Muscle spindles
    Golgi tendon receptors
Hearing
  Sound receptors of cochlea
Equilibrium
  Vestibular receptors
Arterial pressure
  Baroreceptors of carotid sinuses and aorta

Thermoreceptors

Cold
  Cold receptors
Warmth
  ?

Nociceptors

Pain
  Free nerve endings

Electromagnetic Receptors

Vision
  Rods
  Cones

Chemoreceptors

Taste
  Receptors of taste buds
Smell
  Receptors of olfactory epithelium
Arterial oxygen
  Receptors of aortic and carotid bodies
Osmolality
  Probably neurons of supraoptic nuclei
Blood CO_2
  Receptors in or on surface of medulla and in aortic and carotid bodies
Blood glucose, amino acids, fatty acids
  Receptors in hypothalamus

Free nerve endings   Merkel's discs   Tactile hair

Pacinian corpuscle   Meissner's corpuscle   Krause's corpuscle

Ruffini's end-organ   Golgi tendon apparatus   Muscle spindle

Figure 8–1. Several types of somatic sensory nerve endings.

stimulus for which it is designed and yet is almost nonresponsive to normal intensities of the other types of sensory stimuli. Thus, the rods and cones are highly responsive to light but are almost completely nonresponsive to heat, cold, pressure on the eyeballs, or chemical changes in the blood. The osmoreceptors of the supraoptic nuclei in the hypothalamus detect minute changes in the osmolality of the body fluids but have never been known to respond to sound. Finally, pain receptors in the skin are almost never stimulated by usual touch or pressure stimuli but do become highly active the moment tactile stimuli become severe enough to damage the tissues.

Modality of Sensation — Law of Specific Nerve Energies

Each of the principal types of sensation that we can experience — pain, touch, sight, sound, and so forth — is called a *modality* of sensation. Yet, despite the fact that we experience these different modalities of sensation, nerve fibers transmit only impulses. Therefore, how is it that different nerve fibers transmit different modalities of sensation?

The answer to this is that each nerve tract terminates at a specific point in the central nervous system, and the type of sensation felt when a nerve fiber is stimulated is determined by this specific area in the nervous system to which the fiber leads. For instance, if a pain fiber is stimulated, the person perceives pain regardless of what type of stimulus excites the fiber. This stimulus can be electricity, heat, crushing, or stimulation of the pain nerve ending by damage to the tissue cells. Yet, whatever the means of stimulation, the person still perceives pain. Likewise, if a touch fiber is stimulated by exciting a touch receptor electrically or in any other way, the person perceives touch because touch fibers lead to specific touch areas in the brain. Similarly, fibers from the retina of the eye terminate in the vision areas of the brain, fibers from the ear terminate in the auditory areas of the brain, and temperature fibers terminate in the temperature areas.

This specificity of nerve fibers for transmitting only one modality of sensation is called the *law of specific nerve energies*. It is also called the *labelled line principle*.

TRANSDUCTION OF SENSORY STIMULI INTO NERVE IMPULSES

LOCAL CURRENTS AT NERVE ENDINGS — RECEPTOR POTENTIALS AND GENERATOR POTENTIALS

All sensory receptors have one feature in common. Whatever the type of stimulus that excites the receptor, its immediate effect is to change the potential across the receptor membrane. This change is called a *receptor potential*.

Mechanisms of Receptor Potentials. Different receptors can be excited in several different ways to cause receptor potentials: (1) by mechanical deformation of the receptor, which stretches the membrane and opens pores; (2) by application of a chemical to the membrane, which also opens pores; (3) by change of the temperature of the membrane, which alters the permeability of the membrane; or (4) by the effects of electromagnetic radiation such as light on the receptor, which either directly or indirectly changes the membrane characteristics and allows ions to flow through the membrane pores. It will be recognized that these four different means for exciting receptors correspond in general with the different types of known sensory receptors. In all instances, the basic cause of the change in membrane potential is a change in receptor membrane permeability, which allows ions to diffuse more or less readily through the membrane and thereby change the transmembrane potential.

Excitation of the Terminal Nerve Fiber by the Receptor — the Generator Potential. In many in-

stances, the sensory receptor is the termination of a nerve fiber itself, as is true for all the different types of receptors illustrated in Figure 8–1. However, a few receptors are specialized receptor cells that lie adjacent to the nerve endings. For instance, the hair cells of the cochlea and the taste cells of the taste buds are both specialized epithelial cells that develop receptor potentials, the hair cells when sound enters the cochlea and the taste cells when certain chemical substances are present in the mouth. In each instance, the receptor potential is then transferred to terminal nerve fibrils that synapse at the bases of the receptor cells, and it is this transfer of potential to the terminal nerve fibrils that causes action potentials.

In the case of the nerve ending receptors, it is the receptor potential itself that causes generation of action potentials in the nerve fibers. In the case of the specialized receptor cells, it is the transferred potential from the receptor to the nerve endings that causes the action potentials. In either case, the potential that actually causes generation of action potentials is called a *generator potential*. For the nerve ending receptors, the generator potential is the same as the receptor potential, but for the specialized receptor cells the generator potential is only that portion of the receptor potential that is transferred to the nerve endings.

Relationship of the Generator Potential to Action Potentials. When the generator potential rises above the threshold for eliciting action potentials in the terminal nerve fibril, then action potentials begin to appear. This is illustrated in Figure 8–2. Note also that the more the generator potential rises above the threshold level, the greater becomes the action potential frequency. Thus, the generator potential stimulates the terminal nerve fibril in the same way that the excitatory postsynaptic potential stimulates neurons in the central nervous system neuron.

Figure 8–2. Typical relationship between generator potential and action potentials when the generator potential rises above the threshold level.

Illustrative Examples of Receptor Function

The Receptor Potential (Generator Potential) of the Pacinian Corpuscle. The pacinian corpuscle is a very large and easily dissected sensory receptor. For this reason, one can study in detail the mechanism by which tactile stimuli excite it and by which it causes action potentials in the sensory fiber leading from it. Note in Figure 8–1 that the pacinian corpuscle has a central nonmyelinated tip of a nerve fiber extending through its core. Surrounding this fiber are many concentric capsule layers so that compression on the outside of the corpuscle tends to elongate, shorten, indent, or otherwise deform the central core of the fiber, depending on how the compression is applied. The deformation causes a sudden change in membrane potential, as illustrated in Figure 8–3, which is the receptor potential and in this case is also the generator potential that causes generation of action potentials. The receptor potential is believed to result from stretching the nerve fiber membrane, thus increasing its permeability and allowing positively charged sodium ions to leak to the interior of the fiber. This change in local potential causes a local circuit of current flow that spreads along the nerve fiber to its myelinated portion. At the first node of Ranvier, which itself lies inside the capsule of the pacinian corpuscle, the local current flow initiates action potentials in the nerve fiber. That is, the current flow through the node depolarizes it, and this then sets off a typical saltatory transmission of an action potential along the nerve fiber toward the central nervous system, as was explained in Chapter 2.

Relationship Between Stimulus Strength and the Receptor (Generator) Potential. Figure 8–4 illustrates the effect on the amplitude of the receptor (generator) potential caused by progressively stronger mechanical compression applied experimentally to the central core of the pacinian corpuscle. Note that the amplitude increases rapidly at first but then progressively less rapidly at high

Figure 8–4. Relationship of amplitude of generator potential to strength of a stimulus applied to a pacinian corpuscle. (From Loewenstein: *Ann. N.Y. Acad. Sci., 94*:510, 1961.)

stimulus strengths. The maximum amplitude that can be achieved by receptor potentials is around 100 millivolts. That is, a receptor potential can have almost as high a voltage as an action potential.

Relationship of Amplitude of Receptor Potential to Nerve Impulse Rate. The frequency of action potentials in the nerve fiber (impulse rate) is almost directly proportional to the amplitude of the generator potential. This relationship is illustrated in Figure 8–5, which shows the impulse

Figure 8–3. Excitation of a sensory nerve fiber by a generator potential produced in a pacinian corpuscle. (Modified from Loewenstein: *Ann. N.Y. Acad. Sci., 94*:510, 1961.)

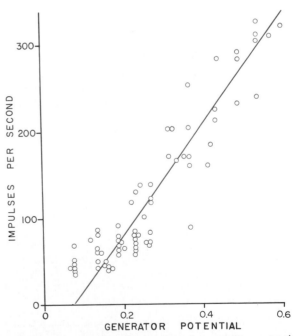

Figure 8–5. Relationship between the generator potential of a muscle spindle and the frequency of sensory impulses transmitted from the spindle. (From Katz: *J. Physiol. [Lond.], 111*:261, 1950.)

rate corresponding to different generator potential amplitudes recorded from a muscle spindle; there is an almost exact proportional relationship. This same relationship between receptor potential and impulse rate is approximately true for most sensory receptors.

ADAPTATION OF RECEPTORS

A special characteristic of all sensory receptors is that they *adapt* either partially or completely to their stimuli after a period of time. That is, when a continuous sensory stimulus is first applied, the receptors respond at a very high impulse rate at first, then progressively less rapidly until finally many of them no longer respond at all.

Figure 8–6 illustrates typical adaptation of certain types of receptors. Note that the pacinian corpuscle adapts extremely rapidly and hair receptors adapt within a second or so, while joint capsule and muscle spindle receptors adapt very slowly.

Furthermore some sensory receptors adapt to a far greater extent than others. For example, the pacinian corpuscles adapt to "extinction" within a few thousandths to a few hundredths of a second, and the hair base receptors adapt to extinction within a second or more. It is probable that all other mechanoreceptors also adapt completely eventually, but some require hours or days to do so for which reason they are frequently called "nonadapting" receptors. The longest measured time for complete adaptation of a mechanoreceptor is about two days for the carotid and aortic baroreceptors.

Some of the other types of receptors, the chemoreceptors and pain receptors for instance, probably never adapt completely. Each of these will be discussed in turn in subsequent chapters.

Mechanisms by Which Receptors Adapt. Adaptation of receptors is an individual property of each type of receptor in much the same way that development of a receptor potential is an individual property. For instance, in the eye, the rods and cones adapt by changing their chemical compositions (which will be discussed in Chapter 19). In the case of the mechanoreceptors, the receptor that has been studied in greatest detail is the pacinian corpuscle. Adaptation occurs in this receptor in two ways. First, the corpuscular structure itself very rapidly adapts to the deformation of the tissue. This can be explained as follows: The pacinian corpuscle is a viscoelastic structure so that when a distorting force is suddenly applied to one side of the corpuscle it is transmitted by the viscous component of the corpuscle directly to the same side of the central core, thus eliciting a receptor potential. However, within a few thousandths to a few hundredths of a second the fluid within the corpuscle redistributes so that the pressure becomes essentially equal all through the corpuscle; this applies an even pressure on all sides of the central core fiber, so that the receptor potential is no longer elicited. Thus, a receptor potential appears at the onset of compression but then disappears within a small fraction of a second.

Then, when the distorting force is removed from the corpuscle, essentially the reverse events occur. The sudden removal of the distortion from one side of the corpuscle allows rapid expansion on that side and a corresponding distortion of the central core occurs once more. Again, within milliseconds, the pressure becomes equalized all through the corpuscle and the stimulus is lost. Thus, the pacinian corpuscle signals the onset of compression and again signals the offset of compression.

The second mechanism of adaptation of the pacinian corpuscle, but a much slower one, results from a process called *accommodation* that occurs in the nerve fiber itself. That is, even if by chance the central core fiber should continue to be excited, as can be achieved after the capsule has been removed and the core is compressed with a stylus, the tip of the nerve fiber itself gradually becomes "accommodated" to the stimulus. This perhaps results from redistribution of ions across the nerve fiber membrane.

Presumably, these same two general mechanisms of adaptation apply to other types of mechanoreceptors. That is, part of the adaptation results from readjustments in the structure of the receptor itself, and part results from accommodation in the terminal nerve fibril.

Function of the Slowly Adapting and Nonadapting Receptors — The "Tonic" Receptors. The slowly adapting receptors (and also the receptors that do not adapt to extinction) continue to trans-

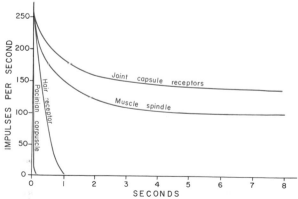

Figure 8–6. Adaptation of different types of receptors, showing rapid adaptation of some receptors and slow adaptation of others.

mit impulses to the brain as long as the stimulus is present (or at least for many minutes or hours). Therefore, they keep the brain constantly apprised of the status of the body and its relation to its surroundings. For instance, impulses from the slowly adapting joint capsule receptors allow the person to "know" at all times the degree of bending of the joints and therefore the positions of the different parts of the body. And impulses from the muscle spindles and Golgi tendon apparatuses allow the central nervous system to know respectively the status of muscle contraction and the load on the muscle tendon at each instant.

Other types of slowly adapting receptors include the receptors of the macula in the vestibular apparatus, the pain receptors, the baroreceptors of the arterial tree, the chemoreceptors of the carotid and aortic bodies, and some of the tactile receptors, such as the Ruffini endings and the Merkel's discs.

Because the slowly adapting receptors can continue to transmit information for many hours, they are also called *tonic* receptors. Many of these slowly adapting receptors would adapt to extinction if the intensity of the stimulus should remain absolutely constant for several hours or days. Fortunately, because of our continually changing bodily state, these receptors can almost never reach a state of complete adaptation.

Function of the Rapidly Adapting Receptors — The Rate Receptors or Movement Receptors or Phasic Receptors. Obviously, receptors that adapt rapidly cannot be used to transmit a continuous signal because these receptors are stimulated only when the stimulus strength changes. Yet they react strongly *while a change is actually taking place.* Furthermore, the number of impulses transmitted is directly related to the *rate at which the change takes place.* Therefore, these receptors are called *rate* receptors, *movement* receptors, or *phasic* receptors. Thus, in the case of the pacinian corpuscle, sudden pressure applied to the skin excites this receptor for a few milliseconds, and then its excitation is over even though the pressure continues. But then it transmits a signal again when the pressure is released. In other words, the pacinian corpuscle is exceedingly important for transmitting information about rapid changes in pressure against the body, but it is useless for transmitting information about constant pressure applied to the body.

Importance of the Rate Receptors–Their Predictive Function. Knowing the rate at which some change in bodily status is taking place, one can predict ahead to the state of the body a few seconds or even a few minutes later. For instance, the receptors of the semicircular canals in the vestibular apparatus of the ear detect the rate at which the head begins to turn when one runs around a curve. Using this information, a person can predict a turn of 10, 30, or some other number of degrees within the next 10 seconds and can adjust the motion of the limbs *ahead of time* to keep from losing balance. Likewise, pacinian corpuscles located in or near the joint capsules help to detect the rates of movement of the different parts of the body. Therefore, when one is running, information from these receptors allows the nervous system to predict ahead of time where the feet will be during any precise fraction of a second, and appropriate motor signals can be transmitted to the muscles of the legs to make any necessary anticipatory corrections in limb position so that the person will not fall. Loss of this predictive function makes it impossible for the person to run.

PSYCHIC INTERPRETATION OF STIMULUS STRENGTH

The ultimate goal of most sensory stimulation is to apprise the psyche of the state of the body and its surroundings. Therefore, it is important that we discuss briefly some of the principles related to the transmission of sensory stimulus strength to the higher levels of the nervous system.

The first question that comes to mind is: How is it possible for the sensory system to transmit sensory experiences of tremendously varying intensities? For instance, the auditory system can detect the weakest possible whisper but can also discern the meanings of an explosive sound only a few feet away, even though the sound intensities of these two experiences can vary almost a trillion-fold; the eyes can see visual images with light intensities that vary as much as a million-fold; or the skin can detect pressure differences of ten thousand- to one hundred thousand-fold.

As a partial explanation of these effects, note in Figure 8–4 the relationship of the generator potential produced by the pacinian corpuscle to the strength of stimulus. At low stimulus strength, very slight changes in stimulus strength increase the potential markedly; while at high levels of stimulus strength, further increases in receptor potential are very slight. Thus, the pacinian corpuscle is capable of accurately measuring extremely minute changes in stimulus strength at low intensity levels and is also capable of detecting much larger changes in stimulus strength at high intensity levels.

The transduction mechanism for detecting sound by the cochlea of the ear illustrates still another method for separating gradations of stimulus intensity. When sound causes vibration at a specific point on the basilar membrane, weak vibration stimulates only those hair cells at the point of maximum vibration. But, as the vibration intensity increases, not only do these hair cells become more intensely stimulated, but still many more hair cells in each direction farther away from the maximum vibratory point also become stimulated. Thus, signals transmitted over progressively increasing numbers of cochlear nerve fibers, as well as increasing intensity of signal strength in each nerve fiber, are two mechanisms by which stimulus strength is transmitted into the central nervous system. These two mechanisms, as well as several others, all of which multiply each other, make it possible for the ear to operate reasonably faithfully at stimulus intensity levels changing almost a trillion-fold.

Importance of the Tremendous Intensity Range of Sensory Reception. Were it not for the tremendous intensity range of sensory reception that we can experience, the various sensory systems would more often than not operate in the wrong range. This is illustrated by the attempts of most persons to adjust the light exposure on a camera without using a light meter. Left to intuitive judgment of light intensity, a person almost always overexposes the film on very bright days and greatly underexposes the film at twilight. Yet, that person's eyes are perfectly capable of discriminating with great detail the surrounding objects in both very bright sunlight and at twilight; the camera cannot do this because of the narrow critical range of light intensity required for proper exposure of film.

JUDGMENT OF STIMULUS STRENGTH

Physiopsychologists have evolved numerous methods for testing one's judgment of sensory stimulus strength, but only rarely do the results from the different methods agree with each other. For instance, one testing method requests selection of a weight that is exactly 100 per cent heavier than another. But the person usually selects a weight that is about 50 per cent heavier instead of 100 per cent heavier. Thus, the weak stimulus is underestimated and the strong stimulus is overestimated. In still another test procedure, a person is given a weight to hold and is then required to select the minimum amount of additional weight that must be added to detect a difference. In this case the person might be holding a 30 gram weight and finds that an additional 1 gram is needed to detect a difference. Then the person holds a 300 gram weight and finds that 10 grams of additional weight are required. In this instance the discriminatory ability is far greater at the low intensity level that at the high intensity level. Thus, the results of these two different types of tests are exactly opposite to each other, which means that the real argument lies in the meaning of the tests themselves. Therefore, at present no real agreement exists as to a proper method for measuring one judgment of stimulus strength. Yet, two principles are widely discussed in the physiopsychology field of sensory interpretation: the *Weber-Fechner principle* and the *power principle*.

The Weber-Fechner Principle — Detection of "Ratio" of Stimulus Strength. In the mid-1800s, Weber first and Fechner later proposed the principle that *gradations of stimulus strength are discriminated approximately in proportion to the logarithm of stimulus strength.* This law is based primarily on one's ability to judge minimal *changes* in stimulus strength. That is, in the second test described in the previous section the person could barely detect a 1 gram increase in weight when holding 30 grams, or a 10 gram increase when holding 300 grams. Thus, the *ratio* of the change in stimulus strength

required for detection of a change remained essentially constant, about 1 to 30, which is what the logarithmic principle means. To express this mathematically,

$$\text{Interpreted signal strength} = \log\,(\text{Stimulus}) + \text{Constant}$$

Because the Weber-Fechner principle offers a ready explanation for the tremendous range of stimulus strength that our nervous system can discern, it unfortunately became widely accepted for all types of sensory experience and for all levels of background sensory intensity. More recently it has become evident that this principle applies mainly to higher intensities of visual, auditory, and cutaneous sensory experience and it applies only poorly to most other types of sensory experience.

Yet, the Weber-Fechner principle is still a good one to remember because it emphasizes that the greater the background sensory stimulus, the greater also must be the additional change in stimulus strength in order for the psyche to detect the change.

The Power Law. Another attempt by physiopsychologists to find a good mathematical relationship between actual stimulus strength and interpretation of stimulus strength is the following formula, known as the power law:

$$\text{Interpreted signal strength} = K \cdot (\text{Stimulus} - k)^y$$

In this formula K and k are constants, and y is the power to which the stimulus strength is raised. The exponent y and the constants K and k are different for each type of sensation.

When this power law relationship is plotted on a graph using double logarithmic coordinates, as illustrated in Figure 8–7, a linear curve can be attained between interpreted stimulus strength and actual stimulus strength over a large range for almost any type of sensory perception. However, as illustrated in the fig-

Figure 8–7. Graphical demonstration of the "power law" relationship between actual stimulus strength and strength that the psyche interprets it to be. Note that the power law does not hold at either very weak or very strong stimulus strengths.

ure, even this power law relationship fails to hold satisfactorily at both very low and very high stimulus strengths.

PHYSIOLOGICAL CLASSIFICATION OF NERVE FIBERS

Some sensory signals need to be transmitted to the central nervous system extremely rapidly, or otherwise the information would be useless. An example of this is the sensory signals that apprise the brain of the momentary positions of the limbs at each fraction of a second during running. It is important that this information be transmitted by way of extremely rapidly conducting nerve fibers. At the other extreme, some types of sensory information, such as that depicting prolonged, aching pain, do not need to be transmitted rapidly at all, so that very slowly conducting fibers will suffice. Fortunately, nerve fibers come in all sizes between 0.2 and 20 microns in diameter — the larger the diameter, the greater the conducting velocity. The range of conducting velocities is between 0.5 and 120 meters per second.

Figure 8–8 gives two different classifications of nerve fibers that are in general use. One of these is a general classification that includes both sensory and motor fibers, including the autonomic nerve fibers as well. The other is a classification of sensory nerve fibers that is used primarily by sensory neurophysiologists.

In the general classification, the fibers are divided into types A and C, and the type A fibers are further subdivided into α, β, γ, and δ fibers.

Type A fibers are the typical myelinated fibers of spinal nerves. Type C fibers are the very small, unmyelinated nerve fibers that conduct impulses at low velocities. These constitute more than half the sensory fibers in most peripheral nerves and also all of the post-ganglionic autonomic fibers.

The sizes, velocities of conduction, and functions of the different nerve fiber types are given in the figure. Note that the very large fibers can transmit impulses at velocities as great as 120 meters per second, a distance in one second that is longer than a football field. On the other hand, the smallest fibers transmit impulses as slowly as 0.5 meter per second, requiring about 2 seconds to go from the big toe to the spinal cord.

Over two-thirds of all the nerve fibers in peripheral nerves are type C fibers. Because of their great number, these can transmit tremendous amounts of information from the surface of the body, even though their velocities of transmission are very slow. Utilization of type C fibers for transmitting this great mass of information represents an important economy of space in the nerves, for use of the larger type A fibers for transmitting all information would require peripheral nerves the size of large ropes and a spinal cord almost as large as the body itself.

Alternate Classification Used by Sensory Physiologists. Certain recording techniques have made it possible to separate the type Aα fibers into two subgroups; and, yet, these same recording techniques cannot distin-

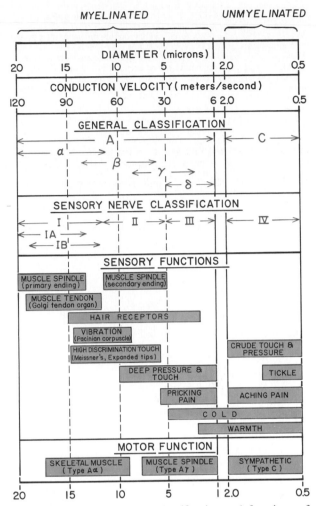

Figure 8–8. Physiological classification and functions of nerve fibers.

guish easily between Aβ and Aγ fibers. Therefore, the following classification is frequently used by sensory physiologists:

Group Ia. Fibers from the annulospiral endings of muscle spindles. (Average about 17 microns in diameter. These are alpha type A fibers in the general classification.)

Group Ib. Fibers from the Golgi tendon organs. (Average about 16 microns in diameter; these also are alpha type A fibers.)

Group II. Fibers from the discrete cutaneous tactile receptors and also from the flower-spray endings of the muscle spindles. (Average about 8 microns in diameter; these are beta and gamma type A fibers in the other classification.)

Group III. Fibers carrying temperature, crude touch, and pricking pain sensations. (Average about 3 microns in diameter; these are delta type A fibers in the other classification.)

Group IV. Unmyelinated fibers carrying pain, itch, temperature, and crude touch sensations. (0.5 to 2 microns in diameter; called type C fibers in the other classification.)

REFERENCES

Anderson, D. J., et al.: Sensory mechanisms in mammalian teeth and their supporting structures. Physiol. Rev., 50:171, 1970.

Anstis, S. M., et al.: Perception. New York, Springer-Verlag, 1978.

Babel, J., et al.: Ultrastructure of the Peripheral Nervous System and Sense Organs. New York, Churchill Livingstone, 1971.

Bate, C. M., et al.: Development of Sensory System. New York, Springer-Verlag, 1978.

Bennett, T. L.: The Sensory World: An Introduction to Sensation and Perception. Monterey, Cal., Brooks/Cole Publishing Co., 1978.

Brown, E., and Deffenbacher, K.: Perception and the Senses. New York, Oxford University Press, 1979.

Brown, M.: Touch Will Tell. New York, Franklin Watts, 1979.

Catton, W. T.: Mechanoreceptor function. Physiol. Rev., 50:297, 1970.

Coren, S., et al.: Sensation and Perception. New York, Academic Press, 1979.

Goldstein, E. B.: Sensation and Perception. Belmont, Cal., Wadsworth Publishing Co., 1980.

Granit, R.: Receptors and Sensory Perception. New Haven, Conn., Yale University Press, 1955.

Gray, J. A. B.: Initiation of impulses at receptors. In Magoun, H. W. (ed.): Handbook of Physiology. Sec. 1, Vol. 1. Baltimore, Williams & Wilkins, 1959.

Halata, Z.: The Mechanoreceptors of the Mammalian Skin. New York, Springer-Verlag, 1975.

Loewenstein, W. R.: The generation of electric activity in a nerve ending. Ann. N.Y. Acad Sci., 81:367, 1959.

Loewenstein, W. R.: Excitation and inactivation in a receptor membrane. Ann. N.Y. Acad. Sci., 94:510, 1961.

Lynn, B.: Somatosensory receptors and their CNS connections. Annu. Rev. Physiol., 37:105, 1975.

McCloskey, D. I.: Kinesthetic sensibility. Physiol. Rev., 58:763, 1978.

Paintal, A. A. (ed.): Morphology and Mechanisms of Chemoreceptors. Delhi, India, Vallabhbhai Patel Chest Institute, University of Delhi, 1976.

Porter, R. (ed.): Studies in Neurophysiology. New York, Cambridge University Press, 1978.

Schmidt, R. F. (ed.): Fundamentals of Sensory Physiology. New York, Springer-Verlag, 1978.

Somjen, G.: Sensory Coding in the Mammalian Nervous System. New York, Appleton-Century-Crofts, 1972.

Thompson, R. F., and Patterson, M. (eds.): Bioelectric Recording Techniques, Part C. Receptor and Effector Processes. New York, Academic Press, 1974.

Wiederhold, M. L.: Mechanosensory transduction in "sensory" and "motile" cilia. Annu. Rev. Biophys. Bioeng., 5:39. 1976.

Wiersma, C. A. G., and Roach, J. L. M.: Principles in the organization of invertebrate sensory systems. In Brookhart, J. M., and Mountcastle, V. B. (eds.): Handbook of Physiology. Sec. 1, Vol. 1. Baltimore, Williams & Wilkins, 1977, p. 1089.

Zimmermann, M.: Neurophysiology of nociception. Int. Rev. Physiol., 10:179, 1976.

9

Somatic Sensations: I. The Mechanoreceptive Sensations

The *somatic senses* are the nervous mechanisms that collect sensory information from the body. These senses are in contradistinction to the *special senses,* which mean specifically sight, hearing, smell, taste, and equilibrium.

CLASSIFICATION OF SOMATIC SENSES

The somatic senses can be classified into three different physiological types: (1) the *mechanoreceptive somatic senses,* stimulated by mechanical displacement of some tissue of the body, (2) the *thermoreceptive. senses,* which detect heat and cold, and (3) the *pain sense,* which is activated by any factor that damages the tissues. This chapter deals with the mechanoreceptive somatic senses, and the following chapter discusses the thermoreceptive and pain senses.

The mechanoreceptive senses include *touch, pressure, vibration,* and *tickle* senses (which are frequently called the *tactile senses*) and the *position sense,* which determines the relative positions and rates of movement of the different parts of the body.

Other Classifications of Somatic Sensations. Different types of somatic sensations are also grouped together in special classes that are not necessarily mutually exclusive, as follows:

Exteroreceptive sensations are those from the surface of the body.

Proprioceptive sensations are those having to do with the physical state of the body, including position sensations, tendon and muscle sensations, pressure sensations from the bottom of the feet, and even the sensation of equilibrium, which is generally considered to be a "special" sensation rather than a somatic sensation.

Visceral sensations are those from the viscera of the body; in using this term one usually refers specifically to sensations from the internal organs.

The *deep sensations* are those that come from the deep tissues, such as from the bone, fasciae, and so forth. These include mainly "deep" pressure, pain, and vibration.

DETECTION AND TRANSMISSION OF TACTILE SENSATIONS

Interrelationship Between the Tactile Sensations of Touch, Pressure, and Vibration. Though touch, pressure, and vibration are frequently classified as separate sensations, they are all detected by the same types of receptors. The only differences among these three are (1) touch sensation generally results from stimulation of tactile receptors in the skin or in tissues immediately beneath the skin, (2) pressure sensation generally results from deformation of deeper tissues, and (3) vibration sensation results from rapidly repetitive sensory signals, but some of the same types of receptors as those for touch and pressure are utilized — specifically the very rapidly adapting types of receptors.

The Tactile Receptors. At least six entirely different types of tactile receptors are known, but many more similar to these also exist. Some of these receptors were illustrated in Figure 8–1 of Chapter 8, and their special characteristics are the following:

First, some *free nerve endings,* which are found everywhere in the skin and in many other tissues, can detect touch and pressure. For instance, even light contact with the cornea of the eye, which contains no other type of nerve ending besides free nerve endings, can nevertheless elicit touch and pressure sensations.

Second, a touch receptor of special sensitivity is *Meissner's corpuscle,* an encapsulated nerve ending that excites a large (type Aβ) myelinated sensory nerve fiber. Inside the capsulation are many whorls of terminal nerve filaments. These receptors are present in the nonhairy parts of the skin (called *glabrous skin*) and are particularly abundant in the fingertips, lips, and other areas of the skin where one's ability to discern spatial characteristics of touch sensations is highly developed. They, along with the expanded tip receptors described subsequently, are mainly responsible for the ability to recognize exactly what point of the body is touched and to recognize the texture of objects touched. Meissner's corpuscles adapt in less than a second after they are stimulated, which means that they are particularly sensitive to movement of very light objects over the surface of the skin and also to low frequency vibration.

Third, the fingertips and other areas that contain large numbers of Meissner's corpuscles also contain large numbers of *expanded tip tactile receptors,* one type of which is *Merkel's discs.* The hairy parts of the skin also contain moderate numbers of expanded tip receptors, even though they have almost no Meissner's corpuscles. These receptors differ from Meissner's corpuscles in that they transmit an initially strong but partially adapting signal and then a continuing weaker signal that adapts only slowly. Therefore, they are responsible for giving steady state signals that allow one to determine continuous touch of objects against the skin. Merkel's discs are usually grouped together in a single receptor organ called the *Iggo dome receptor,* which projects upward against the underside of the epithelium of the skin, as illustrated in Figure 9–1. This causes the epithelium at this point to protrude outward, thus creating a dome. Also note that the entire group of

Merkel's discs is innervated by a single large type of myelinated nerve fiber (type Aβ). Each dome receptor has a diameter averaging only 0.2 mm., and these receptors are extremely sensitive. They probably play a very important role in localizing touch sensations to the specific surface areas of the body.

Fourth, slight movement of any hair on the body stimulates the nerve fiber entwining its base. Thus, each hair and its basal nerve fiber, called the *hair end-organ,* are also a type of touch receptor. This receptor adapts readily and, therefore, like Meissner's corpuscles, detects mainly movement of objects on the surface of the body or initial contact with the body.

Fifth, located in the deeper layers of the skin and also in deeper tissues are many *Ruffini's end-organs,* which are multibranched endings, as described and illustrated in the previous chapter. These endings adapt very little and, therefore, are important for signaling continuous states of deformation of the skin and deeper tissues, such as heavy and continuous touch signals and pressure signals. They are also found in joint capsules and signal the degree of joint rotation.

Sixth, many *pacinian corpuscles,* which were discussed in detail in Chapter 8, lie both beneath the skin and also deep in the tissues of the body. These are stimulated only by very rapid movement of the tissues because these receptors adapt in a few thousandths of a second. Therefore, they are particularly important for detecting tissue vibration or other extremely rapid changes in the mechanical state of the tissues.

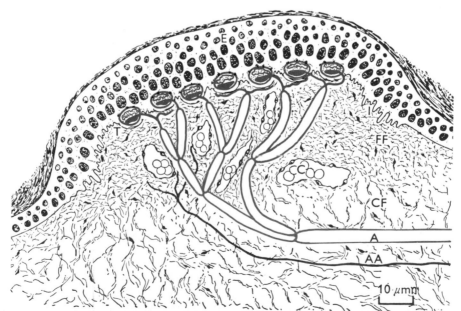

Figure 9–1. The Iggo dome receptor. Note the multiple numbers of Merkel's discs innervated by a single large myelinated fiber and abutting tightly the undersurface of the epithelium (From Iggo and Muir: *J. Physiol., 200*:763, 1969.)

Transmission of Tactile Sensations in Peripheral Nerve Fibers. Almost all the specialized sensory receptors, such as Meissner's corpuscles, Iggo dome receptors, hair receptors, pacinian corpuscles, and Ruffini's endings, transmit their signals in type Aβ nerve fibers that have transmission velocities of 30 to 70 meters per second. On the other hand, free nerve ending tactile receptors transmit signals mainly via the small type Aδ myelinated fibers that conduct at velocities of 5 to 30 meters per second. Some tactile free nerve endings transmit via type C unmyelinated fibers at velocities from a fraction of a meter up to 2 meters per second; these send signals into the spinal cord and lower brain stem, probably subserving mainly the sensation of tickle. Thus, the more critical types of sensory signals — those that help to determine precise localization on the skin, minute gradations of intensity, or rapid changes in sensory signal intensity — are all transmitted in the rapidly conducting types of sensory nerve fibers. On the other hand, the cruder types of signals, such as crude pressure, poorly localized touch, and especially tickle, are transmitted via much slower nerve fibers, fibers that also require much less space than in the nerves.

DETECTION OF VIBRATION

All the different tactile receptors are involved in detection of vibration, though different receptors detect different frequencies of vibration. Pacinian corpuscles can signal vibrations from 60 to 500 cycles per second, because they respond extremely rapidly to minute and rapid deformations of the tissues, and they also transmit their signals over type Aβ nerve fibers, which can transmit more than 1000 impulses per second.

Low frequency vibrations up to 80 cycles per second, on the other hand, stimulate other tactile receptors — especially Meissner's corpuscles, which are less rapidly adapting than pacinian corpuscles.

THE SUBCONSCIOUS "MUSCLE SENSE"

Highly specialized sensory receptors are found in both skeletal muscles and tendons — *muscle spindles* in muscles and *Golgi tendon organs* in tendons. These receptors transmit their signals into the spinal cord, cerebellum, and cerebral cortex to control reflex contraction of the muscles. But, from what is known at present, these signals operate entirely at a subconscious level or almost so. These specialized receptors and reflexes that they subserve will be considered in detail in relation to spinal cord reflexes and control of muscle contraction in Chapter 11.

However, some psychological effects have pointed to the existence of a conscious "muscle sense." For instance, one is capable of determining how heavy an object is, and this has long been believed to be detected by the specialized muscle spindles or tendon organs; but critical experiments have not proved this. Instead, this type of information is probably signaled in two ways: (1) by usual tactile signals in the deep tissues and (2) by signals from the motor portions of the brain indicating intensity of motor signals to the muscles required to lift an object.

TICKLING AND ITCH

The phenomenon of tickling and itch has often been stated to be caused by very mild stimulation of pain nerve endings, because whenever pain is blocked by local anesthesia of a nerve or by compressing the nerve, the phenomenon of tickling and itch also disappears. However, recent neurophysiological studies have demonstrated the existence of very sensitive, rapidly adapting, free nerve endings that elicit only the tickle and itch sensation. Furthermore, these endings are found almost exclusively in the superficial layers of the skin, which is also the only tissue from which the tickle and itch sensation can usually be elicited. Furthermore, exciting itch receptors in animals initiates scratch reflexes, which contrasts with the effect of exciting pain nerve endings that always causes withdrawal reflexes instead.

Therefore, it seems clear that the itch and tickle sensations are transmitted by very small type C, unmyelinated fibers similar to those that transmit the burning type of pain; these fibers, however, are distinctly separate from the pain fibers. Furthermore, the endings of these fibers are readily excited by light mechanoreceptive stimuli, indicating that they are mechanoreceptors in contradistinction to the probable chemoreceptor nature of pain fibers.

The purpose of the itch sensation is presumably to call attention to mild surface stimuli such as a flea crawling on the skin or a fly about to bite, and the elicited signals then lead to scratching or other maneuvers that rid the host of the irritant.

The relief of itch by the process of scratching occurs only when the irritant is removed or when the scratch is strong enough to elicit pain. The pain signals are believed to suppress the itch signals in the cord by the process of inhibition that will be described in the following chapter.

THE DUAL SYSTEM FOR TRANSMISSION OF MECHANORECEPTIVE SOMATIC SENSORY SIGNALS INTO THE CENTRAL NERVOUS SYSTEM

Either all or almost all sensory information from the somatic segments of the body enters the spinal cord through the posterior roots. Immediately after entering the cord, the nerve fibers separate into two major groups: (1) a *dorsal-lemniscal system* that includes the (a) *dorsal columns* and (b) the *spinocervical* tracts located in the *dorsolateral columns;* and (2) the *anterolateral spinothalamic system* located in the anterior and lateral columns. Closely associated with the dorsal-lemniscal system are the dorsal and ventral spinocerebellar tracts, which operate at a subconscious level and transmit sensory information to the cerebellum. These tracts will be discussed in Chapter 13 along with the discussion of cerebellar function.

Comparison of the Dorsal-Lemniscal System with the Anterolateral Spinothalamic System. The distinguishing difference between the dorsal-lemniscal system and the anterolateral spinothalamic system is that the dorsal-lemniscal system is comprised mainly of large myelinated nerve fibers that transmit signals to the brain at velocities of 30 to 110 meters per second while the anterolateral spinothalamic system is comprised of much smaller myelinated fibers (averaging 4 microns in diameter) that transmit impulses at velocities ranging between 10 and 60 meters per second.

Another difference between the two systems is that the dorsal system has a very high degree of spatial orientation of the nerve fibers with respect to their origin on the surface of the body, while the spinothalamic system has a much smaller degree of spatial orientation, with some fibers seeming to have very little orientation at all.

These differences in the two systems immediately characterize the types of sensory information that can be transmitted by the two systems. First, sensory information that must be transmitted rapidly and with temporal fidelity is transmitted in the dorsal-lemniscal system, while that which does not need to be transmitted rapidly is transmitted mainly in the anterolateral spinothalamic system. Second, those sensations that detect fine gradations of intensity are transmitted in the dorsal system, while those that lack the fine gradations are transmitted in the spinothalamic system. And, third, sensations that are discretely localized to exact points in the body are transmitted in the dorsal system, while those transmitted in the spinothalamic system can be localized much less exactly. On the other hand, the spinothalamic system has a special capability that the dorsal system does not have: the ability to transmit a broad spectrum of sensory modalities — pain, warmth, cold, and crude tactile sensations; the dorsal system is limited to mechanoreceptive sensations alone. With this differentiation in mind we can now list the types of sensations transmitted in the two systems.

The Dorsal-Lemniscal System

1. Touch sensations requiring a high degree of localization of the stimulus.
2. Touch sensations requiring transmission of fine gradations of intensity.
3. Phasic sensations, such as vibratory sensations.
4. Sensations that signal movement against the skin.
5. Position sensations.
6. Pressure sensations having to do with fine degrees of judgment of pressure intensity.

The Anterolateral Spinothalamic System

1. Pain.
2. Thermal sensations, including both warm and cold sensations.
3. Crude touch and pressure sensations capable of only crude localizing ability on the surface of the body and having little capability for intensity discrimination.
4. Tickle and itch sensations.
5. Sexual sensations.

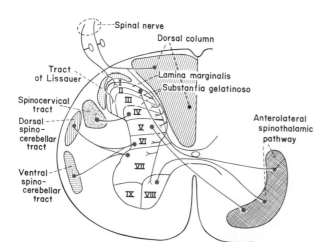

Figure 9–2. Cross section of the spinal cord showing the anatomical laminae I through IX of the cord gray matter and the ascending sensory tracts in the white columns of the spinal cord.

FUNCTION OF THE SPINAL CORD NEURONS IN TRANSMITTING SENSORY SIGNALS

The gray matter of the spinal cord subserves three major functions. First, it is the locus of the integrating system for the spinal cord reflexes, a function that will be discussed in Chapter 11. Second, it functions as the initial processor of incoming sensory signals and as a relay station to relay most of these signals all the way to the brain; it is with this function that we are concerned in this chapter. Third, it is the area for final processing of motor signals transmitted downward from the brain to the muscles. This will be discussed in Chapter 13.

Relay of Sensory Signals in the Spinal Cord. Upon first entering the spinal cord through the posterior roots, as illustrated in Figure 9–2, most of the large, sensory nerve fibers, mainly type Aβ fibers, turn medially toward the dorsal columns. Then they usually divide into two major branches: one ascends upward through the dorsal columns and the other enters the anterior portion of the dorsal horn of the spinal cord gray matter. Also, a large share of the fibers that ascend in the dorsal columns enters the gray matter a few segments farther up the cord. Approximately 25 per cent of them travel the entire distance to the terminus of the dorsal columns at the dorsal column nuclei in the medulla.

In the dorsal horn gray matter, the terminals of these large fibers synapse with second order neurons of two types: (1) local neurons that play an intricate role in the control of spinal cord reflexes, and (2) relay neurons that give rise to long, ascending fiber tracts that transmit sensory information to the brain. Most of the fibers from the relay neurons ascend in the *spinocervical tract* located in the dorsolateral column, as shown in Figure 9–2.

The smaller fibers entering the spinal cord from the posterior roots, in general, take a more lateral pathway than the larger fibers, and they either enter the gray matter of the dorsal horn immediately or either ascend or descend a few segments and then enter the dorsal horn. Most of these fibers terminate on small neurons in the posterior portions of the dorsal horns, and these often give rise to short fibers that terminate somewhere else in the gray matter before the information is finally relayed to the long ascending pathways. Essentially all the sensory information from the smaller fibers eventually enters the anterolateral spinothalamic tract that crosses to the opposite side of the cord in the anterior commissure and then ascends to the brain in the anterolateral white matter.

Processing of Sensory Signals by Spinal Neurons. Most of the sensory information transmitted through the large sensory fibers is transmitted very faithfully, with either no processing or very little processing in the spinal cord. On the other hand, the signals transmitted through the smaller fibers, especially the pain signals, are often subject to a high degree of processing. This occurs mainly in the posterior portions of the dorsal horns, and it consists principally of (1) control of sensitivity of sensory transmission as a result of inhibitory signals transmitted from the brain to the cord, (2) control of sensitivity as a result of collateral signals from other fibers entering the spinal cord through the posterior roots, and (3) summation of signals from adjacent sensory nerves. This will be discussed in more detail in the following chapter in relation to the processing of pain signals.

The Anatomical Laminae of the Spinal Cord Gray Matter. Figure 9–2 illustrates the spinal cord gray matter divided into nine separate laminae. These divisions are based mainly on the types of neurons found within each separate area of the gray matter. Unfortunately, the exact functions of the neurons in the different areas are not fully known. However, the locus of some of the relay neurons for the ascending sensory tracts have been localized to the following laminae:

Spinothalamic tract	Laminae I, IV, V, and VI
Spinocervical tract	Laminae IV, V, and VI
Dorsal and ventral spinocerebellar tracts	Laminae VI and VII
Spinoreticular tract	Laminae VI, VII, and VIII

TRANSMISSION IN THE DORSAL-LEMNISCAL SYSTEM

ANATOMY OF THE DORSAL-LEMNISCAL SYSTEM

Sensory signals are transmitted to the brain by way of two major pathways in the dorsal-lemniscal system: (1) the *dorsal column pathway,* and (2) the *spinocervical pathway.* Until recently it was believed that all the sensory signals transmitted in this system were conducted only in the dorsal columns. However, complete transection of the dorsal columns is now known to cause only partial loss of sensations normally ascribed to the dorsal-lemniscal system, and it has been discovered that a major share of the remaining signals is transmitted in the spinocervical tracts located in the dorsolateral white columns of the cord, as illustrated in Figure 9–2. The routes that both the dorsal column pathway and the spinocervical pathway take to the brain are illustrated in Figure 9–3.

Figure 9–3. The dorsal column and spinocervical pathways for transmitting critical types of tactile signals. (Modified from Ranson and Clark: Anatomy of the Nervous System. Philadelphia, W. B. Saunders Company, 1959.)

Anatomy of the Dorsal Column Pathway. Note in Figure 9–3 that the nerve fibers entering the dorsal columns pass up these columns to the medulla, where they synapse in the *dorsal column nuclei* (the *cuneate* and *gracile nuclei*). From here, *second order neurons* decussate immediately to the opposite side and then pass upward to the thalamus through bilateral pathways called the *medial lemnisci*. Each medial lemniscus terminates in a *ventrobasal complex of nuclei* located in the ventral posterolateral nucleus of the *thalamus*. In its pathway through the hindbrain, the medial lemniscus is joined by additional fibers from the *main sensory nucleus of the trigeminal nerve and from the upper portion of its descending nuclei;* these fibers subserve the same sensory functions for the head that the dorsal column fibers subserve for the body.

From the ventrobasal complex, *third order neurons* project, as shown in Figure 9–4, mainly to the *postcentral gyrus* of the *cerebral cortex* called *somatic sensory area I*. But, in addition, neurons also project to closely associated regions of the cortex behind and in front of the postcentral gyrus. Finally, a few fibers project to the lowermost lateral portion of each parietal lobe, an area called *somatic sensory area II*.

Anatomy of the Spinocervical Pathway. The anatomy of the spinocervical pathway is much less well known than that of the dorsal column pathway. However, many of the large sensory fibers that enter the cord in the dorsal roots soon synapse mainly in lamina IV of the cord gray matter but also in adjacent laminae as well, giving rise to second order fibers that enter the *dorsolateral white columns* and ascend in the spinocervical tract to the cervical region of the cord or even to the medulla. At these points these fibers again synapse either in the dorsal horn of the cord or in medullary nuclei either adjacent to or as part of the *dorsal column nuclei*. Then third order neurons decussate to the opposite side and pass along with the second order neurons of the dorsal column pathway upward to the thalamus through the *medial lemnisci*. Thus, the pathway within the brain parallels that of the dorsal column pathway.

Separation of Sensory Modalities Between the Dorsal Column Pathway and the Spinocervical Pathway

The way in which the nervous system distinguishes among the different modalities of sensation is to transmit the signals of different modalities to the separate central nervous system areas. This separation of modality begins in the spinal cord. It has already been noted that only certain mechanoreceptor modalities are transmitted in the dorsal-lemniscal system while all the other somatic modalities are transmitted in the anterolateral spinothalamic system. However, even within the dorsal system there is an additional degree of separation. The dorsal column pathway transmits mainly signals from rapidly adapting sensory receptors. For instance, it is only through the dorsal column pathway that signals are transmitted from the extremely rapidly adapting pacinian corpuscles. Also, most of the signals from the Meissner's corpuscles and from the hair receptors, both

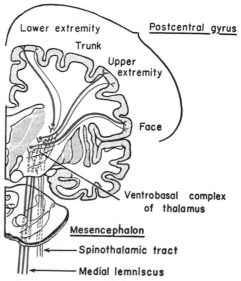

Figure 9–4. Projection of the dorsal-lemniscal system from the thalamus to the somesthetic cortex. (Modified from Brodal: Neurological Anatomy in Relation to Clinical Medicine. New York, Oxford University Press, 1969.)

of which are moderately rapidly adapting receptors, are transmitted through this pathway.

On the other hand, the more slowly adapting signals from the Merkel's discs, from the deep tissue Ruffini end-organs, and from the slowly adapting Ruffini position sense receptors of the joint capsules seem to be transmitted through the spinocervical pathway.

At the level of the cerebral cortex, separation of the mechanoreceptor sensory modalities is also found in somatic sensory area I, as will be discussed later. Therefore, it is presumed that these modalities remain separated throughout their entire pathway from the spinal cord to the cortex.

Spatial Orientation of the Nerve Fibers in the Dorsal-Lemniscal System

One of the distinguishing features of the dorsal-lemniscal system is a distinct spatial orientation of nerve fibers from the individual parts of the body that is maintained throughout. For instance, in the dorsal columns, the fibers from the lower parts of the body lie toward the center, while those that enter the spinal cord at progressively higher segmental levels form successive layers laterally.

The spatial orientation in the spinocervical pathway is less well known. However, stimulation experiments of single fibers within this pathway have shown that the sensory signals diverge very little, indicating a high degree of spatial orientation in this pathway as well.

In the thalamus, the distinct spatial orientation is still maintained, with the tail end of the body represented by the most lateral portions of the ventrobasal complex and the head and face represented in the medial component of the complex. However, because of the crossing of the medial lemnisci in the medulla, the left side of the body is represented in the right side of the thalamus, and the right side of the body is represented in the left side of the thalamus. In a similar manner, the fibers passing to the cerebral cortex also are spatially oriented so that a single part of the cortex receives signals from a discrete area of the body, as is described below.

THE SOMESTHETIC CORTEX

The area of the cerebral cortex to which the sensory signals are projected is called the *somesthetic cortex*. In the human being, this area lies mainly in the anterior portions of the parietal lobes. Two distinct and separate areas are known to receive direct afferent nerve fibers from the relay nuclei of the thalamus; these, called *somatic sensory area I* and *somatic sensory area II,* are illustrated in Figure 9–5. However, somatic sensory area I is so much more important to the sensory functions of the body than is somatic sensory area II that in popular usage, the term

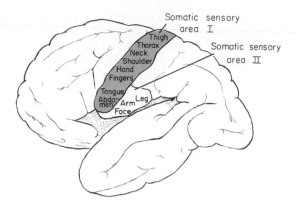

Figure 9–5. The two somesthetic cortical areas, somatic sensory areas I and II.

somesthetic cortex is almost always used to mean area I exclusive of area II. Yet, to keep these two areas separated, we will henceforth refer to them separately as somatic sensory area I and somatic sensory area II.

Projection of the Body in Somatic Sensory Area I. Somatic sensory area I lies in the postcentral gyrus of the human cerebral cortex (in Brodmann areas 3, 1, and 2 immediately behind the central sulcus). A distinct spatial orientation exists in this area for reception of nerve signals from the different areas of the body. Figure 9–6 illustrates a cross-section through the brain at the level of the postcentral gyrus, showing the representations of the different parts of the body in separate regions of somatic sensory area I. Note, however, that

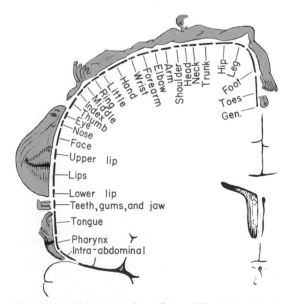

Figure 9–6. Representation of the different areas of the body in the somatic sensory area I of the cortex. (From Penfield and Rasmussen: Cerebral Cortex of Man: A Clinical Study of Localization of Function. New York, Macmillan Company, 1968.)

each side of the cortex receives sensory information exclusively from the opposite side of the body (with the exception of a small amount of sensory information from the same side of the face).

Some areas of the body are represented by large areas in the somatic cortex — the lips by far the greatest of all, followed by the face and thumb — while the entire trunk and lower part of the body are represented by relatively small areas. The sizes of these areas are directly proportional to the number of specialized sensory receptors in each respective peripheral area of the body. For instance, a great number of specialized nerve endings are found in the lips and thumb, while only a few are present in the skin of the trunk.

Note also that the head is represented in the lower or lateral portion of the postcentral gyrus, while the lower part of the body is represented in the medial or upper portion of the postcentral gyrus.

Modality Differentiation in Somatic Sensory Area I.   Not only is there spatial projection of the body in somatic sensory area I but also modality separation of different types of mechanoreceptor signals. Tactile signals stimulate the central and anterior portions of the postcentral gyrus, while two other types of signals stimulate respectively the posterior and very anterior portions of somatic sensory area I. The posterior portion receives signals mainly from the joint receptors that provide the brain with information about position of all parts of the body with respect to each other. The very anterior edge of somatic sensory area I, where it dips deeply into the central sulcus and abuts the primary motor cortex anterior to the central sulcus, receives sensory signals mainly from the muscle spindles. This muscle information seemingly operates at a subconscious level and is probably used almost exclusively to help control the muscles from which the signals derive. This separation of modalities is important because it helps us to understand how the brain dissects different types of information from incoming sensory signals.

Somatic Sensory Area II.   The second cortical area to which somatic afferent fibers project, somatic sensory area II, is a much smaller area that lies posterior and inferior to the lower end of the postcentral gyrus and on the upper wall of the lateral fissure, as shown in Figure 9–5. The degree of localization of the different parts of the body is very poor in this area compared with somatic sensory area I. The face is represented anteriorly, the arms centrally, and the legs posteriorly.

So little is known about the function of somatic sensory area II that it cannot be discussed intelligently. It is known that signals enter this area from both the dorsal system and the spino-reticulo-thalamic system, and that signals reach this area from both sides of the body. Also, stimulation of somatic sensory area II in some instances causes complex body movements, for

which reason it possibly plays a role in sensory control of motor functions.

Excitation of Vertical Columns of Neurons in the Somesthetic Cortex

The cerebral cortex contains *six* separate layers of neurons, and, as would be expected, the neurons in each layer perform functions different from those in other layers. Also, the neurons are arranged functionally in vertical columns extending all the way through the six layers of the cortex, each column having a diameter of about 0.33 to 1 millimeter and containing about 100,000 neuronal cell bodies. Unfortunately, we still know relatively little about the functions of these columns of cells but we are certain about the following facts:

1. The incoming sensory signal excites mainly neuronal layer IV first; then the signal spreads toward the surface of the cortex and also toward the deeper layers.

2. Layers I and II receive a diffuse, nonspecific input from the reticular activating system that can facilitate the whole brain at once; this system will be described in Chapter 14. This input perhaps controls the overall level of excitability of the cortex.

3. The neurons in layers V and VI send axons to other parts of the nervous system — some to other areas of the cortex, some to deeper structures of the brain, such as the thalamus or brain stem, and some even to the spinal cord.

Similar vertical columns of neurons exist in all other areas of the cortex as well as in the somesthetic cortex. In particular, they have been shown to be very important for function of the visual cortex and the motor cortex.

Each vertical column of neurons seems to be able to decipher a specific quality of information from the sensory signal. For instance, in the visual cortex one specific column will detect a line oriented in a particular direction, while an adjacent column will detect a similar line oriented in a slightly different direction. Presumably, in the somesthetic cortex each column detects separate qualities of signals (angles of orientation of rough spots, lengths of rough spots, perhaps roundness of objects, perhaps sharpness of objects, and so forth) from specific surface areas of the body.

Functions of Somatic Sensory Area I

The functional capabilities of different areas of the somesthetic cortex have been determined by selective excision of the different portions. Widespread excision of somatic sensory area I causes loss of the following types of sensory judgment:

1. The person is unable to localize discretely the different sensations in the different parts of the body. However, he or she can localize these sensations very crudely, such as to a particular hand, which indicates that the thalamus or parts of the cerebral cortex not normally considered to be concerned with somatic sensations can perform some degree of localization.

2. He is unable to judge critical degrees of pressure against his body.

3. He is unable to judge exactly the weights of objects.

4. He is unable to judge shapes or forms of objects. This is called *astereognosis.*

5. He is unable to judge texture of materials, for this type of judgment depends on highly critical sensations caused by movement of the skin over the surface to be judged.

6. He is unable to recognize the relative orientation of the different parts of his body with respect to each other.

Note in the above list that nothing has been said about loss of pain. However, in the absence of somatic sensory area I, the appreciation of pain may be altered either in quality or in intensity. But more important, the pain that does occur is poorly localized, indicating that pain localization probably depends mainly upon simultaneous stimulation of tactile stimuli that use the topographical map of the body in somatic sensory area I to localize the source of the pain.

SOMATIC ASSOCIATION AREAS

Brodmann areas 5 and 7 of the cerebral cortex, which are located in the parietal cortex immediately behind somatic sensory area I and above somatic sensory area II, play important roles in deciphering the sensory information that enters the somatic sensory areas. Therefore, these areas are called the *somatic association areas.*

Electrical stimulation in the somatic association area can occasionally cause a person to experience a complex somatic sensation, sometimes even the "feeling" of an object such as a knife or a ball. Therefore, it seems clear that the somatic association area combines information from multiple points in the somatic sensory area to decipher its meaning. This also fits with the anatomical arrangement of the neuronal tracts that enter the somatic association area, for it receives signals from (a) the primary somatic areas, (b) the ventrobasal complex of the thalamus, and (c) adjacent areas of the thalamus which themselves receive input from the ventrobasal complex.

Effect of Removing the Somatic Association Area — Amorphosynthesis. When the somatic association area is removed, the person especially loses the ability to recognize complex objects and complex forms that are felt. In addition, the person loses most of the sense of form of his or her own body. An especially interesting fact is that loss of the somatic association area on one side of the brain causes the person sometimes to be oblivious of the opposite side of the body — that is, to forget that it is there. Likewise, when feeling objects, the person will tend to feel only one side of the object and to forget that the other side even exists. This complex sensory deficit is called *amorphosynthesis.*

CHARACTERISTICS OF TRANSMISSION IN THE DORSAL-LEMNISCAL SYSTEM

Faithfulness of Transmission. The most important functional characteristic of the dorsal-lemniscal system is its *faithfulness* of transmission. That is, each time a point in the periphery is stimulated, a signal ordinarily is transmitted all the way to the somesthetic cortex. Also, if this peripheral stimulus increases in intensity, the intensity of the signal at the cerebral cortex increases proportionately. And, finally, when a discrete area of the body is stimulated, the signal from this area is transmitted to a discrete area of the cerebral cortex. Thus, the dorsal system is adequately organized for transmission of accurate information from the periphery to the sensorium. Furthermore, the responsiveness of this system can be altered only moderately by stimuli from other areas of the nervous system, and it is not depressed to a significant extent even by moderate degrees of general anesthesia; this is quite different for most portions of the spinothalamic pathway.

Basic Neuronal Circuit and Discharge Pattern in the Dorsal-Lemniscal System. The lower part of Figure 9–7 illustrates the basic organization of the neuronal circuit of the dorsal column pathway, showing that at each synaptic stage divergence occurs. However, the upper part of the figure shows that a single receptor stimulus on the skin does not cause all the cortical neurons with which that receptor connects to discharge at the same rate. Instead, the cortical neurons that discharge to the greatest extent are those in a central part of the cortical "field" for each respective receptor. Thus, a weak stimulus causes only the centralmost neurons to fire. A stronger stimulus causes still more neurons to fire, but those in the center still discharge at a considerably more rapid rate than do those farther away from the center.

Two-Point Discrimination. A method frequently used to test tactile capabilities is to determine a person's so-called "two-point discriminatory ability." In this test, two needles are pressed against the skin, and the subject determines whether two points of stimulus are felt or one point. On the tips

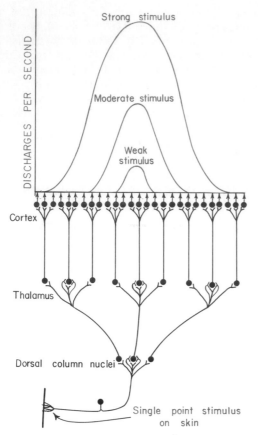

Figure 9–7. Transmission of pinpoint stimulus signal to the cortex.

a valley that allow the sensory cortex to detect the presence of two stimulatory points rather than a single point. However, the capability of the sensorium to distinguish between two points of stimulation is strongly influenced by another mechanism, the mechanism of lateral inhibition, as explained in the following section.

Increase in Contrast in the Perceived Spatial Pattern Caused by Lateral Inhibition. In Chapter 7 it was pointed out that contrast in sensory patterns is increased by inhibitory signals transmitted laterally in the sensory pathway. This effect was illustrated in Figure 7–11 of that chapter.

In the case of the dorsal column system, an excited sensory receptor in the skin transmits not only excitatory signals to the somesthetic cortex but also inhibitory signals laterally to adjacent fiber pathways. These inhibitory signals help to block lateral spread of the excitatory signal, a process called *lateral inhibition* or *surround inhibition*. As a result, the peak of excitation stands out, and much of the surrounding diffuse stimulation is blocked. This effect is illustrated by the two colored curves in Figure 9–8, showing complete separation of the peaks when the intensity of the surround inhibition is very great. Obviously, this mechanism accentuates the contrast between the areas of peak stimulation and the surrounding areas, thus greatly increasing the contrast or sharpness of the perceived spatial pattern.

Transmission of Rapidly Changing and Repetitive Sensations. The dorsal column system is of particular value for apprising the sensorium of rapidly changing peripheral conditions. This system can "follow" changing stimuli up to at least 400 cycles per second and can "detect" changes as

of the fingers a person can distinguish two separate points even when the needles are as close together as 1 to 2 mm. However, on the person's back, the needles must usually be as far apart as 30 to 70 mm. before one can detect two separate points. The reason for this is that there are many specialized tactile receptors in the tips of the fingers in comparison with a small number in the skin of the back. Referring back to Figure 9–6, we can see also that the portions of the body that have a high degree of two-point discrimination have a correspondingly large cortical representation in somatic sensory area I.

Figure 9–8 illustrates the mechanism by which the dorsal column pathway, and the other sensory pathways as well but to a less critical degree, transmit two-point discriminatory information. This figure shows two adjacent points on the skin that are strongly stimulated, and it also shows the small area of the somesthetic cortex (greatly enlarged) that is excited by signals from the two stimulated points. The solid black curve shows the spatial pattern of cortical excitation when both skin points are stimulated simultaneously. Note that the resultant zone of excitation has two separate peaks. It is these two peaks separated by

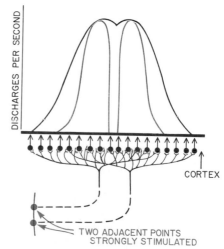

Figure 9–8. Transmission of signals to the cortex from two adjacent pinpoint stimuli. The solid black curve represents the pattern of cortical stimulation without "surround" inhibition, and the two colored curves represent the pattern with "surround" inhibition.

high as 700 cycles. Obviously, very rapid response to a sudden stimulus on the skin allows one to direct attention immediately to any point of contact, which, in turn, allows one to make necessary corrections before damage can be done.

Vibratory Sensation. Because vibratory signals are rapidly repetitive (can be detected as vibration up to 700 cycles per second), they can be transmitted only in the dorsal column pathway and not in the other, more slowly transmitting pathways. For this reason, application of vibration with a tuning fork to different peripheral parts of the body is an important tool used by the neurologist for testing functional integrity of the dorsal columns.

THE POSITION SENSE

The term position sense can be divided into two subtypes: (1) *static position,* which means conscious recognition of the orientation of the different parts of the body with respect to each other, (2) *kinesthesia,* which means conscious recognition of rates of movement of the different parts of the body. The position sensations are transmitted to the sensorium mainly through the dorsallemniscal system. However, special features of the position sense require further explanation.

The Position Sense Receptors. Sensory information from many different types of receptors is used to determine both static position and kinesthesia. These include especially the extensive sensory endings in the joint capsules and ligaments but also receptors in the skin and deep tissues near the joints.

Three major types of nerve endings have been described in the joint capsules and ligaments about the joints. (1) By far the most abundant of these are spray-type *Ruffini endings,* one of which was illustrated in Figure 8–1 of Chapter 8. These endings are stimulated strongly when the joint is suddenly moved; they adapt slightly at first but then transmit a steady signal thereafter. (2) A second type of ending resembling the stretch receptors found in muscle tendons (called *Golgi tendon receptors)* is found particularly in the ligaments about the joints. Though far less numerous than the Ruffini endings, they have essentially the same response properties. (3) A few *pacinian corpuscles* are also found in the tissues around the joints. These adapt extremely rapidly and presumably help to detect *rate of rotation* at the joint.

Detection of Static Position by the Joint Receptors. Figure 9–9 illustrates the excitation of seven different nerve fibers leading from separate joint receptors in the capsule of a cat's knee joint. Note that at 180 degrees of joint rotation one of the receptors is stimulated; then at 150 degrees still another is stimulated; at 140 degrees two are stimulated, and so forth. The information from

Figure 9–9. Responses of seven different nerve fibers from knee joint receptors in a cat at different degrees of rotation. (Modified from Skoglund: *Acta Physiol. Scand.,* Suppl. 124, *36*:1, 1956.)

these joint receptors continually apprises the central nervous system of the momentary rotation of the joint. That is, the rotation determines *which* receptor is stimulated and how much it is stimulated, and from this the brain knows how far the joint is bent.

Detection of Rate of Movement (Kinesthesia) at the Joint. Because pacinian corpuscles are especially adapted for detecting movement of tissues, it is tempting to suggest that rate of movement at the joints is detected by the pacinian corpuscles. However, the number of pacinian corpuscles in the joint tissues is small, for which reason rate of movement at the joint is probably detected mainly in the following way: The Ruffini and Golgi endings in the joint tissues are stimulated very strongly at first by the joint movement, but within a fraction of a second this strong level of stimulation fades to a lower, steady state rate of firing. Nevertheless, this early overshoot in receptor stimulation is directly proportional to the rate of joint movement and is believed to be the signal used by the brain to discern the rate of movement. However, it is likely that the few pacinian corpuscles also play at least some role in this process.

Transmission of Position Sense Signals in the Dorsal-Lemniscal Pathways. In the past it had been believed that essentially all of the position sense signals were transmitted in the dorsal columns. However, on the basis of studies in animals, there is now much reason to believe that many of these signals are transmitted in the spinocervical pathway as well. This is probably especially true of the static position signals, that is, those signals that are slowly adapting and that transmit information about the relative positions of the different parts of the body when the person is not moving.

Processing of Position Sense Information in the Dorsal-Lemniscal Pathways. Despite the faithfulness of transmission of signals from the periphery to the sensory cortex in the dorsal-lemniscal system, there is also some processing of sensory

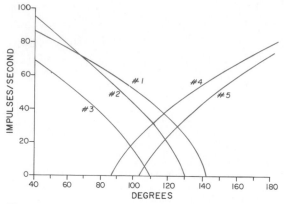

Figure 9–10. Typical responses of five different neurons in the knee joint receptor field of the ventrobasal complex when the knee joint is moved through its range of motion. (The curves were constructed from data in Mountcastle et al.: *J. Neurophysiol., 26*:807, 1963.)

information at lower synaptic levels before it reaches the cerebral cortex. For instance, the signal pattern from static position receptors changes as it passes progressively up the dorsal column system. Figure 9–9 showed that individual joint receptors are stimulated maximally at specific degrees of rotation of the joint, with the intensity of stimulation decreasing on either side of the maximal point for each receptor. However, the static position signal for joint rotation is quite different at the level of the ventrobasal complex of the thalamus, as can be seen by referring to Figure 9–10. This figure shows that the ventrobasal neurons that respond to the joint rotation signal are of two types: (1) those that are maximally stimulated when the joint is at full rotation and (2) those that are maximally stimulated when the joint is at minimal rotation. In each case, as the degree of rotation changes, the rate of stimulation of the neuron either decreases or increases, depending on the direction in which the joint is being rotated. Furthermore, the intensity of neuronal excitation changes over angles of 40 to 60 degrees of angulation in contrast to 20 to 30 degrees for the individual receptors, as was illustrated in Figure 9–9. Thus, the signals from the individual joint receptors are integrated in the space domain by the thalamic neurons, giving a progressively stronger signal as the joint moves in only one direction rather than giving a peaked signal as occurs in stimulation of individual receptors.

TRANSMISSION IN THE ANTEROLATERAL SPINOTHALAMIC SYSTEM

It was pointed out earlier in the chapter that the anterolateral spinothalamic system transmits sen-

sory signals which do not require highly discrete localization of the signal source and also do not require discrimination of fine gradations of intensity. These include pain, heat, cold, crude tactile, tickle and itch, and sexual sensations. In the following chapter pain and temperature sensations will be discussed, while the present chapter is concerned principally with transmission of the tactile sensations.

ANATOMY OF THE ANTEROLATERAL SPINOTHALAMIC PATHWAY

The anterolateral spinothalamic fibers originate mainly in laminae I, IV, V, and VI in the dorsal horns where the small, peripheral, sensory nerve fibers terminate after entering the cord (see Figure 9–2). Then, as illustrated in Figure 9–11, the fibers immediately cross in the anterior commissure of the cord to the opposite anterolateral white column where they turn upward toward the brain. These fibers ascend rather diffusely throughout the anterolateral columns. However, most anatomists still separate this pathway into a ventral spinothalamic tract and a lateral spinothalamic tract as illustrated in Figure 9–11 even though physiologically it

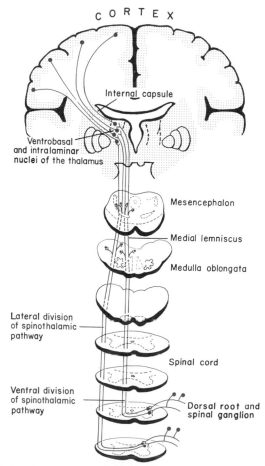

Figure 9–11. The spinothalamic pathways. (Modified from Ranson and Clark: Anatomy of the Nervous System. Philadelphia, W. B. Saunders Company, 1959.)

has been difficult to make this differentiation using electrical recording techniques.

The upper terminus of the anterolateral spinothalamic pathway is mainly two-fold: (1) throughout the *reticular nuclei of the brain stem,* and (2) in two different nuclear complexes of the thalamus, the *ventrobasal complex* and the *intralaminar nuclei.* In general, the tactile signals are transmitted mainly into the ventrobasal complex, and this is probably also true for the temperature signals. On the other hand, only part of the pain signals project to this complex. Instead, most of these enter the reticular nuclei of the brain stem and intralaminar nuclei of the thalamus, as will be discussed in greater detail in the following chapter.

Spinoreticular, Spinotectal, and Paleospinothalamic Pathways. Closely associated with the anterolateral spinothalamic pathway are several other diffuse pathways: (1) the *spinoreticular pathway* that originates in laminae VI, VII, and VIII and terminates in the reticular nuclei of the brain stem; (2) a *spinotectal pathway* that closely parallels the anterolateral spinothalamic pathway but terminates instead in the tectum; and (3) a *paleospinothalamic pathway* that is composed of multiple neurons in series that transmit crude sensory signals from segment to segment of the cord and also upward through the reticular nuclei of the brain stem to the intralaminar nuclei of the thalamus. The functions of all these tracts are not well documented, but they presumably are related to the transmission of crude tactile, thermal, and pain signals and perhaps play either subconscious or mildly conscious roles in controlling the neural functions of the brain stem.

Projection of Spinothalamic Signals from the Thalamus to the Cortex. Spinothalamic signals entering the ventrobasal complex of the thalamus are relayed in association with those from the dorsal-lemniscal system mainly to somatic area I but to a lesser extent to somatic area II. These relayed signals seem to be concerned mainly with tactile sensation, perhaps to a moderate extent with temperature sensation, but probably very little with pain sensation. On the other hand, most of the pain signals seem to be relayed into other areas of the thalamus and into surrounding basal regions of the brain such as the hypothalamus, septal nuclei, and so forth.

Characteristics of Transmission in the Anterolateral Spinothalamic Pathway. In general, the same principles apply to transmission in the anterolateral spinothalamic pathway as in the dorsal-lemniscal system except for the following differences: (a) the velocities of transmission in the spinothalamic pathway are only one-half to one-third those in the dorsal system, ranging between 10 and 60 meters per second; (b) the degree of spatial localization of signals is poor, especially in the pain pathways; (c) the gradations of intensities are also far less acute, most of the sensations being recognized in 10 to 20 gradations of strength rather than as many as 100 gradations for the dorsal system; and (d) the ability to transmit rapidly repetitive sensations is poor.

Thus, it is evident that the anterolateral spinothalamic system is a cruder type of transmission system than the dorsal-lemniscal system. Even so, certain modalities of sensation are transmitted in this system only and not at all in the dorsal-lemniscal system. These are pain, thermal, tickle and itch, and sexual sensations.

SOME SPECIAL ASPECTS OF SENSORY FUNCTION

Function of the Thalamus in Somatic Sensation. When the somesthetic cortex of a human being is destroyed, that person loses most critical tactile sensibilities, but a slight degree of crude tactile sensibility does return. Therefore, it must be assumed that the thalamus has a slight ability to discriminate tactile sensation but functions mainly to relay this type of information to the cortex.

On the other hand, loss of the somesthetic cortex has little effect on one's perception of pain sensation and only a moderate effect on the perception of temperature. Therefore, there is much reason to believe that the thalamus and other associated basal regions of the brain play perhaps the dominant role in discrimination of these sensibilities; it is interesting that these sensibilities appeared very early in the phylogenetic development of animalhood while the critical tactile sensibilities were a late development.

Cortical Control of Sensory Sensitivity. Almost all sensory information that enters the cerebrum, except that from the olfactory system, but including sensory information from the eyes, the ears, the taste receptors, and all the somatic receptors, is relayed through one or another of the thalamic nuclei. Furthermore, the conscious brain is capable of directing its attention to different segments of the sensory system. This function is believed to be mainly achieved through facilitation or inhibition of the cortical receptive areas.

But, in addition, "corticofugal" signals are transmitted from the cortex to the lower relay stations in the sensory pathways to *inhibit* transmission. For instance, corticofugal pathways control the sensitivity of the synapses at all levels of the sensory pathways — in the thalamus, in the brain stem reticular nuclei, in the dorsal column nuclei, and especially in the dorsal horn relay station of the spino-reticulo-thalamic system. Also, similar inhibitory mechanisms are known for the visual, auditory, and olfactory systems, which are discussed in later chapters. Each corticofugal pathway begins in the cortex where the sensory pathway that it controls terminates. Thus, a feedback control loop exists for each sensory pathway.

Obviously, corticofugal control of sensory input could allow the cerebral cortex to alter the threshold for different sensory signals. Also, it might help the brain focus its attention on specific types of information, which is an important and necessary quality of nervous system function.

Automatic Gain Control in the Sensory Pathways, and Enhancement of Contrast. One of the byproducts of corticofugal inhibition is believed to be automatic gain control in many if not most of the sensory pathways.

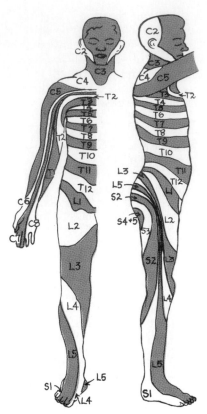

Figure 9–12. The dermatomes. (Modified from Grinker and Sahs: Neurology. Springfield, Ill., Charles C Thomas, 1966.)

That is, when excess sensory signals pass to the brain, recurrent inhibition back to the cord decreases the sensitivity of the sensory pathway. This obviously prevents overloading of the pathway with signals. Also, it helps to preserve contrast in the perception of sensory signals because an excess of signals in the pathway would deluge the cerebral cortex with such a high degree of excitation that it would be impossible to distinguish the highlights from the chaff.

Segmental Fields of Sensation — The Dermatomes. Each spinal nerve innervates a "segmental field" of the skin called a *dermatome*. The different dermatomes are illustrated in Figure 9–12. However, these are shown as if there were distinct borders between the adjacent dermatomes, which is far from true because much overlap exists from segment to segment.

Indeed, because of the great overlap, the posterior roots from an entire segment of the spinal cord can be destroyed without causing significant loss of sensation in the skin.

Figure 9–12 shows that the anal region of the body lies in the dermatome of the most distal cord segment. In the embryo, this is the tail region and is the most distal portion of the body. The legs develop from the lumbar and upper sacral segments rather than from the distal sacral segments, which is evident from the dermatomal map. Obviously, one can use a dermatomal map such as that illustrated in Figure 9–12 to determine the level in the spinal cord at which various cord injuries may have occurred when the peripheral sensations are disturbed.

REFERENCES

Also see bibliographies of Chapters 8 and 10.

Anstis, S. M., *et al.*: Perception. New York, Springer-Verlag, 1978.
Boudreau, J. C., and Tsuchitani, C.: Sensory Neurophysiology: with Special Reference to the Cat. New York, Van Nostrand Reinhold Co., 1973.
Brown, M.: Touch Will Tell. New York, Franklin Watts, 1979.
Coren, S. *et al.*: Sensation and Perception. New York, Academic Press, 1979.
Darian-Smith, I., *et al.*: Posterior parietal cortex: Relations of unit activity to sensorimotor function. *Annu. Rev. Physiol., 41*:141, 1979.
Emmers, R., and Tasker, R. R.: The Human Somesthetic Thalamus. New York, Raven Press, 1975.
Goldstein, E. B.: Sensation and Perception. Belmont, Cal., Wadsworth Publishing Co., 1980.
Gordon, G. (ed.): Active Touch; The Mechanism of Recognition of Objects by Manipulation. New York, Pergamon Press, 1978.
Heath, C. J.: The somatic sensory neurons of pericentral cortex. *In* Porter, R. (ed.): International Review of Physiology: Neurophysiology III. Vol. 17. Baltimore, University Park Press, 1978, p. 193.
Kenshalo, D. R. (ed.): Sensory Function of the Skin of Humans. New York, Plenum Press, 1979.
Lapresle, J., and Haguenau, M.: Anatomico-chemical correlation in focal thalamic lesions. *Z. Neurol., 205*:29, 1973.
Lynn, B.: Somatosensory receptors and their CNS connections. *Annu. Rev. Physiol., 37*:105, 1975.
McCloskey, D. I.: Kinesthetic sensibility. *Physiol. Rev., 58*:763, 1978.
Mountcastle, V. B., et al.: The relation of thalamic cell response to peripheral stimuli varied over an intensive continuum. *J. Neurophysiol., 26*:807, 1963.
Norrsell, U.: Behavioral studies of the somatosensory system. *Physiol. Rev., 60*:327, 1980.
Olton, D. S.: Spatial memory. *Sci. Am., 236*(6):82, 1977.
Perl, E. R., and Boivie, J. G.: Neural substrates of somatic sensations. *In* MTP International Review of Science: Physiology. Vol. 3. Baltimore, University Park Press, 1974, p. 303.
Vallbo, A. B., *et al.*: Somatosensory, proprioceptive, and sympathetic activity in human peripheral nerves. *Physiol. Rev., 59*:919, 1979.
Wall, P. D., and Dubner, R.: Somatosensory pathways. *Annu. Rev. Physiol., 34*:315, 1972.

10

Somatic Sensations: II. Pain, Visceral Pain, Headache, and Thermal Sensations

Many, if not most, ailments of the body cause pain. Furthermore, the ability to diagnose different diseases depends to a great extent on a doctor's knowledge of the different qualities of pain, a knowledge of how pain can be referred from one part of the body to another, how pain can spread from the painful site, and, finally, what the different causes of pain are. For these reasons, the present chapter is devoted mainly to pain and to the physiologic basis of some of the associated clinical phenomena.

The Purpose of Pain. Pain is a protective mechanism for the body; it occurs whenever any tissues are being damaged, and it causes the individual to react to remove the pain stimulus. Even such simple activities as sitting for a long time on the ischia can cause tissue destruction because of lack of blood flow to the skin where the skin is compressed by the weight of the body. When the skin becomes painful as a result of the ischemia, the person shifts weight unconsciously. A person who has lost the pain sense, such as after spinal cord injury, fails to feel the pain and therefore fails to shift weight. This eventually results in ulceration at the areas of pressure unless special measures are taken to move the person from time to time.

QUALITIES OF PAIN

Pain has been classified into three different major types: pricking, burning, and aching pain. Other terms used to describe different types of pain include throbbing pain, nauseous pain, cramping pain, sharp pain, electric pain, and others, most of which are well known to almost everyone.

Pricking pain is felt when a needle is stuck into the skin or when the skin is cut with a knife. It is also often felt when a widespread area of the skin is diffusely but strongly irritated.

Burning pain is, as its name implies, the type of pain felt when the skin is burned. It can be excruciating and is the most likely of the pain types to cause suffering.

Aching pain is not felt on the surface of the body, but, instead, is a deep pain with varying degrees of annoyance. Aching pain of low intensity in widespread areas of the body can summate into a very disagreeable sensation.

It is not necessary to describe these different qualities of pain in great detail because they are well known to all persons. The real problem, and one that is only partially solved, is what causes the differences in quality. It is known, however, that pricking pain results from stimulation of delta type A pain fibers, whereas burning and aching pain results from stimulation of the more primitive type C fibers, which will be discussed later in the chapter.

METHODS FOR MEASURING THE PERCEPTION OF PAIN

The intensity of a stimulus necessary to cause pain can be measured in many different ways, but the most used methods have been pricking the skin with a pin at measured pressures, pressing a solid object against a protruding bone with measured force, pinching the skin, or heating the skin with measured amounts of heat. The latter method has proved to be especially accurate from a quantitative point of view.

Figure 10–1 illustrates the basic principles of a heat apparatus used for measuring pain threshold. An intense light is focused by a large condenser lens onto a black spot painted on the forehead of the subject, and the heat intensity delivered by the light is controlled by a rheostat. In determining the subject's threshold for pain, the intensity of the heat is increased in progressive steps,

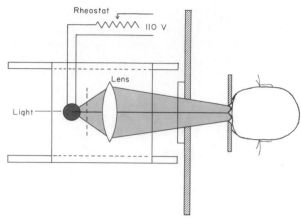

Figure 10–1. Heat apparatus for measuring pain threshold. (From Hardy, Wolff, and Goodell: *J. Clin. Invest, 19*:649, 1940.)

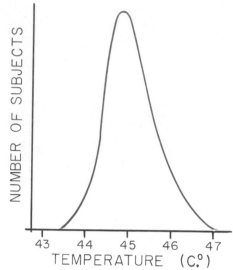

Figure 10–3. Distribution curve obtained from a large number of subjects of the minimal skin temperature that causes pain. (Modified from Hardy: *J. Chronic Dis., 4*:22, 1956.)

and the length of time required for the forehead to heat sufficiently to elicit pain is recorded for each heat intensity. These data are then plotted in the form of a "strength-duration curve" to express pain threshold, as follows.

Strength-Duration Curve for Expressing Pain Threshold. Figure 10–2 illustrates a typical strength-duration curve obtained by using the above procedure for measuring pain threshold. This curve is almost identical with the strength-duration curves discussed in Chapter 10 for stimulation of nerve fibers by electrical currents of increasing intensities. Note that a very intense stimulus applied for only a second elicits a sensation of pain while a stimulus of much less intensity may require many seconds. The lowest intensity of stimulus that will excite the sensation of pain when the stimulus is applied for a prolonged period of time is called the *pain threshold*.

The Intensity of Pain — "JNDs." The increase in stimulus intensity that will barely cause a detectable difference in degree of pain is called a *just noticeable difference* (JND). By applying all different stimulus intensities between the level of no pain at all and the most intense pain that a person can distinguish, it has been found that approximately 22 JNDs can be discerned by the average person.

The Pain Threshold. Figure 10–3 shows graphically the skin temperature at which pain is first perceived by

different persons. By far the greatest number perceive pain when the skin temperature reaches almost exactly 45° C., and almost everyone perceives pain before the temperature reaches 47° C. Indeed, measurements in people as widely different as Eskimos, Indians, and whites have shown little differences in their *thresholds for pain*. However, different people do *react* very differently to pain, as is discussed below.

THE PAIN RECEPTORS AND THEIR STIMULATION

Free Nerve Endings as Pain Receptors. The pain receptors in the skin and other tissues are all free nerve endings. They are widespread in the superficial layers of the *skin* and also in certain internal tissues, such as the *periosteum*, the *arterial walls*, the *joint surfaces*, and the *falx* and *tentorium* of the cranial vault. Most of the other deep tissues are not extensively supplied with pain endings but are weakly supplied; nevertheless, any widespread tissue damage can still summate to cause the aching type of pain in these areas.

Types of Stimuli that Excite Pain Receptors — Mechanical, Thermal, and Chemical. Some pain fibers are excited almost entirely by excessive mechanical stress or mechanical damage to the tissues; these are called *mechanosensitive pain receptors*. Others are sensitive to extremes of heat or cold and therefore are called *thermosensitive pain receptors*. And, still others are sensitive to various chemical substances and are called *chemosensitive pain receptors*. Some of the different chemicals that excite the chemosensitive receptors include *bradykinin, serotonin, histamine, po-*

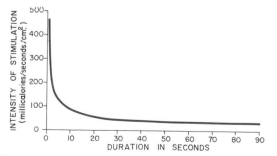

Figure 10–2. Strength-duration curve for depicting pain threshold. (From Hardy: *J. Chronic Dis. 4*:20, 1956.)

tassium ions, acids, prostaglandins, acetylcho-line, and *proteolytic enzymes.*

Though some pain receptors are mainly sensitive to only one of the above types of stimuli, most are sensitive to more than one of the types.

Nonadapting Nature of Pain Receptors.   In contrast to most other sensory receptors of the body the pain receptors adapt either not at all or almost not at all. In fact, under some conditions, the threshold for excitation of the pain fibers becomes progressively lower and lower as the pain stimulus continues, thus allowing these receptors to become progressively more activated with time. This increase in sensitivity of the pain receptors is called *hyperalgesia.*

One can readily understand the importance of this failure of pain receptors to adapt, for it allows them to keep the person apprised of a damaging stimulus that causes the pain as long as it persists.

RATE OF TISSUE DAMAGE AS THE CAUSE OF PAIN

The average critical temperature of 45° C. at which a person first begins to perceive pain is also the temperature at which the tissues begin to be damaged by heat; indeed, the tissues are eventually completely destroyed if the temperature remains at this level indefinitely. Therefore, it is immediately apparent that pain resulting from heat is closely correlated with the ability of heat to damage the tissues.

Furthermore, in studying soldiers who had been severely wounded in World War II, it was found that the majority of them felt little or no pain except for a short time after the severe wound had been sustained. This, too, indicates that *pain generally is not felt after damage has been done* but only *while damage is being done.*

Mechanism by Which Tissue Damage Stimulates Pain Receptors

It has already been pointed out that the tissues contain three different types of pain receptors, those that respond to excessive mechanical stress in the tissues, those that respond to extremes of heat, and those that respond to abnormal chemicals in the tissues. Therefore, all the pain receptors can be stimulated by different types of tissue damage.

Special Importance of Chemical Pain Stimuli During Tissue Damage.   Injection of certain chemical substances under the skin in human beings can cause the highest degrees of pain. Furthermore, extracts from damaged tissues also cause intense pain when injected beneath the normal skin. Among the substances in such ex-

tracts that are especially painful are *bradykinin, histamine, prostaglandins, acids, excesses of potassium ions, serotonin,* and *proteolytic enzymes.* Obviously, many of these substances could cause direct damage to the pain nerve endings, especially the proteolytic enzymes. But some of the other substances, such as bradykinin and some of the prostaglandins, can cause direct extreme stimulation of pain nerve fibers without necessarily damaging them.

Release of the various substances listed above not only stimulates the chemosensitive pain endings but also greatly decreases the threshold for stimulation of the mechanosensitive and thermosensitive pain receptors as well. A widely known example of this is the extreme pain caused by slight mechanical or heat stimuli following tissue damage by sunburn.

Tissue Ischemia as a Cause of Pain.   When blood flow to a tissue is blocked, the tissue becomes very painful within a few minutes. And the greater the rate of metabolism of the tissue, the more rapidly the pain appears. For instance, if a blood pressure cuff is placed around the upper arm and inflated until the arterial blood flow ceases, exercise of the forearm muscles can cause severe muscle pain within 15 to 20 seconds. In the absence of muscle exercise, the pain will not appear for three to four minutes. Cessation of blood flow to the skin, in which the metabolic rate is very low, usually does not cause pain for about 20 to 30 minutes.

The cause of pain in ischemia is yet unknown; however, it is relieved by supplying oxygen to the ischemic tissue. Flow of unoxygenated blood to the tissue will not relieve the pain.

One of the suggested causes of pain in ischemia is accumulation of large amounts of lactic acid in the tissues, formed as a consequence of the anaerobic metabolism (metabolism without oxygen) that occurs during ischemia. However, it is also possible that other chemical agents, such as bradykinin, proteolytic enzymes, and so forth, are formed in the tissues because of cell damage and that these, rather than lactic acid, stimulate the pain nerve endings.

Muscle Spasm as a Cause of Pain.   Muscle spasm is also a very common cause of pain, and it is the basis of many clinical pain syndromes. This pain probably results partially from the direct effect of muscle spasm in stimulating mechanosensitive pain receptors. However, it possibly results also from the indirect effect of muscle spasm in causing ischemia and thereby stimulating chemosensitive pain receptors. The muscle spasm not only compresses the blood vessels and diminishes blood flow but also increases the rate of metabolism in the muscle tissue at the same time, thus making the relative ischemia even greater and creating ideal conditions for release of chemical pain-inducing substances.

TRANSMISSION OF PAIN SIGNALS INTO THE CENTRAL NERVOUS SYSTEM

"Fast" Pain Fibers and "Slow" Pain Fibers. Pain signals are transmitted from the periphery to the spinal cord by small delta type A fibers at velocities between 6 and 30 meters per second and also by type C fibers at velocities between 0.5 and 2 meters per second. When the delta type A fibers are blocked without blocking the C fibers by moderate compression of the nerve trunk, the pricking type of pain disappears. On the other hand, when the type C fibers are blocked without blocking the delta fibers by low concentrations of local anesthetic, the burning and aching types of pain disappear.

Because of this double system of pain innervation, a sudden onset of painful stimulus gives a "double" pain sensation: a fast pricking pain followed a second or so later by a slow burning pain. The pricking pain apprises the person very rapidly of a damaging influence and, therefore, plays an important role in making the person react immediately to remove himself from the stimulus. On the other hand, the slow burning sensation tends to become more and more painful over a period of time. It is this sensation that gives one the intolerable suffering of long-continued pain.

Transmission in the Anterolateral Spinothalamic Pathway. Pain fibers enter the cord through the dorsal roots, ascend or descend one to two segments in the *tract of Lissauer,* and then terminate on neurons in the dorsal horns of the cord gray matter, the type Aδ fibers in laminae I and V and the type C fibers in laminae II and III, also called the substantia gelatinosa. Most of the signals then probably pass through one or more additional short-fibered neurons, the last of which gives rise to long fibers that cross immediately to the opposite side of the cord in the *anterior commissure* and pass upward to the brain via the anterolateral spinothalamic pathway as was described in the previous chapter.

We shall see later that the intensity of pain signals can be modified markedly as they pass through the neuronal synapses of the gray matter of the dorsal horns, especially in response to simultaneous signals transmitted by mechanoreceptor sensory nerve fibers and in response to signals entering the dorsal horns from the brain via corticofugal fibers.

As the pain pathways pass into the brain they separate into two pathways: *the pricking pain pathway* and *the burning pain pathway.*

The Pricking Pain Pathway. Figure 10–4 illustrates that the pricking pain pathway terminates in the ventrobasal complex in close association with the areas of termination of the tactile sensation fibers of both the dorsal-lemniscal system and the spinothalamic system. From here signals are transmitted into other areas of the thalamus and to the somatic sensory cortex, mainly to somatic area I. However, the signals to the cortex are probably important mainly for localizing the pain, not for interpreting it.

The Burning Pain Pathway — Stimulation of the Reticular Activating System. Figure 10–4 also shows that the burning and aching pain fibers terminate in the reticular area of the brain stem and in the intralaminar nuclei of the thalamus, which are themselves an upward extension of the reticular formation protruding among the thalamic specific nuclei. Both the reticular area of the brain stem and the intralaminar nuclei are parts of the reticular activating system. In Chapter 14 we will discuss in detail the functions of this system; briefly, it transmits activating signals into essentially all parts of the brain, especially upward through the thalamus to all areas of the cerebral cortex and also laterally into the basal regions of the brain around the thalamus including very importantly the hypothalamus.

Thus, the burning and aching pain fibers, because they do excite the reticular activating system, have a very potent effect for activating essentially the entire nervous system, that is, to arouse one from sleep, to create a state of excitement, to create a sense of urgency, and to promote

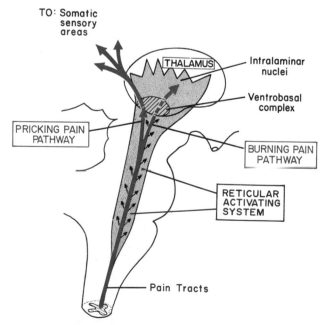

Figure 10–4. Transmission of pain signals into the hindbrain, thalamus, and cortex via the "pricking pain" pathway and the "burning pain" pathway.

defense and aversion reactions designed to rid the person or animal of the painful stimulus.

The signals that are transmitted through the burning pain pathway can be localized only to very gross areas of the body. Therefore, these signals are designed almost entirely for the single purpose of calling one's attention to injurious processes in the body. They create suffering that is sometimes intolerable. Their gradation of intensity is poor; instead, even weak pain signals can summate over a period of time by a process of temporal summation to create an unbearable feeling even though the same pain for short periods of time may be relatively mild.

Function of the Thalamus and Cerebral Cortex in the Appreciation of Pain. Complete removal of the somatic sensory areas of the cerebral cortex does not destroy one's ability to perceive pain. Therefore, it is believed that pain impulses entering only the thalamus and other lower centers cause at least some conscious perception of pain. However, this does not mean that the cerebral cortex has nothing to do with normal pain appreciation; indeed, electrical stimulation of the somesthetic cortical areas causes a person to perceive mild pain in approximately 3 per cent of the stimulations. It is believed that the cortex plays an important role in interpreting the quality of pain even though pain perception might be a function of lower centers.

Localization of Pain in the Body. Most localization of pain probably results from simultaneous stimulation of tactile receptors along with the pain stimulation. However, the pricking type of pain, transmitted through delta type A fibers, can be localized perhaps within 10 to 20 cm. of the stimulated area. On the other hand, the burning and aching types of pain, transmitted through C fibers, are localizable only very grossly, perhaps to a major part of the body such as a limb but certainly not to small areas. This is in keeping with the fact that these fibers terminate extremely diffusely in the hindbrain and thalamus.

Surgical Interruption of Pain Pathways. Often a person has such severe and intractable pain (this often results from rapidly spreading cancer) that it is necessary to relieve the pain. To do this the pain pathway can be destroyed at any one of several different points. If the pain is in the lower part of the body, a *cordotomy* in the upper thoracic region usually relieves the pain at least for a few months. To do this, the spinal cord on the side opposite to the pain is sectioned almost entirely through its anterolateral quadrant, which interrupts the spinothalamic tracts.

Unfortunately, though, the cordotomy is not always successful in relieving the pain for two reasons. First, many of the pain fibers from the upper part of the body do not cross to the opposite side of the spinal cord until they have reached the brain so that the cordotomy does not transsect these fibers. Second, pain frequently returns several months later; indeed, the new pain is often even more objectionable than the original pain. This pain presumably is transmitted in the dorsal half of the cord, but the locus and destination of the fiber pathways are unknown.

An experimental operative procedure to relieve pain is to place lesions in or around the pain-receptive areas of the thalamus to block the pain pathway at this point. It has been claimed that destruction of portions of the intralaminar nuclei in the thalamus can relieve the suffering elicited by pain while still leaving intact one's appreciation of the pricking quality of pain, which remains an important protective mechanism.

THE REACTION TO PAIN AND ITS CONTROL WITHIN THE NERVOUS SYSTEM

It has already been pointed out that the threshold for perceiving pain is determined by the sensitivity of the pain receptors themselves and that this threshold is approximately equal from one person to another. On the other hand, the degree to which each person reacts to pain varies tremendously. Also, the intensity of the pain signals transmitted up the spinal cord to the different pain-receptive areas of the brain can change tremendously under different conditions. This results mainly from activation of a pain inhibiting system, both in the spinal cord and in the brain, that we shall discuss shortly.

Pain causes both reflex motor reactions and psychic reactions. Some of the reflex actions occur in the spinal cord before the pain signals reach the brain, for pain impulses entering the gray matter of the cord can directly initiate "withdrawal reflexes" that remove the body or a portion of the body from the noxious stimulus, as will be discussed in Chapter 11. These primitive spinal cord reflexes, though important in lower animals, are mainly suppressed in the human being by the higher centers of the central nervous system. Yet, in their place, much more complicated and more effective reflexes from the brain are initiated by the pain signals to eliminate the painful stimulus.

The psychic reactions to pain are likely to be far more subtle; they include all the well-known aspects of pain such as anguish, anxiety, crying, depression, nausea, and excess muscular excitability throughout the body. These reactions vary tremendously from one person to another following comparable degrees of pain stimuli.

A PAIN CONTROL ("ANALGESIC") SYSTEM IN THE BRAIN AND SPINAL CORD

Electrical stimulation in several different areas of the brain and spinal cord can greatly reduce or almost block pain signals transmitted in the spinal cord. The most important areas from which this "stimulus-produced analgesia" can be produced include the *periventricular area of the diencephalon* immediately adjacent to the third ventricle, the *periaqueductal gray area* of the brain stem, the *midline raphe nuclei* of the brain stem, and to a lesser extent the *medial forebrain bundle*.

It is believed that this analgesia system operates in the following way: Stimulation in either the periventricular area of the diencephalon or the periaqueductal gray area transmits signals into the midline raphe nuclei. Then, from these nuclei, especially from the *raphe magnus nucleus* in the medulla, fiber tracts pass down the spinal cord to terminate in the dorsal horns, mainly in laminae I, II, and III. It will be recalled that this is the general area of the dorsal horns where the pain sensory fibers from the periphery terminate. It has been shown experimentally that stimulation of the analgesic system will block or suppress transmission of pain impulses through the local neurons of this dorsal horn pain receptive area, most of the block probably occurring in laminae II and III, which is the area called the *substantia gelatinosa*. Stimulation of this analgesic system will suppress pain transmitted by both the type A delta pain fibers and type C fibers as well, but it has almost no effect on the transmission of the other modalities of sensation.

It is very probable that this analgesic system also inhibits brain transmission at other points in the brain pathway, especially in the *reticular nuclei in the brain stem and in the intralaminar nuclei of the thalamus*.

The Brain's Opiate System – the Enkephalins and the Endorphins

A most remarkable research discovery 15 years ago was that injection of morphine in extremely minute quantities either in the periventricular area around the third ventricle of the diencephalon or in the periaqueductal gray area of the brain stem will cause an extreme degree of analgesia. It was immediately assumed that a specific neuronal membrane receptor substance existed in these areas for morphine or morphine-like substances. It was also postulated that substances similar to morphine must exist even normally within a brain analgesic system. This set off a long and intensive search for such morphine-like substances. Finally, only a few years ago two closely related types of compounds with morphine-like actions, called the *enkephalins* and the *endorphins*, were isolated. The enkephalins are found mainly in those areas of the brain associated with pain control, including the periventricular area, the periaqueductal gray, the midline raphe nuclei, the substantia gelatinosa of the dorsal horns in the spinal cord, and the intralaminar nuclei of the thalamus. The endor-

phins have been found in abundance in the hypothalamus and in the pituitary gland.

Therefore, it is now presumed that the enkephalins and the endorphins function as excitatory transmitter substances that activate portions of the brain's analgesic system. Also, infusion of either of these into the cerebrospinal fluid of the third ventricle can lead to analgesia.

Two different types of enkephalins, *met-enkephalin* and *leu-enkephalin*, are found at different points in the analgesic system. Though several different types of endorphins have been isolated, the one that is most potent and presumably most important is *β-endorphin*.

Inhibition of Pain Transmission at the Cord Level by Tactile Signals

Another important landmark in the saga of pain control was the discovery that stimulation of large sensory fibers from the peripheral tactile receptors depresses the transmission of pain signals either from the same area of the body or even from areas sometimes located many segments away. This explains why such simple maneuvers as rubbing the skin near painful areas is often very effective in relieving pain. And it probably also explains why liniments are often useful in the relief of pain. This mechanism and simultaneous psychogenic excitation of the central analgesic system are probably the basis of pain relief by acupuncture.

Treatment of Pain by Electrical Stimulation. Several clinical procedures have been developed recently for suppressing pain by stimulating large sensory nerve fibers. The stimulating electrodes are placed on selected areas of the skin, or on occasion they have been implanted over the spinal cord to stimulate the dorsal sensory columns. And, in a few patients, electrodes have even been placed stereotaxically in the periventricular area of the diencephalon. The patient can then personally control the degree of stimulation. Dramatic relief has been reported in some instances.

The Gating Theory for Pain Control

About a dozen years ago it was proposed that the dorsal horns of the spinal column function as *gates* for controlling entry of pain signals into the pain pathways. And, more specifically, it was proposed that pain signals are constantly balanced against tactile signals, each of these capable of inhibiting the other. It was reasoned that so long as there was excess tactile stimulation, the gates for transmission of pain would be closed, while in the absence of tactile stimulation, pain transmission is unimpeded.

In the intervening years, researchers have now shown that the precise neuronal circuitry proposed for the gating mechanism was mainly incorrect but that slightly different mechanisms for pain sensitivity control do indeed exist. These have been discussed above. Therefore, in a sense, a new concept of pain gating has now been developed, thus supervening the original gating concept but subserving the same function. Yet, it is probably better not to speak in terms of pain gating but instead of pain control.

REFERRED PAIN

Often a person feels pain in a part of his body that is considerably removed from the tissues causing the pain. This pain is called *referred pain*. Usually the pain is initiated in one of the visceral organs and referred to an area of the body surface. Also, pain may originate in a viscus and be referred to another deep area of the body not exactly coincident with the location of the viscus producing the pain. A knowledge of these different types of referred pain is extremely important in diagnosis because many visceral ailments cause no other signs except referred pain.

Mechanism of Referred Pain. Figure 10–5 illustrates the most likely mechanism by which most pain is referred. In the figure, branches of visceral pain fibers are shown to synapse in the spinal cord with some of the same second order neurons that receive pain fibers from the skin. When the visceral pain fibers are stimulated, pain signals from the viscera are then conducted through at least some of the same neurons that conduct pain signals from the skin, and the person has the feeling that the sensations actually originate in the skin itself.

REFERRED PAIN CAUSED BY REFLEX MUSCULAR SPASM

Some types of referred pain are caused secondarily by reflex muscular spasm. For instance, pain in a ureter can cause reflex spasm of the lumbar muscles. Often the

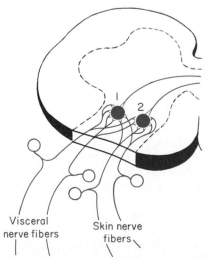

Figure 10–5. Mechanism of referred pain and referred hyperalgesia.

pain from the ureter itself is hardly felt at all, but instead almost all the pain results from spasm of the lumbar muscles.

Many back pains and some types of headache also appear to be caused by muscular spasm, the spasm originating reflexly from much weaker pain signals originating elsewhere in the body.

VISCERAL PAIN

In clinical diagnosis, pain from the different viscera of the abdomen and chest is one of the few criteria that can be used for diagnosing visceral inflammation, disease, and other ailments. In general, the viscera have sensory receptors for no other modalities of sensation besides pain. Also, visceral pain differs from surface pain in several important aspects.

One of the most important differences between surface pain and visceral pain is that highly localized types of damage to the viscera rarely cause severe pain. For instance, a surgeon can cut the gut entirely in two in a patient who is awake without causing significant pain. On the other hand, any stimulus that causes *diffuse stimulation of pain nerve endings* throughout a viscus causes pain that can be extremely severe. For instance, ischemia caused by occluding the blood supply to a large area of gut stimulates many diffuse pain fibers at the same time and can result in extreme pain.

CAUSES OF TRUE VISCERAL PAIN

Any stimulus that excites pain nerve endings in diffuse areas of the viscera causes visceral pain. Such stimuli include ischemia of visceral tissue, chemical damage to the surfaces of the viscera, spasm of the smooth muscle in a hollow viscus, distention of a hollow viscus, or stretching of the ligaments.

Essentially all the true visceral pain originating in the thoracic and abdominal cavities is transmitted through sensory nerve fibers that run in the sympathetic nerves. These fibers are small type C fibers and, therefore, can transmit only burning and aching types of pain. The pathways for transmitting true visceral pain will be discussed in more detail later in this chapter.

Ischemia. Ischemia causes visceral pain in exactly the same way that it does in other tissues, presumably because of the formation of acidic metabolic end-products or tissue degenerative products, such as bradykinin, proteolytic enzymes, or so forth that stimulate the pain nerve endings.

Chemical Stimuli. On occasion, damaging substances leak from the gastrointestinal tract into the peritoneal cavity. For instance, proteolytic acidic gastric juice often leaks through a ruptured gastric or duodenal ulcer. This juice causes widespread digestion of the visceral peritoneum, thus stimulating extremely broad areas of pain fibers. The pain is usually extremely severe.

Spasm of a Hollow Viscus. Spasm of the gut, the gallbladder, a bile duct, the ureter, or any other hollow viscus can cause pain in exactly the same way that spasm of skeletal muscle causes pain. This possibly results from mechanical stimulation of the pain endings. Or its cause might be diminished blood flow to the muscle combined with increased metabolic need of the muscle for nutrients. Thus, *relative* ischemia could develop, which causes severe pain.

Often, pain from a spastic viscus occurs in the form of *cramps*, the pain increasing to a high degree of severity and then subsiding, this process continuing rhythmically once every few minutes. The rhythmic cycles result from rhythmic contraction of smooth muscle. For instance, each time a peristaltic wave travels along an overly excitable spastic gut, a cramp occurs. The cramping type of pain frequently occurs in gastroenteritis, constipation, menstruation, parturition, gallbladder disease, or ureteral obstruction.

Overdistension of a Hollow Viscus. Extreme overfilling of a hollow viscus also results in pain, presumably because of overstretch of the tissues themselves. However, overdistension can also collapse the blood vessels that encircle the viscus, or that pass into its wall, thus perhaps promoting ischemic pain.

Insensitive Viscera

A few visceral areas are almost entirely insensitive to pain of any type. These include the parenchyma of the liver and the alveoli of the lungs. Yet the liver *capsule* is extremely sensitive to both direct trauma and stretch, and the *bile ducts* are also sensitive to pain. In the lungs, even though the alveoli are insensitive, the bronchi and the parietal pleura are both very sensitive to pain.

"PARIETAL" PAIN CAUSED BY VISCERAL DAMAGE

In addition to true visceral pain, some pain sensations are also transmitted from the viscera through nerve fibers that innervate the parietal peritoneum, pleura, or pericardium. The parietal surfaces of the visceral cavities are supplied mainly by spinal nerve fibers that penetrate from the surface of the body inward.

Characteristics of Parietal Visceral Pain. When a disease affects a viscus, it often spreads to the parietal wall of the visceral cavity. This wall, like the skin, is supplied with extensive innervation from the spinal nerves, not from the sympathetic nerves, including the "fast" delta fibers which are different from only "slow" type C fibers in the true visceral pain pathways of the sympathetic nerves. Therefore, pain from the parietal wall of the visceral cavity is frequently very sharp and pricking in quality, though it can also have burning and aching qualities as well if the pain stimulus is diffuse. To emphasize the difference between this pain and true visceral pain, a knife incision through the *parietal* peritoneum is very painful, even though a similar cut through the visceral peritoneum or through a gut is not painful.

LOCALIZATION OF VISCERAL PAIN — THE "VISCERAL" AND THE "PARIETAL" TRANSMISSION PATHWAYS

Pain from the different viscera is frequently difficult to localize for a number of reasons. First, the brain does not know from firsthand experience that the different organs exist, and, therefore, any pain that originates internally can be localized only generally. Second, sensations from the abdomen and thorax are transmitted by two separate pathways to the central nervous system — the *true visceral pathway* and the *parietal pathway*. The true visceral pain is transmitted via sensory fibers of the autonomic nervous system, and the sensations are *referred* to surface areas of the body often far from the painful organ. On the other hand, parietal sensations are conducted *directly* from the parietal peritoneum, pleura, or pericardium, and the sensations are usually *localized directly over the painful area*.

The True Visceral Pathway for Transmission of Pain. Most of the internal organs of the body are supplied by type C pain fibers that pass along the visceral sympathetic nerves into the spinal cord and thence up the anterolateral spinothalamic tract along with the pain fibers from the body's surface. A few visceral pain fibers — those from the distal portion of the colon, from the rectum, and from the bladder — enter the spinal cord through the sacral parasympathetic nerves, and some enter the central nervous system through various cranial nerves. These include fibers in the glossopharyngeal and vagus nerves which transmit pain from the pharynx, trachea, and upper esophagus. Some fibers from the surfaces of the diaphragm as well as from the lower esophagus are also carried in the phrenic nerves.

Localization of Referred Pain Transmitted by the Visceral Pathways. The position in the cord to which visceral afferent fibers pass from each organ depends on the segment of the body from which the organ developed embryologically. For instance, the heart originated in the neck and upper thorax. Consequently, the heart's visceral pain fibers enter the cord all the way from C-3 down to T-5. The stomach had its origin approximately from the seventh to the ninth thoracic segments of the embryo, and consequently the visceral afferents from the stomach enter the spinal cord between these levels. The gallbladder had its origin almost entirely in the ninth thoracic segment, so that the visceral afferents from the gallbladder enter the spinal cord at T-9.

Because the visceral afferent pain fibers are responsible for transmitting referred pain from the viscera, the location of the referred pain on the surface of the body is in the dermatome of the segment from which the visceral organ was originally derived in the embryo. Some of the areas of referred pain on the surface of the body are shown in Figure 10–6.

The Parietal Pathway for Transmission of Abdominal and Thoracic Pain. A second set of pain fibers penetrates inward from the spinal nerves to innervate the parietal peritoneum, parietal pleura, and parietal pericardium. Also, retroperitoneal visceral organs and perhaps portions of the mesentery are innervated to some extent by parietal pain fibers. The kidney, for instance, is supplied by both visceral and parietal fibers.

Pain from the viscera is frequently localized to two surface areas of the body at the same time because of the dual pathways for transmission of pain. Figure 10–7 illustrates dual transmission of pain from an inflamed appendix. Impulses pass from the appendix through the sympathetic visceral pain fibers into the sympathetic chain and then into the spinal cord at approximately T-10 or T-11; this pain is referred to an area around the umbilicus and is of the aching, cramping type. On the other hand, pain impulses also often originate in

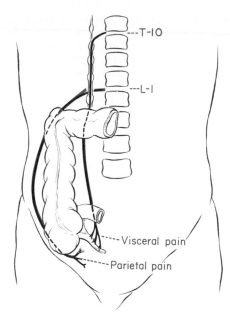

Figure 10–7. Visceral and parietal transmission of pain from the appendix.

the parietal peritoneum where the inflamed appendix touches the abdominal wall, and these impulses pass through the spinal nerves into the spinal cord at a level of approximately L-1 or L-2. This pain is localized directly over the irritated peritoneum in the right lower quadrant of the abdomen and is of the sharp type.

VISCERAL PAIN FROM VARIOUS ORGANS

Cardiac Pain. Almost all pain that originates in the heart results from ischemia secondary to coronary atherosclerosis caused by fat deposits. This pain is referred mainly to the base of the neck, over the shoulders, over the pectoral muscles, and down the arms. Most frequently, the referred pain is on the left side rather than on the right — probably because the left side of the heart is much more frequently involved in coronary disease than is the right side — but occasionally referred pain occurs on the right side of the body as well as on the left.

The pain impulses are conducted through sympathetic nerves passing to the middle cervical ganglia, to the stellate ganglia, and to the first four or five thoracic ganglia of the sympathetic chains. Then the impulses pass into the spinal cord through the second, third, fourth and fifth thoracic spinal nerves.

Direct Parietal Pain from the Heart. When coronary ischemia is extremely severe, such as immediately after a coronary thrombosis, intense cardiac pain frequently occurs directly underneath the sternum simultaneously with pain referred to other areas. This direct pain from underneath the sternum is difficult to explain on the basis of the visceral nerve connections. Therefore, it is highly probable that sensory nerve endings passing from the heart through the pericardial reflections around the great vessels conduct this direct pain.

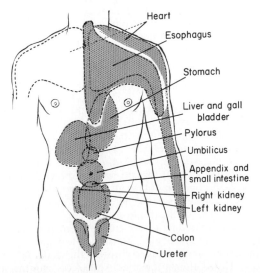

Figure 10–6. Surface areas of referred pain from different visceral organs.

In addition to pain from the heart, other sensations may accompany coronary thrombosis. One of these is a tight, oppressive sensation beneath the sternum. The exact cause of this is unknown, but a possible cause is reflex spasm of blood vessels, bronchioles, or muscles in the chest region.

Relief of Referred Cardiac Pain by Sympathectomy. To interrupt pain impulses from the heart one can either cut the sympathetic nerves that pass from the heart to the sympathetic chains or, as is usually performed, cut nerve fibers as they pass through the sympathetic chains into the spinal cord. Relief of cardiac pain can frequently be accomplished simply by removing the sympathetic chain from T-2 through T-5 on only the left side, but sometimes it is necessary to remove the fibers on both sides in order to obtain satisfactory results.

Esophageal Pain. Pain from the esophagus is usually referred to the pharynx, to the lower neck, to the arms, or to midline chest regions beginning at the upper portion of the sternum and ending approximately at the lower level of the heart. Irritation of the gastric end of the esophagus may cause pain directly over the heart, though the pain has nothing whatever to do with the heart. Such pain may be caused by spasm of the cardia, the area where the esophagus empties into the stomach, which causes excessive dilatation of the lower esophagus, or it may result from chemical, bacterial, or other types of inflammatory irritations.

Gastric Pain. Pain arising in the fundus of the stomach — usually caused by gastritis — is referred to the anterior surface of the chest or upper abdomen, from slightly below the heart to an inch or so below the xyphoid process. This pain is frequently characterized as burning pain; it, or pain from the lower esophagus, causes the condition known as "heartburn."

Most peptic ulcers occur within 1 to 2 inches on either side of the pylorus in the stomach or in the duodenum, and pain from such ulcers is usually referred to a surface point approximately midway between the umbilicus and the xiphoid process. The cause of ulcer pain is almost undoubtedly chemical, because when the acid juices of the stomach are not allowed to reach the pain fibers in the ulcer crater the pain does not exist. This pain is characteristically intensely burning.

Biliary and Gallbladder Pain. Pain from the bile ducts and gallbladder is localized in the midepigastrium almost coincident with pains caused by peptic ulcers. Also, biliary and gallbladder pain is often burning, like that from ulcers, though cramps often occur too.

Biliary disease, in addition to causing pain on the abdominal surface, frequently refers pain to a small area at the tip of the right scapula. This pain is transmitted through sympathetic afferent fibers that enter the ninth thoracic segment of the spinal cord.

Pancreatic Pain. Lesions of the pancreas, such as acute or chronic pancreatitis in which the pancreatic enzymes eat away the pancreas and surrounding structures, promote intense pain in areas both anterior to and behind the pancreas. It should be remembered that the pancreas is located beneath the parietal peritoneum and that it receives many parietal sensory fibers from the posterior abdominal wall. Therefore, the pain is usually localized directly behind the pancreas in the back and is severe and burning in character.

Renal Pain. The kidney, kidney pelvis, and ureters are all retroperitoneal structures and receive most of their pain fibers directly from skeletal nerves. Therefore, pain is usually felt directly behind the ailing structure. However, pain occasionally is referred via visceral afferents to the anterior abdominal wall below and about 2 inches to the side of the umbilicus.

Pain from the bladder is felt directly over the bladder, presumably because the bladder is well innervated by parietal pain fibers. However, pain also is sometimes referred to the groin and testicles because some nerve fibers from the bladder apparently synapse in the cord in association with fibers from the genital areas.

Uterine Pain. Both parietal and visceral afferent pain may be transmitted from the uterus. The low abdominal cramping pains of dysmenorrhea are mediated through the sympathetic afferents, and an operation to cut the hypogastric nerves between the hypogastric plexus and the uterus will in many instances relieve this pain. On the other hand, lesions of the uterus that spread into the adnexa around the uterus, or lesions of the fallopian tubes and broad ligaments, usually cause pain in the lower back or side. This pain is conducted over parietal nerve fibers and is usually sharper in nature rather than the diffuse cramping pain of true dysmenorrhea.

SOME CLINICAL ABNORMALITIES OF PAIN AND OTHER SENSATIONS

HYPERALGESIA

A pain pathway may become excessively excitable; this gives rise to hyperalgesia, which means hypersensitivity to pain. The basic causes of hyperalgesia are: (1) excessive sensitivity of the pain receptors themselves, which is called *primary hyperalgesia,* and (2) facilitation of sensory transmission, which is called *secondary hyperalgesia.*

An example of primary hyperalgesia is the extreme sensitivity of sunburned skin. Secondary hyperalgesia frequently results from lesions in the spinal cord or in the thalamus. Several of these will be discussed in subsequent sections.

THE THALAMIC SYNDROME

Occasionally the posterolateral branch of the posterior cerebral artery, a small artery supplying the posteroventral portion of the thalamus, becomes blocked by thrombosis so that the nuclei of this area of the thalamus degenerate, while the medial and anterior nuclei of the thalamus remain intact. The patient suffers a series of abnormalities, as follows: First, loss of almost all sensations from the opposite side of the body occurs because of destruction of the relay nuclei. Second, ataxia (inability to control movements precisely) may be evident because of loss of position and kinesthetic signals normally relayed through the thalamus to the cortex. Third, after a few weeks to a few months some sensory perception in the opposite side of the body returns, but strong stimuli are usually necessary to elicit this. When the sensations do occur, they are poorly —if at all — localized, almost always very painful, sometimes lancinating, regardless of the type of stimulus applied to the body. Fourth, the person is likely to perceive many affective sensations of extreme unpleasantness or, rarely, extreme pleasantness; the unpleasant ones are often associated with emotional tirades.

The medial nuclei of the thalamus are not destroyed by thrombosis of the artery. Therefore, it is believed that these nuclei become facilitated and give rise to the enhanced sensitivity to pain transmitted through the reticular system as well as to the affective perceptions.

HERPES ZOSTER

Occasionally a virus that is believed to be identical to the chickenpox virus infects a dorsal root ganglion. This causes severe pain in the dermatomal segment normally subserved by the ganglion, thus eliciting a segmental type of pain that circles halfway around the body. The disease is called herpes zoster, and the pain is commonly called "shingles."

There are two possible causes of the pain of herpes zoster. One is that the disease destroys mainly the large mechanoreceptor afferent sensory fibers. This theoretically could reduce the normal inhibitory effect of these fibers on the pain pathway in the substantia gelatinosa of the dorsal horn. Therefore, pain signals could become exacerbated in the absence of this inhibition.

A second possibility is that the irritated neuronal cell bodies of the root ganglion are stimulated to excessive activity and thereby cause the pain.

TIC DOULOUREUX

Lancinating pains occur in some persons over one side of the face in part of the sensory distribution area of the fifth or ninth nerves; this phenomenon is called tic douloureux (or trigeminal neuralgia or glossopharyngeal neuralgia). The pains feel like sudden electric shocks, and they may appear for only a few seconds at a time or they may be almost continuous. Often, they are set off by exceedingly sensitive "trigger areas" on the surface of the face, in the mouth or in the throat — almost always by a mechanoreceptive stimulus instead of a pain stimulus. For instance, when the patient swallows a bolus of food, as the food touches a tonsil it might set off a severe lancinating pain in the mandibular portion of the fifth nerve.

The pain of tic douloureux can usually be blocked by cutting the peripheral nerve from the hypersensitive area. The sensory portion of the fifth nerve is often sectioned immediately inside the cranium, where the motor and sensory roots of the fifth nerve can be separated so that the motor portions, which are needed for many of the jaw movements, are spared while the sensory elements are destroyed. Obviously, this operation leaves the side of the face anesthetic, which in itself may be annoying. Furthermore, it is sometimes unsuccessful, indicating that the lesion might be more central than the nerves themselves.

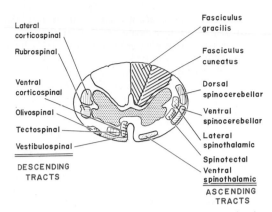

Figure 10–8. Cross-section of the spinal cord, showing principal ascending tracts on the right and principal descending tracts on the left.

THE BROWN-SEQUARD SYNDROME

Obviously, if the spinal cord is transected entirely, all sensations and motor functions distal to the segments of transection are blocked, but if only one side of the spinal cord is transected, the so-called Brown-Séquard syndrome occurs. The following effects of such a transection occur, and these can be predicted from a knowledge of the cord fiber tracts illustrated in Figure 10–8: All motor functions are blocked on the side of the transection in all segments below the level of the transection; yet, only some of the modalities of sensation are lost on the transected side and others are lost on the opposite side. The sensations of pain, heat, and cold are lost on the opposite side of the body in all dermatomes two to six segments below the level of the transection. The sensations that are transmitted only in the dorsal and dorsolateral columns — kinesthetic and position sensations, vibration sensation, discrete localization, and two-point discrimination — are lost entirely on the side of the transection in all dermatomes below the level of the transection. Touch is impaired on the side of the transection because the principal pathway for transmission of light touch, the dorsal columns, is transected. Yet, "crude touch," which is poorly localized, still persists because of transmission in the opposite ventral spinothalamic tract.

HEADACHE

Headaches are actually referred pain to the surface of the head from the deep structures. Many headaches result from pain stimuli arising inside the cranium, but equally as many probably result from pain arising outside the cranium.

HEADACHE OF INTRACRANIAL ORIGIN

Pain-Sensitive Areas in the Cranial Vault. The brain itself is almost totally insensitive to pain. Even cutting or electrically stimulating the somesthetic centers of the cortex only occasionally causes pain; instead, it causes tactile paresthesias on the area of the body represented by the portion of the somesthetic cortex stimulated. Therefore, it is obvious from the outset that much or most of the pain of headache probably is not caused by damage within the brain itself.

On the other hand, *tugging on the venous sinuses, damaging the tentorium,* or *stretching the dura at the base of the brain* can all cause intense pain that is recognized as headache. Also, almost any type of traumatizing, crushing, or stretching stimulus to the *blood vessels of the dura* can cause headache. A very sensitive structure is the middle meningeal artery, and neurosurgeons are careful to anesthetize this artery specifically when performing brain operations under local anesthesia.

Areas of the Head to Which Intracranial Headache Is Referred. Stimulation of pain receptors in the intracranial vault above the tentorium, including the upper surface of the tentorium itself, initiates impulses in the fifth nerve and, therefore, causes referred headache to the front half of the head in the area supplied by the fifth cranial nerve, as illustrated in Figure 10–9.

On the other hand, pain impulses from beneath the tentorium enter the central nervous system mainly through the second cervical nerve, which also supplies the scalp behind the ear. Therefore, subtentorial pain stimuli cause "occipital headache" referred to the posterior part of the head as shown in Figure 10–9.

Types of Intracranial Headache. *Headache of Meningitis.* One of the most severe headaches of all is that resulting from meningitis, which causes inflammation of all the meninges, including the sensitive areas of the dura and the sensitive areas around the venous sinuses. Such intense damage as this can cause extreme headache pain referred over the entire head.

Headache Resulting from Direct Meningeal Trauma. Following a brain operation the patient ordinarily has intense headache for several days to several weeks. Though part of this headache may result from the brain trauma, experiments indicate that most of it results from meningeal irritation.

Another type of meningeal trauma that almost invariably causes headache is the meningeal irritation resulting from brain tumor. Usually, tumor headache is referred to a localized area of the head, the exact area depending on the portion of the meninges affected by the tumor. Since a tumor above the tentorium is likely to refer its pain to the front half of the head and any tumor below the tentorium to the occipital region of the skull, the general location of an intracranial tumor can often be predicted from the area of the headache.

Headache Caused by Low Cerebrospinal Fluid Pressure. Removing as little as 20 ml. of fluid from the spinal canal, particularly if the person remains in the upright position, often causes intense intracranial headache. Removing this quantity of fluid removes the flotation for the brain that is normally provided by the cerebrospinal fluid. Therefore, the weight of the brain stretches the various dural surfaces and thereby elicits the pain which causes the headache.

Migraine Headache. Migraine headache is a special type of headache that is thought to result from abnormal vascular phenomena, though the exact mechanism is unknown.

Migraine headaches often begin with various prodromal sensations, such as nausea, loss of vision in part of the field of vision, visual aura, or other types of sensory hallucinations. Ordinarily, the prodromal symptoms begin half an hour to an hour prior to the beginning of the headache itself. Therefore, any theory that explains migraine headache must also explain these prodromal symptoms.

One of the theories of the cause of migraine headaches is that prolonged emotion or tension causes reflex vasospasm of some of the arteries of the head, including arteries that supply the brain itself. The vasospasm theoretically produces ischemia of portions of the brain, and this is responsible for the prodromal symptoms. Then, as a result of the intense ischemia, something happens to the vascular wall to allow it to become flaccid and incapable of maintaining vascular tone for 24 to 48 hours. The blood pressure in the vessels causes them to dilate and pulsate intensely, and it is supposedly the excessive stretching of the walls of the arteries — including the extracranial arteries such as the temporal artery — that causes the actual pain of migraine headaches. However, it is possible that diffuse after-effects of ischemia in the brain itself are at least partially responsible for this type of headache.

Alcoholic Headache. As many people have experienced, a headache usually follows an alcoholic binge. It is most likely that alcohol, because it is toxic to tissues, directly irritates the meninges and causes intracranial pain.

Headache Caused by Constipation. Constipation causes headache in many persons. Because it has been shown that constipation headache can occur in persons whose spinal cords have been cut, we know that this headache is not caused by nervous impulses from the colon. Therefore, it possibly results from absorbed toxic products or from changes in the circulatory system. Indeed, constipation sometimes does cause temporary loss of plasma into the wall of the gut, and a resulting poor flow of blood to the head could be the cause of the headache.

EXTRACRANIAL TYPES OF HEADACHE

Headache Resulting from Muscular Spasm. Emotional tension often causes many of the muscles of the

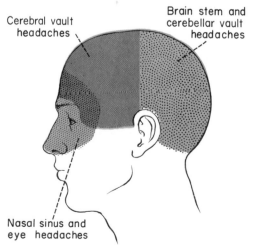

Cerebral vault headaches

Brain stem and cerebellar vault headaches

Nasal sinus and eye headaches

Figure 10–9. Areas of headache resulting from different causes.

head, including especially those muscles attached to the scalp and the neck muscles attached to the occiput, to become spastic, and it is postulated that this is one of the most common causes of headache. The pain of the spastic head muscles supposedly is referred to the overlying areas of the head and gives one the same type of headache as do intracranial lesions.

Headache Caused by Irritation of the Nasal and Accessory Nasal Structures. The mucous membranes of the nose and also of all the nasal sinuses are sensitive to pain, but not intensely so. Nevertheless, infection or other irritative processes in widespread areas of the nasal structures usually cause headache that is referred behind the eyes or, in the case of frontal sinus infection, to the frontal surfaces of the forehead and scalp, as illustrated in Figure 10–9. Also, pain from the lower sinuses — such as the maxillary sinuses — can be felt in the face.

Headache Caused by Eye Disorders. Difficulty in focusing one's eyes clearly may cause excessive contraction of the ciliary muscles in an attempt to gain clear vision. Even though these muscles are extremely small, tonic contraction of them can be the cause of retro-orbital headache. Also, excessive attempts to focus the eyes can result in reflex spasm in various facial and extraocular muscles. Tonic spasm in these muscles is also a possible cause of headache.

A second type of headache originating in the eyes occurs when the eyes are exposed to excessive irradiation by ultraviolet light rays. Watching the sun or the arc of an arc-welder for even a few seconds may result in headache that lasts from 24 to 48 hours. The headache sometimes results from "actinic" irritation of the conjunctivae, and the pain is referred to the surface of the head or retro-orbitally. However, focusing intense light from an arc or the sun on the retina can actually burn the retina, and this could result in headache.

THERMAL SENSATIONS

THERMAL RECEPTORS AND THEIR EXCITATION

The human being can perceive different gradations of cold and heat, progressing from *freezing cold* to *cold* to *cool* to *indifferent* to *warm* to *hot* to *burning hot*.

Thermal gradations are discriminated by at least three different types of sensory receptors: the cold receptors, the warmth receptors, and two sub-types of pain receptors, cold-pain receptors and warmth-pain receptors. The two types of pain receptors are stimulated only by extreme degrees of heat or cold and therefore are responsible, along with the cold and warmth receptors, for "freezing cold" and "burning hot" sensations.

The cold and warmth receptors are located immediately under the skin at discrete but separated points, each having a stimulatory diameter of about 1 mm. In most areas of the body there are 3 to 4 times as many cold receptors as warmth receptors, and the number varies from as great as 15 to 25 cold points per square centimeter in the lips, to 3 to 5 cold points per square centimeter in the finger, and to less than 1 cold point per square centimeter in some broad surface areas of the body — and correspondingly fewer numbers of warmth points.

Though it is quite certain on the basis of psychological tests that there are distinctive warmth nerve endings, these have not yet been identified histologically. They are presumed to be free nerve endings because warmth signals are transmitted over type C nerve fibers at transmission velocities of only 0.4 to 2 meters per second.

On the other hand, a definitive cold receptor has been identified. It is a special, small, type A delta myelinated nerve ending that branches a number of times, the tips of which protrude into the bottom surfaces of basal epidermal cells. Signals are transmitted from these receptors via the delta nerve fibers at velocities up to about 20 meters per second. However, cold sensations are also transmitted in type C nerve fibers, which suggests that some free nerve endings also might function as cold receptors.

Stimulation of Thermal Receptors — Sensations of Cold, Cool, Indifferent, Warm, and Hot. Figure 10–10 illustrates the effects of different temperatures on the responses of four different types of nerve fibers: (1) a cold-pain fiber, (2) a cold fiber, (3) a warmth fiber, and (4) a heat-pain fiber. Note especially that these fibers respond differently at different levels of temperature. For instance, in the *very* cold region only the cold-pain fibers are stimulated (if the skin becomes even colder so that it nearly freezes or actually does freeze, even these fibers cannot be stimulated). As the temperature rises to 10 to 15° C., pain impulses cease, but the cold receptors begin to be stimulated. Then, above about 30° C. the warmth receptors become stimulated while the cold recep-

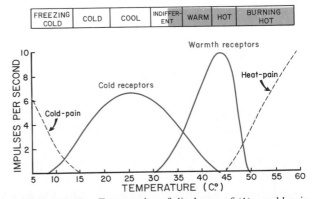

Figure 10–10. Frequencies of discharge of (1) a cold-pain fiber, (2) a cold fiber, (3) a warmth fiber, and (4) a heat-pain fiber. (The responses of these fibers are drawn from original data collected in separate experiments by Zotterman, Hensel, and Kenshalo.)

tors fade out at about 43° C. Finally, at around 45° C., the heat-pain fibers begin to be stimulated.

One can understand from Figure 10–10, therefore, that a person determines the different gradations of thermal sensations by the relative degrees of stimulation of the different types of endings. For instance, at 20° C. only cold endings are stimulated, whereas at 44° C. only warm endings are stimulated; at 35° C. both cold and warm endings are stimulated, and at 60° C. both cold and pain endings are stimulated. One can understand also from this figure why extreme degrees of cold or heat can be painful and why both these sensations, when intense enough, may give almost exactly the same quality of sensations — that is, freezing cold and burning hot sensations feel almost alike; they are both very painful.

Stimulatory Effects of Rising and Falling Temperature — Adaptation of Thermal Receptors. When a cold receptor is suddenly subjected to an abrupt fall in temperature, it becomes strongly stimulated at first, but this stimulation fades rapidly during the first few seconds and progressively more slowly during the next half hour or more. In other words, the receptor adapts to a very great extent; this is illustrated in Figure 10–11, which shows that the frequency of discharge of a cold receptor rose approximately four-fold when the temperature fell suddenly from 32° to 30° C., but in less than a minute the frequency fell about five sixths of the way back to the original control value. Later, the temperature was suddenly raised from 30° to 32° C. The cold receptor stopped firing entirely for a short time, but after adapting returned to its original control level.

Thus, it is evident that the thermal senses respond markedly to *changes in temperature* in addition to being able to respond to steady states of temperature, as was depicted in Figure 10–10.

This means, therefore, that when the temperature of the skin is actively falling, a person feels much colder than when the temperature remains at the same level. Conversely, if the temperature is actively rising the person feels much warmer than he would at the same temperature if it were constant.

The response to changes in temperature explains the extreme degree of heat that one feels on first entering a tub of hot water and the extreme degree of cold felt on going from a heated room to the out-of-doors on a cold day. The adaptation of the thermal senses explains the ability of the person to become accustomed to the new temperature environment.

Mechanism of Stimulation of the Thermal Receptors. It is believed that the thermal receptors are stimulated by changes in their metabolic rates, these changes resulting from the fact that temperature alters the rates of intracellular chemical reactions about 2 times for each 10° C. change. In other words, thermal detection probably results not from direct physical stimulation but instead from chemical stimulation of the endings as modified by the temperature.

Spatial Summation of Thermal Sensations. Because the number of cold or warmth endings in any one surface area of the body is very slight, it is difficult to judge gradations of temperature when small areas are stimulated. However, when a large area of the body is stimulated all at once, the thermal signals from the entire area summate. Indeed, one reaches the maximum ability to discern minute temperature variations when the entire body is subjected to a temperature change all at once. For instance, rapid changes in temperature as little as 0.01° C. can be detected if this change affects the entire surface of the body simultaneously. On the other hand, temperature changes 100 times this great might not be detected when the skin surface affected is only a square centimeter or so in size.

TRANSMISSION OF THERMAL SIGNALS IN THE NERVOUS SYSTEM

In general, thermal signals are transmitted in almost exactly the same pathways as pain signals. On entering the spinal cord, the signals travel for a few segments upward or downward in the *tract of Lissauer* and then terminate mainly in laminae I, II, and III of the dorsal horns. After a small amount of processing by one or more cord neurons, the signals enter long, ascending thermal fibers that cross to the opposite anterolateral spinothalamic tract and terminate in (a) the reticular areas of the brain stem, (b) the ventrobasal complex of the thalamus, and perhaps (c) in the intralaminar nuclei of the thalamus along with pain

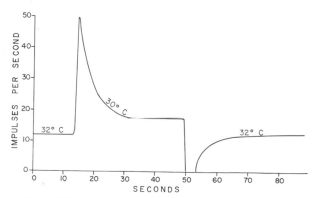

Figure 10–11. Response of a nerve fiber from a cold receptor following, first, instantaneous change in skin temperature from 32° to 30°C. and, second, instantaneous change back to 32°C. Note the adaptation of the receptor and also the higher steady state level of discharge at 30° than at 32°.

signals. A few thermal signals are also relayed to the somesthetic cortex from the ventrobasal complex. Occasionally, a neuron in somatic sensory area I has been found by microelectrode studies to be directly responsive to either cold or warm stimuli in specific areas of the skin. Furthermore, it is known that removal of the postcentral gyrus in the human being reduces the ability to distinguish different gradations of temperature.

REFERENCES

Also see bibliographies following Chapters 7, 8, and 9.

Beaumont, A., and Hughes, J.: Biology of opioid peptides. *Annu. Rev. Pharmacol. Toxicol., 19*:245, 1979.

Bonica, J. J. (ed.): International Symposium on Pain. New York, Raven Press, 1974.

Bonica, J. J., *et al.*: Recent Advances in Pain. Springfield, Ill., Charles C Thomas, 1974.

Bonica. J. J., *et al.* (eds.): Proceedings of the Second World Congress on Pain. New York, Raven Press, 1979.

Brainard, J. B.: Control of Migraine. New York, W. W. Norton & Co., 1979.

Bresler, D. E., and Trubo, R.: Freedom from Pain. New York, Simon and Schuster, 1979.

Casey, K. L.: Pain: A current view of neural mechanisms. *Am. Sci., 61*:194, 1973.

Coren, S., *et al.*: Sensation and Perception. New York, Academic Press, 1979.

Currie, D. J.: Abdominal Pain. Washington, D.C., Hemisphere Publishing Corporation, 1979.

Dalessio, D. J.: Wolff's Headache and Other Head Pain, 3rd Ed. New York, Oxford University Press, 1972.

Fairley, P.: The Conquest of Pain. New York, Charles Scribner's Sons, 1979.

Fields, H. L., and Bashbaum, A. I.: Brainstem control of spinal pain-transmission neurons. *Annu. Rev. Physiol., 40*:217, 1978.

Goldstein, E. B.: Sensation and Perception. Belmont, Cal., Wadsworth Publishing Co., 1980.

Greep, J. M., *et al.* (eds): Pain in Shoulder and Arm. Hingham, Mass., Kluwer Boston, 1979.

Guyton, A. C., and Reeder, R. C.: Pain and contracture in poliomyelitis. *Arch. Neurol. Psychiatr., 63*:954, 1950.

Hardy, J. D.: The nature of pain. *J. Chronic Dis., 4*:22, 1956.

Hardy, J. D., *et al.*: Pain Sensations and Reactions. Baltimore, Williams & Wilkins, 1952.

Herz, A. (ed.): Developments in Opiate Research. New York, Marcel Dekker, 1978.

Hewer, C. L., and Atkinson, R. S. (eds.): Recent Advances in Anaesthesia and Analgesia. Boston, Little, Brown, 1978.

Jacob, J. (ed.): Receptors, New York, Pergamon Press, 1979.

Kenshalo, D. R. (ed.): Sensory Function of the Skin of Humans. New York, Plenum Press, 1979.

Leroy, P. L., *et al.* (eds.): Current Concepts in the Management of Chronic Pain. Miami, Symposia Specialists, 1977.

Lipton, S. (ed.): Persistent Pain: Modern Methods of Treatment. New York, Grune & Stratton, 1977.

Livingston, W. K.: Pain Mechanisms: A Physiologic Interpretation of Causalgia and Its Related States. Wilmington, Del., International Academic Publishers, 1979.

Newman, P. O.: Visceral Afferent Functions of the Nervous System. Monograph of the Physiological Society, No. 25. Baltimore, Williams & Wilkins, 1974.

Perl, E. R., and Boivie, J. G.: Neural substrates of somatic sensation. *In* MTP International Review of Science: Physiology. Vol. 3. Baltimore, University Park Press, 1974, p. 303.

Raskin, N. H., and Appenzeller, O.: Headache. Philadelphia, W. B. Saunders Co., 1980.

Ryan, R. E., and Ryan, R. E., Jr. (eds.): Headache and Head Pain: Diagnosis and Treatment. St. Louis, C. V. Mosby, 1978.

Seltzer, S.: Pain in Dentistry: Diagnosis and Management. Philadelphia, J. B. Lippincott Co., 1978.

Silen, W. (rev.): Cope's Early Diagnosis of the Acute Abdomen. New York, Oxford University Press, 1979.

Simon, E. J., and Hiller, J. M.: The opiate receptors. *Annu. Rev. Pharmacol. Toxicol., 18*:371, 1978.

Snyder, S. H.: Opiate receptors and internal opiates. Sci. Am. *236*(3): 44, 1977.

Snyder, S. H., and Childres, S. R.: Opiate receptors and opioid peptides. *Annu. Rev. Neurosci., 2*:35, 1979.

Swerdlow, M.: Relief of Intractable Pain. New York, American Elsevier Publishing Co., 1974.

Wilson, M. E.: The neurological mechanisms of pain. A review. *Anaesthesia, 29*:407, 1974.

Zimmerman, M.: Neurophysiology of nociception. *Int. Rev. Physiol., 10*:179, 1976.

11

Motor Functions of the Spinal Cord and the Cord Reflexes

In the discussion of the nervous system thus far, we have considered principally the input of sensory information. In the following chapters we will discuss the origin and output of motor signals, the signals that cause muscle contraction and other motor effects throughout the body. Sensory information is integrated at all levels of the nervous system and causes appropriate motor responses, beginning in the spinal cord with relatively simple reflexes, extending into the brain stem with still more complicated responses, and, finally, extending to the cerebrum where the most complicated responses are controlled. The present chapter discusses the control of motor function especially in response to spinal cord reflexes.

Experimental Preparations for Studying Cord Reflexes — The Spinal Animal and the Decerebrate Animal. Normally the functions of the spinal cord are strongly controlled by signals from the brain. Therefore, to study the isolated cord reflexes it is necessary to separate the cord from the higher centers. This is usually done in one of two different types of preparations: (1) the *spinal animal* or (2) the *decerebrate animal.*

The spinal animal is prepared by cutting the spinal cord at any level above the region in which the cord reflexes are to be studied. For a variable period of time, depending upon the phylogenetic level of the animal, as will be discussed later in the chapter, the cord reflexes are deeply depressed immediately after removal of the signals from the brain. However, over a period of minutes, hours, or days in animals and over a period of weeks in the human being, the cord reflexes become progressively more active and can then be studied independently of control by the upper levels of the nervous system. Often the cord reflexes become even more excitable under these conditions than normally.

In the decerebrate preparation, the brain stem is usually transected between the superior and inferior colliculi. Transecting the brain stem at this level removes the voluntary control centers of the forebrain, and it also removes inhibitory influences from the basal ganglia that normally suppress the activities of the lower brain stem and spinal cord; this will be discussed in detail in the following chapter. Removal of this inhibi-

tion causes an immediate increase in the activity of many of the cord reflexes, especially the extensor reflexes that help the animal hold itself up against gravity. This preparation has an advantage over the spinal animal in that many of the cord reflexes are exacerbated even in the acute preparation and, therefore, can be studied immediately, though, of course, lower brain stem reflexes may still interfere with the cord functions.

ORGANIZATION OF THE SPINAL CORD FOR MOTOR FUNCTIONS

The cord gray matter is the integrative area for the cord reflexes and other motor functions. Figure 11–1 shows the typical organization of the cord gray matter in a single cord segment. Sensory signals enter the cord through the sensory roots. After entering the cord, every sensory signal travels to two separate destinations. First, either in the same segment of the cord or in nearby segments, the sensory nerve or its collaterals terminate in the gray matter of the cord and elicit local segmental

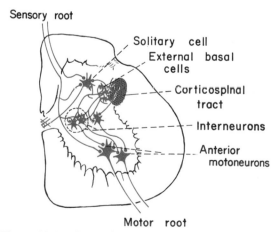

Figure 11–1. Connections of the sensory fibers and corticospinal fibers with the interneurons and anterior motoneurons of the spinal cord.

responses — local excitatory effects, facilitatory effects, reflexes, and so forth. Second, the signals travel to higher levels of the nervous system — to higher levels in the cord itself, to the brain stem, or even to the cerebral cortex. It is these sensory signals that cause the conscious sensory experiences described in the past few chapters.

Each segment of the spinal cord has several million neurons in its gray matter. Aside from the sensory relay neurons already discussed, these neurons are divided into two separate types, the *anterior motoneurons* and the *interneurons* (also called *internuncial cells*).

The Anterior Motoneurons. Located in each segment of the anterior horns of the cord gray matter are several thousand neurons that are 50 to 100 per cent larger than most of the others and are called *anterior motoneurons*. These give rise to the nerve fibers that leave the cord via the anterior roots and innervate the skeletal muscle fibers. The fibers are of two types, the *alpha motoneurons* and the *gamma motoneurons*.

The Alpha Motoneurons. The alpha motoneurons give rise to large, type A alpha ($A\alpha$) nerve fibers ranging from 9 to 20 microns in diameter and passing through the spinal nerves to innervate the skeletal muscle fibers. Stimulation of a single nerve fiber excites from 3 to 2000 skeletal muscle fibers which are collectively called the *motor unit*. Transmission of nerve impulses into skeletal muscles and their stimulation of the muscle fibers were discussed in Chapters 2 through 4.

The Gamma Motoneurons. In addition to the alpha motoneurons that excite contraction of the skeletal muscle fibers, about one-half as many much smaller motoneurons, located along with the alpha motoneurons also in the anterior horns, transmit impulses through type A gamma ($A\alpha$) fibers, averaging 5 microns in diameter, to special skeletal muscle fibers called *intrafusal fibers*. These are part of the *muscle spindle*, which is discussed at length later in the chapter.

The Interneurons. The interneurons are present in all areas of the cord gray matter — in the dorsal horns, in the anterior horns, and in the intermediate areas between these two. These cells are numerous — approximately 30 times as numerous as the anterior motoneurons. They are small and highly excitable, often exhibiting spontaneous activity and capable of firing as rapidly as 1500 times per second. They have many interconnections one with the other, and many of them directly innervate the anterior motoneurons as illustrated in Figure 11–1. The interconnections among the interneurons and anterior motoneurons are responsible for many of the integrative functions of the spinal cord that are discussed in the remainder of this chapter.

Essentially all the different types of neuronal circuits described in Chapter 7 are found in the interneuron pool of cells of the spinal cord, including the *diverging, converging,* and *repetitive-discharge* circuits. In the following sections of this chapter we will see the many applications of these different circuits to the performance of specific reflex acts by the spinal cord.

Only a few incoming sensory signals to the spinal cord or signals from the brain terminate directly on the anterior motoneurons. Instead, most of them are transmitted first through interneurons where they are appropriately processed before stimulating the anterior motoneurons. Thus, in Figure 11–1, it is shown that the corticospinal tract terminates almost entirely on interneurons, and it is through these that the cerebrum transmits most of its signals for control of muscular function.

The Renshaw Cell Inhibitory System. Located also in the ventral horns of the spinal cord in close association with the motoneurons are a large number of small interneurons called *Renshaw cells*. Almost immediately after the motor axon leaves the motoneuron, collateral branches from the axon pass to the adjacent Renshaw cells. These in turn are inhibitory cells that transmit inhibitory signals to the nearby motoneurons. Thus, stimulation of each motoneuron tends to inhibit the surrounding motoneurons, an effect called recurrent inhibition. This effect is probably important for two major reasons:

1. It shows that the motor system utilizes the principle of lateral inhibition to focus, or sharpen, its signals — that is, to allow unabated transmission of the primary signal while suppressing the tendency for signals to spread to adjacent neurons.

2. The peripheral axon of the anterior motoneuron is known to secrete acetylcholine at its nerve endings. Therefore, the ability of collateral nerve endings from the same axon to stimulate the Renshaw cells proves that acetylcholine is one of the central nervous system excitatory transmitters, acting in the same way that it acts as an excitatory transmitter at the neuromuscular junction.

Sensory Input to the Motoneurons and Interneurons

Most of the sensory fibrils entering each segment of the spinal cord terminate on interneurons, but a very small number of large sensory fibers from the muscle spindles terminate directly on the anterior motoneurons. Thus, there are two pathways in the spinal cord that cord reflexes can take: either directly to the anterior motoneuron itself, utilizing a *monosynaptic pathway;* or through one or more interneurons first, before passing to the anterior motoneuron, thus utilizing a *polysynaptic pathway.* The monosynaptic pathway provides an extremely rapid reflex feedback system and is the basis of the very important muscle *stretch reflex* that will be discussed later in the chapter. All other cord reflexes utilize polysynaptic pathways, pathways that can modify the signals tremendously and that can cause complex reflex patterns. For instance, the very important protective reflex called the *withdrawal reflex* (flexor reflex) utilizes this type of pathway.

Multisegmental Connections in the Spinal Cord — The Propriospinal Fibers. More than half of all the nerve fibers ascending and descending in the spinal cord are *propriospinal fibers.* These are fibers that run from one segment of the cord to another. In addition, the terminal fibrils of sensory fibers as they enter the cord branch both up and down the spinal cord, some of the branches transmitting signals only a segment or two in each direction, while others transmit signals many segments. These ascending and descending fibers of the cord provide pathways for the multisegmental reflexes that will be described later in this chapter, including many reflexes that coordinate movements in both the forelimbs and hindlimbs simultaneously.

ROLE OF THE MUSCLE SPINDLE IN MOTOR CONTROL

Muscles and tendons have an abundance of two special types of receptors: (1) *muscle spindles* that detect (a) change in length of muscle fibers and (b) rate of this change in length, and (2) *Golgi tendon organs* that detect the tension applied to the muscle tendon during muscle contraction or muscle stretch.

The signals from these two receptors operate entirely at a subconscious level, causing no sensory perception at all. But they do transmit tremendous amounts of information into the spinal cord, cerebellum, and even the cerebral cortex, thereby helping all these portions of the nervous system to perform their functions for controlling muscle contraction.

RECEPTOR FUNCTION OF THE MUSCLE SPINDLE

Structure and Innervation of the Muscle Spindle. The physiologic organization of the muscle spindle is illustrated in Figure 11–2. Each spindle is built around three to ten small *intrafusal muscle fibers* that are pointed at their ends and are attached to the sheaths of the surrounding *extrafusal* skeletal muscle fibers. The intrafusal fiber is a very small skeletal muscle fiber. However, the central region of each of these fibers has either no or few actin and myosin filaments. Therefore, this central portion does not contract when the ends do. The end portions are excited by the small *gamma efferent* motor nerve fibers described earlier.

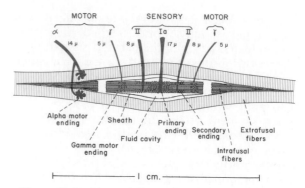

Figure 11–2. The muscle spindle, showing its relationship to the large extrafusal skeletal muscle fibers. Note also both the motor and the sensory innervation of the muscle spindle.

Excitation of the Spindle Receptors

The receptor portion of the muscle spindle is located midway between its two ends where the intrafusal muscle fibers have no contractile elements. As illustrated in Figure 11–2, sensory fibers originate in this area and are stimulated by stretch of this mid-portion of the spindle. One can readily see that there are two different ways in which the muscle spindle receptor can be excited:

1. Stretching the whole muscle in which the muscle spindle is located will obviously stretch the mid-portion of the spindle and therefore excite the receptor.

2. Even if the length of the entire muscle does not change, contraction of the end-portions of the intrafusal fibers will also stretch the mid-portions and therefore excite the receptor.

Two types of sensory endings are found in the receptor area of the muscle spindle. These are:

The Primary Ending. In the very center of the receptor area a large, type Ia fiber encircles the central portions of the intrafusal fibers, forming the so-called *primary ending,* also called the *annulospiral ending.* This nerve fiber averages 17 microns in diameter and transmits sensory signals to the spinal cord at a velocity of about 100 meters per second, as rapidly as any type of sensory nerve fiber in the entire body.

The Secondary Endings. Usually two smaller sensory nerve fibers, type II fibers with an average diameter of 8 microns, innervate the receptor regions on either side of the primary ending, as illustrated in Figure 11–2. These sensory endings are called *secondary endings,* or sometimes they are called *flower spray endings* because in some preparations they look like flower sprays even though they mainly encircle the intrafusal fibers in the same way that the type Ia fiber does.

Division of the Intrafusal Fibers into Nuclear Bag and Nuclear Chain Fibers — Dynamic and Static

Responses of the Muscle Spindle. There are also two different types of intrafusal fibers: (1) *nuclear bag fibers* (one to three), in which a large number of nuclei are congregated into a bag in the central portion of the receptor area, and (2) *nuclear chain fibers* (three to seven), which are about half as large in diameter and half as long as the nuclear bag fibers and have nuclei spread in a chain throughout the receptor area. The primary ending innervates both the nuclear bag intrafusal fibers *and* the nuclear chain fibers. On the other hand, the secondary endings are located almost entirely on the nuclear chain fibers. These relationships are illustrated in Figure 11–3.

Static Response of Both the Primary and the Secondary Receptors. When the receptor portion of the muscle spindle is stretched slowly, the number of impulses transmitted from both the primary and the secondary endings increases almost directly in proportion to the degree of stretch, and the endings continue to transmit these impulses for many minutes. This effect is called the *static response* of the spindle receptors, meaning simply that the receptors continue to transmit their signals for a prolonged period of time.

Dynamic Response of the Primary Endings. The primary ending also exhibits a very strong *dynamic response,* which means that it responds extremely actively to a rapid *rate of change* in length. When the length of a spindle receptor increases only a fraction of a micron, if this increase occurs in a fraction of a second, the primary receptor transmits tremendous numbers of excess impulses into the Ia fiber, but only *while the length is actually increasing.* As soon as the length has stopped increasing, the rate of impulse discharge returns almost back to its original level, except for the small static response that is still present in the signal.

Conversely, when the spindle receptor shortens, this change momentarily decreases the impulse output from the primary ending; as soon as the receptor area has reached its new shortened length, the impulses reappear in the Ia fiber within a fraction of a second. Thus, the primary ending sends extremely strong signals to the central nervous system to apprise it of any change in length of the spindle receptor area.

Since both the primary and the secondary endings innervate the nuclear chain intrafusal fibers, it is assumed that it is these nuclear chain fibers that are responsible for the static response of both the primary and the secondary endings. On the other hand, only the primary endings innervate the nuclear bag fibers. Therefore, it is assumed that the nuclear bag fibers are responsible for the powerful dynamic response.

Control of the Static and Dynamic Responses by the Gamma Efferent Nerves. Some physiologists believe that the gamma efferent nerves to the muscle spindle can be divided into two different types: gamma-dynamic (gamma-d) and gamma-static (gamma-s). The first of these excites mainly the nuclear bag intrafusal fibers and the second excites mainly the nuclear chain intrafusal fibers. When the gamma-d fibers excite the nuclear bag fibers, the dynamic response of the muscle spindle becomes tremendously enhanced, whereas the static response remains very weak or even none at all. On the other hand, stimulation of the gamma-s fibers, which excite mainly the nuclear chain fibers, supposedly enhances the static response while having little influence on the dynamic response. We shall see in subsequent paragraphs that these two different types of responses of the muscle spindle are exceedingly important in different types of muscle control.

Continuous Discharge of the Muscle Spindles Under Normal Conditions. Normally, particularly when there is a slight amount of gamma efferent excitation, the muscle spindles emit sensory nerve impulses all of the time. Stretching the muscle spindles increases the rate of firing, whereas shortening the spindle decreases this rate of firing. Thus, the degree of excitation of the spindles can be either increased or decreased.

THE STRETCH REFLEX (ALSO CALLED MUSCLE SPINDLE REFLEX OR MYOTATIC REFLEX)

From the above description of all the intricacies of the muscle spindle, one can readily see that the spindle is a very complex organ. Its function is manifested in the form of the muscle *stretch reflex* — that is, whenever a muscle is stretched, excitation of the spindles causes reflex contraction of the muscle. And, because of the static and the dynamic types of muscle spindle response, the stretch reflex also consists of a *static reflex* and a *dynamic reflex.*

Neuronal Circuitry of the Stretch Reflex. Figure 11–4 illustrates the basic circuit of the muscle

Figure 11–3. Details of nerve connections to the nuclear bag and nuclear chain muscle spindle fibers. (Modified from Stein: *Physiol. Rev.,* 54:225, 1974, and Boyd: *Philos. Trans. R. Soc. Lond.* [*Biol. Sci.*], 245:81, 1962.)

STRETCH REFLEX

Figure 11–4.   Neuronal circuit of the stretch reflex.

spindle reflex, showing a type Ia nerve fiber originating in a muscle spindle and entering the dorsal root of the spinal cord. It then synapses directly with an anterior motoneuron whose motor nerve fiber transmits an appropriate reflex signal, with almost negligible delay, back to the same muscle containing the muscle spindle.

In addition to the monosynaptic pathway of the Ia muscle spindle nerve fiber synapsing with the anterior motoneuron, collaterals from this fiber, as well as the type II fibers from the secondary spindle endings, terminate on interneurons in the gray matter of the cord, and these in turn transmit more delayed signals to the anterior motoneuron.

The Dynamic Stretch Reflex.   The dynamic stretch reflex is caused by the potent dynamic signal transmitted via the primary endings of the muscle spindles. That is, when a muscle is suddenly stretched, a strong signal is transmitted to the spinal cord, and this causes an instantaneous, very strong reflex contraction of the same muscle from which the signal originated. Thus, the reflex functions to oppose sudden changes in the length of the muscle, because the muscle contraction opposes the stretch.

The Static Stretch Reflex.   Though the dynamic stretch reflex is over within a fraction of a second after the muscle has been stretched to its new length, a much weaker static stretch reflex continues for a prolonged period of time thereafter. This reflex is elicited by the continuous static receptor signals transmitted by both the primary and secondary endings. The importance of the static stretch reflex is that it continues to cause muscle contraction as long as the muscle is maintained at an excessive length (for as long as several hours, but not for days). The muscle contraction in turn opposes the force that is causing the excess length.

The Negative Stretch Reflex.   When a muscle is

suddenly shortened, exactly opposite effects occur. If the muscle is already taut, any sudden release of the load on the muscle that allows it to shorten will elicit both dynamic and static reflex muscle inhibition rather than reflex excitation. Thus, *this negative stretch reflex* opposes the shortening of the muscle in the same way that the positive stretch reflex opposes lengthening of the muscle. Therefore, one can begin to see that the stretch reflex tends to maintain the status quo for the length of a muscle.

Feedback Control of Muscle Length — The Load Reflex

Let us assume that a person's biceps is contracted so that the forearm is horizontal to the earth. Then assume that a five-pound weight is put in the hand. The hand will immediately drop. However, the amount that the hand will drop is determined to a great extent by the degree of activity of the muscle spindle reflex. If the gamma-s fibers to the muscle spindles are strongly stimulated so that the static reflex is very active, even slight lengthening of the biceps, and therefore also of the muscle spindles in the biceps, will cause a strong feedback contraction of the extrafusal skeletal muscle fibers of the biceps. This contraction in turn will limit the degree of fall of the hand, thus automatically maintaining the forearm in a nearly horizontal position. This response is called a *load reflex*.

Effect of Gamma Efferent Stimulation on Increasing the Effectiveness of the Load Reflex.   If the gamma efferent nerves to the static portion of the muscle spindle (the gamma-s fibers) are not stimulated at all, then the spindle sensitivities are greatly depressed, and the effectiveness of the load reflex is almost zero. On the other hand, if these gamma efferents are strongly stimulated so that the static muscle spindle reflex is an extremely potent one, then one would expect the length of the muscle to remain almost exactly constant regardless of the change in load. In many of our muscle activities a particular part of our body often is fixed in a given position, and any attempt to move that part of the body from the position is met by instantaneous reflex resistance. This probably results to a great extent from the load reflex. Furthermore, the fact that we can change the sensitivity of this load reflex by changing the intensity of gamma-s stimulation allows us to make a particular part of the body be either flail or tightly locked in place. To give an example, when a person is threading a needle he tends to fix both of his hands into precise positions, and any extra load applied to either of the two hands will hardly change its position.

The Damping Function of the Dynamic and Static Stretch Reflexes

Another extremely important function of the stretch reflex — indeed, probably just as important as, if not more important than, the load reflex — is the ability of the stretch reflex to prevent some types of oscillation and jerkiness of the body movements. This is a damping, or smoothing, function. An example is the following:

Use of the Damping Mechanism in Smoothing Muscle Contraction. Occasionally, signals from other parts of the nervous system are transmitted to a muscle in a very unsmooth form, first increasing in intensity for a few milliseconds, then decreasing in intensity, then changing to another intensity level, and so forth. When the muscle spindle apparatus is not functioning satisfactorily, the degree of muscle contraction changes jerkily during the course of such a signal. This effect is illustrated in Figure 11–5, which shows an experiment in which a sensory nerve signal entering one side of the cord is transmitted to a motor nerve on the other side of the cord to excite a muscle. In curve A the muscle spindle reflex of the excited muscle is intact. Note that the contraction is relatively smooth even though the sensory nerve is excited at a very slow frequency of 8 per second. Curve B, on the other hand, is the same experiment in an animal whose muscle spindle sensory nerves from the excited muscle had been sectioned three months earlier. Note the very unsmooth muscle contraction. Thus, curve A illustrates very graphically the ability of the damping mechanism of the muscle spindle to smooth muscle contractions even though the input signals to the muscle motor system may themselves be very jerky. This effect can also be called a *signal averaging* function of the muscle spindle reflex.

Function of the Gamma Efferent System in Controlling the Degree of Damping. In the same way that the gamma efferent system can play a potent role in determining the effectiveness of the load reflex, so also can the gamma efferent system determine the degree of damping. For instance, there are times when a person wishes his limbs to move extremely rapidly in response to rapidly changing input signals. Under such conditions, one would wish less damping. On the other hand, there are other times when it is very important that the muscle contractions be very smooth. Under these conditions one would like a high degree of damping. Therefore, even though we are not completely sure how the nervous system can make such changes as this, psychophysiological tests do tell us that our motor system does have such capability to increase or decrease the degree of damping in any given muscle response.

ROLE OF THE MUSCLE SPINDLE IN VOLUNTARY MOTOR ACTIVITY

To emphasize the importance of the gamma efferent system, one needs to recognize that 31 per cent of all the motor nerve fibers to the muscle are gamma efferent fibers rather than large, type A alpha motor fibers. Whenever signals are transmitted from the motor cortex or from any other area of the brain to the alpha motoneurons, almost invariably the gamma motoneurons are stimulated simultaneously, an effect called *co-activation* of the alpha and gamma motor neurons. This causes both the extrafusal and the intrafusal muscle fibers to contract at the same time.

The purpose of contracting the muscle spindle fibers at the same time that the large skeletal muscle fibers contract is probably two-fold: First, it keeps the muscle spindle from opposing the muscle contraction. Second, it also maintans proper damping and proper load responsiveness of the muscle spindle regardless of change in muscle length. For instance, if the muscle spindle should not contract and relax along with the large muscle fibers, the receptor portion of the spindle would sometimes be flail and at other times be overstretched, in neither instance operating under optimal conditions for spindle function.

Possible "Servo" Control of Muscle Contraction by Exciting the Gamma Motor Neurons. Several physiologists have suggested that the muscle spindle reflex can also operate as a servo controller of muscle contraction. A "servo" control system is one in which the major function is not activated directly but instead is activated indirectly in the following way: Suppose that a gamma efferent nerve fiber to a muscle spindle were stimulated.

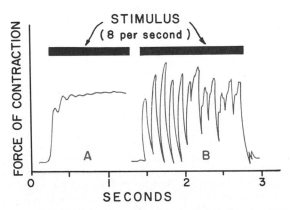

Figure 11–5. Muscle contraction caused by a central nervous system signal under two different conditions: (A) in a normal muscle, and (B) in a muscle whose muscle spindles had been denervated by section of the posterior roots of the cord 82 days previously. Note the smoothing effect of the muscle spindles in Part A.

This would contract the intrafusal fibers and excite the muscle spindle receptors. The signals from these receptors would then pass to the cord and thence back to the large skeletal muscle fibers to cause them to contract also. Thus, an initial contraction of the spindle intrafusal fibers would cause a similar contraction of the surrounding large skeletal muscle fibers.

If such a servo system as this should exist, signals transmitted from the brain downward through the gamma efferent system could cause secondary contractions of the muscles in accordance with the dictates of the muscle spindles. Unfortunately, most of the data indicate that a mechanism such as this probably does not occur to a significant extent. For a system of this type to function properly, it would be necessary to have a static response of the muscle spindles that is very potent and also unchanging. Unfortunately, the static response of the muscle spindles is usually very weak — that is, it has a low gain. Also, it decays very slowly over a period of many minutes to an hour so that changes in length of a muscle spindle could cause only temporary changes in length of the surrounding large skeletal muscle fibers. Therefore, despite the attractiveness of this possible type of muscle control, it is doubtful that it does actually occur in normal function.

Probable Servo-Assist Function of the Muscle Spindle Reflex. It is much more likely that the muscle spindle reflex acts as a servo-assist device than as a pure servo controller. But, first, let us explain what is meant by a "servo-assist mechanism."

When both the alpha and gamma motoneurons are stimulated simultaneously, if the intra- and extrafusal fibers contract equal amounts, the degree of stimulation of the muscle spindles will not change at all — neither increase nor decrease. However, in case the extrafusal muscle fibers contract less than the intrafusal fibers (as might occur when the muscle is contracting against a great load), this mismatch will stretch the receptor portions of the spindles and, therefore, elicit a stretch reflex that will further excite the extrafusal fibers. Thus, failure of the extrafusal fibers to contract to the same degree as the intrafusal fibers contract causes an accessory neuronal signal that increases the degree of stimulation of the extrafusal fibers. This is exactly the same mechanism as that employed by power steering in an automobile. That is, the steering wheel directly turns the front wheels and will do this even when the power steering is not effective. However, if the wheels fail to follow even the slightest extra force applied to the steering wheel, a servo-assist device is activated that applies additional power to turn the wheels.

The servo-assist type of motor function has several important advantages, as follows:

1. It allows the brain to cause a muscle contraction against a load without the brain having to expend much extra nervous energy — instead, the spindle reflex provides most of the nervous energy.

2. It makes the muscle contract almost the desired length even when the load is increased or decreased between successive contractions. In other words, it makes the length of contraction less load-insensitive.

3. It compensates for fatigue or other abnormalities of the muscle itself because any failure of the muscle to provide the proper contraction elicits an additional

muscle spindle reflex stimulus to make the contraction occur.

But, unfortunately, we still do not know how important this probable function of the muscle spindle reflex actually is.

Brain Areas for Control of the Gamma Efferent System

The gamma efferent system is excited primarily by the *bulboreticular facilitatory* region of the brain stem, and secondarily by impulses transmitted into this area from (a) the *cerebellum*, (b) the *basal ganglia*, and even (c) the *cerebral cortex*. Unfortunately, little is known about the precise mechanisms of control of the gamma efferent system. However, since the bulboreticular facilitatory area is particularly concerned with postural contractions, emphasis is given to the possible or probable important role of the gamma efferent mechanism in controlling muscle contraction for positioning the different parts of the body and for damping the movements of the different parts.

In addition to transmitting signals into the spinal cord, the muscle spindle also transmits signals up the cord to the cerebellum and thence into the bulboreticular areas and also as far as the cerebral cortex, as will be discussed in greater detail in Chapter 13. However, both the signals that operate in the spinal cord and those that pass to the brain are entirely subconscious, so that the conscious portion of the brain is never apprised of the immediate changes in length of the muscles. On the other hand, as has already been pointed out in Chapter 9, signals from the position receptors constantly apprise the conscious brain of the positions of the different parts of the body, even though the muscle receptors do not.

CLINICAL APPLICATIONS OF THE STRETCH REFLEX

The Knee Jerk and Other Muscle Jerks. Clinically, a method used to determine the functional integrity of the stretch reflexes is to elicit the knee jerk and other muscle jerks. The knee jerk can be elicited by simply striking the patellar tendon with a reflex hammer; this stretches the quadriceps muscle and initiates a *dynamic stretch reflex* to cause the lower leg to jerk forward. The upper part of Figure 11–6 illustrates a myogram from the quadriceps muscle recorded during a knee jerk.

Similar reflexes can be obtained from almost any muscle of the body either by striking the tendon of the muscle or by striking the belly of the muscle itself. In other words, sudden stretch of muscle spindles is all that is required to elicit a stretch reflex.

The muscle jerks are used by neurologists to assess the degree of facilitation of spinal cord centers. When large numbers of facilitatory impulses are being transmitted from the upper regions of the central nervous system into the cord, the muscle jerks are greatly

Figure 11–6. Myograms recorded from the quadriceps muscle during elicitation of the knee jerk and from the gastrocnemius muscle during ankle clonus.

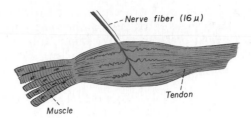

Figure 11–7. Golgi tendon organ.

exacerbated. On the other hand, if the facilitatory impulses are depressed or abrogated, the muscle jerks are considerably weakened or completely absent. These reflexes are used most frequently to determine the presence or absence of muscle spasticity following lesions in the motor areas of the brain. Ordinarily, large lesions in the contralateral motor areas of the cerebral cortex, especially those caused by strokes or brain tumors, cause greatly exacerbated muscle jerks.

Clonus. Under appropriate conditions, the muscle jerks can oscillate, a phenomenon called clonus (see lower myogram, Fig. 11–6). Oscillation can be explained particularly well in relation to ankle clonus, as follows:

If a man standing on his tiptoes suddenly drops his body downward to stretch one of his gastrocnemius muscles, impulses are transmitted from the muscle spindles into the spinal cord. These reflexly excite the stretched muscle, which lifts the body back up again. After a fraction of a second, the reflex contraction of the muscle dies out and the body falls again, thus stretching the spindles a second time. Again a dynamic stretch reflex lifts the body, but this too dies out after a fraction of a second, and the body falls once more to elicit still a new cycle. In this way, the stretch reflex of the gastrocnemius muscle continues to oscillate, often for long periods of time; this is clonus.

Clonus ordinarily occurs only if the stretch reflex is highly sensitized by facilitatory impulses from the brain. For instance, in the decerebrate animal, in which the stretch reflexes are highly facilitated, clonus develops readily. Therefore, to determine the degree of facilitation of the spinal cord, neurologists test patients for clonus by suddenly stretching a muscle and keeping a steady stretching force applied to the muscle. If clonus occurs, the degree of facilitation is certain to be very high.

THE TENDON REFLEX

The Golgi Tendon Organ and Its Excitation. Golgi tendon organs, illustrated in Figure 11–7, lie within muscle tendons immediately beyond their attachments to the muscle fibers. An average of 10 to 15 muscle fibers are usually connected in series with each Golgi tendon organ, and the organ is stimulated by the tension produced by this small bundle of muscle fibers. Thus, the major difference between the functions of the Golgi tendon organ and the muscle spindle is that the spindle detects relative muscle length, and the tendon organ detects muscle *tension.*

The tendon organ, like the primary receptor of the muscle spindle, has both a *dynamic response* and a *static response,* responding very intensely when the muscle tension suddenly increases (the dynamic response), but within a small fraction of a second it settles down to a lower level of steady state firing that is almost directly proportional to the muscle tension (the static response). Thus, the Golgi tendon organs provide the nervous system with instantaneous information of the degree of tension on each small segment of each muscle.

Transmission of Impulses from the Tendon Organ into the Central Nervous System. Signals from the tendon organ are transmitted through large, rapidly conducting type Ib nerve fibers, fibers averaging 16 microns in diameter, only slightly smaller than those from the primary receptors of the muscle spindle. These fibers, like those from the primary receptors, transmit signals both into local areas of the cord and through the spinocerebellar tracts into the cerebellum and through still other tracts to the cerebral cortex. The local signal is believed to excite a single inhibitory interneuron that in turn inhibits the anterior alpha motoneuron. Thus, this local circuit directly inhibits the individual muscle without affecting adjacent muscles. The signals to the brain will be discussed in Chapter 13.

Inhibitory Nature of the Tendon Reflex. When the Goli tendon organs of a muscle are stimulated by increased muscle tension, signals are transmitted into the spinal cord to cause reflex effects in the respective muscle. However, this reflex is entirely inhibitory, the exact opposite to the muscle spindle reflex. Thus, this reflex provides a negative feedback mechanism that prevents the development of too much tension on the muscle.

When tension on the muscle and, therefore, on the tendon becomes extreme, the inhibitory effect from the tendon organ can be so great that it causes sudden relaxation of the entire muscle. This effect is called the *lengthening reaction;* it is probably a protective mechanism to prevent tearing of the muscle or avulsion of the tendon from its attachments to the bone. We know, for instance, that direct electrical stimulation of muscles in the laboratory can frequently cause such destructive effects.

However, possibly as important as this protective reaction is function of the tendon reflex as a part of the overall servo control of muscle contraction in the following manner:

The Tendon Reflex as a Possible Servo Control Mechanism for Muscle Tension. In the same way that the strech reflex possibly operates as a feedback mechanism to control muscle length, the tendon reflex theoretically can operate as a servo feedback mechanism to control muscle tension. That is, if the tension on the muscle becomes too great, inhibition from the tendon organ decreases this tension back to a lower value. On the other hand, if the tension becomes too little, impulses from the tendon organ cease; and the resulting loss of inhibition allows the alpha motoneurons to become active again, thus increasing muscle tension back toward a higher level.

Very little is known at present about the function of or control of this tension servo feedback mechanism, but it is postulated to operate in the following basic manner: Signals from the brain are presumably transmitted to the cord centers to set the gain of the tendon feedback system. This can be done by changing the degree of facilitation of the neurons in the feedback loop. If the gain is high, then this system will be extremely sensitive to signals coming from the tendon organs; on the other hand, lack of excitatory signals from the brain could make the system very insensitive to the signals from the tendon organ. In this way, control signals from higher nervous centers could automatically set the level of tension at which the muscle would be maintained.

Yet, a word of caution: Despite this speculation, the measured feedback gains of the tendon-muscle feedback system have been far too little to prove that it can be very useful as a tension servo controller.

Value of a Servo Mechanism for Control of Tension. An obvious value of a mechanism for setting the degree of muscle tension would be to allow the different muscles to apply a desired amount of force irrespective of how far the muscles contract. An example of this is paddling a boat, in which a person sets the amount of force that he pulls backward on the paddle and maintains that degree of force throughout the entire movement. Were it not for some type of tension feedback mechanism, the same amount of force would not be maintained throughout the stroke because uncontrolled muscles change their force of contraction as their lengths change. One can imagine hundreds of different patterns of muscle function that might require maintenance of constant tension rather than maintenance of constant lengths of the muscles.

THE FLEXOR REFLEX (THE WITHDRAWAL REFLEXES)

In the spinal or decerebrate animal, almost any type of cutaneous sensory stimulus on a limb is likely to cause the flexor muscles of the limb to contract strongly, thereby withdrawing the limb from the stimulus. This is called the flexor reflex.

In its classic form the flexor reflex is elicited most frequently by stimulation of pain endings, such as by pinprick, heat, or some other painful stimulus, for which reason it is also frequently called a *nociceptive reflex,* or simply *pain reflex.* However, even stimulation of the touch receptors can also occasionally elicit a weaker and less prolonged flexor reflex.

If some part of the body besides one of the limbs is painfully stimulated, this part, in a similar manner, will be withdrawn from the stimulus, but the reflex may not be confined entirely to flexor muscles even though it is basically the same type of reflex. Therefore, the many patterns of reflexes of this type in the different areas of the body are called the *withdrawal reflexes*.

Neuronal Mechanism of the Flexor Reflex. The left-hand portion of Figure 11–8 illustrates the neuronal pathways for the flexor reflex. In this instance, a painful stimulus is applied to the hand; as a result, the flexor muscles of the upper arm become reflexly excited, thus withdrawing the hand from the painful stimulus.

The pathways for eliciting the flexor reflex do not pass directly to the anterior motoneurons but, instead, pass first into the interneuron pool of neurons and then to the motoneurons. The shortest possible circuit is a three- or four-neuron arc; however, most of the signals of the reflex traverse many more neurons than this and involve the following basic types of circuits: (1) diverging circuits to spread the reflex to the necessary

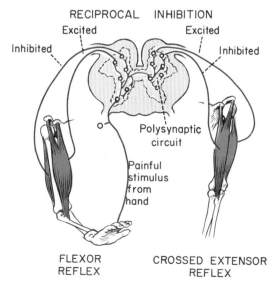

Figure 11–8.   The flexor reflex, the crossed extensor reflex, and reciprocal inhibition.

Figure 11–9. Myogram of a flexor reflex, showing rapid onset of the reflex, an interval of fatigue, and finally after-discharge after the stimulus is over.

muscles for withdrawal, (2) circuits to inhibit the antagonist muscles, called *reciprocal inhibition circuits,* and (3) circuits to cause a prolonged repetitive after-discharge even after the stimulus is over.

Figure 11–9 illustrates a typical myogram from a flexor muscle during a flexor reflex. Within a few milliseconds after a pain nerve is stimulated, the flexor response appears. Then, in the next few seconds the reflex begins to *fatigue,* which is characteristic of essentially all of the more complex integrative reflexes of the spinal cord. Then, soon after the stimulus is over, the contraction of the muscle begins to return toward the base line, but, because of *after-discharge,* will not return all the way for many milliseconds. The duration of the after-discharge depends on the intensity of the sensory stimulus that had elicited the reflex; a weak stimulus causes almost no after-discharge in contrast to an after-discharge lasting for several seconds following a very strong stimulus. Furthermore, a flexor reflex initiated by nonpainful stimuli and transmitted through the large sensory fibers causes essentially no after-discharge, whereas nociceptive impulses transmitted through the small type A fibers and type C fibers cause prolonged after-discharge.

The after-discharge that occurs in the flexor reflex almost certainly results from all three types of repetitive-discharge circuits that were discussed in Chapter 7. Electrophysiological studies indicate that the immediate after-discharge, lasting for about 6 to 8 milliseconds, results from the interneuron repetitive firing mechanism and from the parallel type of circuit, with impulses being transmitted from one interneuron to another to another and all these in turn transmitting their signals successively to the anterior motoneurons. However, the prolonged after-discharge that occurs following strong pain stimuli presumably involves reverberating circuits in the interneurons, these transmitting impulses to the anterior motoneurons sometimes for several seconds after the incoming sensory signal is completely over.

Thus, the flexor reflex is appropriately organized to withdraw a pained or otherwise irritated part of the body away from the stimulus. Furthermore, because of the after-discharge the reflex can hold the irritated part away from the stimulus for as long as 1 to 3 seconds even after the irritation is over. During this time, other reflexes and actions of the central nervous system can move the entire body away from the painful stimulus.

The Pattern of Withdrawal. The pattern of withdrawal that results when the flexor reflex (or the many other types of withdrawal reflexes) is elicited depends on the sensory nerve that is stimulated. Thus, a painful stimulus on the inside of the arm not only elicits a flexor reflex in the arm but also contracts the abductor muscles to pull the arm outward. In other words, the integrative centers of the cord cause those muscles to contract that can most effectively remove the pained part of the body from the object that causes pain. This same principle applies for any part of the body but especially to the limbs, because they have highly developed flexor reflexes.

THE CROSSED EXTENSOR REFLEX

Approximately 0.2 to 0.5 second after a stimulus elicits a flexor reflex in one limb, the opposite limb begins to extend. This is called the *crossed extensor reflex.* Extension of the opposite limb obviously can push the entire body away from the object causing the painful stimulus.

Neuronal Mechanism of the Crossed Extensor Reflex. The right-hand portion of Figure 11–8 illustrates the neuronal circuit responsible for the crossed extensor reflex, showing that signals from the sensory nerves cross to the opposite side of the cord to cause exactly opposite reactions to those that cause the flexor reflex. Because the crossed extensor reflex usually does not begin until 200 to 500 milliseconds following the initial pain stimulus, it is certain that many internuncial neurons are in the circuit between the incoming sensory neuron and the motoneurons of the opposite side of the cord responsible for the crossed extension. Furthermore, after the painful stimulus is removed, the crossed extensor reflex continues for an even longer period of after-discharge than that for the flexor reflex. Therefore, again, it is presumed that this prolonged after-discharge results from reverberatory circuits among the internuncial cells.

Figure 11–10 illustrates a myogram recorded from a muscle involved in a crossed extensor reflex. This shows the relatively long latency before the reflex begins and also the long after-discharge following the end of the stimulus. The prolonged after-discharge obviously would be of

Figure 11–10. Myogram of a crossed extensor reflex, showing slow onset but prolonged after-discharge.

Figure 11–11. Myogram of a flexor reflex, illustrating reciprocal inhibition caused by a stronger flexor reflex in the opposite limb.

benefit in holding the body away from a painful object until other neurogenic reactions could cause the body to move away.

RECIPROCAL INHIBITION AND RECIPROCAL INNERVATION

In the foregoing paragraphs we have pointed out several times that excitation of one group of muscles is often associated with inhibition of another group. For instance, when a stretch reflex excites one muscle, it simultaneously inhibits the antagonist muscles. This is the phenomenon of *reciprocal inhibition,* and the neuronal mechanism that causes this reciprocal relationship is called *reciprocal innervation.* Likewise, reciprocal relationships exist between the two sides of the cord, as exemplified by the flexor and extensor reflexes described above.

Figure 11–11 illustrates a typical example of reciprocal inhibition. In this instance, a moderate but prolonged flexor reflex is elicited from one limb of the body, and while this reflex is still being elicited a still stronger flexor reflex is elicited in the opposite limb, causing reciprocal inhibition of the first limb. Then removal of the strong flexor reflex allows the original reflex to reassume its previous intensity.

FATIGUE OF REFLEXES; REBOUND

Figure 11–9 illustrated that the flexor reflex begins to *fatigue* within a few seconds after its initiation. This is a common effect in most of the cord reflexes as well as many other reflexes of the central nervous system, and it presumably results from progressive fatigue of synaptic transmission in the reflex circuits, a subject that was discussed more fully in Chapter 6.

Another effect closely allied to fatigue is *rebound.* This means that, immediately after a reflex is over, a second reflex of the same type is much more difficult to elicit for a given time thereafter.

However, because of reciprocal innervation, reflexes of the antagonist muscles become even more easily elicited during that same period of time. For instance, if a flexor reflex occurs in a left limb, a second flexor reflex is more difficult to establish for a few seconds thereafter, but a crossed extensor reflex in this same limb will be greatly exacerbated. Rebound is probably one of the important mechanisms by which the rhythmic to-and-fro movements required in locomotion are effected, which are described in more detail later in the chapter.

THE REFLEXES OF POSTURE AND LOCOMOTION

THE POSTURAL AND LOCOMOTIVE REFLEXES OF THE CORD

The Positive Supportive Reaction. Pressure on the footpad of a decerebrate animal causes the limb to extend against the pressure being applied to the foot. Indeed, this reflex is so strong that an animal whose spinal cord has been transected for several months can often be placed on its feet, and the reflex will stiffen the limbs sufficiently to support the weight of the body — the animal will stand in a rigid position. This reflex is called the *positive supportive reaction.*

The positive supportive reaction involves a complex circuit in the interneurons similar to those responsible for the flexor and the crossed-extensor reflexes. Furthermore, the locus of the pressure on the pad of the foot determines the position to which the limb will extend; pressure on one side causes extension in that direction, an effect called the *magnet reaction.* This obviously helps to keep an animal from falling to one side.

The Cord "Righting" Reflexes. When a spinal cat or even a well-recovered young spinal dog is laid on its side, it will make incoordinate movements that indicate that it is trying to raise itself to the standing position. This is called a *cord righting reflex,* and it illustrates that relatively complicated reflexes associated with posture are at least partially integrated in the spinal cord. Indeed, a puppy with a well-healed transected thoracic cord caudal to the cord level for the forelegs can completely right itself from the lying position and can even walk on its hindlimbs. And, in the case of the opossum with a similar transection of the thoracic cord, the walking movements of the hind-limbs are hardly different from those in the normal opossum — except that the hindlimb movements are not synchronized with those of the forelimbs as is normally the case.

Rhythmic Stepping Movements of a Single Limb. Rhythmic stepping movements are frequently observed in the limbs of spinal animals. Indeed, even when the lumbar portion of the spinal cord is separated from the remainder of the cord and a longitudinal section is made down the center of the cord to block neuronal connections between the two limbs, each hind limb can still perform stepping functions. Forward flexion of the limb is followed a second or so later by backward extension. Then flexion occurs again, and the cycle is repeated over and over.

This oscillation back and forth between the flexor and extensor muscles occurs even after the sensory nerves have been cut, and it seems to result mainly from reciprocal inhibition and rebound. That is, the forward flexion of the limb causes reciprocal inhibition of the cord center controlling the extensor muscles, but shortly thereafter the flexion begins to die out; as it does so, *rebound* inhibition of the flexors and reciprocal *rebound* excitation of the extensors cause the leg to move downward and backward. After extension has continued for a time, it, too, begins to die and is followed by reciprocal rebound excitation of the flexor muscles. And the oscillating cycle continues again and again.

The sensory signals from the footpads and from the position sensors around the joints play a strong role in controlling foot pressure and rate of stepping when the foot is allowed to walk along a surface.

Reciprocal Stepping of Opposite Limbs. If the lumbar spinal cord is not sectioned down its center as noted above, every time stepping occurs in the forward direction in one limb, the opposite limb ordinarily steps backward. This effect results from reciprocal innervation between the two limbs.

Diagonal Stepping of All Four Limbs — The "Mark Time" Reflex. If a well-healed spinal animal is held up from the table and its legs are allowed to fall downward as illustrated in Figure 11–12, the stretch on the limbs occasionally elicits stepping reflexes that involve all four limbs. In general, stepping occurs diagonally between the fore- and hindlimbs. That is, the right hindlimb and the left forelimb move backward together while the right forelimb and left hindlimb move forward. This diagonal response is another manifestation of reciprocal innervation, this time oc-

Walking movement

Figure 11–12. Diagonal stepping movements exhibited by a spinal animal.

curring the entire distance up and down the cord between the fore- and hindlimbs. Such a walking pattern is often called a *mark time reflex*.

The Galloping Reflex. Another type of reflex that occasionally develops in the spinal animal is the galloping reflex, in which both forelimbs move backward in unison while both hindlimbs move forward. If stretch or pressure stimuli are applied almost exactly equally to opposite limbs at the same time, a galloping reflex will likely result, whereas unequal stimulation of one side versus the other elicits the diagonal walking reflex. This is in keeping with the normal patterns of walking and of galloping, for, in walking, only one limb at a time is stimulated, and this would predispose to continued walking. Conversely, when the animal strikes the ground during galloping, the limbs on both sides are stimulated approximately equally; this obviously would predispose to further galloping and, therefore, would continue this pattern of motion in contradistinction to the walking pattern.

THE SCRATCH REFLEX

An especially important cord reflex in lower animals is the scratch reflex, which is initiated by the *itch and tickle sensation*. It actually involves two different functions: (1) a *position sense* that allows the paw to find the exact point of irritation on the surface of the body and (2) a *to-and-fro scratching movement*.

Obviously, the scratch reflex, like the stepping movements of locomotion, involves reciprocal innervation circuits that cause oscillation. One of the important discoveries in relation to the to-and-fro movement of the scratch reflex (and also of the stepping movements as described above) is that it can still occur even when all the sensory roots from the oscillating limb are sectioned. In other words, feedback from the limb itself is not necessary to maintain the neuronal oscillation, which means that the oscillation can occur intrinsically as a result of oscillating circuits within the spinal interneurons themselves.

The *position sense* of the scratch reflex is also a highly developed function, for even though a flea might be crawling as far forward as the shoulder of a spinal animal, the hind paw can often find its position. Furthermore, this can be accomplished even though 19 different muscles in the limb must be contracted simultaneously in a precise pattern to bring the paw to the position of the crawling flea. To make the reflex even more complicated, when the flea crosses the midline, the paw stops scratching, but the opposite paw begins the to-and-fro motion and eventually finds the flea.

THE SPINAL CORD REFLEXES THAT CAUSE MUSCLE SPASM

In human beings, local muscle spasm is often observed. The mechanism of this has not been elucidated to complete satisfaction even in experimental animals, but it is known that pain stimuli can cause reflex spasm of local muscles, which presumably is the cause of much if not most of the muscle spasm observed at localized regions of the human body.

Muscle Spasm Resulting from a Broken Bone. One type of clinically important spasm occurs in muscles surrounding a broken bone. This seems to result from the pain impulses initiated from the broken edges of the bone, which cause the muscles surrounding the area to contract powerfully and tonically. Relief of the pain by injection of a local anesthetic relieves the spasm; a general anesthetic also relieves the spasm. One of these procedures is often necessary before the spasm can be overcome sufficiently for the two ends of the bone to be set back into appropriate positions.

Abdominal Muscle Spasm in Peritonitis. Another type of local spasm caused by a cord reflex is the abdominal spasm resulting from irritation of the parietal peritoneum by peritonitis. Here, again, relief of the pain caused by the peritonitis allows the spastic muscle to relax. Almost the same type of spasm often occurs during surgical operations; pain impulses from the parietal peritoneum cause the abdominal muscles to contract extensively and sometimes actually to extrude the intestines through the surgical wound. For this reason deep surgical anesthesia is usually required for intra-abdominal operations.

Muscle Cramps. Still another type of local spasm is the typical muscle cramp. Electromyographic studies indicate that the cause of at least some muscle cramps is the following:

Any local irritating factor or metabolic abnormality of a muscle — such as severe cold, lack of blood flow to the muscle, or overexercise of the muscle — can elicit pain or other types of sensory impulses that are transmitted from the muscle to the spinal cord, thus causing reflex muscle contraction. The contraction in turn stimulates the same sensory receptors still more, which causes the spinal cord to increase the intensity of contraction still further. Thus, a positive feedback mechanism occurs so that a small amount of initial irritation causes more and more contraction until a full-blown muscle cramp ensues. Reciprocal inhibition

of the muscle can sometimes relieve the cramp. That is, if a person purposefully contracts the muscle on the opposite side of the joint from the cramped muscle while at the same time using another hand or leg to prevent movement of the joint, the reciprocal inhibition that occurs in the cramped muscle can at times relieve the cramp immediately.

THE AUTONOMIC REFLEXES IN THE SPINAL CORD

Many different types of segmental autonomic reflexes occur in the spinal cord, most of which are discussed in other chapters. Briefly, these include: (1) changes in vascular tone, resulting from heat and cold, (2) sweating, which results from localized heat at the surface of the body, (3) intestino-intestinal reflexes that control some motor functions of the gut, (4) peritoneointestinal reflexes that inhibit gastric motility in response to peritoneal irritation, and (5) evacuation reflexes for emptying the bladder and the colon. In addition, all the segmental reflexes can at times be elicited simultaneously in the form of the so-called mass reflex as follows:

The Mass Reflex. In a spinal animal or human being, the spinal cord sometimes suddenly becomes excessively active, causing massive discharge of large portions of the cord. The usual stimulus that causes this is a strong nociceptive stimulus to the skin or excessive filling of a viscus, such as overdistention of the bladder or of the gut. Regardless of the type of stimulus, the resulting reflex, called the mass reflex, involves large portions or even all of the cord, and its pattern of reaction is the same. The effects are: (1) a major portion of the body goes into strong flexor spasm, (2) the colon and bladder are likely to evacuate, (3) the arterial pressure often rises to maximal values — sometimes to a mean pressure well over 200 mm. Hg, and (4) large areas of the body break out into profuse sweating. The mass reflex might be likened to the epileptic attacks that involve the central nervous system in which large portions of the brain become massively activated.

The precise neuronal mechanism of the mass reflex is unknown. However, since it lasts for minutes, it presumably results from activation of great masses of reverberating circuits that excite large areas of the cord at once.

SPINAL CORD TRANSECTION AND SPINAL SHOCK

When the spinal cord is suddenly transected, essentially all cord functions, including the cord reflexes, immediately become depressed to the point of oblivion, a reaction called *spinal shock*. The reason for this is that normal activity of the cord neurons depends to a great extent on continual tonic discharges from higher centers, particularly discharges transmitted through the reticulospinal tracts and corticospinal tracts.

After a few hours to a few days or weeks of spinal shock, the spinal neurons gradually regain their excitability. This seems to be a natural characteristic of neurons everywhere in the nervous system — that is, after they lose their source of facilitatory impulses, they increase their own natural degree of excitability to make up for the loss. In most nonprimates, the excitability of the cord centers returns essentially to normal within a few hours to a day or so, but in human beings the return is often delayed for several weeks and occasionally is never complete; or, on the other hand, recovery is sometimes excessive, with resultant hyperexcitability of all or most cord functions.

Some of the spinal functions specifically affected during or following spinal shock are: (1) The arterial blood pressure falls immediately — sometimes to as low as 40 mm. Hg — thus illustrating that sympathetic activity becomes blocked almost to extinction. However, the pressure ordinarily returns to normal within a few days. (2) All skeletal muscle reflexes integrated in the spinal cord are completely blocked during the initial stages of shock. In lower animals, a few hours to a few days are required for these reflexes to return to normal, and in human beings two weeks to several months are usually required. Sometimes, both in animals and people, some reflexes eventually become hyperexcitable, particularly if a few facilitatory pathways remain intact between the brain and the cord while the remainder of the spinal cord is transected. The first reflexes to return are the stretch reflex, followed in order by the progressively more complex reflexes, the flexor reflexes, the postural antigravity reflexes, and remnants of stepping reflexes. (3) The sacral reflexes for control of bladder and colon evacuation are completely suppresed in human beings for the first few weeks following cord transection, but they eventually return.

REFERENCES

Burke, R. E., and Rudonmin, P.: Spinal neurons and synapses. In Brookhart, J. M., and Mountcastle, V. B. (eds.): Handbook of Physiology. Sec. 1, Vol. 1. Baltimore, Williams & Wilkins, 1977, p. 877.

Creed, R. S. et al.: Reflex Activity of the Spinal Cord. New York, Oxford University Press, 1932.

Crowley, W. J.: Neural control of skeletal muscle. In Frohlich, E. D. (ed.): Pathophysiology, 2nd Ed. Philadelphia, J. B. Lippincott Co., 1976, p. 735.

Daube, J. R., et al.: Medical Neurosciences: An Approach to Anatomy, Pathology, and Physiology by Systems and Levels. Boston, Little, Brown, 1978.

Desmedt, J. E. (ed.): Physiological Tremor, Pathological Tremors and Clonus. New York, S. Karger, 1978.

Easton, T. A.: On the normal use of reflexes. Am. Sci., 60:591, 1972.

Gallistel, C. R.: The Organization of Action: A New Synthesis. New York, Halsted Press, 1979.

Granit, R.: Muscular tone, J. Sport Med., 2:46, 1962.

Granit, R., and Pompeiano, O. (eds.): Reflex Control of Posture and Movement. New York, Elsevier Scientific Publishing Co., 1979.

Granit, R., et al.: First supraspinal control of mammalian muscle spindles: extra- and intrafusal co-activation. J. Physiol. (Lond.), 147:385, 1959.

Houk, J. C.: Regulation of stiffness in skeletomotor reflexes. Annu. Rev. Physiol., 41:99, 1979.

Hughes, J. T.: Pathology of the Spinal Cord. Philadelphia, W. B. Saunders Co., 1978.

Hunt, C. C., and Perl, E. R.: Spinal reflex mechanisms concerned with skeletal muscle. Physiol. Rev., 40:538, 1960.

Kostyuk, P. G., and Vasilenko, D.: Spinal interneurons. Annu. Rev. Physiol., 41:115, 1979.

Matthews, P. B. C.: Mammalian Muscle Receptors and Their Central Actions. Baltimore, Williams & Wilkins, 1972.

Merton, P. A.: How we control the contraction of our muscles. Sci. Am., 226:30, 1972.

Orlovsky. G. N.. and Shik. M. L.: Control of locomotion: A neurophysiological analysis of the cat locomotor system. Int. Rev. Physiol., 10:281, 1976.

Pearson, K.: The control of walking. Sci. Am. 235(6):72, 1976.

Peterson, B. W.: Reticulospinal projections to spinal motor nuclei. Annu. Rev. Physiol., 41:127, 1979.

Porter, R.: The neurophysiology of movement performance. In MTP International Review of Science: Physiology. Vol. 3. Baltimore, University Park Press, 1974, p. 151.

Purves, D.: Long-term regulation in the vertebrate peripheral nervous system. Int. Rev. Physiol., 10:125, 1976.

Roaf, R., and Hodkinson, L. J.: The Paralysed Patient. Philadelphia, J. B. Lippincott Co., 1977.

Rogers, M. A.: Paraplegia. Boston, Faber and Faber, 1978.

Sherrington, C. S.: The Integrative Action of the Nervous System. New Haven, Conn., Yale University Press, 1911.

Shik, M. L., and Orlovsky, G. N.: Neurophysiology of Locomotor Automatism. Physiol. Rev., 56:465, 1976.

Stein, P. S. G.: Motor systems with specific reference to the control of locomotion. Annu. Rev. Neurosci., 1:61, 1978.

Stein, R. B.: Peripheral control of movement. Physiol. Rev., 54:215, 1974.

Trieschmann, R. B.: Spinal Cord Injuries. New York, Pergamon Press, 1979.

12

Motor Functions of the Brain Stem and Basal Ganglia — Reticular Formation, Vestibular Apparatus, Equilibrium, and Brain Stem Reflexes

The brain stem is a complex extension of the spinal cord. Collected in it are numerous neuronal circuits to control respiration, cardiovascular function, gastrointestinal function, eye movement, equilibrium, support of the body against gravity, and many special stereotyped movements of the body. Some of these functions — such as control of respiration and cardiovascular functions — are described in special sections of this text. The present chapter deals primarily with the control of whole body movement and equilibrium.

THE RETICULAR FORMATION, AND SUPPORT OF THE BODY AGAINST GRAVITY

Throughout the entire extent of the brain stem — in the medulla, pons, mesencephalon, and even in portions of the diencephalon — are areas of diffuse neurons collectively known as the *reticular formation*. Figure 12–1 illustrates the extent of the reticular formation, showing it to begin at the upper end of the spinal cord and to extend upward through the medulla, pons, and mesencephalon into (a) the central portions of the thalamus, (b) the hypothalamus, and (c) other areas adjacent to the thalamus. The lower end of the reticular formation is continuous with the interneurons of the spinal cord, and, indeed, the reticular formation of the brain stem functions in a

manner quite analogous to many of the functions of the interneurons in the cord gray matter.

Interspersed throughout the reticular formation are both motor and sensory neurons; these vary in size from very small to very large. The small

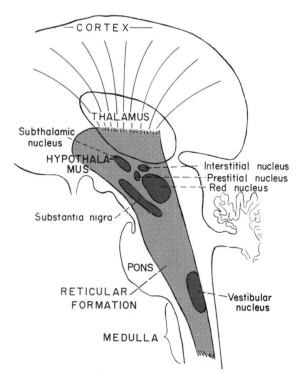

Figure 12–1. The reticular formation and associated nuclei.

148

neurons, which constitute the greater number, have short axons that make multiple connections within the reticular formation itself. The large neurons are mainly motor in function, and their axons often bifurcate almost immediately, with one division extending downward to the spinal cord and the other extending upward to the thalamus or other basal regions of the diencephalon or cerebrum.

The sensory input to the reticular formation is from multiple sources, including: (1) the spinoreticular tracts and collaterals from the spinothalamic tracts, (2) the vestibular nuclei, (3) the cerebellum, (4) the basal ganglia, (5) the cerebral cortex, especially the motor regions, and (6) the hypothalamus and other nearby associated areas.

Though most of the neurons in the reticular formation are evenly dispersed, some of them are collected into *specific nuclei,* some of which are labeled in Figure 12–1. In general, these specific nuclei are not considered to be part of the reticular formation per se even though they do operate in association with it. In most instances they are the loci of "preprogrammed" control of stereotyped movements. As an example, the vestibular nuclei provide preprogrammed attitudinal contractions of the muscles for maintenance of equilibrium, as will be discussed later in the chapter.

EXCITATORY FUNCTION OF THE RETICULAR FORMATION

The reticular formation and the vestibular nuclei, which function in very close association with each other, are both intrinsically excitable, but this excitability is usually held in check by inhibitory signals that flow into this area mainly from the basal ganglia. Also, some areas of the cerebral cortex send inhibitory signals to the reticular formation mainly by way of the basal ganglia. As will be noted later in the chapter when we discuss the decerebrate animal, destruction of the higher portions of the nervous system, the basal ganglia and the cortex, removes this inhibition and allows the reticular formation and vestibular nuclei to become tonically active; this causes rigidity of the antigravity skeletal muscles throughout the body.

On the other hand, when the brain stem is sectioned at a level slightly below the vestibular nuclei, loss of the motor signals normally transmitted from the reticular formation and vestibular nuclei to the spinal cord causes almost all the musculature to become totally flaccid.

Reciprocal Excitation or Inhibition of Antagonist Muscles by the Reticular Formation. Though very little is known about the function of specific areas in the reticular formation, in general stimulation near the midline of the reticular formation causes the flexor muscles on the same side of the body to contract and the extensors to relax. Stimulation in the lateral portions of the reticular formation tends to cause opposite effects, excitation of the extensor muscles and inhibition of the flexors. And at the same time that contraction occurs on one side of the body the same muscle on the opposite side tends to relax while its antagonist contracts. Thus, the phenomenon of reciprocal inhibition is strongly expressed in the reticular formation, as it is in the spinal cord, both for reciprocal control of antagonist pairs of muscles as well as for control of muscles between the two sides of the body.

SUPPORT OF THE BODY AGAINST GRAVITY

When a person or an animal stands, the vestibular nuclei and the closely related nuclei in the reticular formation transmit continuous impulses into the spinal cord and thence to the extensor muscles to stiffen the limbs. This allows the limbs to support the body against gravity. These impulses are transmitted mainly by way of the vestibulospinal and reticulospinal tracts.

However, the degree of activity in the individual extensor muscles is determined by the equilibrium mechanisms. Thus, if an animal begins to fall to one side, the extensor muscles on that side stiffen while those on the opposite side relax. And analogous effects occur when it tends to fall forward or backward.

In essence, then, the vestibular nuclei and the reticular formation provide the nervous energy to support the body against gravity. But other factors, particularly the vestibular apparatuses, control the relative degree of extensor contraction in the different parts of the body, which provides the function of equilibrium.

VESTIBULAR SENSATIONS AND THE MAINTENANCE OF EQUILIBRIUM

THE VESTIBULAR APPARATUS

The vestibular apparatus is the sensory organ that detects sensations concerned with equilibrium. It is composed of a *bony labyrinth* containing the *membranous labyrinth* which is the functional part of the apparatus. The top of Figure 12–2 illustrates the membranous labyrinth; it is composed mainly of the *cochlear duct,* the three *semicircular canals,* and the two large chambers known as the *utricle* and the *saccule.* The cochlear duct is the major sensory area for hearing and has nothing to do with equilibrium. However, the

MEMBRANOUS LABYRINTH

CRISTA AMPULLARIS AND MACULA

Figure 12–2. The membranous labyrinth, and organization of the crista ampullaris and the macula. (From Goss: Gray's Anatomy of the Human Body. Lea & Febiger; modified from Kolmer by Buchanan: Functional Neuroanatomy. Lea & Febiger.)

utricle, the *saccule,* and the *semicircular canals* are all integral parts of the equilibrium mechanism.

The Utricle and the Saccule. Located on the wall of both the utricle and the saccule is a small area slightly over 2 mm. in diameter, called a *macula.* Each of these maculae is a sensory area for detecting the orientation of the head with respect to the direction of gravitational pull or of other acceleratory forces, as will be explained in subsequent sections of this chapter. Each macula is covered by a gelatinous layer in which many small calcium carbonate crystals called *otoconia* are imbedded. Also, in the macula are thousands of *hair cells,* which project *cilia* up into the gelatinous layer. The bases and sides of the hair cells synapse with sensory axons of the vestibular nerve.

Even under resting conditions, most of the nerve fibers leading from the hair cells transmit a continuous series of nerve impulses. Bending the cilia of a hair cell to one side causes the impulse traffic in its nerve fibers to increase markedly; bending the cilia to the opposite side decreases the impulse traffic, often turning it off completely. Therefore, as the orientation of the head in space changes and the weight of the otoconia (whose specific gravity is about 3 times that of the surrounding tissues) bends the cilia, appropriate signals are transmitted to the brain to control equilibrium.

In each macula the different hair cells are oriented in different directions so that some of them are stimulated when the head bends forward, some when it bends backward, others when it bends to one side, and so forth. Therefore, a different pattern of excitation occurs in the macula for each position of the head; it is this "pattern" that apprises the brain of the head's orientation.

The Semicircular Canals. The three semicircular canals in each vestibular apparatus, known respectively as the *superior, posterior,* and *external* (or *horizontal*) *semicircular canals,* are arranged at right angles to each other so that they represent all three planes in space. When the head is bent forward approximately 30 degrees, the two external semicircular canals are located approximately horizontal with respect to the surface of the earth. The superior canals are then located in vertical planes that project *forward and 45 degrees outward,* and the posterior canals are also then in vertical planes but project *backward and 45 degrees outward.* Thus, the superior canal on each side of the head is in a plane parallel to that of the posterior canal on the opposite side of the head, whereas the two external canals on the two sides are located in approximately the same plane.

Each semicircular canal has an enlargement at one of its ends called the *ampulla,* and the canals are filled with fluid called *endolymph.* Flow of this fluid in the canals excites a sensory organ in the ampulla. As illustrated in Figure 12–2, located in each ampulla is a small crest called a *crista ampullaris,* and on top of the crista is a gelatinous mass similar to that in the utricle and known as the *cupula.* Into the cupula are projected hairs from hair cells located along the ampullary crest, and these hair cells in turn are connected to sensory nerve fibers that pass into the *vestibular nerve.* Bending the cupula to one side, caused by flow of fluid in the canal, stimulates the hair cells, while bending in the opposite direction inhibits them. Thus, appropriate signals are sent through the vestibular nerve to apprise the central nervous system of fluid movement in the respective canal.

Directional Sensitivity of the Hair Cells — The Kinocilium. Each hair cell, whether in a macula or a cupula, has a large number of very small cilia plus one very large cilium called the *kinocilium.*

This kinocilium is located to one side of the hair cell, always on the same side of the cell with respect to its orientation on the ampullary crest. This is the cause of the directional sensitivity of the hair cells: namely, stimulation when the cilia are bent toward the kinocilium side and inhibition when bent in the opposite direction.

Neuronal Connections of the Vestibular Apparatus with the Central Nervous System. Figure 12–3 illustrates the central connections of the vestibular nerve. Most of the vestibular nerve fibers end in the vestibular nuclei, which are located approximately at the junction of the medulla and the pons, but some fibers pass without synapsing to the fastigial nuclei, uvula, and flocculonodular lobes of the cerebellum. The fibers that end in the vestibular nuclei synapse with second order neurons that also send fibers into these areas of the cerebellum as well as to the cortex of other portions of the cerebellum, into the vestibulospinal tract, into the medial longitudinal fasciculus, and to other areas of the brain stem, particularly the reticular formation.

Note especially the very close association between the vestibular apparatus, the vestibular nuclei, and the cerebellum. The primary pathway for the reflexes of equilibrium begins in the vestibular nerves and passes next to both the vestibular nuclei and the cerebellum. Then, after much two-way traffic of impulses between these two, signals are sent into the reticular nuclei of the brain stem as well as down the spinal cord via vestibulospinal and reticulospinal tracts. In turn, the signals to the cord control the interplay between facilitation and inhibition of the extensor muscles, thus automatically controlling equilibrium.

The *flocculonodular lobes* of the cerebellum seem to be especially concerned with equilibrium functions of the semicircular canals because destruction of these lobes gives almost exactly the same clinical symptoms as destruction of the semicircular canals themselves. That is, severe injury to either of these structures causes loss of equilibrium during *rapid changes in direction of motion* but does not seriously disturb equilibrium under static conditions, as will be discussed in subsequent sections. It is also believed that the uvula of the cerebellum plays an equally important role in static equilibrium.

Signals transmitted upward in the brain stem from both the vestibular nuclei and the cerebellum via the *medial longitudinal fasciculus* cause corrective movements of the eyes every time the head rotates so that the eyes can remain fixed on a specific visual object. Signals also pass upward (either through this same tract or through reticular tracts) to the cerebral cortex, probably terminating in a primary cortical center for equilibrium located in the parietal lobe deep in the Sylvian fissure, on the opposite side of the fissure wall from the auditory area of the superior temporal gyrus. These signals apprise the psyche of the equilibrium status of the body.

FUNCTION OF THE UTRICLE AND THE SACCULE IN THE MAINTENANCE OF STATIC EQUILIBRIUM

It is especially important that the different hair cells are oriented in all different directions in the maculae of the utricles and saccules so that at different positions of the head, different hair cells become stimulated. The "patterns" of stimulation of the different hair cells apprise the nervous system of the position of the head with respect to the pull of gravity. In turn, the vestibular, cerebellar, and reticular motor systems reflexly excite the appropriate muscles to maintain proper equilibrium.

The maculae in the utricle and saccule function extremely effectively for maintaining equilibrium especially when the head is in the near-vertical position. That is, a person can determine as little as a half-degree of mal-equilibrium when the head leans from the precise upright position. On the other hand, as the head is leaned further and further from the upright, the determination of head orientation by the vestibular sense becomes poorer and poorer. Obviously, extreme sensitivity in the upright position is of major importance for maintenance of precise vertical static equilibrium, which is the most essential function of the vestibular apparatus.

Detection of Linear Acceleration by the Maculae. When the body is suddenly thrust forward — that is, when the body accelerates — the otoconia, which have greater inertia than the surrounding fluids, fall backward on the hair cell cilia, and information of mal-equilibrium is sent into the nervous centers, causing the individual to feel as if he were falling backward. This automatically causes him to lean his body forward until the anterior shift of the otoconia caused by leaning exactly equals the tendency for the otoconia to fall backward. At this point, the nervous system detects a state of proper equilibrium and therefore leans the body no farther forward. As long as the degree of linear acceleration remains constant and

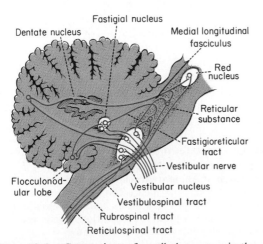

Figure 12–3. Connections of vestibular nerves in the central nervous system.

Dentate nucleus
Fastigial nucleus
Medial longitudinal fasciculus
Red nucleus
Reticular substance
Fastigioreticular tract
Vestibular nerve
Flocculonodular lobe
Vestibular nucleus
Vestibulospinal tract
Rubrospinal tract
Reticulospinal tract

the body is maintained in this forward leaning position, the person falls neither forward nor backward. Thus, the maculae operate to maintain equilibrium during linear acceleration in exactly the same manner as they operate in static equilibrium.

The otoconia *do not* operate for the detection of linear *velocity*. When a runner first begins to run, he must lean far forward to keep from falling over backward because of *acceleration,* but once he has achieved running speed, he would not have to lean forward at all if he were running in a vacuum. When running in air he leans forward to maintain equilibrium only because of the air resistance against his body, and in this instance it is not the otoconia that make him lean but the pressure of the air acting on pressure end-organs in the skin, which initiate the appropriate equilibrium adjustments to prevent falling.

THE SEMICIRCULAR CANALS AND THEIR DETECTION OF ANGULAR ACCELERATION AND ANGULAR VELOCITY

When the head suddenly *begins* to rotate in any direction, the endolymph in the membranous semicircular canals, because of its inertia, tends to remain stationary while the semicircular canals themselves turn. This causes relative fluid flow in the canals in a direction opposite to the rotation of the head.

Figure 12–4 illustrates an *ampulla* of one of the semicircular canals, showing the *cupula* and its embedded hairs bending in the direction of fluid movement. And Figure 12–5 illustrates the discharge signal from a single hair cell in the crista ampullaris when an animal is rotated for 40 sec-

Figure 12–5. Response of a hair cell when a semicircular canal is stimulated first by rotation and then by stopping rotation.

onds, showing that (1) even when the cupula is in its resting position the hair cell emits a tonic discharge of approximately 15 impulses per second; (2) when the animal is rotated, the hairs bend to one side and the rate of discharge increases greatly; and (3) with continued rotation, the excess discharge of the hair cell gradually subsides back to the resting level in about 20 seconds.

The reason for this adaptation of the receptor is that within a second or more of rotation, friction in the semicircular canal causes the endolymph to rotate as rapidly as the semicircular canal itself; then in an additional 15 to 20 seconds the cupula slowly returns to its resting position in the middle of the ampulla because of its own elastic recoil.

When the rotation suddenly stops, exactly the opposite effects take place: the endolymph continues to rotate while the semicircular canal stops. This time the cupula is bent in the opposite direction, causing the hair cell to stop discharging entirely. After another few seconds, the endolymph stops moving, and the cupula returns gradually to its resting position in about 20 seconds, thus allowing the discharge of the hair cell to return to its normal tonic level as shown to the right in Figure 12–5.

Thus, the semicircular canal transmits a positive signal when the head *begins* to rotate and a negative signal when it *stops* rotating. Furthermore, at least some hair cells will always respond to rotation in any plane — horizontal, sagittal, or coronal — for fluid movement always occurs in at least one semicircular canal.

Detection of Angular Acceleration and Angular Velocity. Angular velocity means the rate of rotation; that is, it is the number of revolutions about an axis in a given period of time. Angular acceleration means the rate at which the angular velocity is changing.

The semicircular canals always give a person a feeling of increasing rotation when he begins to rotate or a

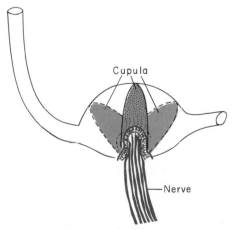

Figure 12–4. Movement of the cupula and its embedded hairs during rotation first in one direction and then in the opposite direction. (Often, the top of the cupula is attached so that it merely bulges in one direction or the other.)

feeling of decreasing rotation when he stops rotating — that is, they give a signal for angular acceleration. Therefore, it is commonly stated that the semicircular canals are primarily a detector of angular acceleration. However, a person also continues to feel that he is rotating for 5 to 15 seconds after he has begun to rotate. That is, he feels angular velocity during this period of time. Therefore, the semicircular canals actually detect a combination of angular acceleration and angular velocity, although the angular velocity effect may last only for 5 to 15 seconds.

Rate of Angular Acceleration Required to Stimulate the Semicircular Canals. The angular acceleration required to stimulate the semicircular canals in the human being averages about 1 degree per second per second. In other words, when one begins to rotate, the velocity of rotation must be as much as 1 degree per second by the end of the first second, 2 degrees per second by the end of the second second, 3 degrees per second by the end of the third second, and so forth, in order for the person barely to detect that the rate of rotation is increasing.

"Predictive" Function of the Semicircular Canals in the Maintenance of Equilibrium. Since the semicircular canals do not detect that the body is off balance in the forward direction, in the side direction, or in the backward direction, one might at first ask: What is the function of the semicircular canals in the maintenance of equilibrium? All they detect is that the person's head is rotating or beginning to rotate or stopping rotation in one direction or another. Therefore, the function of the semicircular canals is not likely to be to maintain static equilibrium or to maintain equilibrium during linear acceleration or when the person is exposed to steady centrifugal forces. Yet loss of function of the semicircular canals causes a person to have very poor equilibrium when attempting to perform *rapid* and *intricate* body movements.

We can explain the function of the semicircular canals best by the following illustration. If a person is running forward rapidly, and then suddenly begins to turn to one side, he falls off balance a second or so later unless appropriate corrections are made *ahead of time*. But, unfortunately, the utricle cannot detect that he is off balance until *after* this has occurred. On the other hand, the semicircular canals will have already detected that the person is turning, and this information can easily apprise the central nervous system of the fact that the person *will* fall off balance within the next second or so unless some correction is made. In other words, the semicircular canal mechanism *predicts ahead of time* that mal-equilibrium is going to occur even before it does occur and thereby causes the equilibrium centers to make appropriate preventive adjustments. In this way, the person need not fall off balance before he begins to correct the situation.

Removal of the flocculonodular lobes of the cerebellum prevents normal function of the semicircular canals but does not prevent normal function of the macular receptors. It is especially interesting in this connection that the cerebellum serves as a "predictive" organ for most of the other rapid movements of the body as well as those having to do with equilibrium. These other functions of the cerebellum are discussed in the following chapter.

VESTIBULAR POSTURAL REFLEXES

Sudden changes in the orientation of an animal in space elicit reflexes that help to maintain equilibrium and posture. For instance, if an animal is suddenly pushed to the right, even before it can fall more than a few degrees its right legs extend instantaneously. In other words, this mechanism *anticipates* that the animal will be off balance in a few seconds and makes appropriate adjustments to prevent this.

Another type of vestibular postural reflex occurs when the animal suddenly falls forward. When this occurs, the forepaws extend forward, the extensor muscles tighten, and the muscles in the back of the neck stiffen to prevent the animal's head striking the ground. This reflex is probably also of importance in locomotion, for, in the case of the galloping horse, the downward thrust of the head can automatically provide reflex thrust of the forelimbs to move the animal forward for the next gallop.

VESTIBULAR MECHANISM FOR STABILIZING THE EYES AND FOR NYSTAGMUS

When a person changes his direction of movement rapidly, or even leans his head sideways, forward, or backward, it would be impossible for him to maintain a stable image on the retinae of his eyes unless he had some automatic control mechanism to stabilize the direction of gaze of the eyes. In addition, the eyes would be of little use in detecting an image unless they remained "fixed" on each object long enough to gain a clear image. Fortunately, each time the head is suddenly angulated, signals from the semicircular canals cause the eyes to angulate in an equal and opposite direction to the angulation of the head. This results from reflexes transmitted from the canals through the *vestibular nuclei,* the *cerebellum,* and the *medial longitudinal fasciculus* to the *ocular nuclei.*

A special example of this stabilization of the eyes occurs when a person begins to rotate. At first the eyes remain glued to the object. But after the head has rotated far to one side, they jump suddenly in the direction of rotation of the head and "fix" on a new object; then they deviate slowly backward again as the rotation proceeds. This sudden jumping motion forward and then slow backward motion is called *nystagmus.* The jumping motion is called the *fast component* of the nystagmus, and the slow movement, the *slow component.*

Nystagmus always occurs automatically when the semicircular canals are stimulated. For instance, if a person's head begins to rotate to the right, backward movement of fluid in the left horizontal canal and forward movement in the right horizontal canal cause the eyes to move slowly to the left; thus, the slow component of nystagmus is initiated by the vestibular apparatuses. But, when the eyes have moved as far to the left as they reasonably can, centers located in the brain stem in close approximation to the nuclei of the abducens nerves cause the eyes to jump suddenly to the right; then the vestibular apparatuses take over once more to move the eyes again slowly to the left.

CLINICAL TESTS FOR INTEGRITY OF VESTIBULAR FUNCTION

Balancing Test. One of the simplest clinical tests for integrity of the equilibrium mechanism is to have the individual stand perfectly still with eyes closed. If there is no longer a functioning static equilibrium system of the utricles, the person will waver to one side or the other and possibly even fall. However, as noted below, some of the proprioceptive mechanisms of equilibrium are occasionally sufficiently well developed to maintain balance even with the eyes closed.

Barany Test. A second test that is frequently performed determines the integrity of the semicircular canals. In this instance the individual is placed in a "Barany chair" and rotated rapidly while placing the head respectively in various planes — first forward, then angulated to one side or the other. By such positioning, each pair of semicircular canals is successively placed in the horizontal plane of rotation. When the rotation of the chair is stopped suddenly, the endolymph, because of its momentum, continues to rotate in the pair of semicircular canals that has been placed in the horizontal plane, causing the cupula to bend in the direction of rotation. As a result, nystagmus occurs, with the slow component in the direction of rotation and the fast component in the opposite direction. Also, as long as the nystagmus lasts (about 15 to 20 seconds) the individual has the sensation that he is rotating in the direction *opposite* to that in which he was actually rotated in the chair. Obviously, this test checks the semicircular canals on both sides of the head at the same time.

Ice Water Test. A clinical test of one vestibular apparatus separately from the other depends on placing ice water in one ear. The external semicircular canal lies adjacent to the ear, and cooling the ear can transfer a sufficient amount of heat from this canal to cool the endolymph. This increases the density of the endolymph, thereby causing it to sink downward and resulting in slight movement of fluid around the semicircular canal. This stimulates the canal, giving the individual a sensation of rotating and also initiating nystagmus. From these two findings one can determine whether the respective semicircular canals are functioning properly. When the semicircular canals are normal, the utricles and saccules are usually normal also, for disease usually destroys the function of all of these components at the same time.

OTHER FACTORS CONCERNED WITH EQUILIBRIUM

The Neck Proprioceptors. The vestibular apparatus detects the orientation and movements *only of the head*.

Therefore, it is essential that the nervous centers also receive appropriate information depicting the orientation of the head with respect to the body as well as the orientation of the different parts of the body with respect to each other. This information is transmitted from the proprioceptors of the neck and body directly into the vestibular and reticular nuclei of the brain stem and also indirectly by way of the cerebellum.

By far the most important proprioceptive information needed for the maintenance of equilibrium is that derived from the *joint receptors of the neck,* for this apprises the nervous system of the orientation of the head with respect to the body. When the head is bent in one direction or the other by bending the neck, impulses from the neck proprioceptors keep the vestibular apparatuses from giving the person a sense of malequilibrium. They do this by transmitting signals that exactly oppose the signals transmitted from the vestibular apparatuses. However, *when the entire body* is changed to a new position with respect to gravity, the impulses from the vestibular apparatuses *are not opposed* by the neck proprioceptors; therefore, the person in this instance does perceive a change in equilibrium status.

The Neck Reflexes. In an animal *whose vestibular apparatuses have been destroyed,* bending the neck causes immediate muscular reflexes called *neck reflexes* occurring especially in the forelimbs. For instance, bending the head forward causes both forelimbs to relax. However, when the vestibular apparatuses are *intact,* this effect does *not* occur because the vestibular reflexes function almost exactly oppositely to the neck reflexes. Thus, if the head is flexed downward, the vestibular reflex tends to extend the forelimbs, while the neck reflexes tend to relax them. Since the equilibrium of the entire body and not of the head alone must be maintained, it is easy to understand that the vestibular and neck reflexes must function oppositely. Otherwise, each time the neck should bend, the animal would immediately fall off balance.

Proprioceptive and Exteroceptive Information from Other Parts of the Body. Proprioceptive information from other parts of the body besides the neck is also necessary for maintenance of equilibrium because appropriate equilibrium adjustments must be made whenever the body is angulated in the chest or abdomen region or elsewhere. Presumably, all this information is algebraically added in the cerebellum, vestibular nuclei, and reticular nuclei of the brain stem, thus causing appropriate adjustments in the postural muscles.

Also important in the maintenance of equilibrium are several types of exteroceptive sensations. For instance, pressure sensations from the footpads can tell one (a) whether his weight is distributed equally between his two feet and (b) whether his weight is more forward or backward on his feet.

Another instance in which exteroceptive information is necessary for maintenance of equilibrium occurs when a person is running. The air pressure against the front of the body signals that a force is opposing the body in a direction different from that caused by gravitational pull; as a result, the person leans forward to oppose this.

Importance of Visual Information in the Maintenance of Equilibrium. After complete destruction of the vestibular apparatuses, and even after loss of most proprioceptive information from the body, a person can still use the visual mechanisms effectively for maintaining equilibrium. Even slight linear or angular movement of the body instaneously shifts the visual images on the retina, and this information is relayed to the equilibrium centers. Many persons with complete destruction of the vestibular apparatus have almost normal equilibrium as long as their eyes are open and as long as they perform all motions slowly. But, when moving rapidly or when the eyes are closed, equilibrium is immediately lost.

Conscious Perception of Equilibrium. A cortical center for conscious perception of the state of equilibrium is believed to lie in the lowest part of the parietal cortex deep in the sylvian fissure, on the medial wall of this fissure opposite to the primary cortical area for hearing. The sensations from the vestibular apparatuses, from the neck proprioceptors, and from most of the other proprioceptors are probably first integrated in the equilibrium centers of the brain stem before being transmitted to the cerebral cortex. Various pathological processes in the vestibular apparatuses or in the vestibular neuronal circuits often affect the equilibrium sensations. Thus, loss of one or both flocculonodular lobes or one or both fastigial nuclei of the cerebellum gives the person a sensation of constant mal-equilibrium for the first few weeks or months after the loss. This probably results because impulses from these cerebellar areas are normally integrated into the subconscious sense of equilibrium by the vestibular and reticular nuclei even before equilibrium information is sent to the cerebral cortex.

FUNCTIONS OF THE RETICULAR FORMATION AND SPECIFIC BRAIN STEM NUCLEI IN CONTROLLING SUBCONSCIOUS, STEREOTYPED MOVEMENTS

Rarely, a child called an *anencephalic monster* is born without brain structures above the mesencephalic region, and some of these children have been kept alive for many months. They are able to perform essentially all the functions of feeding, such as suckling, extrusion of unpleasant food from the mouth, and moving the hands to the mouth to suck the fingers. In addition, they can yawn and stretch. They can cry and follow objects with the eyes and by movements of the head. Also, placing pressure on the upper anterior parts of their legs will cause them to pull to the sitting position.

Therefore, it is obvious that many of the stereotyped motor functions of the human being are integrated in the brain stem. Unfortunately, the loci of most of the different motor control systems have not been found except for the following:

Stereotyped Body Movements. Most movements of the trunk and head can be classified into several simple movements, such as forward flexion, extension, rotation, and turning movements of the entire body. These types of movements are controlled by special nuclei located mainly in the mesencephalic and lower dien-

cephalic region. For instance, *rotational movements* of the head and eyes are controlled by the *interstitial nucleus,* which is illustrated in Figure 12–1. This nucleus lies in close approximation to the *medial longitudinal fasciculus,* through which it transmits a major portion of its control impulses. The *raising movements* of the head and body are controlled by the *prestitial nucleus,* which is located approximately at the juncture of the diencephalon and mesencephalon. On the other hand, the *flexing movements* of the head and body are controlled by the *nucleus precommissuralis* located at the level of the posterior commissure. Finally, the *turning movements* of the entire body, which are much more complicated, involve both the pontile and mesencephalic reticular formation. However, for full expression of the turning movements, the caudate nucleus and the cingulate gyrus of the cerebral cortex are also required. The turning movements can cause an animal or person to continue circling around and around in one direction or the other.

Function of the Red Nucleus. The red nucleus, illustrated in Figure 12–6, is composed of two distinct parts, the *magnocellular portion* and a *small cellular portion.*

The magnocellular nuclei receive impulses both from the *basal ganglia* and from the *prestitial nucleus* and *nucleus commissuralis.* In turn they transmit signals by way of the *rubrospinal tract* into the spinal cord and by way of collaterals from the rubrospinal tract into the *reticular nuclei* of the brain stem. Stimulation of this portion of the red nucleus causes the head and upper trunk to extend backward. Thus, this portion of the red nucleus enters into a particular type of gross body movement concerned with forward and backward deviation of the body axis.

The small cells of the red nucleus are excited principally by impulses from the *cerebellum* through the *cerebellorubral tracts.* In turn, they send impulses mainly into the reticular formation of the brain stem. These tracts are part of the overall cerebellar mechanism for control of motor function, which will be discussed in the following chapter.

Function of the Subthalamic Areas — Forward Progression. Much less is known about function of higher brain stem centers in posture and locomotion than of the lower centers, principally because of the complexity of the neuronal connections. However, it is known that stimulation of centers in or around the subthalamic nuclei can cause rhythmic limb motions, including forward walking reflexes. This does not mean that the individual muscles of walking are controlled from this region but simply that excitation of this region sends "command" signals to activate the cord centers where *pre-programmed* neuronal circuits then cause the actual walking movements.

A cat with its brain transected beneath the thalamus but above the subthalamus can walk in an almost completely normal fashion — so much so that the observer often cannot tell the difference. However, when the animal comes to an obstruction it simply butts its head against the obstruction and tries to keep on walking. Thus, it lacks *purposefulness of locomotion.*

The function of the subthalamic region in walking is frequently described as that of controlling *forward progression.* In the previous chapter we have already noted that a decerebrate animal can stand perfectly well, and also it can make attempts to right itself from the lying position. Unfortunately, though, the decerebrate animal with the brain stem sectioned below the subthalamus cannot force itself to move forward in a normal walking pattern. This seems to be the function of areas either in or somewhere close to the subthalamic nuclei.

MOTOR FUNCTIONS OF THE BASAL GANGLIA

Physiologic Anatomy of the Basal Ganglia. The anatomy of the basal ganglia is so complex and so poorly known in its details that it would be pointless to attempt a complete description at this time. However, Figure 12–6 illustrates the principal structures of the basal ganglia and their multitude of neural connections with other parts of the nervous system. Physiologically, the basal ganglia are considered to be the *caudate nucleus, putamen, globus pallidus, substantia nigra,* and *subthalamus.* However, major portions of the *thalamus, reticular formation,* and *red nuclei* operate in close association with these and are therefore part of the basal ganglial system for motor control.

Some important features of the different pathways illustrated in Figure 12–6 are the following:

1. Numerous nerve pathways pass from the motor portion of the cerebral cortex, particularly from the *motor association areas* in front of the primary motor cortex (also called the premotor areas), to the caudate nucleus and putamen, which together are called the *striate body.* In turn, the caudate nucleus and putamen send numerous fibers to the globus pallidus, substantia nigra, and subthalamus. Then these nuclei send fibers to the ventrolateral and ventroanterior nuclei of the thalamus, and still another set of fibers from these nuclei pass

back to the motor areas of the cerebral cortex. Thus, circular pathways are established from the motor cortical regions to the basal ganglia, the thalamus, and back to the motor regions from which the pathways begin. These circuits obviously could operate as a feedback system of the servo control type, as will be discussed later.

2. Still another circular pathway exists among the basal ganglia themselves, in which signals are transmitted downward from the caudate nucleus and putamen through the globus pallidus to the substantia nigra; then signals return upward from the substantia nigra back to the putamen and caudate nucleus. A special feature of this circuit is that both its downward and upward limbs are probably inhibitory, the downward pathway secreting the transmitter substance *GABA* and the upward pathway from the substantia nigra to the putamen and caudate nucleus secreting *dopamine.* As we shall see, these two pathways play a major role in controlling the intrinsic activity level in the basal ganglia themselves.

3. In the following chapter it will be noted that signals also pass from the motor regions of the cerebral cortex to the pons and then into the cerebellum. In turn, signals from the cerebellum are transmitted back to the motor cortex by way of the ventrolateral nucleus of the thalamus, a nucleus through which many of the basal ganglial signals returning to the cortex also are transmitted. This circuit could allow integration between the basal ganglial feedback signals and the feedback signals from the cerebellum.

4. The basal ganglia have numerous short neuronal connections among themselves. Also, the lower basal ganglia, such as the globus pallidus, substantia nigra, and subthalamus send signals into the lower brain stem, projecting especially onto the reticular nuclei, the red nucleus, and the inferior olive. It is presumably through these pathways that many of the so-called extrapyramidal signals for motor control are transmitted.

5. Large numbers of nerve fibers pass directly from the motor cortex to the reticular nuclei and other nuclei of the brain stem. These bypass the basal ganglia but converge on the same brain stem nuclei that are innervated by the basal ganglia.

FUNCTIONS OF THE DIFFERENT BASAL GANGLIA

Before attempting to discuss the functions of the basal ganglia in human beings, we should speak briefly of the better known functions of these ganglia in lower animals. In birds, for instance, the cerebral cortex is poorly developed while the basal ganglia are highly developed. These ganglia perform essentially all the motor functions, even controlling the voluntary movements in much the same manner that the motor cortex of the human being controls voluntary movements. Furthermore, in the cat, and to a lesser extent in the dog, decortication removes only the discrete types of motor functions and does not interfere with the animal's ability to walk, eat, fight, develop rage, have periodic sleep and wakefulness, and even participate naturally in sexual activities. However, if a major portion of the basal ganglia is

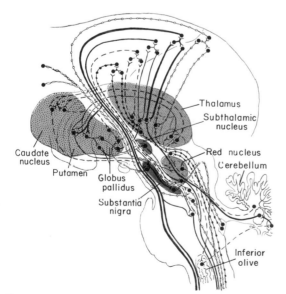

Figure 12–6. Pathways through the basal ganglia and related structures of the brain stem, thalamus, and cerebral cortex. (From Jung and Hassler: Handbook of Physiology, Sec. I, Vol. II. Baltimore, Williams & Wilkins Company, 1960.)

destroyed, only gross stereotyped movements remain, which were discussed above in relation to the mesencephalic animal.

Finally, in the human being, cortical lesions in very young individuals destroy the discrete movements of the body, particularly of the hands and distal portions of the lower limbs, but do not destroy the person's ability to walk crudely, to control equilibrium, or to perform many other subconscious types of movements. However, simultaneous destruction of a major portion of the caudate nuclei almost totally paralyzes the opposite side of the body except for a few stereotyped reflexes integrated in the cord or brain stem.

With this brief background of the overall function of the basal ganglia, we can attempt to dissect the functions of the individual portions of the basal ganglia system, realizing that the system actually operates, along with the motor cortex and cerebellum, as a total unit and that individual functions cannot be ascribed completely to the different parts of the basal ganglia.

Inhibition of Motor Tone by the Basal Ganglia. Though it is wrong to ascribe a single function to all the basal ganglia, nevertheless, one of the general effects of diffuse basal ganglia excitation is to inhibit muscle tone throughout the body. This effect results from inhibitory signals transmitted from the basal ganglia to both the motor cortex and the lower brain stem. Therefore, whenever widespread destruction of the basal ganglia occurs, this causes muscle rigidity throughout the body. For instance, when the brain stem is transected at the mesencephalic level, which removes the inhibitory effects of the basal ganglia, the phenomenon of decerebrate rigidity occurs.

Yet, despite this general inhibitory effect of the basal ganglia, stimulation of specific areas within the basal ganglia can at times elicit positive muscle contractions and at times even complex patterns of movements.

Function of the Caudate Nucleus and Putamen — The Striate Body. The caudate nucleus and putamen, because of their gross appearance on sections of the brain, are together called the *striate body*. They seem to function together to initiate and regulate gross intentional movements of the body. To perform this function they transmit inpulses through two different pathways: (1) into the *globus pallidus* and *substantia nigra*, thence by way of the *thalamus* to the *cerebral cortex,* and finally downward into the spinal cord through the *corticospinal* and *extracorticospinal pathways;* (2) downward through the *globus pallidus* and the *substantia nigra* by way of short axons into the *reticular formation* and finally into the spinal cord mainly through the *reticulospinal tracts*.

In summary, the striate body helps to control gross intentional movements that we normally perform unconsciously. However, this control also involves the motor cortex, with which the striate body is very closely connected.

Function of the Globus Pallidus. It has been suggested that the principal function of the globus pallidus is to provide background muscle tone for intended movements, whether these be initiated by impulses from the cerebral cortex or from the striate body. That is, a person wishing to perform an exact function with one hand, first positions the body, next the legs and arms, and also tenses the muscles of the upper arm. These associated tonic contractions are supposedly initiated by circuits that strongly involve the globus pallidus. Destruction of the globus pallidus removes these attitudinal movements that are necessary to position the hand and, therefore, makes it difficult or impossible for the distal portions of the limbs to perform their more discrete activities.

The globus pallidus is believed to function through two pathways: first, through feedback circuits to the thalamus, to the cerebral cortex, and thence by way of corticospinal and extracorticospinal tracts to the spinal cord; and, second, by way of short axons to the reticular formation of the brain stem and thence mainly by way of the reticulospinal tracts into the spinal cord.

Electrical stimulation of the globus pallidus while an animal is performing a gross body movement will often stop the movement in a static position, the animal holding that position for many seconds while the stimulation continues. This fits with the concept that the globus pallidus is involved in some type of servo feedback motor control system that is capable of locking the different parts of the body into specific positions. Obviously, such a circuit could be extremely important in providing the background body movements and upper limb movements when a person performs delicate tasks with the hands.

CLINICAL SYNDROMES RESULTING FROM DAMAGE TO THE BASAL GANGLIA

Much of what we know about the function of the basal ganglia comes from study of patients with basal ganglia lesions whose brains have undergone pathologic studies after death. Among the different clinical syndromes are:

Chorea. Chorea is a disease in which random uncontrolled movement patterns occur continuously. Normal progression of movements cannot occur; instead, the person may perform one pattern of movement for a few seconds and then suddenly begin another pattern of movement; then still another pattern begins after a few seconds. Because of this peculiar progression of movements, one type of chorea is frequently called *St. Vitus' dance.*

Pathologically, chorea results from *diffuse and widespread damage in the caudate and putamen nuclei.* Especially, the neurons that secrete the inhibitory transmitter GABA are greatly reduced in number or activity. Therefore, the normal inhibitory signals transmitted from the caudate nucleus and putamen into the lower basal ganglia — especially into the globus pallidus and substantia nigra — can no longer hold these lower areas in check. As a result, recurrent signals from these lower areas, probably mainly from the globus pallidus to the thalamus and thence to the motor cortex, elicit trains of successive choreiform movements.

Athetosis. In this disease, slow, writhing movements of a hand, the neck, the face, the tongue, or some other part of the body occur continually. The movements are likely to be wormlike, first with overextension of the hands and fingers, then flexion, then rotary twisting to the side — all these continuing in a slow, rhythmic, repetitive writhing pattern. The contracting muscles exhibit a high degree of spasm, and the movements are enhanced by emotions or by excessive signals from the sensory organs. Furthermore, voluntary movements in the affected area are greatly impaired or sometimes even impossible.

The damage in athetosis is usually found in the *outer portion of the globus pallidus* or in this area and the *striate body*. Athetosis is usually attributed to the interruption of feedback circuits among the basal ganglia, thalamus, and cerebral cortex. The normal feedback circuits presumably allow a constant and rapid interplay between antagonistic muscle groups so that finely controlled static or progressive movements can take place. However, if the feedback circuits are blocked, it is supposed that the detouring impulses may take devious routes through the basal ganglia, thalamus, and motor cortex, causing a succession of abnormal movements.

Hemiballismus. Hemiballismus is an uncontrollable succession of violent movements of large areas of the body. These may occur once every few seconds or sometimes only once in many minutes. For instance, an entire leg might suddenly jerk uncontrollably to full flexion, or the entire trunk might go through an extreme, sudden torsion movement, or an arm might be pulled upward suddenly with great force. Hemiballismus of the legs or trunk causes the person to fall to the ground if walking, and even in bed, the person tosses violently when affected by these powerful and strong intermittent movements. Furthermore, attempts to perform voluntary movements frequently invoke ballistic movements in place of the normal movements.

Hemiballismus of one side of the body results from a *large lesion in the opposite subthalamus*. The smooth, progressive or rhythmic movements of the limbs or other parts of the body normally integrated in this area can no longer occur, but excitatory impulses attempting to evoke such movements elicit instead uncontrollable ballistic movements.

Parkinson's Disease. Parkinson's disease, which is also known as *paralysis agitans,* results almost invariably from *widespread destruction of the substantia nigra,* but often associated with lesions of the *globus pallidus* and other related areas. It is characterized by (1) *rigidity* of the musculature either in widespread areas of the body or in isolated areas, (2) *tremor at rest* of the involved areas in most but not all instances, and (3) a serious *inability to initiate movement,* called *akinesia*.

The cause or causes of these abnormal motor activi-

ties are almost entirely unknown. However, they are almost certainly related to *loss of dopamine secretion* in the caudate nucleus and putamen by the nerve endings of the *nigrostriatal tract*. Destruction of the substantia nigra causes this tract to degenerate and the dopamine normally secreted in the caudate nucleus and putamen no longer to be present. But still present are large numbers of neurons that secrete acetylcholine. These are believed to transmit excitatory signals throughout the basal ganglia. It is also believed that the dopamine from the nigrostriatal pathway normally acts to inhibit these acetylcholine-producing neurons or in some other way to counter their activity. But, in the absence of dopamine secretion, the acetylcholine pathways become overly active, which presumably is the basis for the motor symptoms in Parkinson's disease.

The rigidity in this disease is somewhat different from that which occurs in decerebrate rigidity, for decerebrate rigidity results mainly from hyperactivity of the muscle spindle system, and even slight movement of a muscle is met with rather extreme reflex resistance resulting from feedback through the stretch reflex mechanism. Parkinsonian rigidity, on the other hand, is of a "plastic" type. That is, sudden movement is not met by intense resistance from the stretch reflexes as in the decerebrate type of rigidity, but instead both protagonist and antagonist muscles remain tightly contracted throughout the movement. Therefore, it is believed that the rigidity of Parkinson's disease results to a great extent from excess impulses transmitted in the corticospinal system, thus activating the alpha motor fibers to the muscles, in addition to probable excess activation of the gamma efferent system as well.

Tremor usually, but not always, occurs in Parkinson's disease. Its frequency is normally four to six cycles per second. When the parkinsonian patient performs voluntary movements, the tremor becomes temporarily or partially blocked, presumably because other motor control signals —perhaps from the cerebral cortex and cerebellum —override the abnormal basal ganglial signals.

The mechanism of the tremor in Parkinson's disease is not known. However, a type of treatment that frequently relieves the tremor is surgical destruction of the *ventrolateral nucleus of the thalamus* which is one of the feedback pathways from the basal ganglia to the motor cortex. Therefore, it is presumed that loss of the inhibitory influence of dopamine in the basal ganglia leads to enhanced activity of the cortical-basal ganglial-thalamic-cortical feedback circuit, leading to an oscillation that produces the muscle tremor.

Though the muscle rigidity and the tremor are both distressing to the parkinsonian patient, even more serious is the *akinesia* that occurs in the final stages of the disease. To perform even the simplest of movement, the person must exert the highest degree of concentration, and the mental effort, even mental anguish, that is necessary to make the movement "go" is often almost beyond the patient's willpower. Then, when the movement does occur, it is stiff and often staccato in character instead of occurring with smooth progression. For instance, when a patient begins to perform a discrete voluntary movement with his hands, the automatic "associated" adjustments of the trunk of his body and the upper arm segments do not occur. Instead, he must voluntarily adjust these segments before he can use his hands. Furthermore, a tremendous amount of nervous effort must be made by the voluntary motor control system to overcome "motor stiffness" of his musculature. Thus, the person with Parkinson's disease has a masklike face, showing almost no automatic emotional facial expressions; he is usually bent forward because of his muscle rigidity; and all his movements of necessity are highly deliberate rather than the many casual subconscious movements that are normally a part of our everyday life.

The cause of the akinesia in Parkinson's disease is not known, and again we must resort to theory. It is presumed that *loss of dopamine secretion in the caudate nucleus and putamen by the nigrostriatal fibers* allows excessive activity of the acetylcholine-producing neurons. But normal operation of the basal ganglia requires a balance between both excitatory and inhibitory activities, and loss of this balance, in effect, leads to a functionless basal ganglia system. We have already pointed out that the basal ganglia are responsible for many of the subconscious stereotyped movements of the body, and also responsible even for the background movements of the trunk, legs, neck, and upper arms that are required preliminary to performing the more discrete movements of the hands. If the subconscious and the background movements cannot occur, then other neural mechanisms must be substituted, especially those of the motor cortex and cerebellum. Unfortunately, though, these cannot replace the movements normally controlled by the basal ganglia and certainly cannot function at a subconscious level.

Treatment with L-Dopa and Anticholinergic Drugs. Administration of L-dopa to patients with Parkinson's disease ameliorates most of the symptoms, especially the rigidity and the akinesia, in about two-thirds of the patients. The reason for this seems to be the following: The dopamine secreted in the caudate nucleus and putamen by the nigrostriated fibers is a derivative of L-dopa. When the substantia nigra is destroyed and the person develops Parkinson's disease, the administered L-dopa is believed to substitute for the dopamine no longer secreted by the destroyed neurons. This causes more or less normal inhibition of the basal ganglia and relieves much or most of the akinesia and rigidity.

The same basal ganglia that are inhibited by dopamine are excited by acetylcholine-secreting neurons, as was discussed earlier. Therefore, as would be expected, administration of anticholinergic drugs such as scopolamine can also decrease the level of activity in the basal ganglia and therefore benefit the parkinsonian patient.

Coagulation of the Ventrolateral Nucleus of the Thalamus for Treatment of Parkinson's Disease. In recent years neurosurgeons have treated Parkinson's disease patients, with varying success, by destroying portions of the basal ganglia or of the thalamus. The most prevalent treatment has been widespread destruction of the ventrolateral nucleus of the thalamus, usually by electrocoagulation. Most fiber pathways from the basal ganglia and cerebellum to the cerebral cortex pass through this nucleus so that its destruction blocks many or most of the feedback functions of the basal ganglia and cerebellum. It is presumed that blockage of some of these feedbacks limits the functions of at least certain

basal ganglia and thereby removes the factors that cause especially the tremor of Parkinson's disease.

REFERENCES

Baldessarini, R. J., and Tarsey, D.: Dopamine and the pathophysiology of dyskinesias induced by antipsychotic drugs. *Annu. Rev. Neurosci.*, 3:23, 1980.

Bizzi, E.: The coordination of eye-head movements. *Sci. Am.*, 231(4):100, 1974.

Bobath, B., and Bobath, K.: Motor Development in the Different Types of Cerebral Palsy. London, W. Heinemann Medical Books, 1975.

Brodal, A. (ed.): Basic Aspects of Central Vestibular Mechanisms. New York, American Elsevier Publishing Co., 1971.

Chase, T. N., et al. (eds.): Huntington's Disease. New York, Raven Press, 1979.

Crowley, W. J.: Neural control of skeletal muscle. *In* Frohlich, E. D. (ed.): Pathophysiology, 2nd Ed. Philadelphia, J. B. Lippincott Co., 1976, p. 735.

Denny-Brown, D.: The Basal Ganglia: Their Relation to Disorders of Movement. New York, Oxford University Press, 1962.

Divac, I., and Öberg, R. G. E. (eds.): The Neostriatum. New York, Pergamon Press, 1979.

Duvoisin, R. C.: Parkinson's Disease. New York, Raven Press, 1978.

Elder, H. Y., and Trueman, E. R. (eds.): Aspects of Animal Movement. New York, Cambridge University Press, 1980.

Evarts, E. V.: Brain mechanisms of movement. *Sci. Am. 241*(3):164, 1979.

Fuxe, K., and Calne, D. B. (eds.): Dopaminergic Ergot Derivatives and Motor Function. New York, Pergamon Press, 1979.

Goldberg, J. M., and Fernandez, C.: Vestibular mechanisms. *Annu. Rev. Physiol.*, 37:129, 1975.

Granit, R., and Pompeiano, O. (eds.): Reflex Control of Posture and Movement. New York, Elsevier Scientific Publishing Co., 1979.

Hobson, J. A., and Brazier, M. A. B. (eds.): The Reticular Formation Revisited: Specifying Function for A Nonspecific System. New York, Raven Press, 1980.

Hood, J. D. (ed.): Vestibular Mechanisms in Health and Disease. New York, Academic Press, 1978.

Horn, A. S., et al. (eds.): The Neurology of Dopamine. New York, Academic Press, 1979.

Nauta, W. J. H., and Freitag, M.: The organization of the brain. *Sci. Am.*, 241(3):88, 1979.

Oosterveld, W. J. (ed.): Audio-Vestibular System and Facial Nerve. New York, S. Karger, 1977.

Orlovsky, G. N., and Shik, M. L.: Control of locomotion: A neurophysiological analysis of the cat locomotor system. *Int. Rev. Physiol.*, 10:281, 1976.

Pearson, K.: The control of walking. *Sci. Am.*, 235(6):72, 1976.

Peterson, B. W.: Reticulospinal projections of spinal motor nuclei. *Annu. Rev. Physiol.*, 41:127, 1979.

Precht, W.: Vestibular system. *In* MTP International Review of Science: Physiology. Vol. 3. Baltimore, University Park Press, 1974, p. 81.

Precht, W.: Vestibular mechanisms. *Annu. Rev. Neurosci.*, 2:265, 1979.

Riklan, M.: L-Dopa and Parkinsonism. Springfield, Ill., Charles C Thomas, 1973.

Sarno, J. E., and Sarno, M. T.: Stroke; The Condition and the Patient. New York, McGraw-Hill, 1979.

Sherrington, C. S.: Decerebrate ridigity and reflex coordination of movements. *J. Physiol. (Lond.)*, 22:319, 1898.

Shik, M. L., and Orlovsky, G. N.: Neurophysiology of locomotor automatism. *Physiol. Rev.*, 56:465, 1976.

Stein, P. S. G.: Motor systems with specific reference to the control of locomotion. *Annu. Rev. Neurosci.* 1:61, 1978.

Talbott, R. E., and Humphrey, D. R. (eds.): Posture and Movement. New York, Raven Press, 1979.

Valentinuzzi, M.: The Organs of Equilibrium and Orientation as a Control System. New York, Harwood Academic Publishers, 1980.

Wilson, V., and Jones. G. M.: Mammalian Vestibular Physiology. New York, Plenum Press, 1979.

Wilson, V. J., and Peterson, B. W.: Peripheral and central substrates of vestibulospinal reflexes. *Physiol. Rev.*, 58:80, 1978

Young, L. R.: Cross coupling between effects of linear and angular acceleration on vestibular nystagmus. *Bibl. Ophthalmol.*, 82:116, 1972.

Cortical and Cerebellar Control of Motor Functions

In preceding chapters we have been concerned with many of the subconscious motor activities integrated in the spinal cord and brain stem, especially those responsible for locomotion. In the present chapter we will discuss the control of motor function by the cerebral cortex and cerebellum as well as their relationship to the basal ganglia and the other lower centers. Much of this control is "voluntary" in contradistinction to the subconscious control effected by the lower centers. Yet we will also see that at least some motor functions of the cerebral cortex and cerebellum are not entirely "voluntary."

PHYSIOLOGIC ANATOMY OF THE MOTOR AREAS OF THE CORTEX AND THEIR PATHWAYS TO THE CORD

Figure 13–1 illustrates a broad area of the cerebral cortex called the *sensorimotor cortex* that is concerned either with sensation from the somatic areas of the body or with control of body movement. We have discussed in previous chapters the somesthetic cortex, which constitutes the posterior portion of the sensorimotor cortex. This area plays a major role in controlling the functions of the motor cortex, as we shall see in more detail later in the chapter.

The *motor cortex* lies anterior to the central sulcus. Its posterior portion, as shown in the figure, is characterized by large pyramid-shaped cells. This area is usually referred to simply as area IV which is the number of the area in the Broadmann classification of the cortical areas. It is frequently also called the *primary motor cortex* or the *pyramidal area*. The anterior portion of the motor cortex is usually referred to as area VI because it is mainly composed of area VI in Broadmann's classification. It is also frequently referred to as either the *motor association area* or the *premotor area*.

The Pyramidal Area and the Pyramidal Tract (Corti-cospinal Tract). The area designated in Figure 13–1 by the darker shading contains in each hemisphere of the cortex approximately 34,000 *giant Betz cells,* or *giant pyramidal cells,* for which reason it is called the "pyramidal area." This area also causes motor movements with the least amount of electrical excitation, which explains its other name, the "primary motor cortex."

One of the major pathways by which motor signals are transmitted from all the motor areas of the cortex to the anterior motoneurons of the spinal cord is through the *pyramidal tract,* or *corticospinal tract,* which is illustrated in Figure 13–2. This tract originates in all the shaded areas in Figure 13–1, including both the motor and the somesthetic areas, about 80 per cent from the motor areas and about 20 per cent from the somesthetic regions posterior to the central sulcus. The function of the fibers from the somesthetic cortex is probably not motor, but instead to cause feedback control of sensory input to the nervous system, as was discussed in Chapter 9.

The most impressive fibers in the pyramidal tract are the large myelinated fibers that originate in the giant Betz cells of the pyramidal area. These account for approximately 34,000 large fibers (mean diameter of about 16 microns) in the pyramidal tract from *each* side of the cortex. However, since each corticospinal tract contains more than a million fibers, only 3 per cent of the total number of corticospinal fibers are of this large type. The other 97 per cent are mainly fibers smaller than 4 microns in diameter.

The pyramidal tract passes downward through the *brain stem;* then it decussates mainly to the opposite side to form the *pyramids of the medulla.* By far the majority of the pyramidal fibers then descend in the *lateral corticospinal tracts* of the cord and terminate principally on interneurons at the bases of the dorsal horns of the cord gray matter. A few fibers, however, do not cross to the opposite side but pass ipsilaterally down the cord in the *ventral corticospinal tracts* and then mainly decussate to the opposite side farther down the cord.

Collaterals from the Pyramidal Tract in the Brain. Even before the pyramidal tract leaves the brain, many collaterals are given off as follows:

1. The axons from the giant Betz cells send short

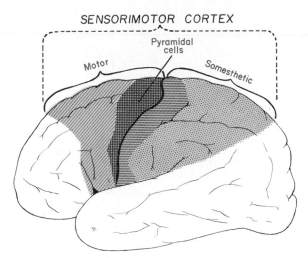

Figure 13–1. Relationship of the motor cortex to the somesthetic cortex.

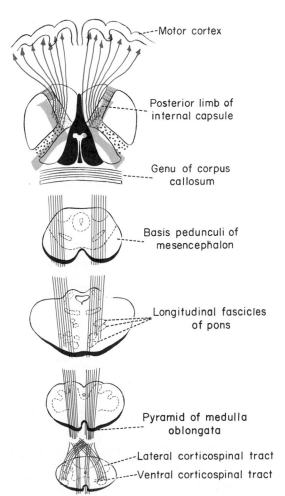

Figure 13–2. The pyramidal tract. (From Ranson and Clark: Anatomy of the Nervous System. Philadelphia, W. B. Saunders Company, 1959.)

collaterals back to the cortex itself. It is believed that these collaterals mainly inhibit adjacent regions of the cortex when the Betz cells discharge, thereby "sharpening" the boundaries of the excitatory signal.

2. A large body of collateral fibers pass into the *striate body,* and *putamen.* From here additional pathways extend through several neurons down the brain stem and then into the spinal cord through the *extrapyramidal tracts,* which are discussed later in the chapter.

3. A moderate number of collaterals pass from the pyramidal tract into the *red nuclei.* From these, additional pathways pass down the cord through the *rubrospinal tract.*

4. A moderate number of collaterals also deviate from the pyramidal tract into the *reticular substance* of the brain stem; from here signals go to the cord via *reticulospinal tracts* and others go to the cerebellum via *reticulocerebellar tracts.*

5. A tremendous number of collaterals synapse in the pontile nuclei, which give rise to the *pontocerebellar fibers.* Thus, whenever signals are transmitted from the motor cortex through the pyramidal tract, simultaneous signals are transmitted into the cerebellar hemispheres.

6. Many collaterals also terminate in the *inferior olivary nuclei,* and from here secondary *olivocerebellar fibers* transmit signals to most areas of the cerebellum.

Thus, the basal ganglia, the brain stem, and the cerebellum all receive strong signals from the pyramidal tract every time a signal is also transmitted down the spinal cord to cause a motor activity.

Importance of the Area Pyramidalis. The giant pyramidal cells of the *area pyramidalis* are very excitable. A single weak electrical shock applied to a focal point in this area is sometimes strong enough to cause a definite motor movement somewhere in the body — for instance, a flick of a finger, deviation of the lip, or some other discrete movement; and a short train of stimuli almost always elicits a movement in some discrete part of the body. In almost no other region of the cortex can one be certain of achieving a motor response with such weak stimuli.

The Extrapyramidal Tracts. The extrapyramidal tracts are, collectively, all the tracts besides the pyramidal tract itself that transmit motor signals from the cortex to the spinal cord. In the above discussion of the collaterals from the pyramidal tract, we have noted some of these extrapyramidal pathways that pass through the striate nuclei, red nuclei, and reticular nuclei of the brain stem. In addition to these collateral fibers from the pyramidal tract, still other fibers course directly from the cortex to these intermediate nuclei. For instance, large numbers of neurons project directly from area VI of the motor cortex into the *caudate nucleus* and then through the *putamen, globus pallidus, subthalamic nucleus, red nucleus, substantia nigra,* and *reticular nuclei of the brain stem* before passing into the spinal cord. The multiplicity of connections within these intermediate nuclei of the basal ganglia and reticular substance was presented in the preceding chapter.

The final pathways for transmission of extrapyramidal signals into the cord are the *reticulospinal tracts,* which lie in both the ventral and lateral columns of the cord, and the *rubrospinal, tectospinal,* and *vestibulospinal tracts.*

THE PRIMARY MOTOR CORTEX OF THE HUMAN BEING

Figure 13–3 illustrates a topographical map of motor and sensory areas in the monkey cortex, showing the left side of the cerebral cortex and, above, a folded-out view of the medial side of the hemisphere as seen from the longitudinal fissure. In the posterior part of this map one sees the two somatic sensory areas, Sm I and Sm II, which were discussed in Chapter 9. Anterior to the central sulcus are illustrated two motor areas. The darkly shaded area, labeled Ms I, is the *primary motor cortex,* while the lightly shaded motor area located on the medial aspect of the frontal lobe, labeled Ms II, is called the *supplemental area,* the function of which is doubtful as we shall discuss later. Note especially in the primary motor cortex the topographical areas from which muscles in different parts of the body can be activated. Note also the very high degree of representation of the hands, feet, and face — especially the digits of the hands and feet. In the human being, the areas representing the hand and also the mouth and tongue are especially enlarged, as we shall see in subsequent figures. Figure 13–4 gives an approximate map of the human brain, showing the points in the primary motor cortex that cause muscle contractions in different parts of the body when

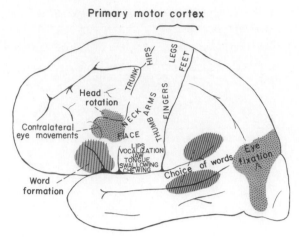

Figure 13–4. Representation of the different muscles of the body in the motor cortex and location of other cortical areas responsible for certain types of motor movements.

electrically stimulated. These have been determined by electrical stimulation of the human brain in patients having brain operations under local anesthesia. Indeed, such stimulation is commonly used by the neurosurgeon to determine the location of the motor cortex, thus permitting avoidance of this area, if possible, during the operation.

Note in the figure that stimulation of the most lateral portions of the motor cortex causes muscular contractions related to swallowing, chewing, and facial movements, while stimulation of the midline portion of the motor cortex where it bends over into the longitudinal fissure causes contraction of the legs, feet, or toes. The spatial organization is similar to that of the somatic sensory cortex I, which was shown in Figure 9–5 of Chapter 9.

Afferent Fibers That Excite the Primary Motor Cortex. The primary motor cortex is stimulated to action by signals from many different sources, including:

1. Subcortical fibers from adjacent regions of the cortex, especially from the somatic sensory areas and from the frontal areas — also subcortical fibers from the visual and auditory cortices.

2. Subcortical fibers that pass through the corpus callosum from the opposite cerebral hemisphere. These fibers connect corresponding areas of the motor cortices in the two sides of the brain.

3. Somatic sensory fibers derived directly from the ventrobasal complex of the thalamus. These transmit mainly cutaneous tactile signals and joint and muscle signals.

4. Tracts from the ventrolateral and ventroanterior nuclei of the thalamus, which in turn receive tracts from cerebellum and the basal ganglia. These tracts provide signals that are necessary for coordination between the functions of the motor cortex, the basal ganglia, and the cerebellum.

5. Fibers from the nonspecific nuclei of the thalamus. These fibers control the general level of excitabili-

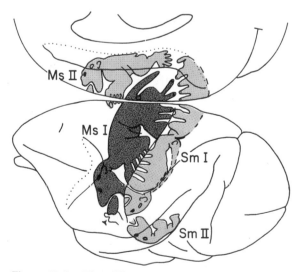

Figure 13–3. The different motor areas of the monkey cortex, illustrating especially the primary motor area (Ms I) located in the precentral gyrus. (The upper portion of the figure illustrates the medial surface of the cerebral hemisphere.) (From Woolsey, *in* Harlow and Woolsey (eds.): Biological and Biochemical Bases of Behavior. University of Wisconsin Press, 1958.)

ty of the motor cortex in the same manner that they also control the general level of excitability of most other regions of the cerebral cortex.

Vertical Columnar Arrangement of the Cells in the Motor Cortex. In Chapters 9 and 20 it is pointed out that the cells in the somatic sensory cortex and the visual cortex — and perhaps in all other parts of the brain as well — are organized in vertical columns of cells. In a like manner, the cells of the motor cortex are also organized in vertical columns — columns 0.5 to 1 mm. in diameter and having perhaps 10,000 to 50,000 neurons in each column.

The columns of cells, in turn, are themselves arranged in six distinct layers, as is the arrangement throughout the cerebral cortex. The functions of these layers from the surface inward are:

Layers I through IV are mainly sensory; that is, they receive afferent fibers from other sources. The fibers from the nonspecific nuclei of the thalamus (from the "reticular activating system" that will be discussed in the following chapter) terminate in layers I and II. These fibers provide general enhancement of the degree of excitability of the cortex when the reticular activating system is stimulated.

Layer IV is the main terminus and layer III the secondary terminus of the specific sensory signals from the thalamus, the signals from the sensory areas of the cortex, the signals from the ventrolateral and ventroanterior nuclei of the thalamus that transmit signals from the cerebellum and the basal ganglia, and the corpus callosal signals from the opposite cerebral hemisphere.

Layers V and VI are the origins of the efferent fibers or "output fibers" from the motor cortex. The large Betz cells that give rise to the long pyramidal tract fibers lie in layer V. Efferent fibers also pass from both layers V and VI to other areas of the brain.

Function of the Columns of Cells. Each column of cells seems to perform a specific motor function, such as stimulating a particular muscle or perhaps stimulating several synergistic muscles. The cells in each column operate both as an integrative and an amplifying system. The integrative function of the column is its ability to combine signals from many different sources and to determine the appropriate output response. Specific cells within a column seem to be responsive to different types of input signals. For instance, some cells respond to somatic sensory signals related to joint movement, others to tactile stimuli, and still others to feedback signals from the cerebellum and basal ganglia. Also, the general level of activation of the motor cortex is provided by signals from the nonspecific nuclei of the thalamus.

The amplifying function of the column of cells allows weak input signals to cause stimulation of large numbers of output neurons. Direct electrical stimulation of a signal output neuron in the motor cortex by means of a micropipette electrode will almost never excite a muscle contraction. Usually as many as 100 pyramidal cells need to be excited simultaneously. Therefore, divergence of the signal within the column provides this needed motive power.

Degree of Representation of Different Muscle Groups in the Primary Motor Cortex. The different muscle groups of the body are not represented equally in the motor cortex. In general, the degree of representation is proportional to the discreteness of movement required of the respective part of the body. Thus, the thumb and fingers have large representations, as is true also of the lips, tongue, and vocal cords. The relative degrees of representation of the different parts of the body are illustrated in Figure 13–5, a figure constructed by Penfield and Rasmussen on the basis of stimulatory charts made of the human motor cortex during hundreds of brain operations.

When barely threshold stimuli are used, only small segments of the peripheral musculature ordinarily contract at a time. In the "finger" and "thumb" regions, which have tremendous representation in the cerebral cortex, threshold stimuli can sometimes cause single muscles or, at times, even single fasciculi of muscles to contract, thus illustrating that a high degree of control is exercised by this portion of the motor cortex over discrete muscular movement.

On the other hand, threshold stimuli in the trunk region of the body might cause as many as 30 to 50 small, closely allied trunk muscles to contract simultaneously, thus illustrating that the motor cortex does not control discrete trunk muscles but instead controls *groups* of muscles. Similarly, threshold stimuli in the lip, tongue, and vocal cord regions of the motor cortex cause contraction of minute muscular areas, whereas stimulation in the leg region ordinarily excites several synergistic muscles at a time, causing some gross movement of the leg. Also, it should be recognized that the

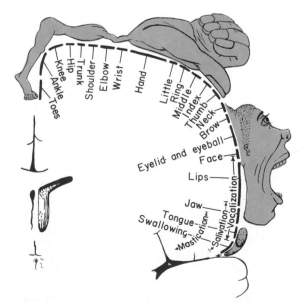

Figure 13–5. Degree of representation of the different muscles of the body in the motor cortex. (From Penfield and Rasmussen: The Cerebral Cortex of Man: A Clinical Study of Localization of Function, New York, Macmillan Company, 1968.)

finger muscles have far more representation in the motor cortex than do the muscles of the upper arm.

COMPLEX MOVEMENTS ELICITED BY STIMULATING THE CORTEX ANTERIOR TO THE MOTOR CORTEX — THE CONCEPT OF A MOTOR ASSOCIATION AREA

Electrical stimulation of the cerebral cortex for distances 1 to 3 centimeters in front of the primary motor cortex will often elicit complex contractions of groups of muscles. Occasionally, vocalization occurs, or rhythmic movements such as alternate thrusting of a leg forward and backward, coordinate moving of the eyes, chewing, swallowing, or contortions of parts of the body into different postural positions.

Some neurophysiologists have called this area the *motor association area* or *premotor cortex* and have ascribed special capabilities to it to control coordinated movements involving many muscles simultaneously. In fact, it is peculiarly organized to perform such a function for the following reasons: (1) It has long subcortical neuronal connections with the sensory association areas of the parietal lobe; (2) It has direct subcortical connections with the primary motor cortex; (3) It connects with areas in the thalamus contiguous with the thalamic areas that connect with the primary motor cortex; and (4) most important of all, it has abundant direct connections with the basal ganglia.

Still another reason for the belief that there is a motor association area (a "premotor cortex") is that damage to this area causes loss of certain coordinate skills, as follows:

Broca's Area and Speech. Note in Figure 13–4 that immediately anterior to the primary motor cortex and immediately above the sylvian fissure is an area labeled "word formation." This region is called *Broca's area*. Damage to it does not prevent a person from vocalizing, but it does make it impossible for the person to speak whole words other than simple utterances such as "no" or "yes." A closely associated cortical area also causes appropriate respiratory function so that respiratory activation of vocal cords can occur simultaneously with the movements of the mouth and tongue during speech. Thus, the activities that are related to Broca's area are highly complex.

The Voluntary Eye Movement Field. Immediately above Broca's area is a locus for controlling eye movements. Damage to this area prevents a person from voluntarily moving the eyes toward different objects. Instead, the eyes tend to lock on specific objects, an effect controlled by signals from the occipital region, as explained in Chapter

20. This frontal area also controls eyelid movements such as blinking.

Head Rotation Area. Still slightly higher in the motor association area, electrical stimulation will elicit head rotation. This area is closely associated with the eye movement field and is presumably related to directing the head toward different objects.

Area for Hand Skills. In the frontal area immediately anterior to the primary motor cortex for the hands and fingers is a region neurosurgeons have called an area for hand skills. That is, when tumors or other lesions cause destruction in this area, the hand movements become incoordinate and nonpurposeful, a condition called *motor apraxia*.

Summary of the Motor Association Area Concept. It is clear that at least some areas anterior to the primary motor cortex can cause complex coordinate movements, such as for speech, for eye movements, for head movements, and perhaps even for hand skills. However, it should be remembered that all these areas are closely connected with corresponding areas in the primary motor cortex, the thalamus, and the basal ganglia. Therefore, the complex coordinate movements almost certainly result from a cooperative effort of all these structures.

EFFECTS OF LESIONS IN THE PRIMARY MOTOR AND MOTOR ASSOCIATION CORTEX

The motor cortex is frequently damaged — especially by the common abnormality called a "stroke," which is caused by loss of blood supply to the cortex. Also, experiments have been performed in animals to remove selectively different parts of the motor cortex.

Ablation of the Area Pyramidalis. Removal of a very small portion of the area pyramidalis (the primary motor cortex — area IV) in a monkey causes paralysis of the represented muscles. If the sublying caudate nucleus and the adjacent motor association area (area VI) are not damaged, gross postural and limb "fixation" movements can still be performed, but the animal loses voluntary control of discrete movements of the distal segments of the limbs — of the hands and fingers, for instance. This does not mean that the muscles themselves cannot contract, but that the animal's ability to control the fine movements is gone.

From these results one can conclude that the area pyramidalis is concerned mainly with voluntary initiation of finely controlled movements. On the other hand, area VI and the deeper motor areas, particularly the basal ganglia, seem to be responsible mainly for the involuntary and postural body movements.

Muscle Spasticity Caused by Ablation of Large Areas of the Motor Cortex — Extrapyramidal Lesions as the Basis of Spasticity. It should be recalled that the motor cortex gives rise to tracts that descend to the spinal cord through both the pyramidal tract and the extrapyramidal tract. These two tracts have opposing effects on the tone of the body muscles. The pyramidal tract causes continuous facilitation and, therefore, a tendency to increase muscle tone throughout the body. On the other hand, the extrapyramidal system transmits inhibitory signals through the basal ganglia and the reticular formation of the brain stem, with resultant inhibition of muscle action. When the motor cortex is destroyed, the balance between these two opposing effects may be altered. If the lesion is located discretely in the area pyramidalis where the large Betz cells lie, there may be a slight degree of muscle flaccidity, but most often very little change in muscle tone results because both pyramidal and extrapyramidal elements are affected about equally. On the other hand, the usual lesion is very large and involves large portions of area VI (the motor association area) and the sensory cortex as well, both anterior and posterior to the area pyramidalis, and both of these regions normally transmit inhibitory signals through the extrapyramidal tracts. Therefore, loss of extrapyramidal inhibition is the dominant feature, thus leading to muscle spasm.

If the lesion involves the basal ganglia as well as the motor cortex itself, the spasm is even more intense because the basal ganglia normally provide very strong inhibition of the brain stem motor centers, and loss of this inhibition further exacerbates the extrapyramidal excitation of the muscles. In patients with strokes, the lesion almost invariably affects both the motor cortex itself and the sublying basal ganglia, so that very intense spasm normally occurs in the muscles of the opposite side of the body.

The muscle spasm that results from damage to the extrapyramidal system is different from the spasticity that occurs in decerebrate rigidity. In decerebrate rigidity the spasm is of the antigravity muscles and is called *extensor spasm.* On the other hand, the spasm resulting from lesions of the extrapyramidal system usually involves the flexors as well, causing intense stiffening of the limbs and other parts of the body.

The Babinski Sign. Destruction of the foot region of the area pyramidalis or transection of the foot portion of the pyramidal tract causes a peculiar response of the foot called the *Babinski sign.* This response is demonstrated when a firm tactile stimulus is applied to the sole of the foot: The great toe extends upward and the other toes fan outward. This is in contradistinction to the normal effect in which all the toes bend downward. Also, the Babinski sign does not occur when the damage is only in the extrapyramidal system. Therefore, the sign is often used clinically to detect damage specifically in the pyramidal portion of the motor control system.

The cause of the Babinski sign is believed to be the following: The pyramidal tract is a major controller of muscle activity for performance of voluntary, purposeful activity. On the other hand, the extrapyramidal system, a much older motor control system, is concerned to a great extent with protection. Therefore, when only the extrapyramidal system is functional, stimuli to the bottom of the feet cause a typical withdrawal protective type of reflex which is expressed ty the upturned great toe and fanning of the other toes. But, when the pyramidal system is also fully functional, it suppresses the protective reflex and instead excites the postural reflexes, including the normal effect of causing downward bending of the toes in response to sensory stimuli from the bottom of the feet.

THE SUPPLEMENTAL MOTOR AREA

Referring again to Figure 13–3, one sees a small area located on the medial side of the frontal lobe, called the *supplemental area.* This area requires considerably stronger electrical stimuli to cause motor activity than does the primary motor area. Also, the movements involve coordinate contraction of many muscles in contradistinction to much more discrete movements elicited from the primary area. Normal function of this area is not known, but strong stimulation is likely to elicit such effects as movement of the head and eyes, vocalization, or yawning. Also, movements are sometimes bilateral rather than unilateral.

STIMULATION OF THE SPINAL MOTONEURONS BY MOTOR SIGNALS FROM THE BRAIN

Figure 13–6 shows several different motor tracts entering a segment of the spinal cord from the brain. The corticospinal tract (pyramidal tract) terminates mainly on small interneurons in the base of the dorsal horns, although as many as 8 per cent may also terminate directly on the anterior motoneurons themselves. From the primary interneurons, most of the motor signals are transmitted through still other interneurons before finally exciting the anterior motoneurons.

Figure 13–6 shows several other descending tracts from the brain, collectively called the *extrapyramidal tracts,* which also carry signals to the anterior motoneurons: (1) the *rubrospinal tract,* (2) the *reticulospinal tracts,* (3) the *tectospinal*

Sensory neurons

Propriospinal tract

INTERNEURONS

Corticospinal tract from
pyramidal cells of cortex

Rubrospinal and reticu-
lospinal tracts

ANTERIOR MOTOR NEURON

MOTOR NERVE

Tectospinal and reticulo-
spinal tracts

Vestibulospinal tract

Figure 13–6. Convergence of all the different motor pathways on the anterior motoneurons.

tract, and (4) the *vestibulospinal tract.* In addition, sensory signals arriving through the *dorsal sensory roots,* as well as signals transmitted from segment to segment of the spinal cord via the *propriospinal tracts,* also stimulate the anterior motoneurons. In general, the extrapyramidal tracts terminate farther anteriorly in the gray matter of the spinal cord than does the corticospinal tract; a larger share of these fibers terminate directly on the anterior motoneurons. Also, some terminate on *inhibitory neurons,* which in turn inhibit the anterior motoneurons, an effect opposite to the excitatory effect of the corticospinal tract.

The corticospinal tract seems to cause very specific muscle contractions; neurophysiological recordings have demonstrated that the intensity of muscle contraction — everything else being equal — is directly proportional to the nervous energy transmitted through the corticospinal tract. On the other hand, some of the extrapyramidal tracts provide less specific muscle contractions. Instead, they provide such effects as general facilitation, general inhibition, or gross postural signals, all of which provide the background against which the corticospinal system operates. Finally, the sensory and propriospinal signals also add their input to the total melee of spinal integration.

Patterns of Movement Elicited by Spinal Cord Centers.   From Chapter 11, recall that the spinal cord can provide specific reflex patterns of movement in response to sensory nerve stimulation. Many of these patterns are also important when the anterior motoneurons are excited by signals from the brain. For instance, the stretch reflex is functional at all times, helping to damp the motor movements initiated from the brain and probably providing at least part of the motive power required to cause the muscle contractions employing the servo-assist mechanism that was described in Chapter 11.

Also, when a brain signal excites an agonist muscle, it is not necessary to transmit an inverse signal to the antagonist at the same time; this transmission will be achieved by the reciprocal innervation circuit that is always present in the cord for coordinating the functions of antagonistic pairs of muscles.

Finally, parts of the other reflex mechanisms such as withdrawal, stepping and walking, scratching, postural mechanisms, and so forth, can be activated by signals from the brain. Thus, very simple signals from the brain can lead, at least theoretically, to many of our normal motor activities, particularly for such functions as walking and the attainment of different postural attitudes of the body.

Inhibition of Sensory Input Signals by Corticospinal Signals.   At times it is important to suppress sensory input from the periphery to prevent its interference with motor activity. Experimental studies have shown that the same corticospinal signals that activate the muscles or muscle groups at the same time inhibit the local cord sensory input to the same muscles. This results from specific inhibitory circuits located in the cord itself at the base of the dorsal horns, through which most of the sensory information feeds. For instance, if pain signals are arriving in the cord from the bottom of the feet and are attempting to cause withdrawal of the feet from a source of pain, nevertheless the cortical signals can still suppress these and allow continued use of the feet for running or other purposes.

THE CEREBELLUM AND ITS MOTOR FUNCTIONS

The cerebellum has long been called a *silent area* of the brain principally because electrical excitation of this structure does not cause any sensation and rarely any motor movement. However, as we shall see, removal of the cerebellum does cause the motor movements to become highly abnormal. The cerebellum is especially vital to the control of very rapid muscular activities such as running, typing, playing the piano, and even talking. Loss of this area of the brain can cause almost total incoordination of these activities even though its loss causes paralysis of no muscles.

But how is it that the cerebellum can be so important when it has no direct control over muscle contraction? The answer to this is that it *monitors and makes corrective adjustments in the motor activities elicited by other parts of the brain*. It receives continuously updated information from the peripheral parts of the body to determine the instantaneous status of each part of the body — its position, its rate of movement, forces acting on it, and so forth. And it is believed that the cerebellum *compares* the actual instantaneous status of each part of the body as depicted by the sensory information with the status that is intended by the motor system. If the two do not compare favorably, then appropriate corrective signals are transmitted instantaneously back into the motor system to increase or decrease the levels of activation of the specific muscles.

Since the cerebellum must make major motor corrections extremely rapidly *during the course of motor movements*, a very extensive and rapidly acting cerebellar input system is required both from the peripheral parts of the body and from the cerebral motor areas. Also, an extensive output system feeding equally as rapidly into the motor system is necessary to provide the necessary corrections of the motor signals.

THE INPUT SYSTEM TO THE CEREBELLUM

For purposes of discussion, the cerebellum is generally divided into three lobes, as illustrated in Figure 13–7: (1) the *flacculonodular lobe;* (2) the *anterior lobe;* and (3) the *posterior lobe.*

The posterior lobe is greatly enlarged in primates, especially so in the human being, forming bilateral protrusions called the *cerebellar hemispheres* (which are illustrated in Figures 13–9 and 13–10). These hemispheres are also known as the *neocerebellum* (new cerebellum) because they represent a phylogenetically new portion of the cerebellum.

The oldest part of the cerebellum is the flocculo-

nodular lobe, which developed in association with the equilibrium apparatus and vestibular nuclei. In the human being, this part of the cerebellum still functions almost entirely in relation to equilibrium, as was described in the previous chapter.

Another part of the cerebellum that is also very old is the entire midline area, 2 to 3 centimeters wide, in both the anterior and posterior lobes, called the *vermis*. In this area most of the nerve signals from the somatic areas of the body terminate. Therefore, this midline structure (the vermis) plays an important role in the integration of subconscious postural mechanisms.

On the other hand, the cerebellar hemispheres are the terminus of most of the signals arriving from the higher levels of the brain, especially from the motor areas of the cerebral cortex.

The Afferent Pathways.   The basic afferent pathways to the cerebellum are also illustrated in Figure 13–7. An extensive and important afferent pathway is the *corticocerebellar pathway,* which originates mainly in the *motor cortex* (but to a lesser extent in the sensory cortex as well) and then passes by way of the *pontile nuclei* and *pontocerebellar tracts* to the contralateral cortex of the cerebellum. In addition, important afferent tracts originate in the brain stem; they include: (a) an extensive *olivocerebellar* tract, which passes from the *inferior olive* to all parts of the cerebellum; this tract is excited by fibers from the *motor cortex*, the *basal ganglia*, widespread areas of the *reticular formation*, and the *spinal cord;* (b) *vestibulocerebellar fibers*, some of which originate in the vestibular apparatus itself and others from the vestibular nuclei; most of these terminate in the *flocculonodular lobe* and *fastigial nucleus* of the cerebellum; and (c) *reticulocerebellar fibers*, which originate in different portions of the reticular formation and terminate mainly in the midline structures (the vermis).

The cerebellum also receives important sensory signals directly from the peripheral parts of the body, which reach the cerebellum by way of the *ventral* and *dorsal spinocerebellar* tracts (which pass ipsilaterally up to the cerebellum, as illustrated in Figure 13–8. The signals transmitted in these tracts originate in the muscle spindles, the Golgi tendon organs, the large tactile receptors of the skin, and the joint receptors, and they apprise the cerebellum of the momentary status of muscle contraction, degree of tension on the muscle tendons, positions and rates of movement of the parts of the body, and forces acting on the surfaces of the body. All this information keeps the cerebellum constantly apprised of the instantaneous physical status of the body.

The spinocerebellar pathways can transmit impulses at velocities over 100 meters per second, which is the most rapid conduction of any pathway in the entire central nervous system. This extremely rapid conduction is also important for the instantaneous appraisal of the cerebellum of changes that take place in the status of the body.

In addition to the signals in the spinocerebellar tracts, other signals are transmitted through the dorsal and dorsolateral columns to the medulla and then relayed from there to the cerebellum. Likewise, signals are transmitted through the *spinoreticular pathway* to the reticular substance of the brain stem and through the

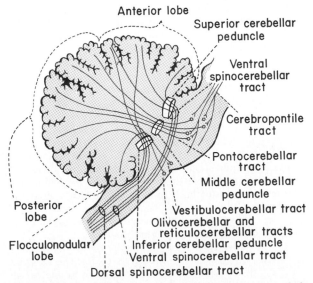

Anterior lobe
Superior cerebellar peduncle
Ventral spinocerebellar tract
Cerebropontile tract
Pontocerebellar tract
Middle cerebellar peduncle
Vestibulocerebellar tract
Olivocerebellar and reticulocerebellar tracts
Inferior cerebellar peduncle
Ventral spinocerebellar tract
Posterior lobe
Flocculonodular lobe
Dorsal spinocerebellar tract

Figure 13–7.   The principal afferent tracts to the cerebellum.

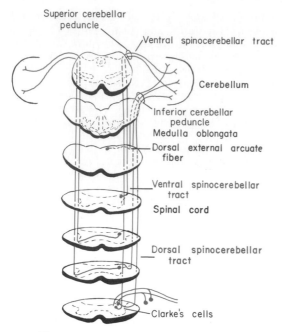

Figure 13–8.   The spinocerebellar tracts.

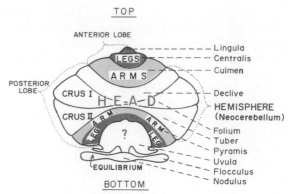

Figure 13–10.   Localization of somatic sensory signals in the cerebellum of the human being.

spino-olivary pathway to the inferior olivary nucleus and then relayed to the cerebellum. Thus, the cerebellum collects continual information about all parts of the body even though it is operating at a subconscious level.

Topographical Localization of Sensory Input to the Cerebellar Cortex.   Because the cerebellum operates in close association both with the motor cortex and with the muscles that are being activated, one would expect separate parts of the cerebellum to be concerned specifically with separate parts of the body. However, it has not been possible to localize the different parts of the body in most areas of the cerebellum. Instead, only a gross representation has been found in the midline

structures. Figure 13–9 illustrates the loci of two different "homunculi" that are believed to have been found in the monkey cerebellar cortex, representing the terminations of somatic sensory fibers from the different parts of the body. Figure 13–10 illustrates the human cerebellum, showing approximate sensory terminations based on anatomical data and extrapolation from animals. However, it should be recognized that these are only gross representations and are based on uncertain data. It should also be noted that no specific somatic representations have been found in the very large cerebellar hemispheres. Even so, many neurophysiologists still believe that point-to-point spatial relationships between these hemispheres and specific stimulatory areas of the cerebral cortex are likely because of the well-known fact that whenever a motor signal is transmitted to the periphery, a signal is transmitted into the cerebral hemispheres at the same time.

OUTPUT SIGNALS FROM THE CEREBELLUM

The Deep Cerebellar Nuclei and the Efferent Pathways.   Located deep in the cerebellar mass are three *deep cerebellar nuclei* — the *dentate, interpositus,* and *fastigial nuclei*. The vestibular nuclei in the medulla also function in some respects as if they were deep cerebellar nuclei because of their direct connections with the cortex of the flocculonodular lobe. These nuclei receive signals from two different sources: (1) the cerebellar cortex, and (2) the sensory afferent tracts to the cerebellum. Each time an input signal arrives in the cerebellum, it goes both to the cerebellar cortex and also directly to the deep nuclei (or the vestibular nuclei) through collateral fibers; then, a short time later, the cerebellar cortex relays its output signals also to the deep nuclei. Thus, all the input signals that enter the cerebellum eventually end in the deep nuclei. We shall discuss this circuit in greater detail below.

Three major efferent pathways lead out of the cerebellum, as illustrated in Figure 13–11:

(1)   A pathway that begins in the *cortex of the two cerebellar hemispheres,* then passes to the *dentate nucleus,* next to the *ventrolateral nucleus of the thalamus,* and finally to the *motor cortex*. This pathway plays an important role in helping to coordinate "voluntary"

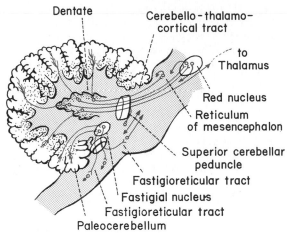

Figure 13–11. Principal efferent tracts from the cerebellum.

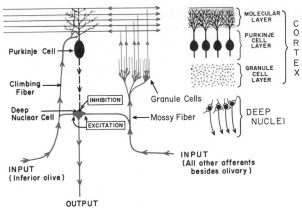

Figure 13–12. Basic neuronal circuit of the cerebellum, showing excitatory pathways in color. At right are the three major layers of the cerebellar cortex and also the deep nuclei.

motor activities initiated by the motor cortex and its associated structures.

(2) A pathway that originates in the *midline structures of the cerebellum* (the *vermis*) and then passes through the *fastigial nuclei* into the *medullary* and *pontile regions of the brain stem*. This circuit functions in close association with the equilibrium apparatus to help control equilibrium and also to control the postural attitudes of the body. It was discussed in detail in the previous chapter in relation to equilibrium.

(3) A pathway that originates in the *intermediate areas* on each side of the cerebellum, between the vermis and the cerebellar hemispheres, then passes (a) through the *nucleus interpositus* to the *ventrolateral nucleus of the thalamus*, and thence to the *motor cortex*, (b) to several *midline structures* of the *thalamus* and thence to the *basal ganglia*, and (c) to the *red nucleus* and *reticular formation* of the upper portion of the brain stem. This circuit functions to coordinate activities between the first two cerebellar output pathways noted above — that is, to help coordinate the interrelationships between subconscious body postural control and conscious command control from the motor cortex.

THE NEURONAL CIRCUIT OF THE CEREBELLUM

The structure of the cerebellar cortex is entirely different from that of the cerebral cortex. Furthermore, each part of the cerebellar cortex has a neuronal organization almost precisely the same as that in all other parts.

The human cerebellum is actually a large folded sheet, approximately 17 cm. wide by 120 cm. long, the folds lying crosswise, as illustrated in Figures 13–9 and 13–10. Each fold is called a *folium*.

The Functional Unit of the Cerebellar Cortex — the Purkinje Cell. The cerebellum has approximately 30 million nearly identical functional units, one of which is illustrated in Figure 13–12. This functional unit centers on the Purkinje cell, of

which there are also 30 million in the cerebellar cortex.

Note to the far right in Figure 13–12 the three major layers of the cerebellar cortex: the *molecular layer*, the *Purkinje cell layer*, and the *granular cell layer*. Then, beneath these layers, the *deep nuclei* are located far within the center of the cerebellar mass.

The Neuronal Circuit of the Functional Unit. As illustrated in Figure 13–12, the output from the functional unit is from a deep nuclear cell. However, this cell is continually under the influence of both excitatory and inhibitory influences. The excitatory influences arise from direct connections with the afferent fibers that enter the cerebellum. The inhibitory influences arise entirely from the Purkinje cells in the cortex of the cerebellum.

The afferent inputs to the cerebellum are of two types, one called the *climbing fiber type* and the other called the *mossy fiber type*. There is one climbing fiber for about 10 Purkinje cells. After sending collaterals to several deep nuclear cells, the climbing fiber projects all the way to the molecular layer of the cerebellar cortex where it makes about 300 synapses with the dendrites of each Purkinje cell. This climbing fiber is distinguished by the fact that a single impulse in it will always cause a single, very prolonged and peculiar oscillatory type of action potential in each Purkinje cell with which it connects. Another distinguishing feature of the climbing fibers is that they all originate in the inferior olive of the medulla.

The mossy fibers also send collaterals to excite the deep nuclear cells. Then these fibers proceed to the granular layer of the cortex where they synapse with hundreds of *granule cells*. These in turn send their very small axons, less than 1 micron in diameter, up to the outer surface of the cerebellar cortex to enter the molecular layers.

Here the axons divide into two branches that extend 1 to 2 millimeters in each direction parallel to the folia. There are literally millions of these *parallel nerve fibers* in each small segment of the cerebellar cortex (there are about 1000 granule cells for every Purkinje cell). It is into this molecular layer that the dendrites of the Purkinje cells project, and 80,000 to 200,000 of these parallel fibers synapse with each Purkinje cell. Yet, the mossy fiber input to the Purkinje cell is quite different from the climbing fiber input because stimulation of a single mossy fiber will never elicit an action potential in the Purkinje cell; instead, large numbers of mossy fibers must be stimulated simultaneously to activate the Purkinje cell. Furthermore, this activation usually takes the form of prolonged facilitation or excitation that, when it reaches threshold for stimulation, causes repetitive Purkinje cell firing of normal, short-duration action potentials rather than the single prolonged action potential occurring in response to the climbing fiber input.

Thus, the Purkinje cells are stimulated by two types of input circuits — one that causes a highly specific output in response to the incoming signal and the other that causes a less specific but tonic type of response. It should be noted that the greater proportion of the afferent input to the cerebellum is of the mossy fiber type because this represents the afferent input from all the cerebellar afferent tracts besides those from the inferior olive.

Balance Between Excitation and Inhibition in the Deep Cerebellar Nuclei. The output signals from the Purkinje cells to the deep nuclei are entirely inhibitory. Therefore, referring again to the circuit of Figure 13–12, *one should note that direct stimulation of the deep nuclear cells by both the climbing and the mossy fibers excites them, whereas the signals arriving from the Purkinje cells inhibit them*. Normally, there is a continual balance between these two effects so that the degree of output from the deep nuclear cell remains relatively constant. On the other hand, in the execution of rapid motor movements, the *timing* of the two effects on the deep nuclei is such that the excitation appears before the inhibition. Then a few milliseconds later inhibition occurs. In this way, very rapid excitatory and inhibitory transient signals can be fed back into the motor pathways to modify motor movements. The inhibitory portions of these signals resemble "delay-line" negative feedback signals of the type that are very effective in providing *damping*. That is, when the motor system is excited, a negative feedback signal occurs after a short delay to stop the muscle movement from overshooting its mark, which is the usual cause of oscillation.

Other Inhibitory Cells in the Cerebellar Cortex. In addition to the granule cells and Purkinje cells, three other types of neurons are also located in the cerebellar cortex: *basket cells, stellate cells,* and *Golgi cells*. All of these are inhibitory cells with very short axons. Both the basket cells and the stellate cells are excited by the parallel fibers in the molecular layer of the cerebellar cortex. These cells in turn cause lateral inhibition of the adjacent Purkinje cells, thus sharpening the signal in the same manner that lateral inhibition sharpens the contrast of signals in many other areas of the nervous system. The Golgi cells are also stimulated by the parallel fibers of the molecular layer, but they inhibit the granule cells instead of the Purkinje cells, possibly functioning as an automatic feedback gain control circuit to prevent overamplification of the input signals.

Special Features of the Cerebellar Neuronal Circuit. A special feature of the cerebellum is that there are no reverberatory pathways in the cerebellar neuronal circuits, so that the input-output signals of the cerebellum are very rapid transients that never persist for long periods of time.

Another special feature is that many of the cells of the cerebellum are constantly active. This is especially true of the deep nuclear cells; they continually send output signals to the other areas of the motor system. The importance of this is that decrease of the nuclear cell firing rate can provide an inhibitory output signal from the cerebellum, while an increase in firing rate can provide an excitatory output signal.

FUNCTION OF THE CEREBELLUM IN CONTROLLING MOVEMENTS

The cerebellum functions in motor control only in association with motor activities initiated elsewhere in the nervous system. These activities may originate in the spinal cord, in the reticular formation, in the basal ganglia, or in motor areas of the cerebral cortex. We will discuss, first, the operation of the cerebellum in association with the spinal cord and lower brain stem for control of postural movements and equilibrium and then discuss its function in association with the motor cortex for control of voluntary movements.

FUNCTION OF THE CEREBELLUM WITH THE SPINAL CORD AND LOWER BRAIN STEM TO CONTROL POSTURAL AND EQUILIBRIUM MOVEMENTS

The cerebellum originated phylogenetically at about the same time that the vestibular apparatus developed. Furthermore, as was discussed in the previous chapter, loss of the flocculonodular lobes of the cerebellum causes extreme disturbance of equilibrium. Yet, we still must ask the question, what role does the cerebellum play in equilibrium that cannot be provided by the other neuronal machinery of the brain stem? A clue is the fact that equilibrium is far more disturbed during performance of rapid motions than during stasis. This suggests that the cerebellum is especially important in controlling the balance between agonist and antagonist muscle contractions during rapid changes in body positions as dictated by the vestibular apparatuses. One of the major problems in controlling this balance is the time required to transmit position signals and kinesthetic signals from the different parts of the body to the brain. Even when utilizing the most rapidly conducting sensory pathways at 120 meters per second, which are indeed utilized by the spinocerebellar system, the delay for transmission from the feet to the brain is still 15 to 20 milliseconds. The feet of a person running rapidly can move as much as 10 inches during this time. Therefore, it is impossible for the brain to know at any given instant during rapid motion the exact position of the different parts of the body.

On the other hand, with appropriate neuronal circuitry, it would be possible for the cerebellum or some other portion of the brain to know how rapidly and in what direction a part of the body was moving 15 to 20 milliseconds previously and then to predict from this information where the parts of the body should be at the present time. And this seems to be one of the major functions of the cerebellum.

As we have already discussed in relation to the neuronal circuitry of the cerebellum, there are abundant sensory pathways from the somatic areas of the body, especially from the muscles, joints, and skin surface, that feed both into the brain stem and into the older areas of the cerebellum — into the flocculonodular lobes through the vestibular nuclei and into the vermis and intermediate areas of the cerebellum through the dorsal and ventral spinocerebellar tracts and reticulocerebellar tracts. Also, the vestibular apparatus is located within a few centimeters of the flocculonodular lobes, allowing no more than a millisecond or so of delay in transmission of the vestibular information.

Therefore, during the control of equilibrium, it is presumed that the extremely rapidly conducted vestibular apparatus information is used in a typical feedback control circuit to provide almost instantaneous correction of postural motor signals as necessary for maintaining equilibrium even during extremely rapid motion, including rapidly changing directions of motion. The feedback signals from the peripheral areas of the body help in this process, but their help is presumably contingent upon some function of the cerebellum to compute positions of the respective parts of the body at any given time, despite the long delay time from the periphery to the cerebellum.

Relationship of Cerebellar Function to the Spinal Cord Stretch Reflex

One major component of cerebellar control of posture and equilibrium is an extreme amount of information transmitted from the muscle spindles to the cerebellum through the dorsal spinocerebellar tracts. In turn, signals are transmitted into the brain stem through the cerebellar fastigial nuclei to stimulate the gamma efferent fibers that innervate the muscle spindles themselves. Therefore, a cerebellar stretch reflex occurs that is similar to but more complex than the spinal cord stretch reflex. It utilizes signals that pass all the way to the cerebellum and back again to the muscles. In general, this reflex adds additional support to the cord stretch reflex, but its feedback time is considerably longer, thus prolonging the effect. It is through this feedback pathway that many of the postural adjustments of the body are believed to occur.

Function of the Cerebellum in Voluntary Muscle Control

In addition to the feedback circuitry between the body periphery and the cerebellum, an almost entirely independent feedback circuitry exists between the motor cortex and the cerebellum. This is illustrated in its simplest form in Figure 13–13 and in a much more complex form, involving the basal ganglia also in the control circuit, in Figure 13–14. Most of the signals of this circuit pass from the motor cortex to the cerebellar hemispheres and then back to the motor cortex again, successively, through the dentate nuclei and ventrolateral nuclei of the thalamus. These circuits are not involved in the control of posture. However, a small component of the feedback to the cortex involves the intermediate areas of the cerebellum lying between the cerebellar hemispheres and the

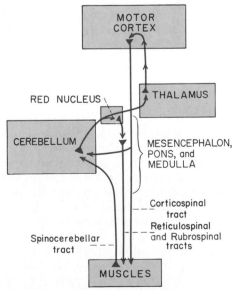

Figure 13–13. Pathways for cerebellar control of voluntary movements.

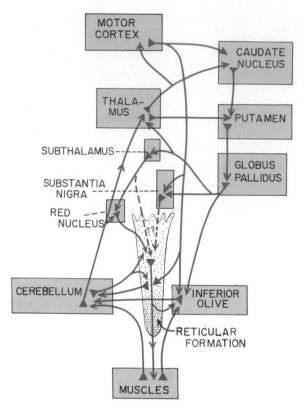

Figure 13–14. Pathways for cerebellar "error" control of involuntary movements.

vermis. This cerebellar area does receive feedback signals from the periphery. Therefore, there is reason to believe that the cerebellum functions in relation to cortical motor control in two ways: (1) by direct feedback circuitry from the motor cortex to the cerebellum, then back to the motor cortex without involving peripheral feedback, and (2) by similar feedback but with the return signals from the cerebellum being modified by conditioning information received from the peripheral parts of the body. Let us discuss the second of these first.

Cerebellar Feedback Control of Cortical Motor Function

There is much reason to believe that the cerebellum operates to provide so-called "error control" in much the same manner as servomechanisms used in (a) various industrial control systems, (b) the control system of the antiaircraft gun, or (c) the control system of the automatic pilot. That is, the motor cortex transmits signals to the periphery to cause a motor function, but at the same time it transmits the same information into the cerebellum. Then the cerebellum seems to compare the "intentions" of the cortex with the "performance" by the parts of the body, and, if the parts

are not moving according to the intentions of the cortex, the "error" between these two is calculated by the cerebellum so that appropriate and immediate corrections can be made. Thus, if the cortex has transmitted a signal intending the limb to move to a particular point, but the limb begins to move too fast and obviously is going to overshoot the point of intention, the cerebellum can initiate "braking impulses" to slow down the movement of the limb and stop it at the point of intention.

Ordinarily, during rapid movements, the motor cortex transmits far more impulses than are needed to perform each intended movement, and the cerebellum therefore must act to inhibit the motor cortex at the appropriate time after the muscle has begun to move. The cerebellum is believed to assess the rate of movement and calculate the length of time that will be required to reach the point of intention. Then appropriate inhibitory impulses are transmitted to the motor cortex to inhibit the agonist muscle and to excite the antagonist muscle. In this way, appropriate "brakes" are applied to stop the movement at the precise point of intention.

Experiments have demonstrated two important characteristics of the cerebellar feedback system:

1. When a person performs a particular act, such as moving a heavy weight rapidly to a new position, at first he is unable to judge the degree of inertia that will be involved in the movement. Therefore, he almost always overshoots the point of intention on his first trial. However, after several trials, he can stop the movement at the precise point. This illustrates that learned knowledge of the inertia of the system is an important feature of the cerebellar feedback mechanism, though it is possible that this learning occurs in the cerebral cortex rather than in the cerebellum.

2. When a rapid movement is made toward a point of intention, the agonist muscle contracts strongly throughout the early course of movement. Then, suddenly, shortly before the point of intention is reached, the agonist muscle becomes completely inhibited while the antagonist muscle becomes strongly excited. Furthermore, the point at which this reversal of excitation occurs depends on the rate of movement and on the previously learned knowledge of the inertia of the system. The faster the movement and the greater the inertia, the earlier the reversal point appears in the course of movement.

Since all these events transpire much too rapidly for the motor cortex to reverse the excitation "voluntarily," it is evident that the excitation of the antagonist muscle toward the end of a movement is an entirely automatic and subconscious function and is not a "willed" contraction of the same nature as the original contraction of the agonist muscle. We shall see below that in patients with serious cerebellar damage, excitation of the antagonist muscles does not occur at the appropriate time but instead always too late. Therefore, it is almost certain that one of the major functions of the cerebellum is automatic excitation of antagonist muscles at the end of a movement while at the same time inhibiting agonist muscles that have started the movement.

The "Damping" Function of the Cerebellum. One of the by-products of the cerebellar feedback mechanism is its ability to "damp" muscular movements. To explain the meaning of "damping" we must first point out that essentially all movements of the body are "pendular." For instance, when an arm is moved, momentum develops, and the momentum must be overcome before the movement can be stopped. And, because of the momentum, all pendular movements have a tendency to overshoot. If overshooting does occur in a person whose cerebellum has been destroyed, the conscious centers of the cerebrum eventually recognize this and initiate a movement in the opposite direction to bring the arm to its intended position. But again the arm, by virtue of its momentum, overshoots, and appropriate corrective signals must again be instituted. Thus, the arm oscillates back and forth past its intended point for several cycles before it finally fixes on its mark. This effect is called an *action tremor,* or *intention tremor.*

However, if the cerebellum is intact, appropriate subconscious signals stop the movement precisely at the intended point, thereby preventing the overshoot and also the tremor. This is the basic characteristic of a damping system. All servocontrol systems regulating pendular elements that have inertia must have damping circuits built into the servomechanisms. In the motor control system of our central nervous system, the cerebellum seems to provide much of this damping function.

Function of the Cerebellum in Prediction. Another important by-product of the cerebellar feedback mechanism is its ability to help the central nervous system predict the future positions of moving parts of the body. Without the cerebellum a person "loses" his or her limbs *when they move rapidly,* indicating that feedback information from the periphery probably must be analyzed by the cerebellum if the brain is to keep up with the motor movements. Thus, the cerebellum detects from the incoming proprioceptive signals the rapidity with which the limb is moving and then seems to predict from this the projected time course of movement. This allows the cerebellum, operating through the cerebellar output circuits to inhibit the agonist muscles and to excite the an-

tagonist muscles when the movement approaches the point of intention.

Without the cerebellum this predictive function is so deficient that *rapidly* moving parts of the body move much farther than the point of intention. This failure to control the distance that the parts of the body move is called *dysmetria,* which simply means poor control of the distance of movement. As would be expected, dysmetria is much more pronounced in rapid movements than in slow movements.

Failure of Smooth "Progression of Movements." One of the most important features of normal motor function is one's ability to progress from one movement to the next in an orderly succession. When the cerebellum becomes dysfunctional and the subconscious ability to predict ahead of time how far the different parts of the body will move in a given time is lost, the person becomes unable also to control the beginning of the next movement. As a result, the succeeding movement may begin much too early or much too late. Therefore, movements such as those required for writing, running, or even talking all become completely incoordinate, lacking completely in the ability to progress in an orderly sequence from one movement to the next.

Extramotor Predictive Functions of the Cerebellum. The cerebellum also plays a role in predicting other events besides movements of the body. For instance, the rates of progression of both auditory and visual phenomena can be predicted. As an example, a person can predict from the changing visual scene how rapidly he is approaching an object. A striking experiment that demonstrates the importance of the cerebellum in this ability is the effect of removing the "head" portion of the cerebellar vermis in monkeys. Such a monkey occasionally charges the wall of a corridor and literally bashes its brains out because it is unable to predict when it will reach the wall.

Unfortunately, we are only now beginning to learn about these extramotor predictive functions of the cerebellum. It is quite possible that the cerebellum provides a "time base," perhaps utilizing time-delay·circuits, against which signals from other parts of the central nervous system can be compared. It is often stated that the cerebellum is especially important in interpreting *spatiotemporal relationships* in sensory information.

Cerebellar Control of Ballistic Movements

We must emphasize again that *feedback* control of motor movements in response to signals from the periphery involves a very long delay time, as much as 15 to 25 milliseconds from the periphery to the motor cortex and at least that much longer back to the periphery, giving a total time interval of 1/30 to 1/20 of a second — far too long for any effective control of extremely rapid movements. The cerebellum does utilize its predictive capability to help overcome this problem, but even so some motor movements are entirely over before any feedback whatsoever can return to the motor cortex. These are called *ballistic* movements. An important example is the saccadic movements of the eyes, in which the eyes jump from one position to the next when reading or when looking at the side of the road while moving in a car, or so forth. The movements are entirely over before any feedback can reach the cerebellum, much less reach the motor cortex. And the same is true of many of the limb movements as well.

Yet, for proper performance of these ballistic movements, the cerebellum is essential. In fact, they are usually disturbed even more than the slower movements when the cerebellum is impaired.

It is believed that mainly the hemispheres of the cerebellum are concerned with these ballistic movements, because the two-way circuits between the motor cortex and these hemispheres provide the most direct and most rapidly functioning pathway between the cortex and cerebellum. Furthermore, this pathway begins mainly in area VI of the motor cortex and returns to area IV. Therefore, there is very little, if any, feed*back* to the point of origin of the signal; instead, this is a feed*forward* circuit.

When the cerebellum is removed, three major changes occur in the ballistic movements: (1) they are slow to begin, (2) the force development is weak, and (3) the movements are slow to turn off. Therefore, it becomes very difficult to perform the very rapid ballistic movements. Furthermore, it is almost impossible to control how far the movement will go because of the difficulty of turning the movement off once it is begun. Thus, in the absence of the cerebellar circuit, the motor cortex has to think very hard to turn ballistic movements on and again has to think hard and take extra time to turn the movement off. Thus, the automatism of ballistic movements is lost.

But, how does the cerebellum function in the control of ballistic movements? We do not know the answer to this. The supposition is: When the motor cortex first initiates the movement, it immediately sends signals to the cerebellum at the same time. The first effect of the signals is to excite the deep cerebellar dentate nuclei, and these immediately send an excitatory signal back to the motor cortex or other motor nuclei to reinforce strongly the onset of the ballistic movement. A few milliseconds later, the signal entering the cerebellum will have had time to go through the delay circuits of the cerebellar cortex and to travel by way of the Purkinje cells back to the dentate nuclei, but this

time inhibiting these rather than exciting them. Therefore, after this given delay time, this automatic delayed inhibitory signal presumably stops the ballistic movement by turning off the agonist muscle and, because of reciprocal innervation, turning on the antagonist at the same time.

If you will reconsider once again the circuitry of the cerebellum as described earlier in the chapter, you will see that it is beautifully organized to perform this biphasic, first excitatory and then delayed, inhibitory function that is required for ballistic movements. You will also see that the time delay circuits of the cerebellar cortex almost undoubtedly are fundamental to this particular ability of the cerebellum.

Function of the Cerebellum in Relation to the Basal Ganglia

It is already clear that proper function of the motor control system requires not only active participation of the motor cortex but also of the cerebellum and basal ganglia. Furthermore, both of these can provide either feed*back* or feed*forward* signals. Yet, their functions are entirely different. Some of the differences are the following:

First, the cerebellum can provide feedback or feedforward signals that last no longer than a few milliseconds at a time. Furthermore, the cerebellum cannot originate motor signals. On the other hand, the basal ganglia can originate signals; they can provide long-term continuous signals to the motor control pathway; they can provide rhythmical patterns of activities; and they can transmit motor control signals into the brain stem and to the muscles sometimes without involving the motor cortex at all.

Second, the basal ganglia are concerned especially with the balance between agonist and antagonist muscle contractions during either static contractions or during smooth progressive contractions. In contrast, the cerebellum is concerned principally with the onset and offset of rapid movements.

Third, the basal ganglia seem to be harbingers of many subconscious stereotyped or even learned programs of movement, either functioning alone or functioning in close association with the cerebral cortex. The cerebellum does not provide such programs of movement. However, whenever the basal ganglial programs involve rapid movements, the cerebellum plays the same role in relation to these movements as it does to the more direct signals from the motor cortex.

CLINICAL ABNORMALITIES OF THE CEREBELLUM

Destruction of small portions of the cerebellar cortex causes no detectable abnormality in motor function. In fact, several months after as much as half the cerebellar cortex has been removed, the motor functions appear to be almost entirely normal — but only as long as the person performs all movements slowly. Thus, the remaining areas of the cerebellum compensate tremendously for loss of part of the cerebellum.

To cause serious and continuous dysfunction of the cerebellum, the cerebellar lesion must usually involve the deep cerebellar nuclei — the *dentate, interpositus,* and *fastigial nuclei* — as well as the cerebellar cortex.

Dysmetria and Ataxia.   Two of the most important symptoms of cerebellar disease are dysmetria and ataxia. It was pointed out above that in the absence of the cerebellum a person cannot predict ahead of time how far movements will go. Therefore, the movements ordinarily overshoot their intended mark. This effect is called *dysmetria,* and it results in incoordinate movements which are called *ataxia.*

Dysmetria and ataxia can also result from lesions in the spinocerebellar tracts, for the feedback information from the moving parts of the body is essential for accurate control of the muscular movements.

Past Pointing.   Past pointing means that in the absence of the cerebellum a person ordinarily moves the hand or some other moving part of the body considerably beyond the point of intention. This probably results from the following effect: The motor cortex normally transmits more impulses to the muscles to perform a given motor function than are actually needed. The cerebellum automatically corrects this by inhibiting the movement after it has begun. However, if the cerebellum is not available to cause this inhibition, the movement ordinarily goes beyond the intended point. Therefore, past pointing is actually a manifestation of dysmetria.

Failure of Progression. *Dysdiadochokinesia.*   When the motor control system fails to predict ahead of time where the different parts of the body will be at a given time, it temporarily "loses" the parts during rapid motor movements. As a result, the succeeding movement may begin much too early or much too late so that no orderly "progression of movement" can occur. One can demonstrate this readily by having a patient with cerebellar damage turn one hand upward and downward at a rapid rate. The patient rapidly "loses" the hand and does not know its position during any portion of the movement. As a result, a series of jumbled movements occurs instead of the normal coordinate upward and downward motions. This is called dysdiadochokinesia.

Dysarthria.   Another instance in which failure of progression occurs is in talking, for the formation of words depends on rapid and orderly succession of individual muscular movements in the larynx, mouth, and respiratory system. Lack of coordination between these and inability to predict either the intensity of the sound or the duration of each successive sound cause jumbled vocalization, with some syllables loud, some weak, some held long, some held for a short interval, and resultant speech that is almost completely unintelligible. This is called dysarthria.

Intention Tremor.   When a person who has lost the cerebellum performs a voluntary act, the muscular movements are jerky; this reaction is called an *intention tremor* or an *action tremor,* and it results from failure of the cerebellar system to damp the motor movements. Tremor is particularly evident when the dentate nuclei or the superior cerebellar peduncle is destroyed, but it is not present when the spinocerebellar tracts from the periphery to the cerebellum are destroyed. This indicates that the feedback pathway from the cerebellum to the motor cortex is a principal pathway for damping of muscular movements.

Cerebellar Nystagmus.   Cerebellar nystagmus is a tremor of the eyeballs that occurs usually when one attempts to fixate the eyes on a scene to the side of the head. This off-center type of fixation results in rapid, tremulous movements of the eyes rather than a steady fixation, and it is probably another manifestation of the failure of damping by the cerebellum. It occurs especially when the flocculonodular lobes are damaged; in this instance it is associated with loss of equilibrium, presumably because of dysfunction of the pathways through the cerebellum from the semicircular canals. Nystagmus resulting from damage to the semicircular canals was discussed in Chapter 12.

Rebound.   If a person with cerebellar disease is asked to contract an arm tightly while the physician holds it back at first and then lets go, the arm will fly back until it strikes the face instead of being automatically stopped. This is called rebound, and it results from loss of the cerebellar component of the stretch reflex. That is, the normal cerebellum ordinarily instantaneously and powerfully sensitizes the spinal cord reflex mechanism whenever a portion of the body begins to move unexpectedly in an unwilled direction. But, without the cerebellum, activation of the antagonist muscles fails to occur, thus allowing overmovement of the limb.

Hypotonia.   Loss of the deep cerebellar nuclei, particularly the dentate nuclei, causes moderate decrease in tone of the peripheral musculature on the side of the lesion, though after several months the motor cortex usually compensates for this by an increase in its intrinsic activity. The hypotonia results from loss of facilitation of the motor cortex and brain stem nuclei by the tonic discharge of the deep nuclei.

SENSORY FEEDBACK CONTROL OF MOTOR FUNCTIONS

Everyone who has ever studied the relationship of the somatic sensory areas to the motor areas of the cortex has been impressed by the close functional interdependence of the two areas. Anatomically, the characteristic pyramidal cells of the motor cortex extend backward into the anterior lip of the postcentral gyrus where they intermingle with large numbers of granule cells of the somatic sensory cortex. Likewise, the granule cells of the sensory cortex extend anteriorly into the precentral gyrus, the *area pyramidalis.* Thus the two areas fade into each other with many somatic sensory fibers actually terminating directly in the motor cortex and some motor signals originating in the sensory cortex.

Furthermore, when a portion of the somatic sensory cortex in the postcentral gyrus is removed, the muscles controlled by the motor cortex immediately anterior to the removed area often lose much of their coordination. This observation illustrates that the somatic sensory area plays a major role in the control of motor functions.

THE SENSORY ENGRAM FOR MOTOR CONTROL

A person performs a motor movement mainly to achieve a purpose. Primarily in the sensory and sensory association areas the person experiences effects of motor movements and records "memories" of the different patterns of motor movements. These are called sensory engrams of the motor movements. Wishing to achieve some purposeful act, one presumably calls forth one of these engrams and then sets the motor system of the brain into action to reproduce the sensory pattern that is laid down in the engram.

The Proprioceptor Feedback Servomechanism for Reproducing the Sensory Engram. In addition to the feedback pathways through the cerebellum, feedback pathways also pass from proprioceptors to the sensory areas of the cerebral cortex and thence back to the motor cortex. And these feedback pathways are capable of modifying the motor response. For instance, as a person learns to cut out a paper doll with scissors, the movements involved in this process cause a particular sequential pattern of proprioceptive impulses to pass to the somatic sensory area. Once this pattern has been "learned" by the sensory cortex, the memory engram of the pattern can be used to activate the motor system to perform the same sequential pattern whenever it is required — even when the person is blindfolded.

To do this, the proprioceptor signals from the fingers, hands, and arms are compared with the engram, and if the two do not match each other, the difference, called the "error," supposedly initiates additonal motor signals that automatically activate appropriate muscles to bring the fingers, hands, and arms into the necessary sequential attitudes for performance of the task. Each successive portion of the engram presumably is projected according to a time sequence, and the motor control system automatically follows from one point to the next so that the fingers go through the precise motions necessary to duplicate the sensory engram of the motor activity.

Thus, one can see that the motor system in this case acts as a *servomechanism*, for it is not the motor cortex itself that controls the pattern of activity to be accomplished. Instead, the pattern is located in the sensory part of the brain, and the motor system merely "follows" the pattern, which is the definition of a servomechanism. If ever the motor system fails to follow the pattern, sensory signals are fed back to the cerebral cortex to apprise the sensorium of this failure, and appropriate corrective signals are transmitted to the muscles.

Other sensory signals besides somesthetic signals are also involved in motor control, particularly visual signals. However, these other sensory systems are often slower to recognize error than is the somatic proprioceptor system. Therefore, when the sensory engram depends on visual feedback for control purposes, the motor movements are usually considerably slowed in comparison with those that depend on somatic feedback.

An extremely interesting experiment that demonstrates the importance of the sensory engram for control of motor movements is one in which a monkey has been trained to perform some complex but slow-moving activity, and then various portions of its cortex are removed. Removal of small portions of the motor cortex that control the muscles normally used for the activity does not prevent the monkey from performing the activity. Instead it automatically uses other muscles in place of the paraylzed ones to perform the same activity. On the other hand, if the corresponding somatic sensory cortex is removed while the motor cortex is left intact, the monkey loses all ability to perform the activity. Thus, this experiment demonstrates that the motor system acts automatically as a servomechanism to use whatever muscles are available to follow the pattern of the sensory engram, and if some muscles are missing, other muscles are substituted automatically. The experiment also demonstrates forcefully that the somatic sensory cortex is essential for performance of some types of "learned" motor activities.

ESTABLISHMENT OF RAPID MOTOR PATTERNS

Many motor activities are performed so rapidly that there is insufficient time for sensory feedback signals to control these activities. For instance, the movements of the fingers during typing occur much too rapidly for somatic sensory signals to be transmitted either to the somatic sensory cortex or even directly to the motor cortex and for these then to control each discrete movement. It is believed that the patterns for control of these rapid coordinate muscular movements are established in the motor system itself, probably involving complex circuitry in the primary motor cortex, in the motor association cortex, the basal ganglia, and even the cerebellum. Indeed, lesions in any of these areas can destroy one's ability to perform rapid coordinated muscular contractions, such as those required during the act of typing, talking, or writing by hand.

Role of Sensory Feedback During Establishment of the Rapid Motor Patterns. Even a highly skilled motor activity can be performed the very first time if it is performed extremely slowly — slowly enough for sensory feedback to guide the movements through each step. However, to be really useful, many skilled motor activities must be performed rapidly. This probably is achieved by successive performance of the same skilled activity until finally an engram for the skilled activity is laid down in the motor control areas of the cortex as well as in the sensory system. This motor engram causes a precise set of muscles to go through a specific sequence of movements required to perform the skilled activity. Therefore, such an engram is called a *pattern of skilled motor function,* and the motor areas are primarily concerned with this.

After a person has performed a skilled activity many times, the motor pattern of this activity can thereafter cause the hand or arm or other part of the body to go through the same pattern of activity again and again, now entirely *without* sensory feedback control. However, even though sensory feedback control is no longer present, the sensory system still determines whether or not the act has been performed correctly. This determination is made in retrospect rather than while the act is being performed. If the pattern has not been performed correctly, information from the sensory system can help to correct the pattern the next time it is performed.

Thus, eventually, hundreds of patterns of different coordinate movements are believed to be laid down in the motor system, and these can be called upon one at a time in different sequential orders to perform literally thousands of complex motor activities.

An interesting experiment that demonstrates the applicability of these theoretical methods of muscular control is one in which the eyes are made to "follow" an object that moves around and around in a circle. At first, the eyes can follow the object only when it moves around the circle slowly, and even then the movements of the eyes are extremely jerky. Thus, sensory feedback is being utilized to control the eye movements for following the object. However, after a few seconds, the eyes begin to follow the moving object rather faithfully, and the rapidity of movement around the circle can be increased to many times per second, and still, the eyes continue to follow the object. Sensory feedback control of each stage of the eye movements at these rapid rates would be completely impossible. Therefore, by this time, the eyes have developed a pattern of movement that is not dependent upon step-by-step sensory feedback. Nevertheless, if the eyes should fail to follow the object around the circle, the sensory system would immediately become aware of this

and presumably could make corrections in the pattern of movement.

INITIATION OF VOLUNTARY MOTOR ACTIVITY

Because of the spectacular properties of the primary motor cortex (the area pyramidalis) and of the instantaneous muscle contractions that can be achieved by stimulating this area, it has become customary to think that the initial brain signals that elicit voluntary muscle contractions begin in the primary motor cortex. However, this almost certainly is far from the truth. Indeed, experiments have shown that the cerebellum and the basal ganglia are activated at almost exactly the same time that the motor cortex is activated, and all of these are activated even *before* the voluntary movement occurs. Furthermore, there is no known mechanism by which the motor cortex can conceive the entire sequential pattern that is to be achieved by the motor movements.

Therefore, we are left with an unanswered question: What is the locus of the initiation of voluntary motor activity? In the following chapter we will learn that the reticular formation of the brain stem and much of the thalamus play essential roles in activating all other parts of the brain. Therefore, it is very likely that these areas provide at least part of the initial signals that lead to subsequent activity in the motor cortex, the basal ganglia, and the cerebellum at the onset of voluntary movement. Here again, we come to a circular question: What is it that initiates the activity in the brain stem and the thalamus? We do know part of the answer to this: The activity is initiated by continual sensory input into these areas, including sensory input from the peripheral receptors of the body and from the cortical sensory storage, or memory, areas. Much of motor activity is almost reflex in nature, occurring instantly after an incoming sensory signal from the periphery. But so-called voluntary activity occurs minutes, hours, or even days after the initiating sensory input — after analysis, storage of memories, recall of the memories, and finally initiation of a motor response. We shall see in Chapter 15 that the control of motor activity is strongly influenced by these prolonged procedures of cerebration. Furthermore, damage to the essential areas of the cerebral cortex for analysis of sensory information leads to serious deficits and abnormalities of voluntary muscle control.

Therefore, for the present, let us conclude that the immediate energy for eliciting voluntary motor activity probably comes from the middle regions of the brain. These, in turn, are under the control of the different sensory inputs, the memory storage areas, and the associated areas of the brain that are devoted to the processes of analysis, a mechanism frequently called *cerebration*.

REFERENCES

Allen, G. I., and Tsukahara, N.: Cerebrocerebellar communication systems. *Physiol. Rev., 54*:957, 1974.

Armstrong, D. M.: The mammalian cerebellum and its contribution to movement control. *In* Porter, R. (ed.): International Review of Physiology: Neurophysiology III. Vol. 17. Baltimore, University Park Press, 1978, p. 239.

Asanuma, H.: Cerebral cortical control of movement. *Physiologist, 16*:143, 1973.

Asanuma, H.: Recent developments in the study of the columnar arrangement of neurons within the motor cortex. *Physiol. Rev., 55*:143, 1975.

Brooks, V. B.,, and Stoney, S. D., Jr.: Motor mechanisms: The role of the pyramidal system in motor control. *Annu. Rev. Physiol., 33*:337, 1971.

Cooper, I. S., *et al.* (eds.): The Cerebellum, Epilepsy, and Behavior. New York, Plenum Press, 1974.

Crowley, W. J.: Neural control of skeletal muscle. *In* Frohlich, E. D. (ed.): Pathophysiology, 2nd Ed. Philadelphia, J. B. Lippincott Co., 1976, p. 735.

Desmedt, J. E. (ed.): Cerebral Motor Control in Man: Long Loop Mechanisms. New York, S. Karger, 1978.

Eccles, J. C.: The Understanding of the Brain. New York, McGraw-Hill, 1973.

Evarts, E. V.: Brain mechanisms in movement. *Sci. Am., 229*:96, 1973.

Evarts, E. V.: Brain mechanisms of movement. *Sci. Am. 241*(3):164, 1979.

Evarts, E. V., and Thach, W. T.: Motor mechanisms of the CNS: Cerebrocerebellar interrelations. *Annu. Rev. Physiol., 31*:451, 1969.

Gallistel, C. R.: The Organization of Action: A New Synthesis. New York, Halsted Press, 1979.

Granit, R.: The Basis of Motor Control. New York, Academic Press, 1970.

Grillner, S.: Locomotion in vertebrates: Central mechanisms and reflex interaction. *Physiol. Rev., 55*:247, 1975.

Llinas, R.: Eighteenth Bowditch lecture. Motor aspects of cerebellar control. *Physiologist, 17*:19, 1974.

Massion, J., and Sasaki, K. (eds.): Cerebro-Cerebellar Interactions. New York, Elsevier/North-Holland, 1979.

McHenry, L. C., Jr.: Cerebral Circulation and Stroke. St. Louis, W. H. Green, 1978.

O'Connell, A. L., and Gardner, E. B.: Understanding the Scientific Bases of Human Movement. Baltimore, Williams & Wilkins. 1972.

Orlovsky, G. N., and Shik, M. L.: Control of locomotion: A neurophysiological analysis of the cat locomotor system. *10*:281, 1976.

Paillard, J.: The patterning of skilled movements. *In* Magoun, H. W. (ed.): Handbook of Physiology. Sec. 1, Vol. 3. Baltimore. Williams & Wilkins, 1960, p. 1679.

Pearson, K.: The control of walking. *Sci. Am., 235*(6):72, 1976.

Penfield, W., and Rasmussen, T.: The Cerebral Cortex of Man. New York, The Macmillan Co., 1950.

Pepper, R. L., and Herman, L. M.: Decay and Interference Effects in the Short-Term Retention of a Discrete Motor Act. Washington, D.C., American Physiological Association, 1970.

Porter, R.: Functions of the mammalian cerebral cortex in movement. *Prog. Neurobiol., 1*:3, 1973.

Porter, R.: The neurophysiology of movement performance. *In* MTP International Review of Science: Physiology. Vol. 3. Baltimore, University Park Press, 1974, p. 151.

Porter, R.: Influences of movement detectors on pyramidal tract neurons in primates. *Annu. Rev. Physiol., 38*:121, 1976.

Shik, M. L., and Orlovsky, G. N.: Neurophysiology of Locomotor Automatism. *Physiol. Rev., 56*:465, 1976.

Stein, P. S. G.: Motor systems with specific reference to the control of locomotion. *Annu. Rev. Neurosci., 1*:61, 1978.

Wilson, D. M.: The flight-control system of the locust. *Sci. Am., 218*:(5):83, 1968.

14

Activation of the Brain — The Reticular Activating System; The Generalized Thalamocortical System; Brain Waves; Epilepsy; Wakefulness and Sleep

We will now consider the many brain functions related to the *reticular activating system*, a system that controls the overall degree of central nervous system activity, including control of wakefulness and sleep, and control of at least part of our ability to direct attention toward specific areas of our conscious minds.

Figure 14–1A illustrates the extent of this system, showing that it begins in the lower brain stem and extends upward through the mesencephalon and thalamus to be distributed throughout the cerebral cortex. Impulses are transmitted from the ascending reticular activating system to the cortex by two different pathways. One pathway passes upward from the brain stem portion of the reticular formation — especially from the mesencephalic region — to the intralaminar, midline, and reticular nuclei of the thalamus and thence through diverse pathways to essentially all parts of the cerebral cortex as well as the basal ganglia. A second and probably much less important pathway is through the subthalamic, hypothalamic, and adjacent areas.

FUNCTION OF THE RETICULAR ACTIVATING SYSTEM IN WAKEFULNESS

Diffuse electrical stimulation in the *mesencephalic, pontile, and upper medullary portions of the reticular formation* — an area discussed in Chapter 12 in relation to the motor functions of the nervous system — causes immediate and marked activation of the cerebral cortex and even causes a sleeping animal to awaken instantaneously. Furthermore, when this mesencephalic portion of the reticular formation is damaged severely, as occurs (a) when a *brain tumor* develops in this region, (b) when serious *hemorrhage* occurs, or (c) in diseases such as *encephalitis lethargica* (sleeping sickness), the person passes into coma and is completely nonsusceptible to normal awakening stimuli.

Function of the Mesencephalic Portion of the Reticular Activating System. Electrical stimuli applied to different portions of the reticular activating system have shown that the mesencephalic portion functions quite differently from the thalamic portion. Electrical stimulation of the mesencephalic portion causes generalized activation of the entire brain, including activation of the cerebral cortex, thalamic nuclei, basal ganglia, hypothalamus, other portions of the brain stem, and even the spinal cord. Furthermore, once the mesencephalic portion is stimulated, the degree of activation throughout the nervous system remains high for as long as a half minute or more after the stimulation is over. Therefore, *it is believed that the mesencephalic portion of the reticular activating system is basically responsible for normal wakefulness of the brain.*

Function of the Thalamic Portion of the Activating System. Electrical stimulation in different areas of the thalamic portion of the activating system (if the stimulation is not too strong) activates specific regions of the cerebral cortex more than others. This is distinctly different from stimu-

A

B

Figure 14–1. (A) The ascending reticular activating system schematically projected on a monkey brain. (From Lindsley: Reticular Formation of the Brain. Little, Brown, and Co.) (B) Convergence of pathways from the cerebral cortex and from the spinal afferent systems on the reticular activating system. (From French, Hernandez-Peon, and Livingston: *J. Neurophysiol., 18*:74, 1955.)

lation in the mesencephalic portion, which activates all the brain at the same time. Therefore, it is believed that the thalamic portion of the activating system has two specific functions: first, it relays most of the diffuse facilitatory signals from the mesencephalon to all parts of the cerebral cortex to cause generalized activation of the cerebrum; second, stimulation of selected points in the thalamic activating system causes specific activation of certain areas of the cerebral cortex in distinction to the other areas. This selective activation of specific cortical areas possibly or probably plays an important role in our ability to direct our attention to certain parts of our mental activity, which is discussed later in the chapter.

THE AROUSAL REACTION — ACTIVATION OF THE RETICULAR ACTIVATING SYSTEM BY SENSORY SIGNALS

When an animal is asleep, the level of activity of the reticular activating system is greatly decreased; yet almost any type of sensory signal can immediately activate the system. For instance, proprioceptive signals from the joints and muscles, pain impulses from the skin, visual signals from the eyes, auditory signals from the ears, or even visceral sensations from the gut can all cause sudden activation of the reticular activating system and therefore arouse the animal. This is called the *arousal reaction.*

Some types of sensory stimuli are more potent than others in eliciting the arousal reaction; the most potent are pain and proprioceptive somatic impulses.

Anatomically, the reticular formation of the brain stem is admirably constructed to perform the arousal functions. It receives tremendous numbers of signals either directly or indirectly from the *spinoreticular tracts,* the *spinothalamic tracts,* the *spinotectal tracts,* the *auditory tracts,* the *visual tracts,* and others, so that almost any sensory stimulus in the body can activate it. The reticular formation in turn can transmit signals both upward into the brain and downward into the spinal cord. Indeed, many of the fibers originating from cells in the reticular formation divide, with one branch of the fiber passing upward and the other branch passing downward, as was explained in Chapter 12.

STIMULATION OF THE RETICULAR ACTIVATING SYSTEM BY THE CEREBRAL CORTEX

In addition to activation of the reticular activating system by sensory impulses, the cerebral cortex can also stimulate this system. Direct fiber pathways pass into the reticular formation, as shown in Figure 14–1B, from almost all parts of the cerebrum but particularly from (1) the *sensorimotor cortex* of the pre- and postcentral gyri, (2) the *frontal cortex,* (3) the *cingulate gyrus,* (4) the *hippocampus* and *other limbic structures,* (5) the *hypothalamus,* and (6) the *basal ganglia.* Because of an exceedingly large number of nerve fibers that pass from the motor regions of the cerebral cortex to the reticular formation, motor activity in particular is associated with a high degree of wakefulness, which partially explains the importance of movement to keep a person awake. However, intense activity of any other part of the cerebrum can also activate the reticular activating system and consequently can cause a high degree of wakefulness.

THE GENERALIZED THALAMOCORTICAL SYSTEM

At this point it is important that we explain some of the interrelationships between the thalamus and the cerebral cortex. The thalamus is the entryway for essentially all sensory nervous signals to the cortex, with the single exception of signals from the olfactory system. In Chapters 9 and 10 we have already discussed the relay of the somatic signals through the *ventrobasal nuclei* of the thalamus to the cerebral cortex, and in Chap-

ters 12 and 13 we traced signals from the cerebellum and basal ganglia through the *ventrolateral* and *ventroanterior thalamic nuclei.* Also, we shall see in Chapters 20, 21, and 22 that all the signals from the visual, auditory, and taste systems are also relayed in the thalamus on their way to the cortex. All these thalamic relay nuclei are called the *specific nuclei of the thalamus;* the combination of these nuclei and their connecting areas in the cortex is called the *specific thalamocortical system.* It is this system of which we usually speak when we discuss the transmission of sensory information to the cerebral cortex.

In addition to the specific thalamocortical system, there is a separate system, partially separated from the specific system, called the *generalized thalamocortical system,* or the *diffuse thalamocortical system,* or the *nonspecific thalamocortical system.* This system is subserved by *diffuse thalamic nuclei* and also by *diffuse fiber projections* from the thalamus to the cortex. The thalamic neurons of this system are, in reality, the uppermost end of the reticular formation, and they are not collected into discrete nuclei as are the neurons of the specific system. Instead, they lie mainly between the specific nuclei or on the outer surface of the thalamus; they are divided into three separate groups: (1) the *intralaminar nuclei,* which are diffuse collections of neurons that lie within the thalamic mass among the specific nuclei; (2) the *periventricular nuclei,* which lie adjacent to the third ventricle and have little organization; and (3) the *reticular nuclei* of the thalamus, which form a thin shell of diffuse neurons that lies over the entire dorsal, anterior, and lateral surfaces of the thalamus and through which all the pathways from the thalamus to the cerebral cortex must pass. All these nuclei make multiple connections with the specific thalamic nuclei. They also project very small fibers to all parts of the cerebral cortex, with the exception of small portions of the temporal lobes that are associated with the limbic system, a very old part of the brain that plays major roles in behavior, emotions, and so forth as will be discussed in Chapter 16.

The generalized system of the thalamus is continuous with the upper end of the reticular formation in the brain stem and receives much of its input from this source. It is also an important terminus of one of the very important somatic sensory pathways, the *paleospinothalamic pathway for pain* — the pathway that transmits the intolerable type of burning, aching pain. This is the same pathway that transmits the major sensory signals into much of the reticular formation of the lower brain stem as well.

Control Functions of the Generalized Thalamocortical System. One can well understand from the above description of the diffuse thalamic nuclei that they lie in propitious locations for affecting the levels of activity of all of the specific nuclei of the thalamus. It is also clear that they are properly located to relay control functions from the mesencephalic reticular formation to the cerebrum, and that they in turn can receive much helpful input information from the specific nuclei of the thalamus. Perhaps most important of all, however, is the fact that these nuclei have a specific capability to control the level of activity in the entire cerebral cortex; this is mediated by signals that play on the cerebral cortex through the diffuse thalamocortical projections.

Effect of the Generalized Thalamic System on Cortical Activity. Activation of the cortex by the generalized thalamic system is entirely different from activation by the specific system. Some of the differences are the following:

1. Stimulation of a specific thalamic nucleus — such as the ventrobasal complex that transmits somatic signals to the somesthetic cortex — activates the cortex within 1 to 2 milliseconds, whereas stimulation of the generalized system causes no activation for approximately the first 25 milliseconds. The activation level builds up over a period of many milliseconds. These differences are illustrated in Figure 14–2.

2. At the end of stimulation, the activation of the cortex by the specific nuclei dies away within another few milliseconds, whereas the activation by the generalized system sometimes continues as an "after-discharge" for as long as 30 seconds.

3. Signals from the specific nuclei to the cortex activate mainly layer IV of the cortex, as was explained in Chapter 49, whereas activation of the generalized thalamic system activates mainly layers I and II of the cortex. Since this latter activation is prolonged and because layers I and II are the loci of many of the dendrites of the deeper

Figure 14–2. Comparison of the response of the visual cortex following stimulation of the lateral geniculate body (record A), which is part of the specific thalamocortical system, with the response of the visual cortex following stimulation of the visual portion of the generalized thalamocortical system (record B). Note in record B the long latent period before appearance of the diffuse response and also the prolonged duration of the response.

cortical neurons, it is supposed that the stimulation by the generalized thalamic system mainly causes partial depolarization of large numbers of dendrites near the surface of the cortex; this in turn causes a generalized increase in the degree of facilitation of the cortex. When the cortex is thus facilitated, specific signals that enter the cortex from other sources are exuberantly received.

4. Stimulation in the generalized thalamic system *facilitates* an *area* of several square centimeters in the cortex, while stimulation at a point in a specific thalamic nucleus *excites* a specific point in the cortex.

In summary, the generalized thalamocortical system controls the overall degree of activity of the cortex. It can at times facilitate activity in regional areas of the cortex distinct from the remainder of the cortex. Collateral signals from this system also control the level of activity in the specific nuclei of the thalamus, the basal ganglia, the hypothalamus, and other structures of the cerebrum as well.

ATTENTION

So long as a person is awake, he has the ability to direct his attention to specific aspects of his mental environment. Furthermore, his degree of attention can change remarkably from (a) almost no attention at all to (b) broad attention to almost everything that is going on, or to (c) intense attention to a minute facet of his momentary mental experience.

Unfortunately, the basic mechanisms by which the brain accomplishes its diverse acts of attention are not known. However, a few clues are beginning to fall into place, as follows:

Reticular Activating System Control of Overall Attentiveness. In exactly the same way that a person can change from a state of sleep to a state of wakefulness, there can be all degrees of wakefulness, from wakefulness in which a person is nonattentive to almost all the surroundings to an extremely high degree of wakefulness in which the person reacts instantaneously to almost any sensory experience. These changes in degree of *overall attentiveness* seem to be caused primarily by changes in activity of the mesencephalic portion of the reticular activating system. Thus, control of the general level of attentiveness is probably exerted by the same mechanism that controls wakefulness, the control center for which is located in the mesencephalon and upper pons.

Function of the Thalamus in Attention. Earlier in the chapter it was pointed out that stimulation of a single specific area in the thalamic portion of the reticular activating system, when the stimulus intensity is not too strong, activates only a small area of the cerebral cortex. Since the cerebral cortex is one of the most important areas of the brain for conscious awareness of our surroundings, one can surmise that the ability of specific thalamic areas to excite specific cortical regions might be one of the mechanisms by which a person can direct attention to specific aspects of the mental environment, whether these be immediate sensory experiences or stored memories.

Relation of Centrifugal Control of Sensory Information to Attention. Nervous pathways extend centrifugally from all sensory areas of the brain toward the lower centers to control the intensity of sensory input to the brain. For instance, the auditory cortex can either inhibit or facilitate signals from the cochlea, the visual cortex can control the signals from the retina in the same way, and the somesthetic cortex can control the intensities of signals from the somatic areas of the body.

Thus, it is likely that activated regions of the cortex control their own sensory input. This is another means by which the brain might direct its attention to specific phases of its mental activity.

POSSIBLE "SEARCHING" AND "PROGRAMMING" FUNCTIONS OF THE BRAIN'S ACTIVATING SYSTEM

At this point it is important to refer back to the analogy drawn in Chapter 6 between the functions of the central nervous system and of a general purpose computer. Almost all complex computers, particularly those that are capable of storing information and then recalling this information at later times, have a control center called a "programming unit" that directs the attention of different parts of the computer to specific information stored in other parts of the computer. It is quite likely that the activating system of the brain operates in much the same way as the programming unit of a computer for the following reasons:

1. The probable ability of the activating system to direct one's attention to specific mental activities is analogous to the ability of the programming unit to call forth information that has been stored in the memory of the computer or to call forth information that is given to the computer at its input, information that is comparable to sensory information in the human being.

2. The programming unit can "find information" when its exact locus is not known. In the computer, this is achieved by dictating certain qualities required of the information and then searching through hundreds or thousands of stored bits of information until the appropriate information is found, a function called *searching*. We know from psychological tests that our own brain can perform this same function, though we do not know how it does so. Yet, since the thalamus perhaps plays a role in directing our attention to stored information in specific areas of the cortex, it is reasonable to postulate that the thalamus, probably operating in conjunction with other basal areas of the brain, plays a major role in this searching operation.

3. The programming unit of a computer determines the sequence of processing of information. Our brain can also control its thoughts in orderly sequence. Here again, mainly on the basis of anatomical considerations and on the basis of the fact that the reticular activating system is the primary controller of cerebral activity, it can be surmised, until we know more about the subject, that the reticular activating system is at least one of the controllers of our sequence of thoughts.

EFFECT OF BARBITURATE ANESTHESIA ON THE RETICULAR ACTIVATING SYSTEM

The barbiturates have a specific depressant effect on the brain stem portion of the reticular activating system. Therefore, barbiturates obviously can either depress brain activity or even cause sleep. Yet it is especially interesting that barbiturate anesthesia does not block transmission in most of the specific sensory systems and also does not entirely block function of the thalamic portion of the reticular activating system. It is probable that many other clinically used anesthetics also have specific depressant effects on the midbrain portion of the reticular activating system and in this way cause general anesthesia.

BRAIN WAVES

Electrical recordings from the surface of the brain or from the outer surface of the head demonstrate continuous electrical activity in the brain. Both the intensity and patterns of this electrical activity are determined to a great extent by the overall level of excitation of the brain resulting from functions in the reticular activating system. The undulations in the recorded electrical potentials, shown in Figure 14–3, are called *brain waves*, and the entire record is called an *electroencephalogram* (EEG).

The intensities of the brain waves on the surface of the scalp range from 0 to 300 microvolts, and their frequencies range from once every few seconds to 50 or more per second. The character of the waves is highly dependent on the degree of activity of the cerebral cortex, and the waves change markedly between the states of wakefulness and sleep.

Much of the time, the brain waves are irregular, and no general pattern can be discerned in the EEG. However, at other times, distinct patterns do appear. Some of these are characteristic of specific abnormalities of the brain, such as epilepsy, which is discussed later. Others occur even in normal persons and can be classified into *alpha, beta, theta,* and *delta waves,* which are all illustrated in Figure 14–3.

Alpha waves are rhythmic waves occurring at a frequency between 8 and 13 per second and are found in the EEG's of almost all normal adult persons when they are awake in a quiet, resting state of cerebration. These waves occur most intensely in the occipital region but can also be recorded at times from the parietal and frontal regions of the scalp. Their voltage usually is about 50 microvolts. During sleep the alpha waves disappear entirely, and when the awake person's atten-

Figure 14–3. Different types of normal electroencephalographic waves.

tion is directed to some specific type of mental activity, the alpha waves are replaced by asynchronous, higher frequency but lower voltage beta waves. Figure 14–4 illustrates the effect on the alpha waves of simply opening the eyes in bright light and then closing the eyes again. Note that the visual sensations cause immediate cessation of the alpha waves and that these are replaced by low voltage, asynchronous beta waves.

Beta waves occur at frequencies of more than 14 cycles per second and as high as 25 and rarely 50 cycles per second. These are most frequently recorded from the parietal and frontal regions of the scalp, and they can be divided into two major types, *beta I* and *beta II*. The beta I waves, which are illustrated in Figure 14–3, have a frequency about twice that of the alpha waves, and these are affected by mental activity in very much the same way as the alpha waves — that is, they disappear and in their place appears an asynchronous but low voltage recording. The beta II waves, on the contrary, appear during activation of the central nervous system or during tension. Thus, one type of beta wave is inhibited by cerebral activity while the other is elicited.

Theta waves have frequencies between 4 and 7 cycles per second. These occur mainly in the parietal and temporal regions in children, but they also occur during emotional stress in some adults, particularly during disappointment and frustration. They can often be brought out in the EEG of a frustrated person by allowing enjoyment of some pleasant experience and then suddenly removing this element of pleasure; this causes approximately 20 seconds of theta waves. These same waves also occur in many brain disorders.

Delta waves include all the waves of the EEG below 3.5 cycles per second and sometimes as low as 1 cycle every 2 to 3 seconds. These occur in deep sleep, in infancy, and in very serious organic brain disease. And

they occur in the cortex of animals that have had subcortical transections separating the cerebral cortex from the thalamus. Therefore, delta waves can occur strictly in the cortex independently of activities in lower regions of the brain.

ORIGIN OF THE DIFFERENT TYPES OF BRAIN WAVES

The discharge of a single neuron or single nerve fiber in the brain cannot be recorded from the surface of the head. Instead, for an electrical potential to be recorded all the way through the skull, large portions of nervous tissue must emit electrical current simultaneously. There are two ways in which this can occur. First, tremendous numbers of nerve fibers can discharge in synchrony with each other, thereby generating very strong electrical currents. Second, large numbers of neurons can partially discharge, though not emit action potentials; furthermore, these partially discharged neurons can give periods of current flow that can undulate with changing degrees of excitability of the neurons. Simultaneous electrical measurements within the brain while recording brain waves from the scalp indicate that it is the second of these that causes the usual brain waves.

To be more specific, the surface of the cerebral cortex is composed almost entirely of a mat of dendrites extending to the surface from neuronal cells in the lower layers of the cortex. When signals impinge on these dendrites, the dendrites become partially discharged. This partially discharged state makes the neurons of the cortex highly excitable — that is, facilitates them, and the negative potential is simultaneously recorded from the surface of the scalp, indicating this high degree of excitability.

One of the important sources of signals to excite the outer dendritic layer of the cerebral cortex is the ascending reticular activating system. Therefore, brain wave intensity is closely related to the degree of activity in either the brain stem or the thalamic portions of the reticular activating system.

Origin of Delta Waves. Transection of the fiber tracts from the thalamus to the cortex, which blocks the reticular activating system fibers, causes delta waves in the cortex. This indicates that some synchronizing mechanism can occur in the cortical neurons themselves — entirely independently of lower structures in the brain — to cause the delta waves.

Delta waves also occur in very deep "slow wave" sleep; and this suggests that the cortex is then released from the activating influences of the reticular activating system, as was explained earlier in the chapter.

Origin of the Alpha Waves. Alpha waves will *not* occur in the cortex without connections with the thalamus. Also, stimulation in the generalized thalamic nuclei often sets up waves in the generalized thalamocortical system at a frequency of between 8 and 13 per second, the natural frequency of the alpha waves. Therefore, it is assumed that the alpha waves result from spontaneous activity in the generalized thalamocortical system, which causes both the periodicity of the alpha waves and the synchronous activation of literally millions of cortical neurons during each wave.

Figure 14–4. Replacement of the alpha rhythm by an asynchronous discharge on opening the eyes.

EFFECT OF VARYING DEGREES OF CEREBRAL ACTIVITY ON THE BASIC RHYTHM OF THE ELECTROENCEPHALOGRAM

There is a general relationship between the degree of cerebral activity and the average frequency of the electroencephalographic rhythm, the average frequency increasing progressively with higher and higher degrees of activity. This is illustrated in Figure 14–5, which shows the existence of delta waves in stupor, surgical anesthesia, and sleep; theta waves in psychomotor states and in infants; alpha waves during relaxed states; and beta waves during periods of intense mental activity. However, during periods of mental activity the waves usually become asynchronous rather than synchronous so that the voltage falls considerably, despite increased cortical activity, as illustrated in Figure 14–4.

CLINICAL USE OF THE ELECTROENCEPHALOGRAM

One of the most important uses of the EEG is to diagnose different types of epilepsy and to find the focus in the brain causing the epilepsy. This is discussed further below. But, in addition, the EEG can be used to localize brain tumors or other space-occupying lesions of the brain and to diagnose certain types of psychopathic disturbances.

Localization of Brain Tumors. There are two means by which brain tumors can be localized. Some brain tumors are so large that they block electrical activity from a given portion of the cerebral cortex, and when this occurs the voltage of the brain waves is considerably reduced in the region of the tumor. However, more frequently a brain tumor compresses the surrounding neuronal tissue and thereby causes abnormal electrical excitation of these surrounding areas; this in turn leads to synchronous discharges of very high voltage waves in the EEG, as shown in the middle two records of Figure 14–6. Localization of the origin of these spikes on the surface of the scalp is a valuable means for locating the brain tumor.

The upper part of Figure 14–6 shows the placement of 16 different electrodes on the scalp, and the lower part of the figure shows the brain waves from four of these electrodes marked in the figure by Xs. Note that in two of these, intense brain waves are recorded and, furthermore, that the two waves are essentially of reverse polarity to each other. This reverse polarity means that the origin of the spikes is somewhere in the area *between* the two respective electrodes. Thus, the excessively excitable area of the brain has been located, and this is a lead to the location of the brain tumor.

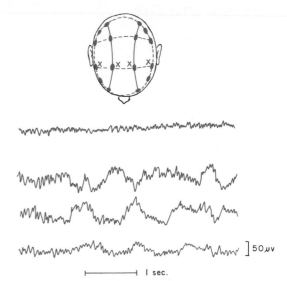

Figure 14–6. Localization of a brain tumor by means of the EEG, illustrating (above) the placement of electrodes and (below) the records from the four electrodes designated by Xs.

Diagnosing Psychopathic Disturbances. Use of brain waves in diagnosing psychopathic abnormalities is generally not very satisfactory because only a few of these cause distinct brain wave patterns. Yet by observing combinations of different types of basic rhythms, reactions of the rhythms to attention, changes of the rhythms during alkalosis caused by forced breathing, the appearance of particular characteristics in the brain waves (such as "spindles" of alpha waves), and so forth, an experienced electroencephalographer can detect at least certain types of psychopathic disturbances. Also, theta waves are frequently found in persons with brain abnormalities.

EPILEPSY

Epilepsy is characterized by uncontrolled excessive activity of either a part or all of the central nervous system. A person who is predisposed to epilepsy has attacks when the basal level of excitability of the nervous system (or of the part that is susceptible to the epileptic state) rises above a certain critical threshold. But, as long as the degree of excitability is held below this threshold, no attack occurs.

Basically, epilepsy can be classified into three major types: *grand mal epilepsy, petit mal epilepsy,* and *focal epilepsy.*

Figure 14–5. Effect of varying degrees of cerebral activity on the basic rhythm of the EEG. (From Gibbs and Gibbs: Atlas of Electroencephalography. Addison-Wesley, 1974.)

GRAND MAL EPILEPSY

Grand mal epilepsy is characterized by extreme neuronal discharges in all areas of the brain — in the cortex, in the deeper parts of the cerebrum, and even in all areas of the reticular activating system. Also, discharges are transmitted from the reticular formation into the spinal cord to cause generalized *tonic convulsions* of the entire body, followed toward the end of the attack by alternating muscular contractions called *tonic-clonic convulsions*. Often the person bites or "swallows" the tongue and usually has difficulty in breathing, sometimes to the extent of developing cyanosis. Also, signals to the viscera frequently cause urination and defecation.

The grand mal seizure lasts from a few seconds to as long as three to four minutes and is characterized by post-seizure depression of the entire nervous system; the person remains in stupor for one to many minutes after the attack is over and then often remains severely fatigued for many hours thereafter.

The middle recording of Figure 14–7 illustrates a typical electroencephalogram from almost any region of the cortex during the tonic phase of a grand mal attack. This illustrates that high voltage, synchronous discharges occur over the entire cortex, having almost the same periodicity as the normal alpha waves. Furthermore, the same type of discharge occurs on both sides of the brain at the same time, illustrating that the abnormal neuronal circuitry responsible for the attack strongly involves the reticular activating system itself.

In experimental animals or even in human beings, grand mal attacks can be initiated by administering neuronal stimulants, such as the well-known drug Metrazol, or they can be caused by insulin hypoglycemia or by the passage of alternating electrical current directly through the brain. Electrical recordings from the thalamus and also from the reticular formation of the brain stem during the grand mal attack show typical high voltage activity in both of these areas similar to that recorded from the cerebral cortex. Furthermore, in an experimental animal, even after transecting the brain stem immediately above the mesencephalon, a typical grand mal seizure can still be induced in the portion of the brain stem beneath the transection.

Presumably, therefore, a grand mal attack is caused by abnormal activation of the reticular activating system itself. The synchronous discharges from this region could result from local reverberating circuits or from reverberation back and forth between the reticular activating system and the cortex.

What Initiates a Grand Mal Attack? Most persons who have grand mal attacks have a hereditary predisposition to epilepsy, a predisposition that occurs in about 1 of every 50 people. In such persons, some of the factors that can increase the excitability of the abnormal "epileptogenic" circuitry enough to precipitate attacks are (1) strong emotional stimuli, (2) alkalosis caused by overbreathing, (3) drugs, (4) fever, or (5) loud noises or flashing lights. Also, even in persons not genetically predisposed, traumatic lesions in almost any part of the brain can cause excess excitability of local brain areas as we shall discuss shortly, and these too can transmit signals into the reticular activating system to elicit grand mal seizures.

What Stops the Grand Mal Attack? The cause of the extreme neuronal overactivity during a grand mal attack is presumed to be massive activation of many reverberating pathways throughout the brain. It is presumed that the major factor, or at least one of the major factors, that stops the attack after a few minutes is the phenomenon of neuronal *fatigue*. However, a second factor is probably *active inhibition* by certain structures of the brain. The change from the tonic type of convulsion to the clonic type during the latter part of the grand mal attack has been suggested to result from partial fatigue of the neuronal system so that some of the excited neurons fade out for a moment, then return to activity after a brief rest, only to fatigue a second time and then a third time, and so forth, until the entire seizure is over. The stupor and fatigue that occur after a grand mal seizure is over are believed to result from the intense fatigue of the neurons following their intensive activity during the grand mal attack.

The *active inhibition* that helps to stop the grand mal attack is believed to result from feedback circuits through inhibitory areas of the brain. The grand mal attack undoubtedly excites such areas as the basal ganglia, which in turn emit many inhibitory impulses into the reticular formation of the brain stem. But the nature of such active inhibition is very much a matter of speculation.

PETIT MAL EPILEPSY

Petit mal epilepsy is closely allied to grand mal epilepsy in that it too almost certainly involves the reticular activating system, but probably the thalamocortical portion rather than the mesencephalic portion. It is characterized by 3 to 30 seconds of unconsciousness during which the person has several twitchlike contractions of the muscles, usually in the head region — especially blinking of the eyes; this is followed by return of consciousness and resumption of previous activities. The patient may have one such attack in many months or in rare instances may have a rapid series of attacks, one following the other. However, the usual course is for the petit mal attacks to appear in late childhood and then to disappear entirely by the age of 30. On occasion, a petit mal epileptic attack will initiate a grand mal attack.

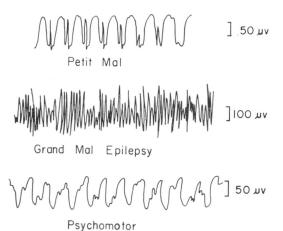

Petit Mal   ] 50 μv

Grand Mal Epilepsy   ] 100 μv

Psychomotor   ] 50 μv

Figure 14–7. Electroencephalograms in different types of epilepsy.

The brain wave pattern in petit mal epilepsy is illustrated by the first record of Figure 14–7, which is typified by a *spike and dome pattern*. The spike portion of this recording is almost identical to the spikes that occur in grand mal epilepsy, but the dome portion is distinctly different. The spike and dome can be recorded over most or all of the cerebral cortex, illustrating that the seizure involves the reticular activating system of the brain.

However, the petit mal attack can sometimes also cause motor twitches or at other times short intervals of psychomotor disturbances. These specific effects suggest that at least some petit mal attacks originate in focal regions of the diffuse thalamic nuclei, possibly in the thalamic intralaminar nuclei.

FOCAL EPILEPSY

Focal epilepsy can involve almost any part of the brain, either localized regions of the cerebral cortex or deeper structures of both the cerebrum and brain stem. And almost always, focal epilepsy results from some localized organic lesion or functional abnormality, such as a scar that pulls on the neuronal tissue, a tumor that compresses an area of the brain, a destroyed area of brain tissue, or congenitally deranged local circuitry. Lesions such as these can promote extremely rapid discharges in the local neurons, and when the discharge rate rises above approximately 1000 per second, synchronous waves begin to spread over the adjacent cortical regions. These waves presumably result from *localized reverberating circuits* that gradually recruit adjacent areas of the cortex into the discharge zone. The process spreads to adjacent areas at a rate as slow as a few millimeters a minute to as fast as several centimeters per second. When such a wave of excitation spreads over the motor cortex, it causes a progressive "march" of muscular contractions throughout the opposite side of the body, beginning most characteristically in the mouth region and marching progressively downward to the legs, but at other times marching in the opposite direction. This is called *jacksonian epilepsy*.

A focal epileptic attack may remain confined to a single area of the brain, but in many instances the strong signals from the convulsing cortex or other part of the brain excite the mesencephalic portion of the reticular activating system so greatly that a grand mal epileptic attack ensues as well.

One type of focal epilepsy is the so-called *psychomotor seizure*, which may cause (1) a short period of amnesia, (2) an attack of abnormal rage, (3) sudden anxiety, discomfort, or fear, (4) a moment of incoherent speech or mumbling of some trite phrase, or (5) a motor act to attack someone, to rub the face with the hand, or so forth. Sometimes the person cannot remember his activities during the attack, but at other times he will have been conscious of everything that he had been doing but unable to control it. Attacks of this type characteristically involve part of the limbic portion of the brain, such as the hippocampus, the amygdala, the septum, or the temporal cortex.

The lower tracing of Figure 14–7 illustrates a typical electroencephalogram during a psychomotor attack, showing a low frequency rectangular wave with a frequency between 2 and 4 per second and with superimposed 14 per second waves.

The electroencephalogram can often be used to localize abnormal spiking waves originating in areas of organic brain disease that might predispose to focal epileptic attacks. Once such a focal point is found, surgical excision of the focus frequently prevents future epileptic attacks.

SLEEP AND WAKEFULNESS

Sleep is defined as a state of unconsciousness from which a person can be aroused by appropriate sensory or other stimuli. Therefore, the unconsciousness caused by deep anesthesia, by total inactivity of the reticular activating system in diseased states (coma), and by excessive activity of the reticular activating system as occurs in grand mal epilepsy would not be considered to be sleep. However, coma and anesthesia do have many characteristics similar to those of deep sleep.

Two Different Types of Sleep. There are two different ways in which sleep can occur. First, it can result from decreased activity in the reticular activating system; this is called *slow wave sleep* because the brain waves are very slow. Second, sleep can result from abnormal channeling of signals in the brain even though brain activity may not be significantly depressed; this is called *paradoxical sleep* or *desynchronized sleep*.

Most of the sleep during each night is of the slow wave variety; this is the deep, restful type of sleep that the person experiences after having been kept awake for the previous 24 to 48 hours. On the other hand, short episodes of paradoxical sleep usually occur at intervals during each night, and this type of sleep may have purposeful functions that will be discussed later.

SLOW WAVE SLEEP

Slow wave sleep is frequently called by different names, such as *deep restful sleep, dreamless sleep, delta wave sleep,* or *normal sleep.* However, we shall see later that paradoxical sleep is also normal and that it has some characteristics of deep sleep.

Electroencephalographic Changes as a Person Falls Asleep. Beginning with wakefulness and proceeding to deep slow wave sleep, the electroencephalogram changes as follows:

1. Alert wakefulness — low voltage, high frequency beta waves showing desynchrony, as illustrated by the second record in Figure 14–3;

2. Quiet restfulness — predominance of alpha waves; a type of "synchronized" brain waves;

3. Light sleep — slowing of the brain waves mainly to theta or low-voltage variety, but interspersed with spindles of alpha waves called *sleep spindles* that last for a few seconds at a time;

4.   Deep slow wave sleep — high voltage delta waves occurring at a rate of 1 to 2 per second, as illustrated by the fourth record of Figure 14–3.

In paradoxical sleep the brain waves change to still a different pattern approaching that of normal wakefulness, as will be discussed below.

Origin of the Delta Waves in Sleep.   When the fiber tracts between the thalamus and the cortex are transected, delta waves are generated in the isolated cortex, indicating that this type of wave probably occurs intrinsically in the cortex when it is not being driven from below. Therefore, it is assumed that the degree of activity in the reticular activating system has fallen to a level too low to maintain normal excitability of the cortex so that the cortex then becomes its own pacemaker.

Characteristics of Deep Slow Wave Sleep.   Most of us can understand the characteristics of deep slow wave sleep by remembering the last time that we were kept awake for more than 24 hours and then the deep sleep that occurred within 30 minutes to an hour after going to sleep. This sleep is dreamless, exceedingly restful, and is associated with a decrease in both peripheral vascular tone and also most of the other vegetative functions of the body as well. There is also a 10 to 30 per cent decrease in blood pressure, respiratory rate, and basal metabolic rate.

PARADOXICAL SLEEP (REM SLEEP)

In a normal night of sleep, bouts of paradoxical sleep lasting 5 to 20 minutes usually appear on the average every 90 minutes, the first such period occurring 80 to 100 minutes after the person falls asleep. When the person is extremely tired, the duration of each bout of paradoxical sleep is very short, and it may even be absent. On the other hand, as the person becomes more rested through the night, the duration of the paradoxical bouts greatly increases.

There are several very important characteristics of paradoxical sleep:

1.   It is usually associated with active dreaming.

2.   The person is even more difficult to arouse than during deep slow wave sleep.

3.   The muscle tone throughout the body is exceedingly depressed, indicating strong inhibition of the spinal projections from the reticular activating system.

4.   The heart rate and respiration usually become irregular, which is characteristic of the dream state.

5.   Despite the extreme inhibition of the peripheral muscles, a few irregular muscle movements occur. These include, in particular, rapid movements of the eyes; consequently, paradoxi-

cal sleep has often been called *REM sleep*, for "rapid eye movements."

6.   The electroencephalogram shows a desynchronized pattern of low voltage beta waves similar to those that occur during wakefulness. Therefore, this type of sleep is also frequently called *desynchronized sleep,* meaning desynchronized brain waves.

In summary, paradoxical sleep is a type of sleep in which the brain is quite active. However, the brain activity is not channeled in the proper direction for the persons to be aware of their surroundings and therefore to be awake.

BASIC THEORIES OF SLEEP AND WAKEFULNESS

Role of the Reticular Activating System in Sleep and Wakefulness.   From the discussion of the reticular activating system earlier in the chapter, it should already be clear that stimulation of this system produces the state of wakefulness. But, what causes sleep? In deep, slow wave sleep, transmission of signals from the reticular activating system to the cortex is greatly diminished, indeed almost absent. Therefore, slow wave sleep presumably results from decreased activity of the reticular activating system.

On the other hand, paradoxical sleep is, as its name implies, paradoxical because some areas of the cerebrum are quite active despite the state of sleep. Therefore, it is assumed that this type of sleep results from a curious mixture of activation of some brain regions while other regions are still suppressed.

Yet, the questions that must be answered before we will understand wakefulness and sleep are: (1) What are the mechanisms that activate the reticular activating system during wakefulness? And (2) what suppresses this system during sleep?

Neuronal Centers, Transmitters, and Mechanisms That Cause Wakefulness

Most of the factors that can cause wakefulness have already been discussed in relation to the reticular activating system. However, let us quickly review these:

1.   Stimulation of the medial portion of the reticular formation, especially in the mesencephalon and upper pons, will cause intense wakefulness.

2.   Widespread stimulation of sensory nerves throughout the body will also cause wakefulness. These nerves transmit strong signals into the mesencephalic portion of the reticular activating system.

3.   Stimulation of most areas of the cerebral

cortex will also cause a high level of wakefulness. These areas also transmit strong signals into both the mesencephalic and thalamic portions of the reticular activating system.

4. Stimulation in certain regions of the hypothalamus, especially in the lateral regions, can also cause extreme degrees of wakefulness. Here again, strong signals are known to be transmitted into the reticular activating system.

5. It is believed that excitation of the area in the pons called the *locus ceruleus* is especially important in maintaining activity in the reticular activating system. The locus ceruleus lies bilaterally immediately beneath the floor of the fourth ventricle. It is a collection of neurons that is considered to be part of the reticular formation though these neurons perform specific functions as follows: The nerve fibers from this area are distributed widely throughout other portions of the reticular formation and throughout almost all areas of the diencephalon and cerebrum as well. They all secrete *norepinephrine* at their endings. It is believed that this norepinephrine in some way plays a role in the wakefulness process. It has been suggested that dopamine and epinephrine, both of which are very similar to norepinephrine, might also contribute to wakefulness because neurons in closely allied regions of the brain stem secrete these transmitter substances and seem to be activated, in many instances, along with the norepinephrine system.

Effect of Lesions in the Wakefulness Areas. Lesions in the mesencephalic portion of the reticular activating system or in fiber pathways leading upward from this area through the diencephalon, if large enough, will invariably lead to coma from which the person cannot be aroused with any type of stimuli.

Also, very discrete lesions located bilaterally in the locus ceruleus will cause a type of sleep that closely resembles natural sleep.

Neuronal Centers, Transmitters, and Mechanisms That Can Cause Sleep

Stimulation of several specific areas of the brain can produce sleep with characteristics very near to those of natural sleep. Some of these are the following:

1. The most conspicuous stimulation area for causing almost natural sleep is the raphe nuclei in the pons and medulla. These are a thin sheet of nuclei located in the midline. Nerve fibers from these nuclei spread widely in the reticular formation and also upward into the thalamus, hypothalamus, and most areas of the limbic cortex. In addition, they extend downward into the spinal cord, terminating in the posterior horns where they can inhibit incoming pain signals, as was discussed in Chapter 10. It is also known that the endings of fibers from these raphe neurons secrete *serotonin*. Therefore, it is assumed that serotonin is the major transmitter substance associated with production of sleep.

2. Stimulation of several other regions in the lower brain stem and diencephalon can also lead to sleep, including (a) the rostral part of the hypothalamus, mainly in the suprachiasmal area, and (b) an occasional area in the diffuse nuclei of the thalamus.

Effect of Lesions in the Sleep-Promoting Centers. Discrete lesions in the raphe nuclei lead to a high state of wakefulness. This is also true of bilateral lesions in the mediorostral suprachiasmal portion of the anterior hypothalamus. In both instances, the reticular activating system seems to become released from inhibition. Indeed, the lesions of the anterior hypothalamus can sometimes cause such intense wakefulness that the animal actually dies of exhaustion.

Other Possible Transmitter Substances Related to Sleep. Experiments have shown that the cerebrospinal fluid and also the blood of animals that have been kept awake for several days contain a substance or substances that cause sleep when injected into the ventricular system of an animal. One of these substances is a small polypeptide with a molecular weight of less than 500. When cerebrospinal fluid containing this sleep-producing substance or substances is injected into the third ventricle, almost natural sleep occurs within a few minutes, and the animal may then stay asleep for several hours. Therefore, it is possible that prolonged wakefulness causes progressive accumulation of a sleep factor in the brain stem or in the cerebrospinal fluid that leads to sleep.

The Cycle Between Sleep and Wakefulness

The above discussions have merely identified neuronal areas, transmitters, and mechanisms that are related either to wakefulness or to sleep. However, they have not explained the cyclic, reciprocal operation of the sleep-wakefulness cycle. It is quite possible that this is caused by a free running intrinsic oscillator within the brain stem that cycles back and forth between the sleep and wakefulness centers, the wakefulness centers presumably activating the reticular activating system, and the sleep centers inhibiting this system.

However, there is much reason to believe that feedback signals from the cerebral cortex and also from the peripheral nerve receptors might also play a very important role in causing the sleep-wakefulness rhythm. One reason for believing this is that interruption of all the sensory nerve tracts leading from the periphery to the reticular activating system will cause the animal to go to sleep permanently. Also, as explained above, stimulation of the cerebral cortex will cause powerful activation of the reticular activating system.

Therefore, a very likely mechanism for causing the rhythmicity of the sleep-wakefulness cycle is the following:

When the reticular activating system is completely rested and the sleep centers are not activated, the wakefulness centers then presumably begin spontaneous activity. This in turn excites both the cerebral cortex and the peripheral nervous system. Next, positive feedback signals come from both of these areas back to the reticular activating system to activate it still further. Thus, once the wakefulness state begins, it has a natural tendency to sustain itself.

However, after the brain remains activated for many hours, even the neurons within the activating system presumably will fatigue, or other factors might activate the sleep centers. Consequently, the positive feedback cycle between the reticular activating system and the cortex, and also that between the reticular activating system and the periphery, will begin to fade. As soon as a few of the neurons in the reticular activating system become inactive, this also eliminates part of the feedback stimulus to the other neurons as well. Therefore, these too become inactive, the process spreading rapidly through the neurons and leading to rapid transition from the wakefulness state to the sleep state.

Then, one could postulate that during sleep the excitatory neurons of the reticular activating system gradually become more and more excitable because of the prolonged rest, while the inhibitory neurons of the sleep centers become less excitable, thus leading to a new cycle of wakefulness.

This theory obviously can explain the rapid transitions from sleep to wakefulness and from wakefulness to sleep. It can also explain arousal, the insomnia that occurs when a person's mind becomes preoccupied with a thought, the wakefulness that is produced by bodily activity, and many other conditions that affect the person's state of sleep or wakefulness.

PHYSIOLOGICAL EFFECTS OF SLEEP

Sleep causes two major types of physiological effects: first, effects on the nervous system itself and, second, effects on other structures of the body. The first of these seems to be by far the more important, for any person who has a transected spinal cord in the neck shows no physiological effects in the body beneath the level of transection that can be attributed to a sleep and wakefulness cycle; that is, lack of sleep and wakefulness causes neither significant harm to the

bodily organs nor even any deranged function. On the other hand, lack of sleep certainly does affect the functions of the central nervous system.

Prolonged wakefulness is often associated with progressive malfunction of the mind and behavioral activities of the nervous system. We are all familiar with the increased sluggishness of thought that occurs toward the end of a prolonged wakeful period, but in addition, a person can become irritable or even psychotic following forced wakefulness for prolonged periods of time. Therefore, one can assume that sleep in some way not presently understood restores both normal sensitivities of and normal "balance" among the different parts of the central nervous system. This might be likened to the "rezeroing" of electronic analog computers after prolonged use, for all computers of this type gradually lose their "base line" of operation; it is reasonable to assume that the same effect occurs in the central nervous system, because overuse of some neurons during wakefulness could easily throw all these out of balance with the remainder of the nervous system. Therefore, in the absence of any definitely demonstrated functional value of sleep, we might postulate, on the basis of known psychological changes that occur with prolonged wakefulness, that sleep performs this rezeroing function for the nervous system to re-establish the natural balance among the neuronal centers.

Even though, as pointed out above, wakefulness and sleep have not been shown to be necessary for somatic functions of the body, the cycle of enhanced and depressed nervous excitability that follows the cycle of wakefulness and sleep does have moderate effects on the peripheral body. For instance, there is enhanced sympathetic activity during wakefulness and also enhanced numbers of impulses to the skeletal musculature to increase muscle tone. Conversely, during sleep, sympathetic activity decreases while parasympathetic activity occasionally increases, and the muscle tone becomes almost nil. Therefore, arterial blood pressure falls, pulse rate decreases, skin vessels dilate, activity of the gastrointestinal tract sometimes increases, muscles fall into a completely relaxed state, and overall basal metabolic rate of the body falls by 10 to 30 per cent.

REFERENCES

Arkin, J. S., *et al.* (eds.): The Mind in Sleep. New York, Halsted Press, 1978.

Begleiter, H. (ed.): Evoked Brain Potentials and Behavior. New York, Plenum Press, 1979.

Block, G. D., and Page, T. L.: Circadian pacemakers in the nervous system. *Annu. Rev. Neurosci., 1*:19, 1978.

Buser, P.: Higher functions of the nervous system. *Annu. Rev. Physiol., 38*:217, 1978.

Buser, P. A., and Rougeul-Buser, A. (eds.): Cerebral Correlates of Conscious Experience. New York, Elsevier/North-Holland, 1978.

Cartwright, R. D.: A Primer on Sleep and Dreaming. Reading, Mass., Addison-Wesley Publishing Co., 1978.

Diehl, L. W.: Treatment of Complicated Epilepsies in Adults: A Clinical-Statistical Study. New York, S. Karger, 1978.

Drucker-Colín, R., et al. (eds.): The Functions of Sleep. New York, Academic Press, 1979.

Edelman, G. M., and Mountcastle, V. B.: The Mindful Brain. Cambridge, Mass., MIT Press, 1978.

Enright, J. T.: The Timing of Sleep and Wakefulness: On the Substructure and Dynamics of the Circadian Pacemakers Underlying the Wake-Sleep Cycle. New York, Springer-Verlag, 1979.

Fröscher, W.: Treatment of Status Epilepticus. Baltimore, University Park Press, 1978.

Gillin, J. C., et al.: The neuropharmacology of sleep and wakefulness. Annu. Rev. Pharmacol. Toxicol., 18:563, 1978.

Glaser, G. H., et al. (eds.): Antiepileptic Drugs. New York, Raven Press, 1980.

Goldberg, P., and Kaufman, D.: Natural Sleep. Emmaus, Pa., Rodale Press, 1978.

Guilleminault, C., and Dement, W. C. (eds.): Sleep Apnea Syndromes. New York, A. R. Liss, 1978.

Hector, M. L.: EEG Recording. Boston, Butterworths, 1979.

Hobson, J. A., and Brazier, M. A. B. (eds.): The Reticular Formation Revisited: Specifying Function for a Nonspecific System. New York, Raven Press, 1980.

Ito, M., et al. (eds.): Integrative Control Functions of the Brain. New York, Elsevier/North-Holland, 1978.

Klass, D. W., and Daly, D. C. (eds.): Current Practice of Clinical Electroencephalography. New York, Raven Press, 1979.

Kool, K. A., et al.: Fundamentals of Electroencephalography. Hagerstown, Md., Harper & Row, 1978.

Livingston, R. B.: Neural integration. In Frohlich, E. D. (ed.): Pathophysiology, 2nd Ed. Philadelphia, J. B. Lippincott Co., 1976, p. 681.

Livingston, R. B.: Sensory Processing, Perception, and Behavior. New York, Raven Press, 1978.

Moore, R. Y., and Bloom, F. E.: Central catecholamine neuron systems: Anatomy and physiology of the norepinephrine and epinephrine systems. Annu. Rev. Neurosci., 2:113, 1979.

Newmark, M. E., and Penry, J. K.: Photosensitivity and Epilepsy: A Review. New York, Raven Press, 1979.

Newmark, M. E., and Penry, J. K.: Genetics of Epilepsy: A Review. New York, Churchill Livingstone, 1980.

O'Keefe, J., and Nadel, L.: The Hippocampus as a Cognitive Map. New York, Oxford University Press, 1978.

Pappenheimer, J. R.: The sleep factor. Sci. Am., 235(2):24, 1976.

Passouant, P., and Oswald, I. (eds.): Pharmacology of the States of Alertness. New York, Pergamon Press, 1979.

Plum, F., and Posner, J. B.: The Diagnosis of Stupor and Coma, 3rd Ed. Philadelphia, F. A. Davis, 1980.

Prince, D. A.: Neurophysiology of epilepsy. Annu. Rev. Neurosci., 1:395, 1978.

Regan, D.: Electrical responses evoked from the human brain. Sci. Am., 241(6):134, 1979.

Roth, S. H.: Physical mechanisms of anesthesia. Annu. Rev. Pharmacol. Toxicol., 19:159, 1979.

Schneider, A. M., and Tarshis, B.: An Introduction to Physiological Psychology. New York, Random House, 1979.

Singer, W.: Control of thalamic transmission by corticofugal and ascending reticular pathways in the visual system. Physiol. Rev., 57:386, 1977.

Spiegel, R.: Sleep and Sleeplessness in Advanced Age. Jamaica, N.Y., Spectrum Publications, 1979.

Stern, R. M., et al.: Psychophysiological Recording. New York, Oxford University Press, 1980.

Wada, J. A. (ed.): Modern Perspectives in Epilepsy: Proceedings of the Inaugural Symposium of the Canadian League Against Epilepsy. St. Albans, Vt., Eden Press, 1978.

15

The Cerebral Cortex and Intellectual Functions of the Brain

It is ironic that we know least about the mechanisms of the cerebral cortex of almost all parts of the brain, even though it is by far the largest portion of the nervous system. Yet, we do know the effects of destruction or of specific stimulation of various portions of the cortex, and still more is known from electrical recordings from the cortex or from the surface of the scalp. In the early part of the present chapter the facts known about cortical functions are discussed and then some basic theories of the neuronal mechanisms involved in thought processes, memory, analysis of sensory information, and so forth are presented briefly.

PHYSIOLOGIC ANATOMY OF THE CEREBRAL CORTEX

The functional part of the cerebral cortex is comprised mainly of a thin layer of neurons 2 to 5 mm. in thickness, covering the surface of all the convolutions of the cerebrum and having a total area of about one-quarter square meter. The total cerebral cortex probably contains about 100 billion neurons.

Figure 15–1 illustrates the typical structure of the cerebral cortex, showing successive layers of different types of cells. Most of the cells are of three types: *granular, fusiform,* and *pyramidal,* the latter named for their characteristic pyramidal shape. To the right in Figure 15–1 is illustrated the typical organization of nerve fibers within the different layers of the cortex. Note particularly the large number of horizontal fibers extending between adjacent areas of the cortex, but note also the vertical fibers that extend to and from the cortex to lower areas of the brain stem or to distant regions of the cerebral cortex through long "association" bundles of fibers.

Neurohistologists have divided the cerebral cortex into almost 100 different areas which have slightly different architectural characteristics. Yet in all these different areas except the hippocampal region there still

persist representations of all the six major layers of the cortex. To the untrained histologist, only five major architectural types of cortex can be distinguished as follows: Type 1 contains large numbers of pyramidal cells with few granular cells and, therefore, is often called the *agranular cortex.* At the other extreme, type 5 contains almost no pyramidal cells but is filled with closely packed granule cells and is called the *granular cortex.* Types 2, 3, and 4 have intermediate characteris-

Figure 15–1. Structure of the cerebral cortex, illustrating: *I,* molecular layer; *II,* external granular layer; *III,* layer of pyramidal cells; *IV,* internal granular layer; *V,* large pyramidal cell layer; *VI,* layer of fusiform or polymorphic cells. (From Ranson and Clark (after Brodmann): Anatomy of the Nervous System. Philadelphia, W. B. Saunders Company, 1959.)

192

Figure 15–2. Structurally distinct areas of the human cerebral cortex. (From Brodmann, modified by Buchanan: Functional Neuroanatomy. Lea & Febiger, 1966.)

tics containing graded proportions of pyramidal and agranular cells.

The agranular cortex, which contains large numbers of pyramidal cells, is characteristic of the motor areas of the cerebral cortex, while the granular cortex, containing almost no pyramidal cells, is characteristic of the primary sensory areas. The other three intermediate types of cortex are characteristic of the association areas between the primary sensory and motor regions.

Figure 15–2 shows a map of cortical areas classified on the basis of histological studies by Brodmann. This classification provides a basis for discussion of functional areas of the brain, even though different architectural types of cortex often have similar functions.

Anatomical Relationship of the Cerebral Cortex to the Thalamus and Other Lower Centers. All areas of the cerebral cortex have direct afferent and efferent connections with the thalamus. Figure 15–3 shows the areas of the cerebral cortex connected with specific parts of the thalamus. These connections are in *two* directions, both from the thalamus to the cortex and then from the cortex back to essentially the same area of the thalamus. Furthermore, when the thalamic connections are cut, the functions of the corresponding cortical area become

entirely or almost entirely abrogated. Therefore, the cortex operates in close association with the thalamus and can almost be considered both anatomically and functionally to be a large outgrowth of the thalamus; for this reason the thalamus and the cortex together are called the *thalamocortical system,* as was explained in the previous chapter. Also, all pathways from the sensory organs to the cortex pass through the thalamus, with the single exception of the sensory pathways of the olfactory tract.

FUNCTIONS OF CERTAIN SPECIFIC CORTICAL AREAS

Studies in human beings by neurosurgeons have shown that some specific functions are localized to certain general areas of the cerebral cortex. Figure 15–4 gives a map of some of these areas as determined by Penfield and Rasmussen from electrical stimulation of the cortex or by neurological examination of patients after portions of the cortex had been removed. The lightly shaded areas are *primary sensory areas,* while the darkly shaded area is the *voluntary motor area* (also called *primary motor area*) from which muscular movements can be elicited with relatively weak electrical stimuli. These primary sensory and motor areas have highly specific functions, while other areas of the cortex perform more general functions that we call association or cerebration.

SPECIFIC FUNCTIONS OF THE PRIMARY SENSORY AREAS

The primary sensory areas all have certain functions in common. For instance, somatic sensory areas, visual sensory areas, and auditory sensory areas all have spatial localizations of

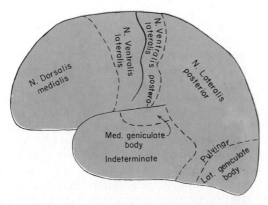

Figure 15–3. Areas of the cerebral cortex that connect with specific portions of the thalamus. (Modified from Elliott: Textbook of the Nervous System. J. B. Lippincott Co.)

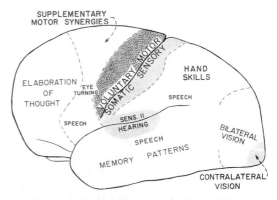

Figure 15–4. Functional areas of the human cerebral cortex as determined by electrical stimulation of the cortex during neurosurgical operations and by neurological examinations of patients with destroyed cortical regions. (From Penfield and Rasmussen: The Cerebral Cortex of Man: A Clinical Study of Localization of Function. New York, Macmillan Company, 1968.)

signals from the peripheral receptors (which are discussed in detail in Chapters 9, 20, and 21).

Electrical stimulation of the primary sensory areas in the parietal lobes in awake patients elicits relatively uncomplicated sensations. For instance, in the somatic sensory area the patient expresses feelings of tingling in the skin, numbness, mild "electric" feeling, or, rarely, mild degrees of temperature sensations. And these sensations are localized to discrete areas of the body in accord with the spatial representation in the somatic sensory cortex, as described in Chapter 9. Therefore, it is believed that the primary somatic sensory cortex analyzes only the simple aspects of sensations and that analysis of intricate patterns of sensory experience requires also adjacent parts of the parietal lobes called the *sensory association areas*.

Electrical stimulation of the primary visual cortex in the occipital lobes causes the person to see flashes of light, bright lines, colors, or other simple visions. Here again, the visual images are localized to specific regions of the visual fields in accord with the portion of the primary visual cortex stimulated, as described in Chapter 20. But the visual cortex alone is not capable of complete analysis of complicated visual patterns; for this, the visual cortex must operate in association with adjacent regions of the occipital cortex, the *visual association areas*.

Electrical stimulation of the auditory cortex in the temporal lobes causes a person to hear a simple sound which may be weak or loud, have low or high frequency, or have other uncomplicated characteristics, such as a squeak or even an undulation. But never are words or any other fully intelligible sound heard. Thus, the primary auditory cortex, like the other primary sensory areas, can detect the individual elements of auditory experience but cannot analyze complicated sounds. Therefore, the primary auditory cortex alone is not sufficient to give one even the usual auditory experiences; these can be achieved, however, when the primary area operates together with the *auditory association areas* in adjacent regions of the temporal lobes.

Despite the inability of the primary sensory areas to analyze the incoming sensations fully, when these areas are destroyed, the ability of the person to utilize the respective sensations usually suffers drastically. For instance, loss of the primary visual cortex in one occipital lobe causes a person to become blind in the ipsilateral halves of both retinae, and loss of the primary visual cortices in both hemispheres causes total blindness. Likewise, loss of both primary auditory cortices causes almost total deafness. Loss of the postcentral gyri causes *depression* of somatic sensory sensations — though not total loss — presumably because of additional cortical representation of these sensations in other cortical areas: somatic sensory area II and the motor cortex, for example. (In animals far down the phylogenetic scale, loss of the visual and auditory cortices may have little effect on vision and hearing, and even an anencephalic human infant having no brain above the mesencephalon detects some visual scenes in the absence of the visual cortex, for such a child can observe a moving object and even follow it by movement of the eyes and head.)

Therefore, we can summarize the functions of the primary sensory areas of the human cerebral cortex in the following way: The lower centers of the brain relay a large part of the sensory signals to the cerebral cortex for analysis. In turn, the primary sensory areas transmit the results of their analyses back to the lower centers and to other regions of the cerebral cortex, as is discussed later in the chapter.

THE SENSORY ASSOCIATION AREAS

Around the borders of the primary sensory areas are regions called *sensory association areas* or *secondary sensory areas*. In general, these areas extend 1 to 5 centimeters in one or more directions from the primary sensory areas; each time a primary area receives a sensory signal, secondary signals spread, after a delay of a few milliseconds, into the respective association area as well. Part of this spread occurs directly from the primary area through subcortical fiber tracts, but a major part also occurs in the thalamus, beginning in the sensory relay nuclei, passing next to corresponding *thalamic association areas*, and then traveling to the association cortex.

The general function of the sensory association areas is to provide a higher level of interpretation of the sensory experiences. The general areas for the interpretative functions for somatic, visual, and auditory experiences are illustrated in Figure 15–5.

Destruction of the sensory association areas greatly reduces the capability of the brain to analyze different characteristics of sensory experiences. For instance, damage in the temporal lobe below and behind the primary auditory area in the "dominant hemisphere" of the brain often causes a person to lose his ability to understand words or other auditory experiences even though he hears them.

Likewise, destruction of the visual association area in Brodmann's areas 18 and 19 of the occipital lobe in the dominant hemisphere (see Figure 15–2), or the presence of a brain tumor or other lesion in these areas, does not cause blindness or prevent normal activation of the primary visual cortex but does greatly reduce the person's ability to inter-

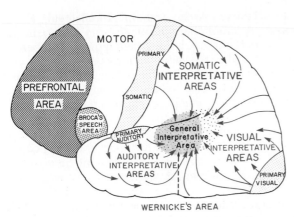

Figure 15–5. Organization of the somatic, auditory, and visual association areas into a general mechanism for interpretation of sensory experience. All of these feed into the *general interpretative area* located in the postero-superior portion of the temporal lobe and the angular gyrus. Note also the prefrontal area, and Broca's speech area.

pret what is seen. Such a person often loses the ability to recognize the meanings of words, a condition that is called *word blindness* or *dyslexia*.

Finally, destruction of the somatic sensory association area in the parietal cortex posterior to primary somatic area I causes the person to lose spatial perception for location of the different parts of the body. In the case of the hand that has been "lost," the skills of the hand are greatly reduced. Thus, this area of the cortex seems to be necessary for interpretation of somatic sensory experiences.

The functions of the association areas are described in more detail in Chapter 9 for somatic, in Chapter 20 for visual, and in Chapter 21 for auditory experiences.

INTERPRETATIVE FUNCTION OF THE POSTERIOR SUPERIOR TEMPORAL LOBE — THE GENERAL INTERPRETATIVE AREA (OR WERNICKE'S AREA)

The somatic, visual, and auditory association areas, which can actually be called "interpretative areas," all meet one another in the posterior part of the superior temporal lobe and in the anterior part of the angular gyrus where the temporal, parietal, and occipital lobes all come together. This area of confluence of the different sensory interpretative areas is especially highly developed in the dominant side of the brain — the *left side* in right-handed persons — and it plays the greatest single role of any part of the cerebral cortex in the higher levels of brain function that we call *cerebration*. Therefore, this region has frequently been

called by different names suggestive of the area having almost global importance: the *general interpretative area*, the *gnostic area*, the *knowing area*, the *tertiary association area*, and so forth. The temporal portion of the general interpretative area is also called *Wernicke's area* in honor of the neurologist who first described its special significance in intellectual processes.

Following severe damage in the general interpretative area, a person might hear perfectly well and even recognize different words but still might be unable to arrange these words into a coherent thought. Likewise, the person may be able to read words from the printed page but be unable to recognize the thought that is conveyed. In addition, the person has similar difficulties in understanding the higher levels of meaning of somatic sensory experiences, even though there is no loss of sensation itself.

Electrical stimulation in the posterior superior temporal lobe of the conscious patient occasionally causes a highly complex thought. This is particularly true when the stimulatory electrode is passed deep enough into the brain to approach the corresponding connecting areas of the thalamus. The types of thoughts that might be experienced include memories of complicated visual scenes that one might remember from childhood, auditory hallucinations such as a specific musical piece, or even a discourse by a specific person. For this reason it is believed that complicated memory patterns involving more than one sensory modality are stored at least partially in the temporal lobe. This belief is in accord with the importance of the general interpretative area in interpretation of the complicated meanings of different sensory experiences.

The angular gyrus portion of the general interpretative area is especially important for interpretation of visual information. If this region is destroyed while the temporal lobe portion of this interpretative area (Wernicke's area) is still intact, the person can still interpret both auditory and somatic experiences as usual, but the stream of visual experiences passing into the general interpretative area from the visual cortex is mainly blocked. Therefore, the person may be able to see words and even know they are words but, nevertheless, not be able to interpret their meanings. This is the condition called *dyslexia*.

Let us again emphasize the global importance of the general interpretative area for most intellectual functions of the brain. Loss of this area in an adult usually leads thereafter to a lifetime of almost demented existence.

The Dominant Hemisphere. The general interpretative functions of Wernicke's area and of the angular gyrus, and also the functions of the speech and motor control areas, are usually much more highly developed in one cerebral hemisphere than in the other. This is called the *dominant hemisphere*. In at least 9 of 10 persons the left hemisphere is the dominant one. At birth, Wernicke's area of the brain is often as much as 50 per cent larger in the left hemisphere than in the right. Therefore, it is easy to understand why the left side of the brain might become dominant over the right side. However, if for some reason the dominant Wernicke's area is removed in early childhood, the opposite side of the brain can develop full dominant characteristics.

A theory that can explain the capability of one hemisphere to dominate the other hemisphere is the following:

The attention of the "mind" seems to be directed to one portion of the brain at a time, as was explained in the preceding chapter. Presumably, because its size is usually larger at birth, the left temporal lobe normally begins to be used to a greater extent than the right, and, thenceforth, because of the tendency to direct one's attention to the better developed region, the rate of learning in the cerebral hemisphere that gains the first start increases rapidly while that in the opposite side remains slight. Therefore, in the normal human being, one side becomes dominant over the other.

In more than 9 of 10 persons the left temporal lobe and angular gyrus become dominant, and in the remaining one tenth of the population either both sides develop simultaneously to have dual dominance, or, more rarely, the right side alone becomes highly developed.

Usually associated with the dominant temporal lobe and angular gyrus is dominance of certain portions of the somesthetic cortex and motor cortex for control of voluntary motor functions. For instance, as is discussed later in the chapter, the premotor speech area (Broca's area), located far laterally in the intermediate frontal area, is almost always dominant also on the left side of the brain. This speech area causes the formation of words by exciting simultaneously the laryngeal muscles, the respiratory muscles, and the muscles of the mouth.

Though the interpretative areas of the temporal lobe and angular gyrus, as well as many of the motor areas, are highly developed in only a single hemisphere, they are capable of receiving sensory information from both hemispheres and are also capable of controlling motor activities in both hemispheres, utilizing mainly fiber pathways in the *corpus callosum* for communication between the two hemispheres. This unitary, cross-feeding organization prevents interference between the two sides of the brain; such interference, obviously, could create havoc with both thoughts and motor responses.

Role of Language in Function of the General Interpretative Area and in Intellectual Functions. A major share of our sensory experience is converted into their language equivalent before being stored in the memory areas of the brain and before being processed for other intellectual purposes. For instance, when we read a book, we do not store the visual images of the words but, instead, store the words themselves in language form. Also, the information is usually converted to language form before its meaning is discerned.

The sensory area of the dominant hemisphere for interpretation of language is closely associated with the primary hearing area located in the auditory association areas of the temporal lobe. This locus probably results from the fact that the first introduction to language is by way of hearing. Later in life, when visual perception of language through the medium of reading develops, the visual information is then presumably channeled into the already developed language regions of the dominant temporal lobe. This probably also explains why the general interpretative area of the brain is more closely allied with the auditory association areas than with other sensory areas of the cortex.

Wernicke's Area in the Nondominant Hemisphere. When Wernicke's area in the dominant hemisphere is destroyed, the person normally loses almost all intellectual functions associated with language or symbolism, such as ability to read, ability to perform mathematical operations, and even the ability to think through logical problems. However, other types of interpretative capabilities, some of which undoubtedly utilize the temporal lobe and angular gyrus regions of the opposite hemisphere, are retained. Psychological studies in patients with damage to their nondominant hemispheres have suggested that this hemisphere may be especially important for understanding and interpreting music, nonverbal visual experiences, spatial relationships between the person and the surroundings, and probably also interpreting many somatic experiences related to use of the limbs and hands. Thus, even though we speak of the "dominant" hemisphere, this dominance is primarily for language- or symbolism-related intellectual functions; the opposite hemisphere can actually be dominant for some other types of intelligence.

An Area for Recognition of Faces

An interesting type of brain abnormality called *prosophenosia* is the inability to recognize faces. This occurs in persons who have extensive damage on the medial undersides of both occipital lobes and along the medioventral surfaces of the temporal lobes as illustrated in Figure 15–6. Loss of these face recognition areas, strangely enough, results in very little other abnormality of brain function.

One wonders why so much of the cerebral cortex should be reserved for the simple task of face recognition. However, when it is remembered that most of our daily tasks involve associations with other people, one can see the importance of this intellectual function.

FACIAL-RECOGNITION AREA

TEMPORAL LOBE

FRONTAL LOBE

Figure 15–6. Facial-recognition areas located on the underside of the brain in the medial occipital and temporal lobes. (From Geschwind: *Sci. Amer. 241*:180, 1979. © 1970 by Scientific American, Inc. All rights reserved.)

The occipital portion of this area is contiguous with the primary visual cortex, and the temporal portion is closely associated with the limbic system that has to do with emotions, brain activation, and control of one's behavioral response to the environment.

THE PREFRONTAL AREAS

The prefrontal areas are those portions of the frontal lobes that lie anterior to the motor regions, as shown in Figure 15–5. For years, this part of the cortex has been considered to be the locus of the higher intellect of the human being, principally because the main difference between the brain of monkeys and that of human beings is the great prominence of the human prefrontal areas. Yet efforts to show that the prefrontal cortex is more important in higher intellectual functions than other portions of the cortex have not been successful. Indeed, destruction of the posterior temporal lobe and angular gyrus region in the dominant hemisphere causes infinitely more harm to the intellect than does destruction of both prefrontal areas.

Psychological studies in lower animals have shown that all portions of the cortex not immediately associated with either sensory or motor functions are important in the ability of an animal to learn complicated information — such as a rat's learning to run through a maze — and that all the different areas are approximately equipotent in this regard. Therefore, the importance of the prefrontal areas to the human being is perhaps mainly that they supply much additional cortical area in which cerebration can take place.

Yet, the prefrontal areas do seem to have some specific functions that are all their own. One of these has to do with control of some types of behavior, especially choice of behavioral options for each social or physical situation. For this purpose, the prefrontal areas transmit signals into the limbic areas of the brain, as will be described in the following two chapters. Some of the other possible functions of the prefrontal lobes include:

Prevention of Distractibility by the Prefrontal Areas — Importance for Sequencing Thoughts. One of the outstanding characteristics of a person who has lost the prefrontal areas is the ease with which he can be *distracted* from a sequence of thoughts. Likewise, in lower animals whose prefrontal areas have been removed, the ability to concentrate on psychological tests is almost completely lost. The human being without prefrontal areas is still capable of performing many intellectual tasks, such as answering short questions and performing simple arithmetic computations (such as $9 \times 6 = 54$), thus illustrating that the basic intellectual activities of the cerebral cortex are still intact without the prefrontal areas.

Yet if concerted *sequences* of cerebral functions are required of the person, he becomes completely disorganized. Therefore, the prefrontal areas seem to be important in keeping the mental functions directed toward goals.

Elaboration of Thought, Prognostication, and Performance of Higher Intellectual Functions by the Prefrontal Areas. Another function that has been ascribed to the prefrontal areas by psychologists and neurologists is *elaboration of thought*. This means simply an increase in depth and abstractness of the different thoughts. Psychological tests have shown that prefrontal lobectomized lower animals presented with successive bits of sensory information fail to store these bits in memory — probably because they are distracted so easily that they cannot hold thoughts long enough for storage to take place. If the prefrontal areas are intact, many such successive bits of information can be stored in all areas of the brain and can be called forth again and again during the subsequent periods of cerebration. This postulated ability of the prefrontal areas to cause storage — even though it be temporary — of many types of information simultaneously, and then perhaps also to cause recall of this information, could well explain the many functions of the brain that we associate with higher intelligence, such as the abilities to (1) prognosticate, (2) plan for the future, (3) delay action in response to incoming sensory signals so that the sensory information can be weighed until the best course of response is decided, (4) consider the consequences of motor actions even before these are performed, (5) solve complicated mathematical, legal, or philosophical problems, (6) correlate all avenues of information in diagnosing rare diseases, and (7) control one's activities in accord with moral laws.

Effects of Destruction of the Prefrontal Areas

The person without prefrontal areas ordinarily acts precipitously in response to incoming sensory signals, such as reacting angrily to slight provocations. Also, he is likely to lose many or most of his morals; he has little embarrassment in relation to his excretory, sexual, and social activities; and he is prone to quickly changing moods of sweetness, hate, joy, sadness, exhilaration, and rage. In short, he is a highly *distractible* person with lack of ability to pursue long and complicated thoughts.

THOUGHTS, CONSCIOUSNESS, AND MEMORY

Our most difficult problem in discussing consciousness, thoughts, memory, and learning is that we do not know the neural mechanism of a thought. We know that destruction of large portions of the cerebral cortex does not prevent a person from having thoughts, but it does reduce the *degree* of awareness of the surroundings. On the other hand, destruction of far smaller portions of the thalamus and especially of the mesencephalic portion of the reticular activating system can cause tremendously decreased awareness or even complete unconsciousness.

Each thought almost certainly involves simultaneous signals in portions of the cerebral cortex, thalamus, limbic system, and reticular formation of the brain stem. Some crude thoughts probably depend almost entirely on lower centers; the thought of pain is probably a good example, for electrical stimulation of the human cortex rarely elicits anything more than the mildest degrees of pain, while stimulation of certain areas of the hypothalamus and mesencephalon in animals apparently causes excruciating pain. On the other hand, a type of thought pattern that requires mainly the cerebral cortex is that involving vision, because loss of the visual cortex causes complete inability to perceive visual form or color.

Therefore, we might formulate a definition of a thought in terms of neural activity as follows: A thought probably results from the momentary "pattern" of stimulation of many different parts of the nervous system at the same time, probably involving most importantly the cerebral cortex, the thalamus, the limbic system, and the upper reticular formation of the brain stem. This is called the *holistic theory* of thoughts. The stimulated areas of the limbic system, thalamus, and reticular formation perhaps determine the general nature of the thought, giving it such qualities as pleasure, displeasure, pain, comfort, crude modalities of sensation, localization to gross areas of the body, and other general characteristics. On the other hand, the stimulated areas of the cortex probably determine the discrete characteristics of the thought (such as specific localization of sensations on the body and of objects in the fields of vision), discrete patterns of sensation (such as the rectangular pattern of a concrete block wall or the texture of a rug), and other individual characteristics that enter into the overall awareness of a particular instant.

MEMORY AND TYPES OF MEMORY

If we accept the above approximation of what constitutes a thought, we can see immediately that the mechanism of memory must be equally as complex as the mechanism of a thought, for, to provide memory, the nervous system must re-create the same spatial and temporal pattern (the "holistic" pattern) of stimulation in the central nervous system at some future date. Though we cannot explain in detail what a memory is, we do know some of the basic psychological and neuronal processes that probably lead to the process of memory.

All of us know that all degrees of memory occur, some memories lasting a few seconds and others lasting hours, days, months, or years. Possibly all these types of memory are caused by the same mechanism operating to different degrees of fulfillment. Yet, it is also possible that different mechanisms of memory do exist. Indeed, most physiologists classify memory into from two to four different types. For the purpose of the present discussion, we will use the following classification:

1. *Sensory memory;*
2. *Short-term memory* or *primary memory;*
3. *Long-term memory,* which itself can be divided into *secondary memory* and *tertiary memory.*

The basic characteristics of these types of memory are the following:

Sensory Memory. Sensory memory means the ability to retain sensory signals in the sensory areas of the brain for a very short interval of time following the actual sensory experience. Usually these signals remain available for analysis for several hundred milliseconds but are replaced by new sensory signals in less than one second. Nevertheless, during the short interval of time that the instantaneous sensory information remains in the brain it can continue to be used for further processing; most important, it can be "scanned" to pick out the important points. Thus, this is the initial stage of the memory process.

Short-Term Memory (Primary Memory). Short-term memory (or primary memory) is the memory of a few facts, words, numbers, letters, or other bits of information for a few seconds to a minute or more at a time. This is typified by a person's memory of the digits in a telephone number for a short period of time after he has looked up the number in the telephone directory. This type of memory is usually limited to about seven bits of information, and when new bits of information are put into this *short-term store,* older information is displaced. Thus, if a person looks up a second telephone number, the first is usually lost. One of the most important features of short-term memory is that the information in this memory store is instantaneously available so that the person does not have to search through his mind for it as he does for information that has been put away in the long-term memory stores.

Long-Term Memory. Long-term memory is the storage in the brain of information that can be recalled at some later time — many minutes, hours, days, months, or years later. This type of memory has been called *fixed memory, permanent memory,* and several other names. Long-term memory is also usually divided into two different types, *secondary memory* and *tertiary memory,* the characteristics of which are the following:

A *secondary memory* is a long-term memory that is stored with either a weak or only a moderately strong memory trace. For this reason it is easy to forget and it is sometimes difficult to recall. Furthermore, the time required to search for the information is relatively long. This type of memory can last from several minutes to several years. When the memories are so weak that they will last for only a few minutes to a few days, they are also frequently called *recent memory.*

A *tertiary memory* is a memory that has become so well ingrained in the mind that the memory can usually last the lifetime of the person. Furthermore, the very strong memory traces of this type of memory make the stored information available within a split second. This type of memory is typified by one's knowledge of his own name, by his ability to recall immediately the numbers from 1 to 10, the letters of the alphabet, and the words that he uses in speech, and also by the memory of his own precise physical structure and of his very familiar immediate surroundings.

PHYSIOLOGICAL BASIS OF MEMORY

Despite the many advances in neurophysiology during the past half century, we still cannot explain what is perhaps the most important function of the brain: its capability for memory. Yet, physiological experiments are beginning to generate conceptual theories of the means by which memory could occur. Some of these are discussed in the following few sections.

Possible Mechanisms for Short-Term Memory. Short-term memory requires a neuronal mechanism that can hold specific information signals for a few seconds to at most a minute or more. Several such mechanisms are the following:

Reverberating Circuit Theory of Short-Term Memory. When a tetanizing electrical stimulus is applied directly to the surface of the cerebral cortex and then is removed after a second or more, the local area excited by this stimulus continues to emit rhythmic action potentials for short periods of time. This effect is believed to result from local reverberating circuits, the signals passing through a multistage circuit of neurons in the local area of the cortex itself or perhaps back and forth between the cortex and the thalamus.

It is postulated that sensory signals reaching the cerebral cortex can set up similar reverberating oscillations and that these could be the basis for short-term memory. Then, as the reverberating circuit fatigues, or as new signals interfere with the reverberations, the short-term memory fades away.

One of the principal observations in support of this theory is that any factor that causes a general disturbance of brain function, such as sudden fright, a very loud noise, or any other sensory experience that attracts the person's undivided attention immediately erases the short-term memory. The memory cannot be recalled when the disturbance is over unless a portion of this memory had already been placed into the long-term memory store, as will be discussed in subsequent sections.

Post-Tetanic Potentiation Theory of Short-Term Memory. In most parts of the nervous system, including even the anterior motoneurons of the spinal cord, tetanic stimulation of a synapse for a few seconds causes increased excitability of the synapse for a few seconds to a few hours.

If during this time the synapse is stimulated again, the stimulated neuron responds much more vigorously than normally, a phenomenon called *post-tetanic potentiation.* This is obviously a type of memory that depends on change in the excitability of the synapse, and it could be the basis for short-term memory. Recent experiments suggest that this phenomenon might result from increased permeability of the synaptic knob membranes to calcium ions, which will be discussed in a later section.

DC Potential Theory of Short-Term Memory. Another change that often occurs in neurons following a period of excitation is a prolonged decrease in the membrane potential of the neuron lasting for from seconds to minutes. Because this changes the excitability of the neuron, it could be the basis for short-term memory. Such changes in neuronal potentials are called *DC potentials* or sometimes *electrotonic potentials*. Measurements in the cerebral cortex show that such potentials occur especially in the superficial dendritic layers of the cortex, indicating that the process of short-term memory could result from changes in dendritic membrane potentials.

Mechanism of Long-Term Memory, Enhancement of Synaptic Transmission Facility

Long-term memory means the ability of the nervous system to recall thoughts long after initial elicitation of the thoughts is over. We know that long-term memory does not depend on continued activity of the nervous system, because the brain can be totally inactivated by cooling, by general anesthesia, by hypoxia, by ischemia, or by any other method and yet memories that have been previously stored are still retained when the brain becomes active once again. Therefore, it is assumed that long-term memory must result from

some actual alterations of the synapses, either physical or chemical.

Many different theories have been offered to explain the synaptic changes that cause long-term memory. Among the most important of these are:

1. Anatomical Changes in the Synapses. Cajal, almost a century ago, discovered that the number of terminal fibrils ending on neuronal cells and dendrites in the cerebral cortex increases with age. Conversely, physiologists have shown that inactivity of regions of the cortex causes thinning of the cortex: for instance, thinning of the primary visual cortex in animals that have lost their eyesight. Also, intense activity of a particular part of the cortex can cause excessive thickening of the cortical shell in that area alone. This has been demonstrated especially in the visual cortex of animals subjected to repeated visual experiences. Finally, some neuroanatomists have observed electron micrographic changes in presynaptic terminals that have been subjected to intense and prolonged activity.

All these observations have led to a widely held belief that fixation of memories in the brain results from anatomical changes in the synapses themselves: perhaps changes in numbers of presynaptic terminals, perhaps in sizes of the terminals, or perhaps in the sizes and conductivities of the dendrites. Such anatomical changes could cause permanent or semipermanent increase in the degree of facilitation of specific neuronal circuits, thus allowing signals to pass through the circuits with progressive ease the more often the memory trace is used. This obviously would explain the tendency for memories to become more and more deeply fixed in the nervous system the more often they are recalled or the more often the person repeats the sensory experience that leads to the memory trace.

Another variant of the anatomical theory is that in early life an excess of synaptic connections is made, and those synapses that are active continue to remain functional, while the others eventually degenerate. Thus, the pattern of synaptic transmission could be established by destroying unused synapses rather than by enhancing the used ones. This theory fits the finding that unused synapses and even unused neurons often disappear completely.

2. Physical or Chemical Changes in the Presynaptic Terminal or the Postsynaptic Membrane. Recent studies in the large snail *Aplysia* have uncovered a mechanism of memory that results from either a physical or chemical change of the presynaptic terminal. This mechanism, illustrated in Figure 15–7, works in the following way: There are two separate presynaptic terminals, one of which ends on the subsequent neuron

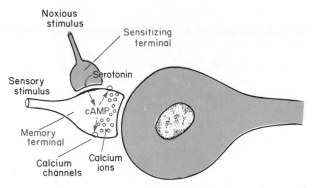

Figure 15–7. A memory system that has been discovered in the snail *Aplysia*.

and the other of which ends on the first presynaptic terminal. In the figure these are called the *memory terminal* and the *sensitizing terminal*. When the memory terminal is stimulated repeatedly but without stimulating the sensitizing terminal, signal transmission at first is very great, but this becomes less and less intense with repeated stimulation until transmission almost ceases. This phenomenon is called *habituation*. It is a type of memory that causes the neuronal circuit to lose its response to repeated events that are insignificant. On the other hand, if a noxious stimulus excites the sensitizing terminal at the same time that the memory terminal is stimulated, then, instead of the transmitted signal becoming progressively weaker, the ease of transmission becomes much stronger and will remain strong for hours, days, or even weeks, even without further stimulation of the sensitizing terminal. Thus, the noxious stimulus causes the memory pathway to become facilitated for weeks thereafter. It is especially interesting that only a few repeated action potentials are required to cause either habituation or sensitization. However, once habituation has occurred, the synapses can become sensitized very rapidly with only a few sensitizing signals.

At the molecular level, the habituation effect in the memory terminal results from progressive closure of calcium channels of the terminal membrane. As a result, much smaller than normal amounts of calcium diffuse into this terminal when action potentials occur, and much less transmitter is therefore released because calcium entry is the stimulus for transmitter release (as was discussed in Chapter 6).

In the case of sensitization, excess amounts of cyclic AMP are believed to develop inside the memory terminal and this opens increased numbers of calcium channels, which correspondingly enhances signal transmission.

Other variants of sensitized synaptic transmission have also been suggested, such as increased amounts of receptor protein in the postsynaptic

membrane, decreased rate of destruction of transmitter substance, and so on.

3. Theoretical Function of RNA in Memory. The discovery that DNA and RNA can act as codes to control reproduction, which in itself is a type of memory from one generation to another, plus the fact that these substances, once formed in a cell, tend to persist for the lifetime of the cell, has led to the theory that nucleic acids might be involved in memory changes of the neurons, changes that could last for the lifetime of the person. In addition, biochemical studies have shown an increase in RNA in some active neurons. Yet, a mechanism by which RNA could cause facilitation of synaptic transmission has not been found. Therefore, this theory seems to be based mainly on analogy rather than on factual evidence. The only possible supporting evidence is that several research workers have claimed that long-term memory will not occur to a significant extent when the chemical processes for formation of RNA are blocked. Since RNA is required to promote most anatomical or physical changes in the synapses, however, these observations could support almost any type of theory for long-term memory.

Summary. The theory that seems most likely at present for explaining long-term memory is that some actual anatomical, physical, or chemical change occurs in the synaptic knobs themselves or in the postsynaptic neurons, these changes permanently facilitating the transmission of impulses at the synapses. If all the synapses are thus facilitated in a thought circuit, this circuit can be re-excited by any one of many diverse incoming signals at later dates, thereby causing memory. The overall facilitated circuit is called a *memory engram* or a *memory trace*.

Consolidation of Long-Term Memory

If a memory is to last in the brain so that it can be recalled days later, it must become "consolidated" — that is, the synapses must become permanently facilitated. This process requires 5 to 10 minutes for minimal consolidation and an hour or more for maximal consolidation. For instance, if a strong sensory impression is made on the brain but is then followed within a minute or so by an electrically induced brain convulsion, the sensory experience will not be remembered at all. Likewise, brain concussion, sudden application of deep general anesthesia, and other effects that temporarily block the dynamic function of the brain can prevent consolidation.

However, if the same sensory stimulus is impressed on the brain and the strong electrical shock is delayed for more than 5 to 10 minutes, at least part of the memory trace will have become established. If the shock is delayed for an hour, the memory will have become fully consolidated.

The process of consolidation and the time required for consolidation can probably be explained by the phenomenon of *rehearsal* of the short-term memory as follows:

Role of Rehearsal in Transference of Short-Term Memory into Long-Term Memory. Psychological studies have shown that rehearsal of the same information again and again accelerates and potentiates the degree of transfer of short-term memory into long-term memory, and therefore also accelerates and potentiates the process of consolidation. The brain has a natural tendency to rehearse newfound information, and especially to rehearse newfound information that catches the mind's attention. Therefore, over a period of time the important features of sensory experiences become progressively more and more fixed in the long-term memory stores. This explains why a person can remember small amounts of information studied in depth far better than large amounts of information studied only superficially. And it also explains why a person who is wide-awake will consolidate memories far better than will a person who is in a state of mental fatigue.

Codifying of Memories During the Process of Consolidation. One of the most important features of the process of consolidation is that memories to be placed permanently into the long-term memory storehouse are first codified into different classes of information. During this process similar information is recalled from the long-term storage bins and is used to help process the new information. The new and old are compared for similarities and for differences, and part of the storage process is to store the information about these similarities and differences rather than simply to store the information unprocessed. Thus, during the process of consolidation, the new memories are not stored randomly in the brain, but instead are stored in direct association with other memories of the same type. This is obviously necessary if one is to be able to scan the memory store at a later date to find the required information.

Change of Long-Term Secondary Memory into Long-Term Tertiary Memory — Role of Rehearsal. Rehearsal also plays an extremely important role in changing the weak trace type of long-term memory, called secondary memory, into the strong trace type, called tertiary memory. That is, each time a memory is recalled or each time the same sensory experience is repeated, a more and more indelible memory trace develops in the brain. The memory finally becomes so deeply fixed in the brain that it can be recalled within a fraction of a second and it will also last for a lifetime, both of which are the characteristics of long-term tertiary memory.

Role of Specific Parts of the Brain in the Memory Process

Role of the Hippocampus for Rehearsal, Codification, and Consolidation of Memories — Anterograde Amnesia. Persons who have had both hippocampi (or other associated limbic structures) removed have essentially normal memory for information stored in the brain prior to removal of the hippocampi. However, after loss of these structures, these persons have very little capability for transferring short-term memory into long-term memory. That is, they do not have the ability to separate out the important information, to codify it, to rehearse it, and to consolidate it in the long-term memory store. Therefore, these persons develop serious *anterograde amnesia,* meaning simply inability to establish new memories.

Other types of lesions that frequently give anterograde amnesia include lesions of (1) the mammillary bodies, (2) the anterior nuclei of the thalamus, (3) the anterior columns of the fornix, or (4) the dorsal medial nuclei of the thalamus.

Retrograde Amnesia. Retrograde amnesia means inability to recall memories from the long-term memory storage bins even though the memories are known to be still there. Usually when a person develops retrograde amnesia, the degree of amnesia for recent events is likely to be much greater than for events of the distant past, though even the distant memories are usually affected at least to some extent.

In most persons who have hippocampal lesions and resultant anterograde amnesia, there is also some degree of retrograde amnesia, which suggests that these two types of amnesia are at least partially related and that hippocampal lesions can cause both. However, it has also been claimed that damage in some thalamic areas can lead specifically to retrograde amnesia without significant anterograde amnesia. This perhaps can be explained by the fact that the thalamus probably plays a major role in directing the person's attention to information in different parts of the memory storehouse, as was discussed in the previous chapter. Thus, the thalamus could easily play important roles in codifying, storing, and recalling memories.

ANALYTICAL OPERATIONS OF THE BRAIN

Thus far, we have considered the approximate nature of thoughts and possible mechanisms by which memory and learning can occur. Now we need to consider the mechanisms by which the brain performs complex intellectual operations, such as the analysis of sensory information and the establishment of abstract thoughts. About these mechanisms we know almost nothing, but experiments along these lines have established the following important facts: First, the brain can focus its attention on specific types of information (which was discussed in the preceding chapter). Second, the different qualities of each set of information signals are split away from the central signal and are transmitted to multiple areas of the brain. Third, the brain compares new information with old information in its memory loci. And, fourth, the brain determines patterns of stimulation.

Analysis of Information by Splitting its Qualities. When sensory information enters the nervous system, one of the first steps in its analysis is to transmit the signal to separate parts of the brain that are selectively adapted for detecting specific qualities. For instance, if the hand is placed on a hot stove, (a) pain information is sent through the spinoreticular and spinothalamic tracts into the reticular formation of the brain stem and into certain thalamic and hypothalamic nuclei, (b) tactile information is sent through the dorsal and dorsolateral column systems to the somesthetic cortex, giving the cortex a detailed description of the part of the hand that is touching the hot stove, and (c) position sense information from the muscles and joints is sent to the cerebellum, the reticular formation, and to higher centers of the brain to give momentary information of the position of the hand. Thus, the different qualities of the overall information are dissected and transmitted to different parts of the brain. On the basis of analyses in all these parts of the brain, motor responses to the incoming sensory information are formulated.

One can see that different centers of the brain react to specific qualities of information — the reticular formation and certain regions of the thalamus and hypothalamus to pain, regions of the mesencephalon and hypothalamus to the affective nature of the sensation (that is, whether it is pleasant or unpleasant), the somatic cortex to the localization of sensation, other areas to kinesthetic activities, and others to visual, auditory, gustatory, olfactory, and vestibular information.

Analysis of New Information by Comparison with Memories. We all know that new sensory experiences are immediately compared with previous experiences of the same or similar types. For instance, this is the way we recognize a person whom we know. Yet, it still remains a mystery how we can make these comparisons. One theory suggests that if the new pattern of stimulation matches the memory trace, some interaction between the two gives the person a sense of recognition.

Analysis of Patterns. In analyzing information, the brain depends to a great extent on "patterns" of stimulation. For instance, a square is detected as a square regardless of its position or angle of rotation in the visual field. Likewise, a series of parallel bars is detected as parallel bars regardless of their orientation, or a fly is detected as a fly whether it is seen in the peripheral or central field of vision. We can extend the same logic to the somatic sensory areas, for a person can detect a cube simply by feeling whether it be in an upright, horizontal, or angulated position. Also, it can be detected even by one's feet even though one's feet may have never felt a cube before.

Processing of Information so That Patterns Can Be Determined. Beautiful examples of the ability of the brain to process information for determination of patterns have been discovered in relation to the visual system. In Chapter 20 we shall point out that the retina itself processes visual information to a great extent even before it is transmitted into the brain. For instance, the neuronal circuits in the retina are organized to detect lines or boundaries between light and dark areas. That is, the visual scene is "differentiated" by this mechanism, bringing out strongly the contrasts of the scene but de-emphasizing the flat areas. This explains why a few lines drawn on a paper can give one the impression of a person's appearance. Certainly the lines do not represent the actual picture of a person, but they do give the visual cortex the same pattern of contrasts that one's own visual system would give.

One can see, therefore, that the visual cortex utilizes transformed types of information to point up the most striking characteristics of the visual scene while neglecting unimportant information. Then, the patterns of the visual scene can be extracted from this "preselected" information.

FUNCTION OF THE BRAIN IN COMMUNICATION

One of the most important differences between the human being and lower animals is the facility with which human beings can communicate with one another. Furthermore, because neurological tests can easily assess the ability of a person to communicate with others, we know perhaps more about the sensory and motor systems related to communication than about any other segment of cortical function. Therefore, we will review rapidly the function of the cortex in communication, and from this one can see immediately how the principles of sensory analysis and motor control apply to this art.

There are two aspects to communication: first, the *sensory aspect,* involving the ears and eyes, and, second, the *motor aspect,* involving vocalization and its control.

Sensory Aspects of Communication. We noted earlier in the chapter that destruction of portions

SPEAKING A HEARD WORD

MOTOR CORTEX

ARCUATE FASCICULUS

BROCA'S AREA

PRIMARY AUDITORY AREA

WERNICKE'S AREA

SPEAKING A WRITTEN WORD

MOTOR CORTEX

BROCA'S AREA

PRIMARY VISUAL AREA

ANGULAR GYRUS

WERNICKE'S AREA

Figure 15–8.   Brain pathways for (a) perception of the heard word and then speaking the same word, and (b) perception of the written word and then speaking the same word. (From Geschwind: *Sci. Amer. 241*:180, 1979. © 1979 by Scientific American, Inc. All rights reserved.)

of the *auditory* and *visual association areas* of the cortex can result in inability to understand the spoken word or the written word. These effects are called, respectively, *auditory receptive aphasia* and *visual receptive aphasia* or, more commonly, *word deafness* and *word blindness* (also called *dyslexia*). On the other hand, some persons are perfectly capable of understanding either the spoken word or the written word but are unable to interpret the thought that each expresses. This results most frequently when *Wernicke's area* in the *posterior portion of the superior temporal gyrus* in the dominant hemisphere is damaged or destroyed. This is considered to be *general sensory aphasia* or *general agnosia*.

Motor Aspects of Communication. *Sensory Aphasia.* The process of speech involves (a) formation in the mind of thoughts to be expressed and choice of the words to be used, then (b) the actual act of vocalization. The formation of thoughts and choice of words is principally the function of the sensory areas of the brain, for a person who has a destructive lesion in the same *Wernicke's area* in the *posterior superior temporal lobe* that is involved in general sensory aphasia also has inability to formulate intelligible thoughts to be communicated. And at other times the thoughts can be formulated, but the person is unable to put together the appropriate words to express the thought. These inabilities to formulate thoughts and word sequences are called *sensory aphasias* or, in honor of the neurologist who first delimited the brain area responsible, *Wernicke's aphasia.*

Motor Aphasia. Often a person is perfectly capable of deciding what he wishes to say, and he is capable of vocalizing, but he simply cannot make his vocal system emit words instead of noises. This effect, called *motor aphasia,* almost always results from damage to *Broca's speech area,* which lies in the *premotor* facial region of the cortex — about 95 per cent of the time in the left hemisphere, as illustrated in Figure 15–5. Therefore, we assume that the *skilled motor patterns* for control of the larynx, lips, mouth, respiratory system, and other accessory muscles of articulation are all controlled in this area.

Articulation. Finally, we have the act of articulation itself, which means the muscular movements of the mouth, tongue, larynx, and so forth, that are responsible for the actual emission of sound. The *facial and laryngeal regions of the motor cortex* activate these muscles, and the *cerebellum, basal ganglia,* and *sensory cortex* all help to control the muscle contractions by feedback mechanisms described in Chapter 13. Destruction of these regions can cause either total or partial inability to speak distinctly.

Summary. Figure 15–8 illustrates two principal pathways for communication. The upper half of the figure shows the pathway involved in speaking a heard word. This sequence is the following: (1) reception in the primary auditory area of the sound signals that encode the word; (2) interpretation of the word in Wernicke's area; (3) determination also in Wernicke's area that the word is to be spoken; (4) transmission of signals from Wernicke's area to Broca's area via the *arcuate fasciculus;* (5) activation of the skilled motor programs in Broca's area for control of word formation; and (6) transmission of appropriate signals into the motor cortex to control the speech muscles.

The lower figure illustrates the comparable steps in speaking a written word. The initial receptive area for the word is in the primary visual area rather than in the primary auditory area. Then the word information passes through early stages of interpretation in the *angular gyrus region* and finally reaches its full level of recognition in Wernicke's area. From here, the sequence is the same as for speaking a heard word.

FUNCTION OF THE CORPUS CALLOSUM AND ANTERIOR COMMISSURE TO TRANSFER THOUGHTS, MEMORIES, AND OTHER INFORMATION TO THE OPPOSITE HEMISPHERE

Fibers in the *corpus callosum* connect the respective cortical areas of the two hemispheres with each other except for the anterior portions of the temporal lobes; these temporal areas, including especially the *amygdala,* are interconnected by fibers that pass through the *anterior commissure.* Because of the tremendous number of fibers in the corpus callosum, it obviously was assumed that this massive structure must have some important function to correlate activities of the two cerebral hemispheres. However, after cutting the corpus callosum in experimental animals, it was difficult to discern changes in brain function. Therefore, for a long time the function of the corpus callosum was a mystery.

Yet, properly designed psychological experiments have demonstrated the extremely important functions of the corpus callosum and anterior commissure. These can be explained best by recounting one of the experiments. A monkey is first prepared by cutting the corpus callosum and splitting the optic chiasm longitudinally. Then it is taught to recognize different types of objects with its right eye while its left eye is covered. Next, the right eye is covered and the monkey is tested to determine whether or not its left eye can recognize the same object. The answer to this is that the left eye *cannot* recognize the object. Yet, on repeating the same experiment in another monkey with the optic chiasm split but the corpus callosum intact, it is found invariably that recognition in one hemisphere of the brain creates recognition also in the opposite hemisphere.

Thus, one of the functions of the corpus callosum and the anterior commissure is to make information stored in the cortex of one hemisphere available to the corresponding cortical area of the opposite hemisphere. Two important examples of such cooperation between the two hemispheres are:

1. Cutting of the corpus callosum blocks transfer of information from the general interpretative area of the dominant hemisphere to the motor cortex on the opposite side of the brain. Therefore, the intellectual functions of the brain, located primarily in the dominant hemisphere, lose their control over the right motor cortex and therefore also of the voluntary motor functions of the left hand and arm even though the usual subconscious movements of the left hand and arm are completely normal.

2. Cutting of the corpus callosum prevents transfer of somatic and visual information from the right hemisphere into the general interpretative area of the dominant hemisphere. Therefore, somatic and visual information from the left side of the body frequently fails to reach the general interpretative area of the brain and, therefore, cannot be used for decision making.

3. Finally, a teen-aged boy whose corpus callosum had been completely sectioned, but whose anterior commissure was not sectioned, recently was found to have two entirely separate conscious portions to his brain. Only the left half of his brain could understand the spoken word, because it was the dominant hemisphere. On the other hand, the right side of the brain could understand the written word and could elicit a motor response to it without the left side of the brain ever knowing why the response was performed. Yet, the effect was somewhat different when an emotional response was evoked in the right side of the brain, because in this case a subconscious emotional response was felt in the left side of the brain as well. This undoubtedly occurred because the limbic areas in the two sides of the brain were still communicating with each other through anterior commissural fibers interconnecting the amygdalas. For instance, when the command "kiss" was written for the right half of his brain to see, the boy immediately and with full emotion, said "No way!" But, when questioned why he said this, he could not explain. Thus, the two halves of the brain have independent capabilities for consciousness, memory storage, communication, and control of motor activities. The corpus callosum is required for the two sides to operate cooperatively, and the anterior commissure plays an important role in unifying the emotional responses of the two brain sides.

REFERENCES

Bannister, R. (rev.): Brain's Clinical Neurology. New York, Oxford University Press, 1978.

Bekhtereva, N. P.: The Neurophysiological Aspects of Human Mental Activity. New York, Oxford University Press, 1978.

Benson, D. F.: Aphasia, Alexia, and Agraphia. New York, Churchill Livingstone, 1979.

Benton, A. L., and Pearl, D.: Dyslexia: An Appraisal of Current Knowledge. New York, Oxford University Press, 1978.

Bloodstein, O.: Speech Pathology: An Introduction. Boston, Houghton Mifflin, 1979.

Buser, P.: Higher functions of the nervous system. Annu. Rev. Physiol., 38:217, 1978.

Corning, W. C., et al. (eds.): Invertebrate Learning. Vol. 3. New York, Plenum Press, 1974.

Daniloff, R., et al.: The Physiological Bases of Verbal Communication. Englewood Cliffs, N.J., Prentice-Hall, 1980.

Darley, F. L., et al. (eds.): Evaluation of Appraisal Techniques in Speech and Language Pathology. Reading, Mass., Addison-Wesley Publishing Co., 1979.

De Silva, F. H. L., and Arnolds, D.E.A.T.: Physiology of the hippocampus and related structures. Annu. Rev. Physiol., 40:185, 1978.

Desmedt, J. E. (ed.): Language and Hemispheric Specialization in Man; Cerebral Event-Related Potentials. New York, S. Karger, 1977.

Deutsch, J. A. (ed.): The Physiological Basis of Memory. New York, Academic Press, 1972.

DiCara, L. V.: Learning mechanisms. In Frohlich, E. D. (ed.): Pathophysiology, 2nd Ed. Philadelphia, J. B. Lippincott Co., 1976, p. 757.

Dimond, S. J.: Neuropsychology: A Textbook of Systems and Psychological Functions of the Human Brain. Boston, Butterworths, 1979.

Edelman, G. M., and Mountcastle, V. B.: The Mindful Brain: Cortical Organization and the Group-Selective Theory of Higher Brain Function. Cambridge, Mass., MIT Press, 1978.

Eggert, G. H.: Wernicke's Works on Aphasia: A Sourcebook and Review. The Hague, Mouton, 1977.

Gazzaniga, M. (ed.): Neuropsychology. New York, Plenum Press, 1978.

Geschwind, N.: The apraxias: Neural mechanisms of disorders of learned movement. Am. Sci., 63:188, 1975.

Geschwind, N.: Specializations of the human brain. Sci. Am., 241(3):180, 1979.

Herron, J. (ed.): Neuropsychology of Left-Handedness. New York, Academic Press, 1979.

Hixon, T. J., et al. (eds.): Introduction to Communicative Disorders. Englewood Cliffs, N. J., Prentice-Hall, 1980.

Hubel, D. H.: The brain. Sci. Am., 241(3):44, 1979.

Johns, D. F. (ed.): Clinical Management of Neurogenic Communicative Disorders. Boston, Little, Brown, 1978.

Kandel, E. R.: Neuronal plasticity and the modification of behavior. In Brookhart, J. M., and Mountcastle, V. B. (eds.): Handbook of Physiology. Sec. 1, Vol. 1. Baltimore, Williams & Wilkins, 1977, p. 1137.

Kandel, E. R.: A Cell-Biological Approach to Learning. Bethesda, Md., Society for Neuroscience, 1978.

Lehmann, D., and Callaway, E. (eds.): Event-Related Potentials in Man: Applications and Probes. New York, Plenum Press, 1979.

Levinthal, C. F.: The Physiological Approach in Psychology. Englewood Cliffs, N.J., Prentice-Hall, 1979.

Moskowitz, B. A.: The acquisition of language. Sci. Am., 239(5):92, 1978.

Nebes, R. D.: Hemispheric specialization in commissurotomized man. Psychol. Bull., 81:1, 1974.

Olton, D. S.: Spatial memory. Sci. Am., 236(6):82, 1977.

Ordy, J. M., and Brizzee, K. R. (eds.): Sensory Systems and Communication in the Elderly. New York, Raven Press, 1979.

Russell, I. S., and vanHof, M. W. (eds.): Structure and Function of Cerebral Commissures. Baltimore, University Park Press, 1978.

Schiefelbusch, R. L., et al. (eds.): Language Intervention Strategies. Baltimore, University Park Press, 1978.

Siegel, R. K.: Hallucinations. Sci. Am., 237(4):132, 1977.

Smith, J. H. (ed.): Psychoanalysis and Language. New Haven, Conn., Yale University Press, 1978.

Sperry, R. W.: Changing concepts of consciousness and free will. Perspect. Biol. Med., 20:9, 1976.

Stein, D. G., and Rosen, J. J.: Learning and Memory. New York, The Macmillan Co., 1974.

Steklis, H. D., and Raleigh, M. J. (eds.): Neurobiology of Social Communication in Primates: An Evolutionary Perspective. New York, Academic Press, 1979.

Terry, R. D., and Davies, P.: Dementia of the Alzheimer type. Annu. Rev. Neurosci., 3:77, 1980.

Uttal, W. R.: The Psychobiology of Mind. New York, Halsted Press, 1978.

Vellutino, F. R.: Dyslexia: Theory and Research. Cambridge, Mass., MIT Press, 1979.

16

Behavioral Functions of the Brain: The Limbic System, Role of the Hypothalamus, and Control of Vegetative Functions of the Body

Behavior is a function of the entire nervous system, not of any particular portion. Even the discrete cord reflexes are an element of behavior, and the wakefulness and sleep cycle discussed in Chapter 14 is certainly one of the most important of our behavioral patterns. However, in this chapter we will deal with those special types of behavior associated with emotions, subconscious motor and sensory drives, and the intrinsic feelings of punishment and pleasure. These functions of the nervous system are performed mainly by subcortical structures located in the basal regions of the brain.

The word "limbic" means "border," and the original usage of the term *limbic system* was to describe the brain structures that lie in the border region between the hypothalamus and its related structures, on the one hand, and the cerebral cortex. However, as we have learned more about the functions of the hypothalamus and the limbic system, it has become clear that they function together as a total system. Therefore, the term limbic system has now been expanded in common usage to mean this entire basal system of the brain that mainly controls the person's emotional behavior and drive.

The hypothalamus and its related structures also control many internal conditions of the body as well as aspects of behavior — such conditions as body temperature, osmolality of the body fluids, the drives to eat and drink, body weight, and so forth. These internal functions are collectively called *vegetative functions* of the body, and their control is obviously closely related to behavior.

FUNCTIONAL ANATOMY OF THE LIMBIC SYSTEM; ITS RELATION TO THE HYPOTHALAMUS

Figure 16–1 illustrates the anatomical structures of the limbic system and its relationship to the hypothalamus, showing these to be an interconnected complex of basal brain elements. Located in the midst of all these is the hypothalamus, which is considered by many anatomists to be a separate structure from the remainder of the limbic system but which, from a physiological point of view, is one of the central elements of the system. Therefore, Figure 16–2 illustrates schematically this key position of the hypothalamus in the limbic system and shows that surrounding it are the other subcortical structures of the limbic system, including the *preoptic area*, the *septum*, the *paraolfactory area*, the *epithalamus*, the *anterior nuclei of the thalamus*, portions of the *basal ganglia*, the *hippocampus*, and the *amygdala*.

Surrounding the subcortical limbic areas is the *limbic cortex* composed of a ring of cerebral cortex (a) beginning in the *orbitofrontal area* on the ventral surface of the frontal lobes, (b) extending upward in front of and over the corpus callosum onto the medial aspect of the cerebral hemisphere to the *cingulate gyrus*, and finally (c) passing behind the corpus callosum and downward onto the ventromedial surface of the temporal lobe to the *hippocampal gyrus, pyriform area,* and *uncus*. Thus, on the medial and ventral surfaces of each cerebral hemisphere is a ring of *paleocortex* that surrounds a group of deep structures intimately associated with overall behavior and with emotions. In turn, this ring of paleocortex functions as a two-way communication and association linkage between the *neocortex* and the lower limbic structures.

It is also important to recognize that many of the

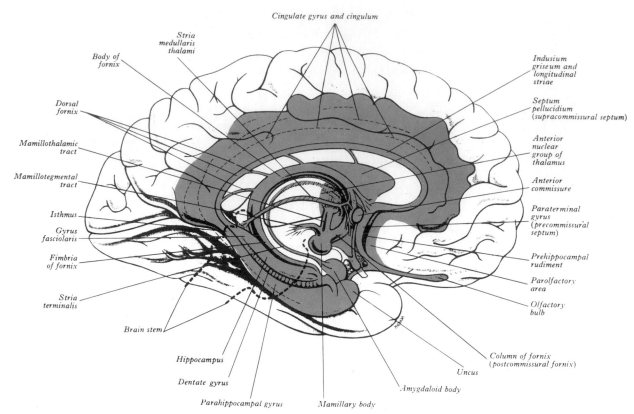

Figure 16–1. Anatomy of the limbic system illustrated by the shaded areas of the figure (From Warwick and Williams: Gray's Anatomy, 35th Brit. Ed. London, Longman Group Ltd., 1973.)

behavioral functions elicited from the hypothalamus and from other limbic structures are mediated through the reticular formation of the brain stem. It was pointed out in Chapters 12 and 14 that stimulation of the excitatory portion of the reticular formation can cause high degrees of somatic excitability; in Chapter 17 we will see that most of the signals for control of the autonomic nervous system either originate in or are transmitted from higher centers through nuclei located in the brain stem reticular formation.

Therefore, from a physiological point of view the reticular formation is a very important part of the limbic system even though anatomically it is considered to be a separate entity. A very important route of communication between the limbic system and the reticular formation is the *medial forebrain bundle* that extends from the septal and orbitofrontal cortical regions downward through the hypothalamus to the reticular formation. This bundle carries fibers in both directions, forming a trunk-line communication system. A second route of communication is through short pathways among the reticular formation, the thalamus, the hypothalamus, and most of the other contiguous areas of the basal brain.

THE HYPOTHALAMUS, THE MAJOR OUTPUT PATHWAY OF THE LIMBIC SYSTEM

Note in Figure 16–2 that the hypothalamus lies in the very middle of the limbic system. It also has communicating pathways with all levels of this system. In turn, it and its closely allied structures, the *septum* and the *mammillary bodies*, send output signals in two directions, (1) downward through the brain stem mainly into the reticular formation of the mesencephalon, pons, and medulla, and (2) upward toward many areas of the

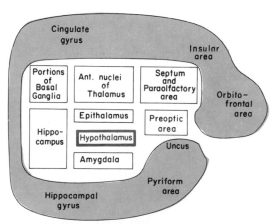

Figure 16–2. The limbic system.

cerebrum, especially the anterior thalamus and the limbic cortex. In addition, the hypothalamus indirectly affects cerebral cortical function very dramatically through activation or inhibition of the reticular activating system that originates in the brain stem.

Thus, the hypothalamus (along with its closely related structures) is the principal motor output pathway of the limbic system. It in turn controls most of the vegetative functions of the body as well as many aspects of emotional behavior. Let us discuss first the vegetative control functions and then return to the behavioral control functions to see how these operate together.

VEGETATIVE CONTROL FUNCTIONS OF THE HYPOTHALAMUS

The different hypothalamic mechanisms for controlling the vegetative functions of the body are so important that they, along with the functions that they control, are discussed in many different chapters throughout this text. For instance, the role of the hypothalamus in arterial pressure regulation is discussed in Chapter 23 and temperature regulation in Chapter 24. However, to illustrate the organization of the hypothalamus as a functional unit, let us summarize the more important of its vegetative functions here as well.

Figure 16–3 shows an enlargement of the hypothalamus, which represented only a small area in Figure 16–1. Please take a few minutes to study this diagram, especially to read the multiple vegetative activities that are stimulated or inhibited when respective centers are stimulated. In addi-

tion to those centers that are illustrated, a large *lateral hypothalamic* area overlies the illustrated areas on each side of the hypothalamus. The lateral areas are especially important in controlling thirst, hunger, and many of the emotional drives.

A word of caution must be issued for studying this diagram, however, for the areas that cause specific activities are not nearly so discrete as shown in the figure. The illustrated areas are merely those from which the functions are likely to be elicited. Also, it is not known whether the effects noted in the figure result from activation of specific control nuclei or whether they result merely from activation of fiber tracts leading from control nuclei located elsewhere. For instance, stimulation of the posterior hypothalamus, through which many of the fiber pathways from other portions of the hypothalamus pass, can at times elicit many functions believed to be controlled primarily by other hypothalamic nuclei. With this caution in mind, we can give the following general description of the vegetative control functions of the hypothalamus.

Cardiovascular Regulation. Stimulation of different areas throughout the hypothalamus can cause every known type of neurogenic effect in the cardiovascular system, including increased arterial pressure, decreased arterial pressure, increased heart rate, and decreased heart rate. In general, stimulation in the *posterior* and *lateral hypothalamus* increases the arterial pressure and heart rate, while stimulation in the *preoptic area* often has opposite effects, causing a decrease in both heart rate and arterial pressure. These effects are transmitted mainly through the cardiovascular control centers in the reticular substance of the medulla and pons.

Regulation of Body Temperature. Large areas in the anterior portion of the hypothalamus, especially in the *preoptic area,* are concerned with regulation of body

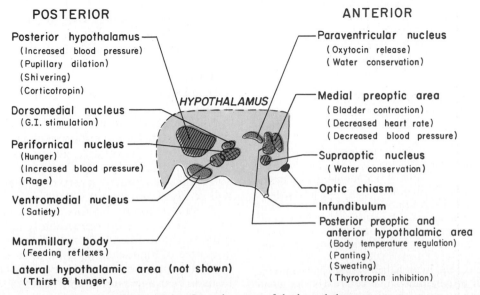

Figure 16–3. Control centers of the hypothalamus.

temperature. An increase in the temperature of the blood flowing through these areas increases their activity, while a decrease in temperature decreases their activity. In turn, these areas control the mechanisms for increasing or decreasing body temperature, as discussed in Chapter 24.

Regulation of Body Water. The hypothalamus regulates body water in two separate ways, by (1) creating the sensation of thirst, which makes an animal drink water, and (2) controlling the excretion of water into the urine. An area called the *thirst center* is located in the lateral hypothalamus. When the electrolytes inside the neurons of this center become too concentrated, the animal develops an intense desire to drink water; it will search out the nearest source of water and drink enough to return the electrolyte concentration of the thirst center to normal.

Control of renal excretion of water is vested mainly in the *supraoptic nuclei.* When the body fluids become too concentrated, the neurons of this area become stimulated. The nerve fibers from these neurons project into the posterior pituitary gland where they secrete a hormone called *antidiuretic hormone.* This hormone is then absorbed into the blood and acts on the collecting ducts of the kidneys to cause massive reabsorption of water, thereby decreasing the loss of water into the urine. These functions are especially important in controlling the water in the body.

Regulation of Uterine Contractility and of Milk Ejection by the Breasts. Stimulation of the *paraventricular nuclei* causes its neuronal cells to secrete the hormone *oxytocin.* This in turn causes increased contractility of the uterus and also contraction of the myoepithelial cells that surround the alveoli of the breasts, which then causes the alveoli to empty the milk through the nipples. At the end of pregnancy, especially large quantities of oxytocin are secreted, and this secretion helps to promote labor contractions that expel the baby. Also, when a baby suckles the mother's breast, a reflex signal from the nipple to the hypothalamus causes oxytocin release, and the oxytocin then performs the necessary function of expelling the milk through the nipples so that the baby can nourish itself. These functions are an essential part of the lactation process.

Gastrointestinal and Feeding Regulation. Stimulation of several areas of the hypothalamus causes an animal to experience extreme hunger, a voracious appetite, and an intense desire to search for food. The area most associated with hunger is the *lateral hypothalamic area.* On the other hand, damage to this causes the animal to lose desire for food, sometimes causing lethal starvation.

A center that opposes the desire for food, called the *satiety center,* is located in the *ventromedial nucleus.* When this center is stimulated, an animal that is eating food suddenly stops eating and shows complete indifference to the food. On the other hand, if this area is destroyed, the animal cannot be satiated, but instead, its hypothalamic hunger centers become overactive so that it has a voracious appetite, resulting in tremendous obesity.

Another area of the hypothalamus that enters into the overall control of gastrointestinal activity is the *mammillary bodies* that activate many feeding reflexes, such as licking the lips and swallowing.

Hypothalamic Control of the Anterior Pituitary Gland. Stimulation of certain areas of the hypothalamus also causes the anterior pituitary gland to secrete its hormones. This subject will be discussed in detail in Chapter 25 in relation to the overall control of the endocrine glands, but, briefly, the basic mechanism of the control of the anterior pituitary is the following:

The adenohypophysis receives its blood supply mainly from veins that flow into the anterior pituitary sinuses from the lower part of the hypothalamus. As the blood courses through the hypothalamus before reaching the anterior pituitary, *neurosecretory substances* are secreted into the blood by various hypothalamic nuclei. They are then transported in the blood to the anterior pituitary where they act on the glandular cells to cause release of the anterior pituitary hormones.

Stimulation of the following areas of the hypothalamus has been said to cause secretion of specific anterior pituitary hormones: (1) preoptic and anterior hypothalamic nuclei, thyrotropin that controls secretion of the thyroid hormones; (2) posterior hypothalamus and median eminence of the infundibulum, corticotropin that causes secretion of adrenocortical hormones; (3) median eminence, follicle-stimulating hormone, and anterior hypothalamus, luteinizing hormone, the two of which cause secretion of the gonadotropic hormones. Other nuclei of the hypothalamus control the secretion of growth hormone and prolactin by the anterior pituitary gland, the first of these accelerating body growth and the second causing lactation.

Summary. A number of discrete areas of the hypothalamus have now been found that control specific vegetative functions. However, these areas are still poorly delimited, so much so that the above separation of different areas for different hypothalamic functions is partially artificial.

BEHAVIORAL FUNCTIONS OF THE HYPOTHALAMUS AND ASSOCIATED LIMBIC STRUCTURES

Aside from the vegetative functions of the hypothalamus, experiments have shown that stimulation of or lesions in the hypothalamus often have profound effects on emotional behavior of animals or human beings.

In animals, the effects of stimulation are the following:

1. Stimulation in the *lateral hypothalamus* not only causes thirst and eating as discussed above in relation to the vegetative functions but also increases the general level of activity of the animal, sometimes leading to overt rage and fighting as will be discussed subsequently.

2. Stimulation of the *most medial portion of the medial hypothalamus* immediately adjacent to the third ventricle (or also stimulation of the central gray area of the mesencephalon that is continuous with this portion of the hypothalamus) usually leads to fear and punishment reactions.

3. Stimulation of the *lateral portion of the medial hypothalamus,* the area lying between the two

areas discussed above, can elicit a number of different hypothalamic drives. In the most anterior portion, stimulation is most likely to increase sexual drive. Immediately behind this area, in the *preoptic hypothalamus,* is the area for control of body temperature. Next, in the anterior hypothalamus is an area that increases the drive mainly for drinking, but to some extent for eating. A little further posteriorly, the drive converts mainly to excessive eating, and, finally, at the very posterior of this mid-zone of the hypothalamus, the sex drive again becomes most prominent.

Lesions in the hypothalamus, in general, cause the opposite effects. For instance:

1. Bilateral lesions in the lateral hypothalamus will decrease drinking and eating almost to zero, often leading to lethal starvation, as was discussed above in relation to the vegetative functions of the lateral hypothalamus. But these lesions cause extreme *passivity* of the animal as well, with loss of most of its overt activities.

2. Bilateral lesions of the ventromedial areas of the hypothalamus cause exactly opposite effects: excessive drinking and eating, as well as hyperactivity and often contiguous savagery along with frequent bouts of extreme rage on the slightest provocation.

Lesions or stimulation in other regions of the limbic system, especially the amygdala, the septal area, and areas in the mesencephalon, often also cause effects similar to those elicited directly from the hypothalamus. We will discuss some of these in more detail later.

The Reward and Punishment (or Pleasure and Pain) Function of the Limbic System

From the above discussion it is already clear that the hypothalamus and other limbic structures are particularly concerned with the affective nature of sensory sensations — that is, whether the sensations are *pleasant* or *painful.* These affective qualities are also called *reward* and *punishment* or *satisfaction* and *aversion.* Electrical stimulation of certain regions pleases or satisfies the animal, whereas electrical stimulation of other regions causes terror, pain, fear, defense, escape reactions, and all the other elements of punishment. Obviously, these two oppositely responding systems greatly affect the behavior of the animal.

Reward Centers. Figure 16–4 illustrates a technique that has been used for localizing the specific reward and punishment areas of the brain. In this figure a lever is placed at the side of the cage and is arranged so that depressing the lever makes electrical contact with a stimulator. Electrodes are placed successively at different areas in the brain so that the animal can stimulate the area by pressing the lever. If stimulating the particular

Figure 16–4. Technique for localizing reward and punishment centers in the brain of a monkey.

area gives the animal a sense of reward, then it will press the lever again and again, sometimes as much as 10,000 to 15,000 times per hour. Furthermore, when offered the choice of eating some delectable food as opposed to the opportunity to stimulate the reward center, it often chooses the electrical stimulation.

By using this procedure, the major reward centers have been found to be located in the septum and hypothalamus, primarily *along the course of the medial forebrain bundle* and in both the *lateral and the ventromedial nuclei of the hypothalamus.* It is strange that the lateral nuclei should be included among the reward areas — indeed it is one of the most potent reward areas of all — because even stronger stimuli in this area can cause rage. But this is true in many areas, with weaker stimuli giving a sense of reward and stronger ones, a sense of punishment.

Less potent reward centers, which are probably secondary to the major ones in the septum and hypothalamus, are found in the amygdala, certain areas of the thalamus and basal ganglia, and finally extending downward into the basal tegmentum of the mesencephalon.

Punishment Centers. The apparatus illustrated in Figure 16–4 can also be connected so that pressing the lever turns off rather than turns on an electrical stimulus. In this case, the animal will not turn the stimulus off when the electrode is in one of the reward areas, but when it is in certain other areas it immediately learns to turn it off. Stimulation in these areas causes the animal to show all the signs of displeasure, fear, terror, and punishment. Furthermore, prolonged stimulation for 24 hours or more causes the animal to become severely sick and actually leads to death.

By means of this technique, the principal centers for pain, punishment, and escape tendencies have been found in the *central gray area surrounding the aqueduct of Sylvius in the mesencephalon* and extending upward into the *periventricular structures of the hypothalamus and thalamus*.

The extent of the punishment areas in the limbic system is only one-seventh as great as the reward areas. Even so, it is particularly interesting that stimulation in the punishment centers can frequently inhibit the reward and pleasure centers completely, illustrating that punishment and fear can take precedence over pleasure and reward.

Importance of Reward and Punishment in Behavior. Almost everything that we do depends on reward and punishment. If we are doing something that is rewarding, we continue to do it; if it is punishing, we cease to do it. Therefore, the reward and punishment centers undoubtedly constitute one of the most important of all the controllers of our bodily activities, our motivations, and so forth.

Importance of Reward and Punishment in Learning and Memory — Habituation or Reinforcement. Animal experiments have shown that a sensory experience causing neither reward nor punishment is remembered hardly at all. Electrical recordings have shown that new and novel sensory stimuli always excite the cerebral cortex. But repetition of the stimulus over and over leads to almost complete extinction of the cortical response if the sensory experience does not elicit either a sense of reward or punishment. Thus, the animal becomes *habituated* to the sensory stimulus, and thereafter ignores this stimulus.

If the stimulus causes either reward or punishment rather than indifference, however, the cortical response becomes progressively more and more intense with repetitive stimulation instead of fading away, and the response is said to be *reinforced*. Thus, an animal builds up strong memory traces for sensations that are either rewarding or punishing but, on the other hand, develops complete habituation to indifferent sensory stimuli. Therefore, it is evident that the reward and punishment centers of the midbrain have much to do with selecting the information that we learn.

Effect of Tranquilizers on the Reward and Punishment Centers. Administration of a tranquilizer, such as chlorpromazine, inhibits both the reward and punishment centers, thereby greatly decreasing the affective reactivity of the animal. Therefore, it is presumed that tranquilizers function in psychotic states by suppressing many of the important behavioral areas of the hypothalamus and its associated regions of the brain.

Rage

An emotional pattern that involves the hypothalamus and has been well characterized is the *rage pattern*. This can be described as follows:

Strong stimulation of the punishment centers of the brain, especially the *periventricular areas of the hypothalamus,* causes the animal to (1) develop a defense posture, (2) extend its claws, (3) lift its tail, (4) hiss, (5) spit, (6) growl, and (7) develop pilo-erection, wide-open eyes, and dilated pupils. Furthermore, even the slightest provocation causes an immediate savage attack. This is approximately the behavior that one would expect from an animal being severely punished, and it is a pattern of behavior that is called *rage*.

Stimulation of the more rostral areas of the punishment areas — in the midline preoptic areas — causes mainly fear and anxiety, associated with a tendency for the animal to run away.

In the normal animal the rage phenomenon is held in check mainly by counterbalancing activity of the lateral portions of the ventromedial nuclei of the hypothalamus. This is the area of the hypothalamus that lies between the punishment centers adjacent to the third ventricle, on the one hand, and, on the other hand, the lateral nuclei of the hypothalamus that provides some of the very strong behavioral drives.

In addition, the hippocampus, the amygdala, and the anterior portions of the limbic cortex, especially the anterior limbic cortex of the subcallosal area and of the anterior temporal lobe, transmit signals that help to suppress the rage phenomenon. Conversely, if these portions of the limbic system are damaged or destroyed, the animal (also the human being) becomes far more susceptible to bouts of rage.

Placidity and Tameness. Exactly the opposite emotional behavioral patterns occur when the reward centers are stimulated: placidity and tameness.

Function of the Hypothalamus and Other Limbic Areas in Sleep, Wakefulness, Alertness, and Excitement

Stimulation of regions of the hypothalamus dorsal to the mammillary bodies greatly excites the reticular activating system and therefore causes wakefulness, alertness, and excitement. In addition, the sympathetic nervous system becomes excited in general, increasing the arterial pressure, causing pupillary dilatation, and enhancing other activities associated with sympathetic activity.

On the other hand, stimulation in the septum, in the anterior hypothalamus, or in isolated points of the thalamic portions of the reticular activating system often inhibits the mesencephalic portion of the reticular activating system, causing somnolence and sometimes actual sleep. Thus, the hypothalamus and other limbic structures indirectly contribute much to the control of the degree of excitement and alertness.

SPECIFIC FUNCTIONS OF OTHER PARTS OF THE LIMBIC SYSTEM

FUNCTIONS OF THE AMYGDALA

The amygdala is a complex of nuclei located immediately beneath the medial surface of the cerebral cortex in the pole of each temporal lobe, and it has abundant direct connections with the hypothalamus. In lower animals, this complex is concerned primarily with association of olfactory stimuli with stimuli from other parts of the brain. Indeed, it is pointed out in Chapter 22 that one of the major divisions of the olfactory tract leads directly to a portion of the amygdala called the *corticomedial nuclei* that lie immediately beneath the cortex in the pyriform area of the temporal lobe. However, in the human being, another portion of the amygdala, the *basolateral nuclei,* has become much more highly developed than the olfactory portion and plays very important roles in many behavioral activities not generally associated with olfactory stimuli.

The amygdala receives impulses from all portions of the limbic cortex, from the orbital surfaces of the frontal lobes, from the cingulate gyrus, from the hippocampal gyrus, and from the neocortex of the temporal, parietal, and occipital lobes, especially from the auditory and visual association areas. Because of these multiple connections, the amygdala has been called the ''window'' through which the limbic system sees the place of the person in the world. In turn, the amygdala transmits signals (a) back into these same cortical areas, (b) into the hippocampus, (c) into the septum, (d) into the thalamus, and (e) especially into the hypothalamus.

Effects of Stimulating the Amygdala. In general, stimulation in the amygdala can cause almost all the same effects as those elicited by stimulation of the hypothalamus, plus still other effects. The effects that are mediated through the hypothalamus include (1) increases or decreases in arterial pressure, (2) increases or decreases in heart rate, (3) increases or decreases in gastrointestinal motility and secretion, (4) defecation and micturition, (5) pupillary dilatation or, rarely, constriction, (6) pilo-erection, (7) secretion of the various anterior pituitary hormones, including especially the gonadotropins and corticotropin.

Aside from these effects mediated through the hypothalamus, amygdala stimulation can also cause different types of involuntary movement. These include (1) tonic movements, such as raising the head or bending the body, (2) circling movements, (3) occasionally clonic, rhythmic movements, and (4) different types of movements associated with olfaction and eating, such as licking, chewing, and swallowing.

In addition, stimulation of certain amygdaloid nuclei can, rarely, cause a pattern of rage, escape, punishment, and fear similar to the rage pattern elicited from the hypothalamus as described above. And stimulation of other nuclei can give reactions of reward and pleasure.

Finally, excitation of still other portions of the amygdala can cause sexual activities that include erection, copulatory movements, ejaculation, ovulation, uterine activity, and premature labor.

Effects of Bilateral Ablation of the Amygdala — the Klüver-Bucy Syndrome. When the anterior portions of both temporal lobes are destroyed in a monkey, this not only removes the temporal cortex but also the amygdalas that lie deep in these parts of the temporal lobes. This causes a combination of changes in behavior called the Klüver-Bucy syndrome, which includes (1) excessive tendency to examine objects orally, (2) loss of fear, (3) decreased aggressiveness, (4) tameness, (5) changes in dietary habits, even to the extent that a herbivorous animal frequently becomes carnivorous, (6) sometimes psychic blindness, and (7) often excessive sex drive. The characteristic picture is of an animal that is not afraid of anything, has extreme curiosity about everything, forgets very rapidly, has a tendency to place everything in its mouth and sometimes even tries to eat solid objects, and, finally, often has a sex drive so strong that it attempts to copulate with immature animals, animals of the wrong sex, or animals of a different species.

Though similar lesions in human beings are rare, afflicted persons respond in a mannner not too different from that of the monkey.

Overall Function of the Amygdala. The amygdala seems to be a behavioral awareness area that operates at a semiconscious level. It also seems to project into the limbic system one's present status in relation both to surroundings and thoughts. Based on this information, the amygdala is believed to help pattern the person's behavioral response so that it is appropriate for each occasion.

FUNCTIONS OF THE HIPPOCAMPUS

The hippocampus is an elongated structure composed of a modified type of cerebral cortex. In fact it is that portion of the temporal lobe cortex that folds inward to form the ventral surface of the inferior horn of the lateral ventricle. One end of the hippocampus abuts the amygdaloid nuclei, and it also fuses along one of its borders with the hippocampal gyrus, which is the cortex of the ventromedial surface of the temporal lobe.

The hippocampus has numerous connections with most portions of the sensory cortex as well as with the basic structures of the limbic system — the amygdala, the hypothalamus, the septum, and the mammillary bodies. Almost any type of sensory experience causes instantaneous activation of different parts of the hippocampus, and the hippocampus in turn distributes many outgoing signals to the hypothalamus and other parts of the limbic system, especially through the *fornix.* Thus, the hippocampus, like the amygdala, is an additional channel through which incoming sensory signals can lead to appropriate limbic reactions, but perhaps for different purposes as we shall see later.

Like other limbic structures, stimulation of different

areas in the hippocampus can cause almost any one of different behavioral patterns, such as rage, passivity, excess sex drive, or so forth.

Another feature of the hippocampus is that very weak electrical stimuli can cause local epileptic seizures that persist for many seconds after the stimulation is over, suggesting that the hippocampus can perhaps give off prolonged output signals even under normal functioning conditions. During the hippocampal seizures, the person experiences various psychomotor effects, including olfactory, visual, auditory, tactile, and other types of hallucinations that cannot be suppressed even though the person has not lost consciousness and knows these hallucinations to be unreal. Probably one of the reasons for this hyperexcitability of the hippocampus is that it is composed of a different type of cortex from that elsewhere in the cerebrum, having only three neuronal layers instead of the six layers found elsewhere.

Effect of Bilateral Removal of the Hippocampi — Inability to Learn. The hippocampi have been removed or destroyed bilaterally in a few human beings. These persons can perform most previously learned activities satisfactorily. However, they can learn essentially nothing new. In fact, they cannot even learn the names or the faces of persons with whom they come in contact every day. Yet, they can remember for a moment or so what transpires during the course of their activities. Thus, they do have a type of short-term memory even though their ability to establish new long-term memories is either completely or almost completely abolished, which is the phenomenon called *anterograde amnesia* that was discussed in the previous chapter.

Destruction of the hippocampi also causes some deficit in previously learned memories (retrograde amnesia), a little more so for recent memories than for memories of the distant past.

Theoretical Function of the Hippocampus in Learning. The hippocampus originated as part of the olfactory cortex. In the very lowest animals it plays essential roles in determining whether the animal will eat a particular food, whether the smell of a particular object suggests danger, whether the odor is sexually inviting, and in making other decisions that are of life and death importance. Thus, very early in the development of the brain, the hippocampus presumably became the critical decision-making neuronal mechanism, determining the importance and type of importance of the incoming sensory signals. Presumably, as the remainder of the brain developed, the connections from the other sensory areas into the hypothalamus have continued to utilize this decision-making capability.

Earlier in this chapter (and also in the previous chapter), it was pointed out that reward and punishment play a major role in determining the importance of information and especially whether or not the information will be stored in memory. A person rapidly becomes habituated to indifferent stimuli but learns assiduously any sensory experience that causes either pleasure or punishment. Yet, what is the mechanism by which this occurs? It has been suggested that the hippocampus acts as the encoding mechanism for translating short-term memory into long-term memory — that is, it translates the short-term memory signals into an appropriate form so that they can be stored in long-term memory and also transmits an additional signal to the long-term memory storage area directing that storage shall take place.

Whatever the mechanism, without the hippocampi *consolidation* of long-term memories does not take place. This is especially true for verbal information, perhaps because the temporal lobes, in which the hippocampi are located, are particularly concerned with verbal information.

FUNCTION OF THE LIMBIC CORTEX

Probably the most poorly understood portion of the entire limbic system is the ring of cerebral cortex called the *limbic cortex* that surrounds the subcortical limbic structures. This cortex functions as a transitional zone through which signals are transmitted from the remainder of the cortex into the limbic system. Therefore, it is presumed that the limbic cortex functions as a cerebral *association area for control of behavior*.

Stimulation of the different regions of the limbic cortex has failed to give any real idea of their functions. However, as is true of so many other portions of the limbic system, essentially all the behavioral patterns that have already been described can also be elicited by stimulation in different portions of the limbic cortex. Likewise, ablation of a few limbic cortical areas can cause persistent changes in an animal's behavior, though ablation in most areas has little effect. Some of the areas that have been noted to cause specific changes include:

Ablation of the Temporal Cortex. When the temporal cortex is ablated bilaterally, the amygdala is almost invariably damaged as well. This was discussed earlier, and it was pointed out that the Klüver-Bucy syndrome occurs. The animal develops consummatory behavior especially, investigates any and all objects, has intense sex drives toward inappropriate animals or even inanimate objects, and loses all fear — thus develops tameness as well.

Ablation of the Posterior Orbital Frontal Cortex. Bilateral removal of the posterior portion of the orbital frontal cortex often causes an animal to develop insomnia and an intense degree of motor restlessness, becoming unable to sit still but moving about continually.

Ablation of the Subcallosal Gyri. The subcallosal gyri are the portions of the limbic cortex that turn downward and under the corpus callosum on the medial portions of the frontal lobes. Destruction of these gyri bilaterally releases the rage centers of the septum and hypothalamus from an inhibitory influence. Therefore, the animal can become vicious and much more subject to fits of rage than normally.

Summary. Until further information is available, it is perhaps best to state that the cortical regions of the limbic system occupy intermediate associative positions between the functions of the remainder of the cerebral cortex and the functions of the subcortical limbic structures for control of behavioral patterns. Thus, in the insular and anterior temporal cortex one especially finds gustatory and olfactory associations. In the hippocampal gyri there is a tendency for complex auditory associations and also complex thought associations derived from the general interpretative areas of the posterior temporal lobes. In the cingulate cortex, there is reason to believe that sensorimotor associations occur. And, finally, the orbitofrontal cortex presumably aids in the analytical functions of the prefrontal lobes.

FUNCTION OF SPECIFIC CHEMICAL TRANSMITTER SYSTEMS FOR BEHAVIOR CONTROL

Recently it has become apparent that some of the synaptic chemical transmitter substances of the brain play especially important roles in behavior. Though this field is only beginning to be explored, the chemical transmitter systems that seem to be especially important are the following:

The Norepinephrine System. In Chapter 14 it was pointed out that large numbers of norepinephrine-secreting neurons are located in the reticular formation, especially in the locus ceruleus, and that they send fibers upward through the reticular activating system to essentially all parts of the diencephalon and cerebrum. One area of the hypothalamus that is especially activated by the norepinephrine system is the ventromedial nuclei that can block many of the drives such as eating, drinking, sex, and so forth when stimulated. Therefore, at the same time that the norepinephrine system activates the cerebral cortex, it also seems to block these other drives that might compete with the higher levels of cerebration.

It is believed that overstimulation of the norepinephrine system is the cause of the manic phase of the manic-depressive psychosis. And, conversely, there is much reason to believe that depressed activity of this system is the basis of the depression stage of the manic-depressive syndrome. Drugs that decrease norepinephrine removal from the synapses are frequently very effective both in increasing the activity of the norepinephrine system and also in the treatment of depression psychoses.

The Dopamine System. In Chapter 12 the dopaminergic neurons located in the substantia nigra and projecting to the striate portion of the basal ganglia were discussed. This system exerts an important continuous restraint on basal ganglia activity.

In addition to projecting to the basal ganglia, these dopaminergic fibers also project to other basal regions of the brain, especially into two areas of the hypothalamus — the area immediately adjacent to the third ventricle and also the lateral hypothalamus. Stimulation of this system especially increases the activity of the lateral hypothalamus, producing enhanced drives for eating and some other types of activity such as fighting. Conversely, destruction of the dopamine system has almost exactly the same effects as destroying the two lateral hypothalami, causing the animal to lose its desire to eat and also decreasing its aversive drives.

It has already been pointed out in Chapter 12 that destruction of the substantia nigral dopamine system causes Parkinson's disease. However, during treatment of Parkinson's disease with L-dopa, which in turn releases dopamine, patients sometimes develop schizophrenic symptoms, indicating that excess dopaminergic activity can cause dissociation of a person's drives and thought patterns. The phenothiazine tranquilizers depress the dopamine system and also are effective in the treatment of many patients with schizophrenia.

The Serotonin System. Located in the medial raphe nuclei of the medulla is a system of serotonin-secreting neurons. Many of the nerve fibers of this system spread downward into the cord where they reduce the input level of pain signals, as was explained in Chapter 50. However, the fibers also spread upward into the reticular formation and into other basal areas of the brain to suppress the activity of the reticular activating system, as well as other brain activity. Thus, this system can promote sleep, as was discussed in Chapter 14. The drug p-chlorophenylalanine inhibits the formation of serotonin, and it can cause prolonged wakefulness in animals. The drug LSD (lysergic acid diethylamide) is also known to act as an antagonist against some functions of serotonin. Its propensity to cause dissociation of both behavioral and mental activities is well known.

The Enkephalin-Endorphin System. Very little is yet known about the behavioral functions of the enkephalin-endorphin system. However, the probable role of this system for suppression of pain was discussed in Chapter 10. It presumably has many other activities as well, because it is secreted in many areas of the brain stem and thalamus.

Effects of the General Hormones on Behavior. Several of the general hormones have specific effects on behavior. Some of these are:

Thyroid hormone increases the overall *metabolism of the body* and increases overall activity of the nervous system as well.

Both *testosterone* in the male and estrogen in the female increase *libido*. Also, injection of a minute quantity of estrogen into the anterior hypothalamus of some lower animals will cause estrous behavior (heat). The sex drive of the human female seems to be increased near the time of ovulation when estrogen secretion is high.

A small, 6 or 7 amino acid *fragment of ACTH,* when injected into the brain of an animal, can cause *intense fear.*

Injection of *norephinephrine,* or excess secretion of norepinephrine or epinephrine by the adrenal medullae, increases the overall activity of the brain, which is essentially the same effect as stimulating the reticular activating system.

Thus, it is becoming clear that various chemical and transmitter systems play important roles in determining an animal's behavior. Furthermore, abnormalities of some of the brain's chemical transmitter systems seem to be the bases of some of the common psychoses.

PSYCHOSOMATIC EFFECTS OF THE BEHAVIORAL SYSTEM

We are all familiar with the fact that abnormal function in the central nervous system can frequently lead to serious dysfunction of the different somatic organs of the body. This is also true in experimental animals. Indeed, prolonged electrical stimulation in the punishment regions of the brain can actually lead to severe sickness of the animal, culminating in death within 24 to 48 hours. We need, therefore, to discuss briefly the mechanisms by which stimulatory effects in the brain can affect the peripheral organs. Ordinarily, this occurs through three routes: (1) through the motor nerves to the skeletal muscles throughout the body, (2) through the autonomic nerves to the different internal organs of the body, and (3) through the hormones secreted by the pituitary gland in response to nervous activity in the hypothalamus, as will be explained in Chapter 25.

Psychosomatic Disorders Transmitted Through the Skeletal Nervous System. Abnormal psychic states can greatly alter the degree of nervous stimulation to the skeletal musculature throughout the body and thereby increase or decrease the skeletal muscular tone. During states of excitement the general skeletal muscular tone as well as sympathetic tone normally increases, whereas during somnolent states skeletal muscular and sympathetic activity both decrease greatly. In neurotic and psychotic states, such as anxiety, tension, and mania, generalized overactivity of both the muscles and sympathetic system often occurs throughout the body. This in turn results in intense feedback from the muscle proprioceptors to the reticular activating system, and the norepinephrine and epinephrine circulating in the blood as a result of the sympathetic activity also excite the reticular activating system, all of which undoubtedly help to maintain an extreme degree of wakefulness and alertness that characterizes these emotional states. Unfortunately, though, the wakefulness prevents adequate sleep and also leads to progressive bodily fatigue and mental dissociations.

Transmission of Psychosomatic Effects Through the Autonomic Nervous System. Many psychosomatic abnormalities result from hyperactivity of either the sympathetic or parasympathetic system. In general, hyperactivity of the sympathetic system occurs in many areas of the body at the same time rather than in focal areas, and the usual effects are (1) increased heart rate — sometimes with palpitation of the heart, (2) increased arterial pressure, (3) constipation, and (4) increased metabolic rate. On the other hand, parasympathetic signals are likely to be much more focal. For instance, stimulation of specific areas in the dorsal motor nuclei of the vagus nerves can cause more or less specifically (1) increased or decreased heart rate or palpitation of the heart, (2) esophageal spasm, (3) increased peristalsis in the upper gastrointestinal tract, or (4) increased hyperacidity of the stomach with resultant development of peptic ulcer. Stimulation of the sacral region of the parasympathetic system, on the other hand, is likely to cause extreme colonic glandular secretion and peristalsis with resulting diarrhea. One can readily see, then, that emotional patterns controlling the sympathetic and parasympathetic centers of the hypothalamus and lower brain stem can cause wide varieties of peripheral psychosomatic effects.

Psychosomatic Effects Transmitted Through the Anterior Pituitary Gland. Electrical stimulation of the posterior hypothalamus increases the secretion of corticotropin by the anterior pituitary gland (as explained earlier in the chapter) and therefore indirectly increases the output of adrenocortical hormones. One of the effects of this is a gradual increase in stomach hyperacidity because of the effect of glucocorticoids on stomach secretion. Over a prolonged period of time this obviously could lead to peptic ulcer, which is a well-

known effect of hypersecretion by the adrenal cortex. Likewise, activity in the anterior hypothalamus increases the pituitary secretion of thyrotropin, which in turn increases the output of thyroxine and leads to an elevated basal metabolic rate. It is well known that different types of emotional disturbances can lead to thyrotoxicosis (as will be explained in Chapter 25), this presumably resulting from overactivity in the anterior hypothalamus.

From these examples, therefore, it is evident that many types of psychosomatic diseases of the body can be caused by abnormal control of anterior pituitary secretion.

REFERENCES

Akiskal, H. (ed.): Affective Disorders: Special Clinical Forms. Philadelphia, W. B. Saunders Co., 1979.

Bargmann, W., *et al.* (eds.): Neurosecretion and Neuroendocrine Activity: Evolution, Structure and Function. New York, Springer-Verlag, 1978.

Belmaker, R. H., and vanPragg, H. (eds.): Mania, An Evolving Concept. Jamaica, N. Y., Spectrum Publications, 1980.

Bentley, D., and Konishi, M.: Neural control of behavior. *Annu. Rev. Neurosci., 1*:35, 1978.

Bourne, G. H., *et al.* (eds.): Neuronal Cells and Hormones. New York, Academic Press, 1978.

Bowsher, D.: Mechanisms of Nervous Disorder: An Introduction. Philadelphia, J. B. Lippincott Co., 1978.

CIBA Foundation Symposium: Functions of the Septo-Hippocampal System. New York, Elsevier/Excerpta Medica/North-Holland, 1978.

Cooper, D. G.: The Language of Madness. London, Allen Lane, 1978.

Cotman, C. W., and McGaugh, J. L.: Behavioral Neuroscience. New York, Academic Press, 1979.

DeFeudis, F. V., and DeFeudis, P. A. F.: Elements of the Behavioral Code. New York, Academic Press, 1977.

Depue, R. A. (ed.): The Psychobiology of the Depressive Disorders: Implications For the Effects of Stress. New York, Academic Press, 1979.

De Silva, F. H. L., and Arnolds, D. E. A. T.: Physiology of the hippocampus and related structures. *Annu. Rev. Physiol., 40*:185, 1978.

DiCara, L. V.: Learning mechanisms. *In* Frohlich, E. D. (eds.): Pathophysiology, 2nd Ed. Philadelphia, J. B. Lippincott Co., 1976, p. 757.

Ehrlich, Y. H. (ed.): Modulators, Medicators, and Specifiers in Brain Function. New York, Plenum Press, 1979.

Elde, R., and Hökfelt, T.: Localization of hypophysiotropic peptides and other biologically active peptides within the brain. *Annu. Rev. Physiol., 41*:587, 1979.

Ferrendelli, J. A., and Gurvitch, G. (eds.): Aspects of Behavioral Neurobiology. Bethesda, Md., Society of Neuroscience, 1977.

Fink, G., and Geffen, L. B.: The hypothalamo-hypophysial system: Model for central peptidergic and monoaminergic transmission. *In* Porter, R. (ed.): International Review of Physiology: Neurophysiology III. Vol. 17. Baltimore, University Park Press, 1978, p. 1.

Fink, M.: Convulsive Therapy: Theory and Practice. New York, Raven Press, 1979.

Fuxe, K. (ed.): Peptidergic Neuron. New York, Plenum Press, 1979.

Gershon, M. D.: Biochemistry and physiology of serotonergic transmission. *In* Brookhart, J. M., and Mountcastle, V. B. (eds.): Handbook of Physiology. Sec. 1, Vol. 1. Baltimore, Williams & Wilkins, 1977, p. 573.

Greist, J. H., and Greist, T. H.: Antidepressant Treatment in Primary Care. Baltimore, Williams & Wilkins, 1979.

Guillemin, R.: Neuroendocrine interrelations. *In* Bondy, P. K., and Rosenberg, L. E. (eds.): Metabolic Control and Disease, 8th Ed. Philadelphia, W. B. Saunders Co., 1980, p. 1155.

Guroff, G.: Molecular Neurobiology. New York, Marcel Dekker, 1979.

Jeffcoate, S. L., and Hutchinson, J. S. M. (eds.): The Endocrine Hypothalamus. New York, Academic Press, 1978.

Jones, N. B., and Reynolds, V.: Human Behaviour and Adaptation. New York, Halsted Press, 1978.

Kelly, D.: Anxiety and Emotions: Physiological Basis and Treatment. Springfield, Ill., Charles C Thomas, 1979.

Lederis, K., and Veale, W. L. (eds.): Current Studies of Hypothalamic Function, 1978. New York, S. Karger, 1978.

Legg, N. J. (ed.): Neurotransmitter Systems and Their Clinical Disorders. New York, Academic Press, 1978.

Livingston, K. E., and Hornykiewicz, O. (eds.): Limbic Mechanism. New York, Plenum Press, 1978.

Livingston, R. B.: Neural integration. In Frohlich, E. D. (ed.): Pathophysiology, 2nd Ed. Philadelphia, J. B. Lippincott Co., 1976, p. 681.

Mandel, P., and DeFeudis, F. V. (eds.): GABA — Biochemistry and CNS Functions. New York, Plenum Press, 1979.

McFadden, D. (ed.): Neural Mechanisms in Behavior. New York, Springer-Verlag, 1980.

McGuigan, F. J.: Psychophysiological Measurement of Covert Behavior. New York, Halsted Press, 1979.

Morgane, P. J., and Panksepp, J. (eds.): Anatomy of the Hypothalamus. New York, Marcel Dekker, 1979.

Morgane, P. J., and Panksepp, J. (eds.): Handbook of the Hypothalamus. New York, Marcel Dekker, 1979.

Norrsel, U.: Behavioral studies of the somatosensory system. Physiol. Rev., 60:327, 1980

Obata, K.: Biochemistry and physiology of amino acid transmitters. In Brookhart, J. M., and Mountcastle, V. B. (eds.): Handbook of Physiology. Sec. 1, Vol. 1. Baltimore, Williams & Wilkins, 1977, p. 625.

Pepeu, G., et al. (eds.): Receptors for Neurotransmitters and Peptide Hormones, New York, Raven Press, 1980.

Plotnik, R., and Mollenauer, S.: Brain and Behavior: An Introduction to Physiological Psychology. San Francisco, Canfield Press, 1978.

Rimm, D. C., and Masters, J. C.: Behavior Therapy: Techniques and Empirical Findings, 2nd Ed. New York, Academic Press, 1979.

Routtenberg, A.: The reward system of the brain. Sci. Am., 239 (5):154, 1978.

Sachar, E. J., and Baron, M.: The biology of affective disorders. Annu. Rev. Neurosci., 2:505, 1979.

Sadoul, P. (ed.): Muscular Exercise in Chronic Lung Disease. New York, Pergamon Press, 1979.

Schou, M., and Strömgren, E. (eds.): Origin, Prevention, and Treatment of Affective Disorders. New York, Academic Press, 1979.

Shopsin, B. (ed.): Manic Illness. New York, Raven Press, 1979.

Snyder, S.: Biological Aspects of Mental Disorder. New York, Oxford University Press, 1980.

Sowers, J. R. (ed.): Hypothalamic Hormones. Stroudsburg, Pa., Dowden, Hutchinson & Ross, 1980.

Tipton, K. F. (ed.): Neurochemistry and Biochemical Pharmacology. Baltimore, University Park Press, 1978.

Tolis, G., et al. (eds.): Clinical Neuroendocrinology. New York, Raven Press, 1979.

Vale, W., Rivier, C., and Brown, M.: Regulatory peptides of the hypothalamus. Annu. Rev. Physiol., 39:473, 1977.

Van Ree, J. M., and Terenius, L. (eds.): Characteristics and Function of Opioids. New York, Elsevier/North Holland, 1978.

Wassermann, G. D.: Neurobiological Theory of Psychological Phenomena. Baltimore, University Park Press, 1978.

Way, E. L. (ed.): Endogenous and Exogenous Opiate Agonists and Antagonists. New York, Pergamon Press, 1979.

Weiner, R. I., and Ganong, W. F.: Role of brain monoamines and histamine in regulation of anterior pituitary secretion. Physiol. Rev., 58:905, 1978.

17

The Autonomic Nervous System; The Adrenal Medulla

The portion of the nervous system that controls the visceral functions of the body is called the *autonomic nervous system*. This system helps to control arterial pressure, gastrointestinal motility and secretion, urinary bladder emptying, sweating, body temperature, and many other activities, some of which are controlled almost entirely and some only partially by the autonomic nervous system.

GENERAL ORGANIZATION OF THE AUTONOMIC NERVOUS SYSTEM

The autonomic nervous system is activated mainly by centers located in the *spinal cord, brain stem,* and *hypothalamus.* Also, portions of the cerebral cortex and especially of the limbic system can transmit impulses to the lower centers and in this way influence autonomic control. Often the autonomic nervous system operates by means of *visceral reflexes.* That is, sensory signals enter the centers of the cord, brain stem, or hypothalamus, and these in turn transmit appropriate reflex responses back to the visceral organs to control their activities.

The autonomic impulses are transmitted to the body through two major subdivisions called the *sympathetic* and *parasympathetic systems,* the characteristics and functions of which follow.

PHYSIOLOGIC ANATOMY OF THE SYMPATHETIC NERVOUS SYSTEM

Figure 17–1 illustrates the general organization of the sympathetic nervous system, showing one of the two *paravertebral sympathetic chains* to the side of the spinal column and nerves extending to the different internal organs. The sympathetic nerves originate in the spinal cord between the segments T-1 and L-2 and pass from here first into the sympathetic chain, thence to the

tissues and organs that are stimulated by the sympathetic nerves.

Preganglionic and Postganglionic Sympathetic Neurons. The sympathetic nerves are different from skeletal motor nerves in the following way: Each motor pathway from the cord to a skeletal muscle is comprised of a single fiber. Each sympathetic pathway, on the other hand, is comprised of two fibers, a *preganglionic*

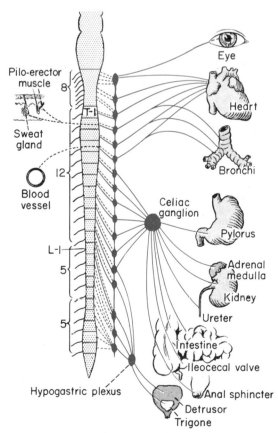

Figure 17–1. The sympathetic nervous system. Dashed lines represent postganglionic fibers in the gray rami leading into the spinal nerves for distribution to blood vessels, sweat glands, and pilo-erector muscles.

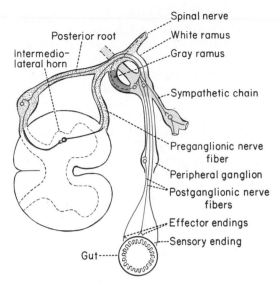

Figure 17–2. Nerve connections between the spinal cord, sympathetic chain, spinal nerves, and peripheral sympathetic nerves.

neuron and a *postganglionic neuron*. The cell body of a preganglionic neuron lies in the *intermediolateral horn* of the spinal cord, and its fiber passes, as illustrated in Figure 17–2, through an *anterior root* of the cord into a *spinal nerve*.

Immediately after the spinal nerve leaves the spinal column, the preganglionic sympathetic fibers leave the nerve and pass through the *white ramus* into one of the *ganglia* of the *sympathetic chain*. Then the course of the fibers can be one of the following three: (1) It can synapse with postganglionic neurons in the ganglion that it enters. (2) It can pass upward or downward in the chain and synapse in one of the other ganglia of the chain. Or (3) it can pass for variable distances through the chain and then through one of the nerves radiating outward from the chain, finally terminating in an *outlying sympathetic ganglion*.

The postganglionic neuron, therefore, can originate either in one of the sympathetic chain ganglia or in one of the outlying ganglia. From either of these two sources, the postganglionic fibers then travel to their destinations in the various organs.

Sympathetic Nerve Fibers in the Skeletal Nerves. Many of the postganglionic fibers pass back from the sympathetic chain into the spinal nerves through *gray rami* (see Fig. 17–2) at all levels of the cord. These pathways are made up of type C fibers that extend to all parts of the body in the skeletal nerves. They control the blood vessels, sweat glands, and piloerector muscles of the hairs. Approximately 8 per cent of the fibers in the average skeletal nerve are sympathetic fibers, a fact that indicates their importance.

Segmental Distribution of Sympathetic Nerves. The sympathetic pathways originating in the different segments of the spinal cord are not necessarily distributed to the same part of the body as the spinal nerve fibers from the same segments. Instead, the *sympathetic fibers from T-1 generally pass up the sympathetic chain into the head; from T-2 into the neck; T-3, T-4, T-5, and T-6*

into the thorax; T-7, T-8, T-9, T-10, and T-11 into the abdomen; T-12, L-1, and L-2 into the legs. This distribution is only approximate and overlaps greatly.

The distribution of sympathetic nerves to each organ is determined partly by the position in the embryo at which the organ originates. For instance, the heart receives many sympathetic nerves from the neck portion of the sympathetic chain because the heart originates in the neck of the embryo. Likewise, the abdominal organs receive their sympathetic innervation from the lower thoracic segments because the primitive gut originates in this area.

Special Nature of the Sympathetic Nerve Endings in the Adrenal Medullae. Preganglionic sympathetic nerve fibers pass, without synapsing, all the way from the intermediolateral horn cells of the spinal cord, through the sympathetic chains, through the splanchnic nerves, and finally into the adrenal medullae. There they end directly on special cells that secrete epinephrine and norepinephrine directly into the circulatory blood. These secretory cells embryologically are derived from nervous tissue and are analogous to postganglionic neurons; indeed, they even have rudimentary nerve fibers, and it is these fibers that secrete the hormones.

PHYSIOLOGIC ANATOMY OF THE PARASYMPATHETIC NERVOUS SYSTEM

The parasympathetic nervous system is illustrated in Figure 17–3, showing that parasympathetic fibers leave the central nervous system through several of the crani-

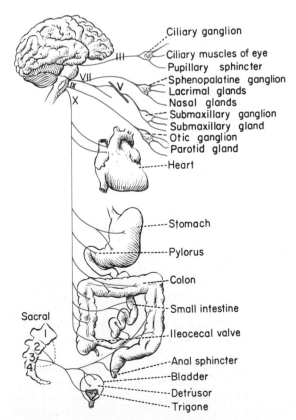

Figure 17–3. The parasympathic nervous system.

al nerves, the second and third sacral spinal nerves, and occasionally the first and fourth sacral nerves. About 75 per cent of all parasympathetic nerve fibers are in the vagus nerves, passing to the entire thoracic and abdominal regions of the body. Therefore, a physiologist speaking of the parasympathetic nervous system is thinking mainly of the two vagus nerves. The vagus nerves supply parasympathetic nerves to the heart, the lungs, the esophagus, the stomach, the small intestine, the proximal half of the colon, the liver, the gallbladder, the pancreas, and the upper portions of the ureters.

Parasympathetic fibers in the *third nerve* flow to the pupillary sphincters and ciliary muscles of the eye. Fibers from the *seventh nerve* pass to the lacrimal, nasal, and submaxillary glands, and fibers from the *ninth nerve* pass to the parotid gland.

The sacral parasympathetic fibers congregate in the form of the *nervi erigentes,* also called the *pelvic nerves,* which leave the sacral plexus on each side of the cord and distribute their peripheral fibers to the descending colon, rectum, bladder, and lower portions of the ureters. Also, this sacral group of parasympathetics supplies fibers to the external genitalia to cause various sexual reactions.

Preganglionic and Postganglionic Parasympathetic Neurons. The parasympathetic system, like the sympathetic, has both preganglionic and postganglionic neurons, but, except in the case of a few cranial parasympathetic nerves, the *preganglionic fibers* pass uninterrupted to the organ that is to be excited by parasympathetic impulses. In the wall of the organ are located the *postganglionic neurons* of the parasympathetic system. The preganglionic fibers synapse with these; then short postganglionic fibers, 1 millimeter to several centimeters in length, leave the neurons to spread in the substance of the organ. This location of the parasympathetic postganglionic neurons in the visceral organ itself is quite different from the arrangement of the sympathetic ganglia, for the cell bodies of the sympathetic postganglionic neurons are almost always located in ganglia of the sympathetic chain or in various other discrete ganglia in the abdomen rather than in the excited organ itself.

BASIC CHARACTERISTICS OF SYMPATHETIC AND PARASYMPATHETIC FUNCTION

CHOLINERGIC AND ADRENERGIC FIBERS — SECRETION OF ACETYLCHOLINE OR NOREPINEPHRINE BY THE POSTGANGLIONIC NEURONS

The sympathetic and parasympathetic nerve endings secrete one of the two synaptic transmitter substances, *acetylcholine* or *norepinephrine*. Those fibers that secrete acetylcholine are said to be *cholinergic*. Those that secrete norepinephrine are said to be *adrenergic,* a term derived from *adrenalin,* which is the British name for epinephrine.

All preganglionic neurons are cholinergic in both the sympathetic and parasympathetic nervous systems. Therefore, acetylcholine or acetylcholine-like substances, when applied to the ganglia, will excite both sympathetic and parasympathetic postganglionic neurons.

The postganglionic neurons of the parasympathetic system are also all cholinergic. On the other hand, most of the postganglionic sympathetic neurons are adrenergic, though this is not entirely so because the sympathetic nerve fibers to the sweat glands and to a few blood vessels are cholinergic.

Thus, in general, the terminal nerve endings of the parasympathetic system secrete acetylcholine, and most of the sympathetic nerve endings secrete norepinephrine. These hormones, in turn, act on the different organs to cause the respective parasympathetic and sympathetic effects. Therefore, these substances are often called respectively *parasympathetic* and *sympathetic mediators.* These are molecular structures of acetylcholine and norepinephrine:

Mechanism of Secretion of Acetylcholine and Norepinephrine by Autonomic Nerve Endings. Some of the autonomic nerve endings, especially those of the parasympathetic nerves, are similar to but much smaller in size than those of the skeletal neuromuscular junction. However, most of the sympathetic nerve fibers merely touch the effector cells of the organs that they innervate as they pass by; in some instances they terminate in connective tissue located adjacent to the cells that are to be stimulated. Where these filaments pass over or near the effector cells, they usually have bulbous enlargements called *varicosities,* and it is in these varicosities that the transmitter vesicles of acetylcholine and norepinephrine are found. Also in the varicosities are large numbers of mitochondria to supply the ATP required to energize acetylcholine or norepinephrine synthesis.

When an action potential spreads over the terminal fibers, the depolarization process increases the permeability of the fiber membrane to calcium ions, thus allowing these to diffuse in moderate numbers into the nerve terminals. There they interact with the vesicles adjacent to the membrane, causing them to fuse with the nerve membrane and to empty their contents to the exterior. Thus, the transmitter substance is secreted.

Synthesis of Acetylcholine, Its Destruction After Secretion, and Duration of Action. Acetylcholine is synthesized in the terminal endings of cholinergic nerve fibers. Most of this synthesis probably occurs in the axoplasm, and the acetylcholine is then transported to the interior of the vesicles. The basic chemical reaction of this synthesis is the following:

$$\text{Acetyl-CoA} + \text{Choline} \xrightarrow{\textit{choline acetyl transferase}} \text{Acetylcholine}$$

Once the acetylcholine has been secreted by the cholinergic nerve ending, most of it is split into acetate ion and choline by the enzyme *acetylcholinesterase* that is present both in the terminal nerve ending itself and on the surface of the receptor organ. Thus, this is the same mechanism of acetylcholine destruction that occurs at the neuromuscular junctions of skeletal nerve fibers. The choline that is formed is in turn transported back into the terminal nerve ending where it is used again for synthesis of new acetylcholine. Though most of the acetylcholine is usually destroyed within a fraction of a second after its secretion, it sometimes persists for as long as several seconds, and a small amount also diffuses into the surrounding fluids. These fluids contain a different type of cholinesterase called *serum cholinesterase* that destroys the remaining acetylcholine within another few seconds. Therefore, the action of acetylcholine released by cholinergic nerve fibers usually lasts for a few seconds at most.

Synthesis of Norepinephrine, Its Removal, and Duration of Action. Synthesis of norepinephrine begins in the axoplasm of the terminal nerve endings of adrenergic nerve fibers but is completed inside the vesicles. The basic steps are the following:

1. Tyrosine $\xrightarrow{\textit{hydroxylation}}$ DOPA

2. DOPA $\xrightarrow{\textit{decarboxylation}}$ Dopamine

3. Transport of dopamine into the vesicles

4. Dopamine $\xrightarrow{\textit{hydroxylation}}$ Norepinephrine

In the adrenal medulla this reaction goes still one step further to form epinephrine, as follows:

5. Norepinephrine $\xrightarrow{\textit{methylation}}$ Epinephrine

Following secretion of norepinephrine by the terminal nerve endings, it is removed from the secretory site in three different ways: (1) re-uptake into the adrenergic nerve endings themselves by an active transport process — accounting for removal of 50 to 80 per cent of the secreted norepinephrine; (2) diffusion away from the nerve endings into the surrounding body fluids and thence into the blood — accounting for removal of most of the remainder of the norepinephrine; and (3) destruction by enzymes to a slight extent (one of these enzymes is *monoamine oxidase,* which is found in the nerve endings themselves, and another is *catechol-O-methyl transferase,* which is present diffusely in all tissues).

Ordinarily, the norepinephrine secreted directly in a tissue by adrenergic nerve endings remains active for only a few seconds, illustrating that its re-uptake and diffusion away from the tissue are rapid. However, the norepinephrine and epinephrine secreted into the body by the adrenal medullae remain active until they diffuse into some tissue where they are destroyed by catechol-O-methyl transferase; this occurs mainly in the liver. Therefore, when secreted into the blood, both norepinephrine and epinephrine remain very active for 10 to 30 seconds, followed by decreasing activity thereafter for one to several minutes.

RECEPTOR SUBSTANCES OF THE EFFECTOR ORGANS

The acetylcholine, norepinephrine, and epinephrine secreted by the autonomic nervous system all stimulate the effector organs by first reacting with receptor substances in the effector cells. The receptor in most instances is in the cell membrane and is a protein molecule. The most likely mechanism for function of the receptor is that the transmitter substance first binds with the receptor and this causes a basic change in the molecular structure of the receptor compound. Because the receptor is in integral part of the cell membrane, this structural change often alters the permeability of the cell membrane to various ions — for instance, to allow rapid influx of sodium, chloride, or calcium ions into the cell or to allow rapid efflux of potassium ions out of the cell. These ionic changes then usually alter the membrane potential, sometimes eliciting action potentials (as occurs in smooth muscle cells) and at other times causing electrotonic effects on the cells (as occurs on glandular cells) to produce the responses. The ions themselves have direct effects within the receptor cells, such as the effect of calcium ions to promote smooth muscle contraction.

Another way that the receptor can function, besides changing the membrane permeability, is to activate an enzyme in the cell membrane and this enzyme in turn promotes chemical reactions within the cell. For instance, epinephrine increases the activity of *adenyl cyclase* in some cell membranes, and this then causes the formation of cyclic AMP at the inner surfaces of the membranes; the cyclic AMP then initiates many intracellular activities.

The Acetylcholine Receptors — "Muscarinic" and "Nicotinic" Receptors. Acetylcholine activates two different types of receptors. These are called *muscarinic* and *nicotinic* receptors. The reason for these names is that muscarine, a poison from toadstools, also activates the muscarinic receptors but will not activate the nicotinic receptors, whereas nicotine will activate only the other receptors; acetylcholine activates both of them.

The muscarinic receptors are found in all the effector cells stimulated by the postganglionic neurons of the parasympathetic nervous system as well as those stimulated by the postganglionic cholinergic neurons of the sympathetic system.

The nicotinic receptors are found in the synapses between the pre- and postganglionic neurons of both the sympathetic and parasympathetic systems and also in the membranes of skeletal muscle fibers at the neuromuscular junction (discussed in Chapter 4).

An understanding of the two different types of receptors is especially important because specific drugs are frequently used in the practice of medicine to stimulate or to block one or the other of the two types of receptors.

The Adrenergic Receptors — "Alpha" and "Beta" Receptors. Research experiments using different drugs (called *sympathomimetic drugs*) to mimic the action of norepinephrine on sympathetic effector organs have shown that there are two major types of adrenergic receptors, called *alpha receptors* and *beta receptors*. (The beta receptors in turn are divided into *beta_1* and *beta_2* receptors because certain drugs affect some beta receptors but not all.)

Norepinephrine and epinephrine, both of which are secreted by the adrenal medulla, have somewhat different effects in exciting the alpha and beta receptors. Norepinephrine excites mainly alpha receptors but excites the beta receptors to a very slight extent as well. On the other hand, epinephrine excites both types of receptors approximately equally. Therefore, the relative effects of norepinephrine and epinephrine on different effector organs is determined by the types of receptors in the organs. Obviously, if they are all beta receptors, epinephrine will be the more effective excitant.

Table 17–1 gives the distribution of alpha and beta receptors in some of the organs and systems controlled by the sympathetics. Note that certain alpha functions are excitatory while others are inhibitory. Likewise, certain beta functions are excitatory and others are inhibitory. Therefore, alpha and beta receptors are not necessarily associated with excitation or inhibition but simply with the affinity of the hormone for the receptors in a given effector organ.

A synthetic hormone chemically similar to epinephrine and norepinephrine, *isopropyl norepinephrine,* has an extremely strong action on beta receptors but essentially no action on alpha receptors. Later in the chapter we will discuss various drugs that can mimic the adrenergic actions of epinephrine and norepinephrine or that will block specifically the alpha or beta receptors.

EXCITATORY AND INHIBITORY ACTIONS OF SYMPATHETIC AND PARASYMPATHETIC STIMULATION

Table 17–2 lists the effects on different visceral functions of the body caused by stimulating the parasympathetic and sympathetic nerves. From this table it can be seen that *sympathetic stimulation causes excitatory effects in some organs but inhibitory effects in others. Likewise, parasympathetic stimulation causes excitation in some organs but inhibition in others.* Also, when sympathetic stimulation excites a particular organ, parasympathetic stimulation often inhibits it, illustrating that the two systems occasionally act reciprocally to each other. However, most organs are dominantly controlled by one or the other of the two systems.

There is no generalization one can use to explain whether sympathetic or parasympathetic stimulation will cause excitation or inhibition of a particular organ. Therefore, to understand sympathetic and parasympathetic function, one must learn the functions of these two nervous systems as listed in Table 17–2. Some of these functions need to be clarified in still greater detail as follows:

EFFECTS OF SYMPATHETIC AND PARASYMPATHETIC STIMULATION ON SPECIFIC ORGANS

The Eye. Two functions of the eye are controlled by the autonomic nervous system: These are the pupillary opening and the focus of the lens. Sympathetic stimulation contracts the meridional *fibers of the iris* and, therefore, dilates the pupil, while parasympathetic stimulation contracts the *circular muscle of the iris* to constrict the pupil. The parasympathetics that control the pupil are reflexly stimulated when excess light enters the eyes; this reflex reduces the pupillary opening and decreases the amount of light that strikes the retina. On the other hand, the sympathetics become stimulated during periods of excitement and, therefore, increase the pupillary opening at these times.

Focusing of the lens is controlled almost entirely by the parasympathetic nervous system. The lens is normally held in a flattened state by tension of its radial

TABLE 17–1. ADRENERGIC RECEPTORS AND FUNCTION

Alpha Receptor	Beta Receptor
Vasoconstriction	Vasodilatation (β_2)
Iris dilatation	Cardioacceleration (β_1)
Intestinal relaxation	Increased myocardial strength (β_1)
Intestinal sphincter contraction	Intestinal relaxation (β_2)
Pilomotor contraction	Uterus relaxation (β_2)
Bladder sphincter contraction	Bronchodilatation (β_2)
	Calorigenesis (β_2)
	Glycogenolysis (β_2)
	Lipolysis (β_1)
	Bladder relaxation (β_2)

TABLE 17–2. AUTONOMIC EFFECTS ON VARIOUS ORGANS OF THE BODY

Organ	Effect of Sympathetic Stimulation	Effect of Parasympathetic Stimulation
Eye: Pupil	Dilated	Constricted
Ciliary muscle	Slight relaxation	Contracted
Glands: Nasal	Vasoconstriction and slight	Stimulation of thin, copious
Lacrimal	secretion	secretion (containing many enzymes
Parotid		for enzyme-secreting glands)
Submaxillary		
Gastric		
Pancreatic		
Sweat glands	Copious sweating (cholinergic)	None
Apocrine glands	Thick, odoriferous secretion	None
Heart: Muscle	Increased rate	Slowed rate
	Increased force of contraction	Decreased force of atrial contraction
Coronaries	Dilated (β_2); constricted (α)	Dilated
Lungs: Bronchi	Dilated	Constricted
Blood vessels	Mildly constricted	? Dilated
Gut: Lumen	Decreased peristalsis and tone	Increased peristalsis and tone
Sphincter	Increased tone	Relaxed
Liver	Glucose released	Slight glycogen synthesis
Gallbladder and bile ducts	Relaxed	Contracted
Kidney	Decreased output	None
Bladder: Detrusor	Relaxed	Excited
Trigone	Excited	Relaxed
Penis	Ejaculation	Erection
Systemic blood vessels:		
Abdominal	Constricted	None
Muscle	Constricted (adrenergic α)	None
	Dilated (adrenergic β)	
	Dilated (cholinergic)	
Skin	Constricted	None
Blood: Coagulation	Increased	None
Glucose	Increased	None
Basal metabolism	Increased up to 100%	None
Adrenal cortical secretion	Increased	None
Mental activity	Increased	None
Piloerector muscles	Excited	None
Skeletal muscle	Increased glycogenolysis	None
	Increased strength	

ligaments. Parasympathetic excitation contracts the *ciliary muscle,* which releases this tension and allows the lens to become more convex. This causes the eye to focus on objects near at hand. The focusing mechanism is discussed in Chapters 18 and 20 in relation to function of the eyes.

The Glands of the Body. The *nasal, lacrimal, salivary,* and many *gastrointestinal glands* are all strongly stimulated by the parasympthetic nervous system, resulting in copious quantities of secretion. The glands of the alimentary tract most strongly stimulated by the parasympathetics are those of the upper tract, especially those of the mouth and stomach. The glands of the small and large intestines are controlled principally by local factors in the intestinal tract itself and not by the autonomic nerves.

Sympathetic stimulation has a slight direct effect on glandular cells in causing formation of a concentrated secretion. However, it also causes vasoconstriction of the blood vessels supplying the glands and in this way often reduces their rates of secretion.

The *sweat glands* secrete large quantities of sweat when the sympathetic nerves are stimulated, but no effect is caused by stimulating the parasympathetic nerves. However, the sympathetic fibers to most sweat glands are *cholinergic* (except for a few adrenergic fibers to palms of the hand and the soles of the feet), in contrast to most other sympathetic fibers, which are adrenergic. Furthermore, the sweat glands are stimulated primarily by centers in the hypothalamus that are usually considered to be parasympathetic centers. Therefore, sweating could be called a parasympathetic function.

The *apocrine glands* secrete a thick, odoriferous secretion as a result of sympathetic stimulation, but they do not react to parasympathetic stimulation. Furthermore, the apocrine glands, despite their close embryological relationship to sweat glands, are controlled by adrenergic fibers rather than by cholinergic fibers and are controlled by the sympathetic centers of the central nervous system rather than by the parasympathetic centers.

The Gastrointestinal System. The gastrointestinal system has its own intrinsic set of nerves known as the *intramural plexus.* However, both parasympathetic and sympathetic stimulation can affect gastrointestinal activity — parasympathetic especially. Parasympathetic stimulation, in general, increases the overall degree of activity of the gastrointestinal tract by promoting peristalsis and relaxing the sphincters, thus allowing rapid propulsion of contents along the tract. This propulsive effect is associated with simultaneous increases in rates of secretion by many of the gastrointestinal glands, which was described above.

Normal function of the gastrointestinal tract is not very dependent on sympathetic stimulation. However, in some diseases, strong sympathetic stimulation inhibits peristalsis and increases the tone of the sphincters. The net result is greatly slowed propulsion of food through the tract.

The Heart. In general, sympathetic stimulation increases the overall activity of the heart. This is accomplished by increasing both the rate and force of the heartbeat. Parasympathetic stimulation causes mainly the opposite effects, decreasing the overall activity of the heart. To express these effects in another way, sympathetic stimulation increases the effectiveness of the heart as a pump, while parasympathetic stimulation decreases its pumping capability. However, sympathetic stimulation unfortunately also greatly increases the metabolism of the heart while parasympathetic stimulation decreases its metabolism and allows the heart a degree of rest.

Systemic Blood Vessels. Most blood vessels, especially those of the abdominal viscera and the skin of the limbs, are constricted by sympathetic stimulation. Parasympathetic stimulation generally has almost no effects on blood vessels but does dilate vessels in certain restricted areas such as in the blush area of the face. Under some conditions, the beta stimulatory function of the sympathetics causes vascular dilatation, especially when drugs have paralyzed the sympathetic alpha effects.

Effect of Sympathetic and Parasympathetic Stimulation on Arterial Pressure. The arterial pressure is caused by propulsion of blood by the heart and by resistance to flow of this blood through the blood vessels. In general, sympathetic stimulation increases both propulsion by the heart and resistance to flow, which can cause the pressure to increase greatly.

On the other hand, parasympathetic stimulation decreases the pumping by the heart, which lowers the pressure a moderate amount, though not nearly so much as the sympathetics can increase the pressure.

The Lungs. In general, the structures in the lungs do not have extensive sympathetic or parasympathetic innervation. Therefore, most effects of stimulation are mild. Sympathetic stimulation can dilate the bronchi and mildly constrict the blood vessels. On the contrary, parasympathetic stimulation can cause mild constriction of the bronchi and can perhaps mildly dilate the vessels.

Effects of Sympathetic and Parasympathetic Stimulation on Other Functions of the Body. Because of the great importance of the sympathetic and parasympathetic control systems, these are discussed many times in this text in relation to a myriad of body functions that are not considered in detail here. In general, most of the entodermal structures, such as the ducts of the liver, the gallbladder, the ureter, and the bladder, are inhibited by sympathetic stimulation but excited by parasympathetic stimulation. Sympathetic stimulation also has metabolic effects, causing release of glucose from the liver, increase in blood glucose concentration, increase in glycogenolysis in muscle, increase in muscle strength, increase in basal metabolic rate, and increase in mental activity. Finally, the sympathetics and parasympathetics are involved in the execution of the male and female sexual acts, as will be explained in Chapter 25.

FUNCTION OF THE ADRENAL MEDULLAE

Stimulation of the sympathetic nerves to the adrenal medullae causes large quantities of epinephrine and norepinephrine to be released into the circulating blood, and these two hormones in turn are carried in the blood to all tissues of the body. On the average, approximately 80 per cent of the secretion is epinephrine and 20 per cent is norepinephrine, though the relative proportions of these change considerably under different physiological conditions.

The circulating epinephrine and norepinephrine have almost the same effects on the different organs as those caused by direct sympathetic stimulation, except that *the effects last about 10 times as long* because these hormones are removed from the blood slowly.

The circulating norepinephrine causes constriction of essentially all the blood vessels of the body; it causes increased activity of the heart, inhibition of the gastrointestinal tract, dilation of the pupils of the eyes, and so forth.

Epinephrine causes almost the same effects as those caused by norepinephrine, but the effects differ in the following respects: First, epinephrine has a greater effect on cardiac activity than norepinephrine. Second, epinephrine causes only weak constriction of the blood vessels of the muscles in comparison with a much stronger constriction that results from norepinephrine. Since the muscle vessels represent a major segment of all vessels of the body, this difference is of special importance because norepinephrine greatly increases the total peripheral resistance and thereby greatly elevates arterial pressure, whereas epinephrine raises the arterial pressure to a lesser extent but increases the cardiac output considerably more because of its effect on the heart and veins.

A third difference between the actions of epinephrine and norepinephrine relates to their effects on tissue metabolism. Epinephrine probably has several times as great a metabolic effect as norepinephrine. Indeed, the epinephrine secreted by the adrenal medullae increases the metabolic rate of the body often to as much as 100 per cent above normal, in this way increasing the activity and excitability of the whole body. It also increases the rate of other metabolic activities, such as glycogenolysis in the liver and muscle and glucose release into the blood.

In summary, stimulation of the adrenal medullae causes the release of hormones that have almost the same effects throughout the body as direct sympathetic stimulation, except that the effects are greatly prolonged, up to a minute or two after the stimulation is over. The only significant differences are caused by the epinephrine in the secretion, which increases the rate of metabolism and cardiac output to a greater extent than is caused by direct sympathetic stimulation.

Value of the Adrenal Medullae to the Function of the Sympathetic Nervous System.   Usually, when any part of the sympathetic nervous system is stimulated, the entire system, or at least major portions of it, is stimulated at the same time. Therefore, norepinephrine and epinephrine are almost always released by the adrenal medullae at the same time that the different organs are being stimulated directly by the sympathetic nerves. Therefore, the organs are actually stimulated in two different ways simultaneously, directly by the sympathetic nerves and indirectly by the medullary hormones. The two means of stimulation support each other, and either can usually substitute for the other. For instance, destruction of the direct sympathetic pathways to the organs does not abrogate excitation of the organs because norepinephrine and epinephrine are still released into the circulating fluids and indirectly cause stimulation. Likewise, total loss of the two adrenal medullae usually has little significant effect on the operation of the sympathetic nervous system because the direct pathways can still perform almost all the necessary duties. Thus, the dual mechanism of sympathetic stimulation provides a safety factor, one mechanism substituting for the other when the second is missing.

Another important value of the adrenal medullae is the capability of epinephrine and norepinephrine to stimulate structures of the body that are not innervated by direct sympathetic fibers. For instance, the metabolic rate of every cell of the body is increased by these hormones, especially by epinephrine, even though only a small proportion of all the cells in the body are innervated directly by sympathetic fibers.

RELATIONSHIP OF STIMULUS RATE TO DEGREE OF SYMPATHETIC AND PARASYMPATHETIC EFFECT

A special difference between the autonomic nervous system and the skeletal nervous system is the low frequency of stimulation required for full activation of autonomic effectors. In general, only one impulse every second or so suffices to maintain normal sympathetic or parasympathetic effect, and full activation occurs when the nerve fibers discharge 10 to 20 times per second. This compares with full activation in the skeletal ner-

vous system at about 75 to 200 impulses per second.

SYMPATHETIC AND PARASYMPATHETIC "TONE"

The sympathetic and parasympathetic systems are continually active, and the basal rates of activity are known, respectively, as *sympathetic tone* or *parasympathetic tone*.

The value of tone is that it allows a single nervous system to increase or to decrease the activity of a stimulated organ. For instance, sympathetic tone normally keeps almost all the blood vessels of the body constricted to approximately half their maximum diameter. By increasing the degree of sympathetic stimulation, the vessels can be constricted even more; but, on the other hand, by inhibiting the normal tone, the vessels can be dilated. If it were not for the continual sympathetic tone, the sympathetic system could cause only vasoconstriction, never vasodilatation.

Another interesting example of tone is that of the parasympathetics in the gastrointestinal tract. Surgical removal of the parasympathetic supply to the gut by cutting the vagi can cause serious and prolonged gastric and intestinal "atony," thus illustrating that in normal function the parasympathetic tone to the gut is strong. This tone can be decreased by the brain, thereby inhibiting gastrointestinal motility, or it can be increased, thereby promoting increased gastrointestinal activity.

Tone Caused by Basal Secretion of Norepinephrine and Epinephrine by the Adrenal Medullae.   The normal resting rate of secretion by the adrenal medullae is about 0.2 μgm./kg./min. of epinephrine and about 0.05 μgm./kg./min. of norepinephrine. These quantities are considerable — indeed, enough to maintain the blood pressure almost up to the normal value even if all direct sympathetic pathways to the cardiovascular system are removed. Therefore, it is obvious that much of the overall tone of the sympathetic nervous system results from basal secretion of epinephrine and norepinephrine in addition to the tone that results from direct sympathetic stimulation.

Effect of Loss of Sympathetic or Parasympathetic Tone Following Denervation.   Immediately after a sympathetic or parasympathetic nerve is cut, the innervated organ loses its sympathetic or parasympathetic tone. In the case of the blood vessels, for instance, cutting the sympathetic nerves results immediately in almost maximal vasodilatation. However, over several days or weeks, the *intrinsic tone* in the smooth muscle of the vessels increases, usually restoring almost normal vasoconstriction.

Essentially the same events occur in most effector organs whenever sympathetic or parasympathetic tone is lost. That is, intrinsic compensation soon develops to return the function of the organ almost to its normal basal level. However, in the parasympathetic system, the compensation sometimes requires many months. For instance, loss of parasympathetic tone to the heart increases the heart rate from 90 to 160 beats per minute in a dog, and this will still be about 120 beats six months later.

DENERVATION SUPERSENSITIVITY OF SYMPATHETIC AND PARASYMPATHETIC ORGANS FOLLOWING DENERVATION

During the first week or so after a sympathetic or parasympathetic nerve is destroyed, the innervated organ becomes more and more sensitive to injected norepinephrine or acetylcholine, respectively. This effect is illustrated in Figure 17–4; the blood flow in the forearm before removal of the sympathetics was 200 ml. per minute, and a test dose of norepinephrine caused only a slight depression in flow. Then the stellate ganglion was removed, and normal sympathetic tone was lost. At first, the blood flow rose markedly because of the lost vascular tone, but over a period of days to weeks the blood flow returned almost to normal because of progressive increase in intrinsic tone of the vascular musculature itself, thus compensating for the loss of sympathetic tone. Another test dose of norepinephrine was then administered and the blood flow decreased much more than before, illustrating that the blood vessels had become about two to four times as responsive to norepinephrine as previously. This phenomenon is called *denervation supersensitivity*. It occurs in both sympathetic and parasympathetic organs and to a far greater extent in some organs than in others, often increasing the response as much as 10- to 50-fold.

Mechanism of Denervation Supersensitivity. The cause of denervation supersensitivity is only partially known. Part of the answer is probably that the number of receptors in the postsynaptic membranes of the effector cells increases — sometimes many-fold — when norepinephrine or acetylcholine are no longer released at the synapses. Therefore, when these hormones appear in the circulating blood, the effector reaction is vastly enhanced.

THE AUTONOMIC REFLEXES

It is mainly by means of autonomic reflexes that the autonomic nervous system regulates visceral functions. Throughout this text the functions of these reflexes are discussed in relation to individual organ systems, but, to illustrate their importance, a few are presented here briefly.

Cardiovascular Autonomic Reflexes. Several reflexes in the cardiovascular system help to control the arterial blood pressure, cardiac output, and heart rate. One of these is the *baroreceptor reflex,* which is described in Chapter 23 along with other cardiovascular reflexes. Briefly, stretch receptors called *baroreceptors* are located in the walls of the major arteries, including the carotid arteries and the aorta. When these become stretched by high pressure, signals are transmitted to the brain stem, where they inhibit the sympathetic impulses to the heart and blood vessels, which allows the arterial pressure to fall back toward normal.

The Gastrointestinal Autonomic Reflexes. The uppermost part of the gastrointestinal tract and also the rectum are controlled principally by autonomic reflexes. For instance, the smell of appetizing food initiates signals from the nose to the vagal, glossopharyngeal, and salivary nuclei of the brain stem. These in turn transmit signals through the parasympathetic nerves to the secretory glands of the mouth and stomach, causing secretion of digestive juices even before food enters the mouth. And when fecal matter fills the rectum at the other end of the alimentary canal, sensory impulses inititated by stretching the rectum are sent to the sacral portion of the spinal cord, and a reflex signal is retransmitted through the parasympathetics to the distal parts of the colon; these result in strong peristaltic contractions that empty the bowel.

Other Autonomic Reflexes. Emptying of the bladder is controlled in the same way as emptying the rectum; stretching of the bladder sends impulses to the sacral cord, and this in turn causes contraction of the bladder as well as relaxation of the urinary sphincters, thereby promoting micturition.

Also important are the sexual reflexes which are initiated by both psychic stimuli from the brain and stimuli from the sexual organs. Impulses from these sources converge on the sacral cord and, in the male, result, first, in erection, mainly a parasympathetic function, and then in ejaculation, a sympathetic function.

Other autonomic reflexes include reflex contributions to the regulation of pancreatic secre-

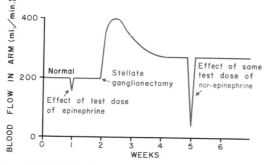

Figure 17–4. Effect of sympathectomy on blood flow in the arm, and the effect of a test dose of norepinephrine before and after sympathectomy, showing sensitization of the vasculature to norepinephrine.

tion, gallbladder emptying, urinary excretion, sweating, blood glucose concentration, and many other visceral functions, all of which are discussed in detail at other points in this text.

MASS DISCHARGE OF THE SYMPATHETIC SYSTEM VERSUS DISCRETE CHARACTERISTICS OF PARASYMPATHETIC REFLEXES

Large portions of the sympathetic nervous system often become stimulated simultaneously, a phenomenon called *mass discharge*. This characteristic of sympathetic action is in keeping with the usually diffuse nature of sympathetic function, such as overall regulation of arterial pressure or of metabolic rate.

However, in a few instances sympathetic activity does occur in isolated portions of the system. The most important of these are: (1) In the process of heat regulation, the sympathetics control sweating and blood flow in the skin without affecting other organs innervated by the sympathetics. (2) During muscular activity in some animals, cholinergic vasodilator fibers of the skeletal muscles are stimulated independently of all the remainder of the sympathetic system. (3) Many "local reflexes" involving the spinal cord but usually not the higher nervous centers affect local areas. For instance, heating a local skin area causes local vasodilatation and enhanced local sweating, while cooling causes the opposite effects.

In contrast to the sympathetic system, most reflexes of the parasympathetic system are very specific. For instance, parasympathetic cardiovascular reflexes usually act only on the heart to increase or decrease its rate of beating. Likewise, parasympathetic reflexes frequently cause secretion mainly in the mouth or, in other instances, secretion mainly in the stomach glands. Finally, the rectal emptying reflex does not affect other parts of the bowel to a major extent.

Yet there is often association between closely allied parasympathetic functions. For instance, though salivary secretion can occur independently of gastric secretion, these two often also occur together, and pancreatic secretion frequently occurs at the same time. Also, the rectal emptying reflex often initiates a bladder emptying reflex, resulting in simultaneous emptying of both the bladder and rectum. Conversely, the bladder emptying reflex can help to initiate rectal emptying.

"ALARM" OR "STRESS" FUNCTION OF THE SYMPATHETIC NERVOUS SYSTEM

From the above discussions of the sympathetic nervous system, one can already see that mass sympathetic discharge in many different ways increases the capability of the body to perform vigorous muscle activity. Let us quickly summarize these ways:

1. increased arterial pressure
2. increased blood flow to active muscles concurrent with decreased blood flow to organs that are not needed for rapid activity
3. increased rates of cellular metabolism throughout the body
4. increased blood glucose concentration
5. increased glycolysis in muscle
6. increased muscle strength
7. increased mental activity
8. increased rate of blood coagulation

The sum of these effects permits the person to perform far more strenuous physical activity than would otherwise be possible. Since it is physical *stress* that usually excites the sympathetic system, it is frequently said that the purpose of the sympathetic system is to provide extra activation of the body in states of stress: this is often called the sympathetic stress *reaction*.

The sympathetic system is also strongly activated in many emotional states. For instance, in the state of *rage,* which is elicited mainly by stimulating the hypothalamus, signals are transmitted downward through the reticular formation and spinal cord to cause massive sympathetic discharge, and all of the sympathetic events listed above ensue immediately. This is called the sympathetic *alarm reaction*. It is also frequently called the *fight or flight reaction* because an animal in this state decides almost instantly whether to stand and fight or to run. In either event, the sympathetic alarm reaction makes the animal's subsequent activities extremely vigorous.

MEDULLARY, PONTINE, AND MESENCEPHALIC CONTROL OF THE AUTONOMIC NERVOUS SYSTEM

Many areas in the reticular substance of the medulla, pons, and mesencephalon, as well as many special nuclei (see Fig. 17-5), control different autonomic functions such as arterial pressure, heart rate, glandular secretion in the upper part of the gastrointestinal tract, gastrointestinal peristalsis, the degree of contraction of the urinary bladder, and many others. The control of each of these is discussed in detail at appropriate points in this text. Suffice it to point out here that the most important factors controlled in the lower brain stem are arterial pressure, heart rate, and respiration. Indeed, transection of the brain stem at the midpontine level allows normal basal control of arterial pressure to continue as before but prevents its modulation by higher nervous centers, particularly the hypothalamus. On the other hand, transection immediately below the medulla causes

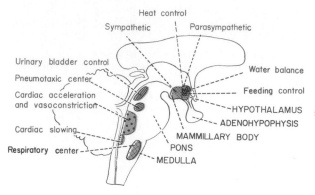

Figure 17–5. Autonomic control centers of the brain stem.

the arterial pressure to fall to about one-half normal for several hours or several days after the transection.

Closely associated with the cardiovascular regulatory centers in the medulla is the medullary center for regulation of respiration discussed in detail in Chapter 23. Though this is not considered to be an autonomic function, it is one of the *involuntary* functions of the body.

Control of Lower Brain Stem Autonomic Centers by Higher Areas. Signals from the hypothalamus and even from the cerebrum can affect the activities of almost all the lower brain stem autonomic control centers. For instance, stimulation in appropriate areas of the hypothalamus can activate the medullary cardiovascular control centers strongly enough to increase the arterial pressure to more than double normal. Likewise, other hypothalamic centers can control body temperature, increase or decrease salivation and gastrointestinal activity, or cause bladder emptying. To a great extent the autonomic centers in the lower brain stem are relay stations for control activities initiated at higher levels of the brain.

In the previous chapter it was also pointed out that many of the behavioral responses of an animal are mediated through the hypothalamus, reticular formation, and the autonomic nervous system. Indeed, the higher areas of the brain can alter the function of the whole autonomic nervous system or of portions of it strongly enough to cause severe autonomic-induced disease, such as peptic ulcer, constipation, heart palpitation, and even heart attacks.

PHARMACOLOGY OF THE AUTONOMIC NERVOUS SYSTEM

DRUGS THAT ACT ON ADRENERGIC EFFECTOR ORGANS — THE SYMPATHOMIMETIC DRUGS

From the foregoing discussion, it is obvious that intravenous injection of norepinephrine causes essentially the same effects throughout the body as sympathetic stimulation. Therefore, norepinephrine is called a *sympathomimetic,* or *adrenergic, drug.* Other sympathomimetic drugs are *epinephrine, methoxamine,* and many others. These differ from each other in the degree to which they stimulate different sympathetic effector organs and in their duration of action. Norepinephrine and epinephrine have actions as short as 1 to 2 minutes, while the actions of most other commonly used sympathomimetic drugs last 30 minutes to 2 hours.

Important drugs that stimulate specific adrenergic receptors but not the others are:

$$phenylephrine — \alpha \text{ receptors}$$
$$isoproterenol — \beta \text{ receptors}$$
$$salbutamol — \text{only } \beta_2 \text{ receptors}$$

Drugs That Cause Release of Norepinephrine from Nerve Endings. Certain drugs have a sympathomimetic action in an indirect manner rather than by directly exciting adrenergic effector organs. These drugs include ephedrine, tyramine, and amphetamine. Their effect is to cause release of norepinephrine from its storage vesicles in the sympathetic nerve endings. The norepinephrine in turn causes the sympathetic effects.

Drugs That Block Adrenergic Activity. Adrenergic activity can be blocked at several different points in the stimulatory process as follows:

1. The synthesis and storage of norepinephrine in the sympathetic nerve endings can be prevented. The best known drug that causes this effect is *reserpine.*

2. Release of norepinephrine from the sympathetic endings can be blocked. This is caused by *guanethidine.*

3. The *alpha* receptors can be blocked. Two drugs that cause this effect are *phenoxybenzamine* and *phentolamine.*

4. The beta receptors can be blocked. A drug that blocks all beta receptors is *propranolol.* One that blocks only beta₁ receptors is *practolol.*

5. Sympathetic activity can be blocked by drugs that block transmission of nerve impulses through the autonomic ganglia. These are discussed in the following section, but the most important drug for blockade of both sympathetic and parasympathetic transmission through the ganglia is *hexamethonium.*

DRUGS THAT ACT ON CHOLINERGIC EFFECTOR ORGANS

Parasympathomimetic Drugs (Muscarinic Drugs). Acetylcholine injected intravenously usually does not cause exactly the same effects throughout the body as parasympathetic stimulation because the acetylcholine is destroyed by cholinesterase in the blood and body fluids before it can reach all the effector organs. Yet a number of other drugs that are not so rapidly destroyed can produce typical parasympathetic effects, and these are called parasympathomimetic drugs.

Two commonly used parasympathomimetic drugs are *pilocarpine* and *methacholine*. These act directly on the muscarinic type of cholinergic receptors.

Parasympathomimetic drugs act on the effector organs of cholinergic *sympathetic* fibers also. For instance, these drugs cause profuse sweating. Also, they cause vascular dilatation in some organs, this effect occurring even in vessels not innervated by cholinergic fibers.

Drugs That Have a Parasympathetic Potentiating Effect. Some drugs do not have a direct effect on parasympathetic effector organs but do potentiate the effects of the naturally secreted acetylcholine at the parasympathetic endings. These are the same drugs as those listed in Chapter 4 that potentiate the effect of acetylcholine at the neuromuscular junction — that is, *neostigmine, physostigmine,* and *diisopropyl fluorophosphate.* These inhibit acetylcholinesterase, thus preventing rapid destruction of the acetylcholine liberated by the parasympathetic nerve endings. As a consequence, the quantity of acetylcholine acting on the effector organs progressively increases with successive stimuli, and the degree of action also increases.

Drugs That Block Cholinergic Activity at Effector Organs. *Atropine* and similar drugs, such as *homatropine* and *scopolamine,* block the action of acetylcholine on the muscarinic type of cholinergic effector organs. However, these drugs do not affect the nicotinic action of acetylcholine on the postganglionic neurons or on skeletal muscle.

DRUGS THAT STIMULATE THE POSTGANGLIONIC NEURONS – "NICOTINIC DRUGS"

The preganglionic neurons of both the parasympathetic and sympathetic nervous systems secrete acetylcholine at their endings, and the acetylcholine in turn stimulates the postganglionic neurons. Therefore, injected acetylcholine can also stimulate the postganglionic neurons of both systems, thereby causing both sympathetic and parasympathetic effects in the body. *Nicotine* is a drug that can also stimulate postganglionic neurons in the same manner as acetylcholine because the neuronal membranes contain *nicotinic receptors,* but it cannot directly stimulate the autonomic effector organs, which have muscarinic receptors as explained earlier in the chapter. Therefore, drugs that cause autonomic effects by stimulating the postganglionic neurons are frequently called nicotinic drugs. Some drugs, such as *acetylcholine* itself and *methacholine,* have both nicotinic and muscarinic actions, whereas pilocarpine has only muscarinic actions.

Nicotine excites both the sympathetic and parasympathetic systems at the same time, resulting in strong sympathetic vasoconstriction in the abdominal organs and limbs, but at the same time resulting in parasym-pathetic effects, such as increased gastrointestinal activity and, sometimes, slowing of the heart.

Ganglionic Blocking Drugs. Many important drugs block impulse transmission from the preganglionic neurons to the postganglionic neurons, including *tetraethyl ammonium ion, hexamethonium ion,* and *pentolinium.* These inhibit impulse transmission in both the sympathetic and parasympathetic systems simultaneously. They are often used for blocking sympathetic activity but rarely for blocking parasympathetic activity, because the sympathetic blockade usually far overshadows the effects of parasympathetic blockade. The ganglionic blocking drugs have been especially important in reducing arterial pressure in patients with hypertension.

REFERENCES

Aviado, D. M., *et al.* (eds.): Pharmacology of Ganglionic Transmission. New York, Springer-Verlag, 1979.

Axelrod, J.: Neurotransmitters. *Sci. Am., 230*(6):58, 1974.

Bhagat, B. D.: Mode of Action of Autonomic Drugs. Flushing, N.Y., Graceway Publishing Company, 1979.

Black, I. B.: Regulation of autonomic development. *Annu. Rev. Neurosci., 1*:183, 1978.

Brooks, C. M., *et al.* (eds.): Integrative Functions of the Autonomic Nervous System. Tokyo, University of Tokyo Press, 1979.

Carrier, O., Jr.: Pharmacology of the Peripheral Autonomic Nervous System. Chicago, Year Book Medical Publishers, 1972.

Collier, B.: Biochemistry and physiology of cholinergic tranmission. *In* Brookhart, J. M., and Mountcastle, V. B. (eds.): Handbook of Physiology. Sec. 1, Vol. I. Baltimore, Williams & Wilkins, 1977, p. 463.

DeQuattro, V., *et al.*: Anatomy and biochemistry of the sympathetic nervous system. *In* DeGroot, L. J., *et al.* (eds.): *Endocrinology.* Vol. 2. New York, Grune & Stratton, 1979, p. 1241.

Eränkö, O.: Small intensely fluorescent (SIF) cells and nervous transmission in sympathetic ganglia. *Annu. Rev. Pharmacol. Toxicol., 18*:417, 1978.

Geffen, L. B., and Jarrott, B.: Cellular aspects of catecholaminergic neurons. *In* Brookhart, J. M., and Mountcastle, V. B. (eds.): Handbook of Physiology. Sec. 1, Vol. 1. Baltimore, Williams & Wilkins, 1977, p. 521.

Guyton, A. C., and Gillespie, W. M., Jr.: Constant infusion of epinephrine: Rate of epinephrine secretion and destruction in the body. *Am. J. Physiol., 165*:319, 1951.

Guyton, A. C., and Reeder, R. C.: Quantitative studies on the autonomic actions of curare. *J. Pharmacol. Exp. Ther., 98*:188, 1950.

Haber, E., and Wrenn, S.: Problems in identification of the beta-adrenergic receptor. *Physiol. Rev., 56*:317, 1976.

Hayward, J. N.: Functional and morphological aspects of hypothalamic neurons. *Physiol. Rev., 57*:574, 1977.

Kalsner, S. (ed.): Trends in Autonomic Pharmacology. Baltimore, Urban & Schwarzenberg, 1979.

Kunos, G.: Adrenoceptors. *Annu. Rev. Pharmacol. Toxicol., 18*:291, 1978.

Landsberg, L., and Young, J. B.: Catecholamines and the adrenal medulla. *In* Bondy, P. K., and Rosenberg, L. E. (eds.): Metabolic Control and Disease, 8th Ed. Philadelphia, W. B. Suunders Co., 1980, p. 1621.

Levitzki, A.: Catecholamine receptors. *In* Adrian, R. H., *et al.* (eds.): Reviews of Physiology, Biochemistry, and Pharmacology. New York, Springer-Verlag, 1978, p. 1.

Mason, C. A., and Bern, H. A.: Cellular biology of the neurosecretory neuron. *In* Brookhart, J. M., and Mountcastle, V. B. (eds.): Handbook of Physiology. Sec. 1, Vol. 1. Baltimore, Williams & Wilkins, 1977, p. 651.

Miyahara, M., and Simpson, F. O.: Adrenoreceptor blockers in cardiovascular therapy. *In* Hayase, S., and Murao, S. (eds.): Cardiology: Proceedings of the VIII World Congress of Cardiology, Tokyo, 1978. New York, Elsevier/North-Holland, 1979, p. 460.

Moore, R. Y., and Bloom, F. E.: Central catecholamine neuron systems: Anatomy and physiology of the dopamine system. *Annu. Rev. Neurosci., 1*:129, 1978.

Morgane, P. J., and Panksepp, J. (eds.): Handbook of the hypothalamus. New York, Marcel Dekker, 1979.

Paton, D. M. (ed.): The Release of Catecholamines from Adrenergic Neurons. New York, Pergamon Press, 1979.

Patterson, P. H.: Environmental determination of autonomic neurotransmitter functions. *Annu. Rev. Neurosci., 1*:1, 1978.

Rémond, A., and Izard, C. (eds.): Electrophysiological Effects of Nicotine. New York, Elsevier/North Holland, 1979.

Robinson, R.: Tumours That Secrete Catecholamines: A Study of Their Natural History and Their Diagnosis. New York, John Wiley & Sons, 1980.

Simon, P. (ed.): Neurotransmitters. New York, Pergamon Press, 1979.

Szabadi, E., *et al.*: Recent Advances in the Pharmacology of Adrenoceptors. New York, Elsevier/North-Holland, 1978.

Tǔcek, S. (eds.): The Cholinergic Synapse. New York, Elsevier/North-Holland, 1979.

Usdin, E., *et al.* (eds.): Catecholamines: Basic and Clinical Frontiers. New York, Pergamon Press, 1979.

von Euler, U. S.: Noradrenaline. Springfield, Ill., Charles C Thomas, 1956.

Westfall, T. C.: Local regulation of adrenergic neurotransmission. *Physiol. Rev., 57*:659, 1977.

Wolf, S. G.: Neural control of visceral function. *In* Frohlich, E. D. (ed.): Pathophysiology, 2nd Ed. Philadelphia, J. B. Lippincott Co., 1976, p. 711.

Part III
THE SPECIAL SENSES

18

The Eye:
I. Optics of Vision

PHYSICAL PRINCIPLES OF OPTICS

Before it is possible to understand the optical system of the eye, the student must be thoroughly familiar with the basic physical principles of optics, including the physics of refraction, a knowledge of focusing, depth of focus, and so forth. Therefore, in the present study of the optics of the eye, a brief review of these physical principles is first presented, and then the optics of the eye is discussed.

REFRACTION OF LIGHT

The Refractive Index of a Transparent Substance. Light rays travel through air at a velocity of approximately 300,000 kilometers per second but much slower through transparent solids and liquids. The refractive index of a transparent substance is the *ratio* of the velocity of light in air to that in the substance. Obviously, the refractive index of air itself is 1.00.

If light travels through a particular type of glass at a velocity of 200,000 kilometers per second, the refractive index of this glass is 300,000 divided by 200,000, or 1.50.

Refraction of Light Rays at an Interface Between Two Media with Different Refractive Indices. When light waves traveling forward in a beam, as shown in the upper part of Figure 18–1, strike an interface that is perpendicular to the beam, the waves enter the second refractive medium without deviating in their course. The only effect that occurs is decreased velocity of transmission. On the other hand, as illustrated in the lower part of Figure 18–1, if the light waves strike an angulated interface, the light waves bend if the refractive indices of the two media are different from each other. In this particular figure the light waves are leaving air, which has a refractive index of 1.00, and are entering a block of glass having a refractive index of 1.50. When the beam first strikes the angulated interface, the lower edge of the beam enters the glass ahead of the upper edge. The wave front in the upper portion

of the beam continues to travel at a velocity of 300,000 kilometers per second while that which has entered the glass travels at a velocity of 200,000 kilometers per second. This causes the upper portion of the wave front to move ahead of the lower portion so that it is no longer vertical but is angulated to the right. Because *the direction in which light travels is always perpendicular to the wave front,* the direction of travel of the light beam now bends downward.

The bending of light rays at an angulated interface is known as *refraction*. Note particularly that the degree of refraction increases as a function of (1) the ratio of the two refractive indices of the two transparent media and (2) the degree of angulation between the interface and the entering wave front.

APPLICATION OF REFRACTIVE PRINCIPLES TO LENSES

The Convex Lens. Figure 18–2 shows parallel light rays entering a convex lens. The light rays passing

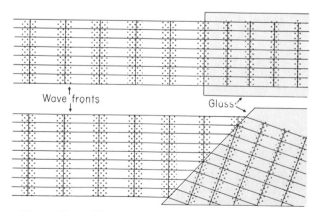

Figure 18–1. Wave fronts entering *(top)* a glass surface perpendicular to the light rays and *(bottom)* a glass surface angulated to the light rays. This figure illustrates that the distance between waves after they enter the glass is shortened to approximately two-thirds that in air. It also illustrates that light rays striking an angulated glass surface are refracted.

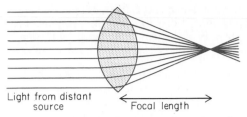

Figure 18–2. Bending of light rays at each surface of a convex spherical lens, showing that parallel light rays are focused to a point focus.

through the center of the lens strike the lens exactly perpendicular to the lens surfaces and therefore pass through the lens without being refracted at all. Toward either edge of the lens, however, the light rays strike a progressively more angulated interface. Therefore, the outer rays bend more and more toward the center. Half of the bending occurs when the rays enter the lens and half as they exit from the opposite side.

Thus, parallel light rays entering an appropriately formed convex lens come to a single point focus at some distance beyond the lens.

The Concave Lens. Figure 18–3 shows the effect of a concave lens on parallel light rays. The rays that enter the very center of the lens strike an interface that is absolutely perpendicular to the beam and, therefore, do not refract at all. The rays at the edge of the lens enter the lens ahead of the rays toward the center. This is opposite to the effect in the convex lens, and it causes the peripheral light rays to *diverge* away from the light rays that pass through the center of the lens.

Thus, the concave lens *diverges* light rays, while the convex lens *converges* light rays.

Spherical Versus Cylindrical Lenses. Figure 18–4 illustrates both a convex *spherical* lens and a convex *cylindrical* lens. Note that the convex cylindrical lens bends light rays from the two sides of the lens but not from either the top or the bottom. Therefore, parallel light rays are bent to a focal *line*. On the other hand, light rays that pass through the spherical lens are refracted at all edges of the lens toward the central ray, and all the rays come to a focal *point*.

The cylindrical lens is well illustrated by a test tube full of water. If the test tube is placed in a beam of sunlight and a piece of paper is brought progressively

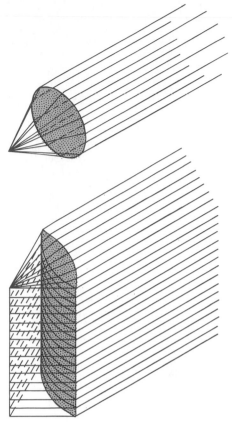

Figure 18–4. *Top:* Point focus of parallel light rays by a spherical convex lens. *Bottom:* Line focus of parallel light rays by a cylindrical convex lens.

closer to the tube, a certain distance will be found at which the light rays come to a focal line. On the other hand, the spherical lens is illustrated by an ordinary magnifying glass. If such a lens is placed in a beam of sunlight and a piece of paper is brought progressively closer to the lens, the light rays will impinge on a common focal point at an appropriate distance.

Concave cylindrical lenses *diverge* light rays in only one plane in the same manner that *convex* cylindrical lenses *converge* light rays in one plane.

Figure 18–5 shows two convex cylindrical lenses at right angles to each other. The vertical cylindrical lens causes convergence of the light rays that pass through the two sides of the lens. The horizontal lens converges the top and bottom rays. Thus, all the light rays come to a single point focus. In other words, *two cylindrical lenses crossed at right angles to each other perform the same function as one spherical lens of the same refractive power.*

FOCAL LENGTH OF THE CONVEX LENS

The distance from a convex lens at which parallel rays converge to a common focal point is the *focal length* of the lens. The diagram at the top of Figure 18–6 illustrates this focusing of parallel light rays. In the middle diagram of Figure 18–6, the light rays that enter the convex lens are not parallel but are diverging because

Figure 18–3. Bending of light rays at each surface of a concave spherical lens, illustrating that parallel light rays are diverged by a concave lens.

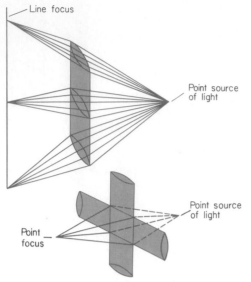

Figure 18–5. Two cylindrical convex lenses at right angles to each other, illustrating that one lens converges light rays in one plane and the other lens converges light rays in the plane at right angles. The two lenses combined give the same point focus as that obtained with a spherical convex lens.

the origin of the light is a point source not far away from the lens itself. The rays striking the center of the lens pass through the lens without any refraction as pointed out above. And the rays striking the edges are refracted toward the center. However, because these rays are diverging outward from the point source, it can be seen from the diagram that they do not come to a point focus at the same distance away from the lens as do parallel

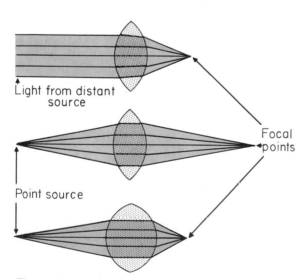

Figure 18–6. The upper two lenses of this figure have the same strength, but the light rays entering the top lens are parallel, while those entering the second lens are diverging; the effect of parallel versus diverging rays on the focal distance is illustrated. The bottom lens has far more refractive power than either of the other two lenses, illustrating that the stronger the lens the nearer to the lens is the point focus.

rays. In other words, when rays of light that are already diverging enter a convex lens, the distance of focus on the other side of the lens is farther from the lens than is the case when the entering rays are parallel to each other.

In the lower diagram of Figure 18–6 are shown light rays that also are diverging toward a convex lens that has far greater curvature than that of the upper two lenses of the figure. In this diagram the distance from the lens at which the light rays come to a focus is exactly the same as that from the lens in the first diagram, in which the lens was less convex but the rays entering it were parallel. This illustrates that both parallel rays and diverging rays can be focused at the same distance behind a lens provided that the lens changes its convexity. It is obvious that the nearer the point source of light is to the lens, the greater is the divergence of the light rays entering the lens and the greater must be the curvature of the lens to cause focusing at the same distance.

The relationship of focal length of the lens, distance of the point source of light, and distance of focus is expressed by the following formula:

$$\frac{1}{f} = \frac{1}{a} + \frac{1}{b}$$

in which f is the focal length of the lens, a the distance of the point source of light from the lens, and b the distance of focus from the lens.

FORMATION OF AN IMAGE BY A CONVEX LENS

The upper drawing of Figure 18–7 illustrates a convex lens with two point sources of light to the left. Because light rays from any point source pass through the center of a convex lens without being refracted in either direction, the light rays from each point source of light are shown to come to a point focus behind the lens *directly in line with the point source and the center of the lens.*

Any object in front of the lens is in reality a mosaic of point sources of light. Some of these points are very bright, some are very weak, and they vary in color. The light rays from each point source of light that enter the very center of the convex lens pass directly through this lens without any of the rays bending. Furthermore, the light rays that enter the edges of the lens come to focal points behind the lens in line with the rays that pass through the center. Therefore, every point source of light on the object comes to a separate point focus on the opposite side of the lens. If all portions of the object are the same distance in front of the lens, all the focal points behind the lens will fall in a common plane a certain distance behind the lens. If a white piece of paper is placed at this distance, one can see an image of the object, as is illustrated in the lower portion of Figure 18–7. However, this image is upside down with respect to the original object, and the two lateral sides of the image are reversed with respect to the original. This is the method by which the lens of a camera focuses light rays on the camera film.

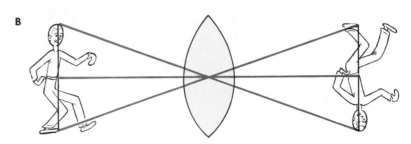

Figure 18–7. A, Two point sources of light focused at two separate points on the opposite side of the lens. B, Formation of an image by a convex spherical lens.

MEASUREMENT OF THE REFRACTIVE POWER OF A LENS – THE DIOPTER

The more a lens bends light rays, the greater is its "refractive power." This refractive power is measured in terms of *diopters*. The refractive power of a convex lens is equal to 1 meter divided by its focal length. Thus a spherical lens has a refractive power of +1 diopter if it converges parallel light rays to a focal point 1 meter beyond the lens, as illustrated in Figure 18–8. If the lens is capable of bending parallel light rays twice as much as a lens with a power of +1 diopter, it is said to have a strength of +2 diopters, and, obviously, the light rays come to a focal point 0.5 meter beyond the lens. A lens capable of converging parallel light rays to a focal point only 10 cm. ($^1/_{10}$ meter) beyond the lens has a refractive power of +10 diopters.

The refractive power of concave lenses cannot be stated in terms of the focal distance beyond the lens because the light rays diverge rather than focusing to a point. Therefore, the power of a concave lens is stated in terms of its ability to diverge light rays in comparison with the ability of convex lenses to converge light rays. That is, if a concave lens diverges light rays the same

amount that a 1 diopter convex lens converges them, the concave lens is said to have a dioptric strength of –1. Likewise, if the concave lens diverges the light rays as much as a +10 diopter lens converges them, it is said to have a strength of –10 diopters.

Note particularly that concave lenses can "neutralize" the refractive power of convex lenses. Thus, placing a 1 diopter concave lens immediately in front of a 1 diopter convex lens results in a lens system with zero refractive power.

The strengths of cylindrical lenses are computed in the same manner as the strengths of spherical lenses. If a cylindrical lens focuses parallel light rays to a line focus 1 meter beyond the lens, it has a strength of +1 diopter. On the other hand, if a cylindrical lens of a concave type *diverges* light rays as much as a +1 diopter cylindrical lens *converges* them, it has a strength of –1 diopter.

THE OPTICS OF THE EYE

THE EYE AS A CAMERA

The eye, as illustrated in Figure 18–9, is optically equivalent to the usual photographic camera, for it has a lens system, a variable aperture system (the

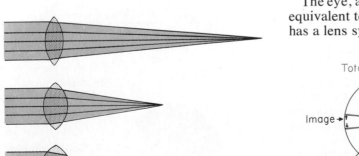

Figure 18–8. Effect of lens strength on the focal distance.

Figure 18–9. The eye as a camera. The numbers are the refractive indices.

pupil), and a retina that corresponds to the film. The lens system of the eye is composed of (1) the interface between air and the anterior surface of the cornea, (2) the interface between the posterior surface of the cornea and the aqueous humor, (3) the interface between the aqueous humor and the anterior surface of the lens, and (4) the interface between the posterior surface of the lens and the vitreous humor. The refractive index of air is 1; the cornea, 1.38; the aqueous humor, 1.33; the lens (on the average), 1.40; and the vitreous humor, 1.34.

The Reduced Eye. If all the refractive surfaces of the eye are algebraically added together and then considered to be one single lens, the optics of the normal eye may be simplified and represented schematically as a "reduced eye." This is useful in simple calculations. In the reduced eye, a single lens is considered to exist with its central point 17 mm. in front of the retina and to have a total refractive power of approximately 59 diopters when the lens is accommodated for distant vision.

The anterior surface of the cornea provides about 48 diopters of the eye's total dioptric strength for three reasons: (1) the refractive index of the cornea is markedly different from that of air; (2) the surface of the cornea is farther away from the retina than are the surfaces of the eye lens; and (3) the curvature of the cornea is reasonably great.

The posterior surface of the cornea is concave and actually acts as a concave lens, but, because the difference in refractive index of the cornea and the aqueous humor is slight, this posterior surface of the cornea has a refractive power of only about −4 diopters, which neutralizes only a small part of the refractive power of the other refractive surfaces of the eye.

The total refractive power of the crystalline lens of the eye when it is surrounded by fluid on each side is only 15 diopters of the total refractive power of the eye's lens system. If this lens were removed from the eye and then surrounded by air, its refractive power would be about 150 diopters. Thus, it can be seen that the lens inside the eye is not nearly so powerful as it would be outside the eye. The reason for this is that the fluids surrounding the lens have refractive indices not greatly different from the refractive index of the lens itself, the smallness of the differences greatly decreasing the amount of light refraction at the lens interfaces. But the importance of the crystalline lens is that its curvature, and therefore also its strength, can be changed to provide accommodation, which will be discussed later in the chapter.

Formation of an Image on the Retina. In exactly the same manner that a glass lens can focus an image on a sheet of paper, the lens system of the eye can also focus an image on the retina. The image is inverted and reversed with respect to the object. However, the mind perceives objects in the upright position despite the upside-down orientation on the retina because the brain is trained to consider an inverted image as the normal.

THE MECHANISM OF ACCOMMODATION

The refractive power of the crystalline lens of the eye can be voluntarily increased from 15 diopters to approximately 29 diopters in young children; this is a total "accommodation" of 14 diopters. To do this, the shape of the lens is changed from that of a moderately convex lens to that of a very convex lens. The mechanism of this is the following:

Normally, the lens is composed of a strong elastic capsule filled with viscous, proteinaceous, but transparent fibers. When the lens is in a relaxed state, with no tension on its capsule, it assumes a spherical shape, owing entirely to the elasticity of the lens capsule. However, as illustrated in Figure 18–10, approximately 70 ligaments attach radially around the lens, pulling the lens edges toward the edge of the choroid. These ligaments are constantly tensed by the elastic pull of their attachments to the choroid, and the tension on the ligaments causes the lens to remain relatively flat under normal resting conditions of the eye. At the insertions of the ligaments in the choroid is the ciliary muscle, which has two sets of smooth muscle fibers, the *meridional fibers* and the *circular fibers*. The meridional fibers extend from the corneoscleral junction to the insertions of the ligaments in the choroid approximately 2 to 3 mm. behind the corneoscleral junction. When

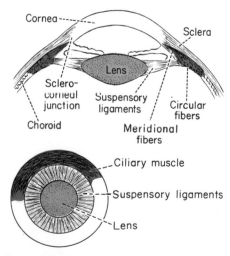

Figure 18–10. Mechanism of accommodation.

these muscle fibers contract, the insertions of the ligaments are pulled forward, thereby releasing a certain amount of tension on the crystalline lens. The circular fibers are arranged circularly all the way around the eye so that when they contract a sphincter-like action occurs, decreasing the diameter of the circle of ligament attachments and allowing the ligaments to pull less on the lens capsule.

Thus, contraction of both sets of smooth muscle fibers in the ciliary muscle relaxes the ligaments to the lens capsule, and the lens assumes a more spherical shape, like that of a balloon, because of elasticity of its capsule. When the ciliary muscle is completely relaxed, the dioptric strength of the lens is as weak as it can become. On the other hand, when the ciliary muscle contracts as strongly as possible, the dioptric strength of the lens becomes maximal.

Autonomic Control of Accommodation. The ciliary muscle is controlled mainly by the parasympathetic nervous system but also to a slight extent by the sympathetic system, as will be discussed in Chapter 20. Stimulation of the parasympathetic fibers to the eye contracts the ciliary muscle, which in turn relaxes the ligaments of the lens and increases its refractive power. With an increased refractive power, the eye is capable of focusing on objects that are nearer to it than is an eye with less refractive power. Consequently, as a distant object moves toward the eye, the number of parasympathetic impulses impinging on the ciliary muscle must be progressively increased for the eye to keep the object constantly in focus. (Sympathetic stimulation has a weak effect in relaxing the ciliary muscle but this plays almost no role in the normal accommodation mechanism, the neurology of which will be discussed in Chapter 20.)

Presbyopia. As a person grows older, the lens loses its elastic nature and becomes a relatively solid mass, probably because of progressive denaturation of the lens proteins. Therefore, the ability of the lens to assume a spherical shape progressively decreases, and the power of accommodation decreases from approximately 14 diopters shortly after birth to approximately 2 diopters at the age of 45 to 50. Thereafter, the lens may be considered to be almost totally nonaccommodating, a condition known as "presbyopia."

Once a person has reached the state of presbyopia, each eye remains focused permanently at an almost constant distance; this distance depends on the physical characteristics of each individual's eyes. Obviously, the eyes can no longer accommodate for both near and far vision. Therefore, to see clearly both in the distance and nearby, an older person must wear bifocal glasses with the upper segment normally focused for far-seeing and the lower segment focused for near-seeing.

THE PUPILLARY APERTURE

A major function of the iris is to increase the amount of light that enters the eye during darkness and to decrease the light in bright light. The reflexes for controlling this mechanism will be considered in the discussion of the neurology of the eye in Chapter 20. The amount of light that enters the eye through the pupil is proportional to the area of the pupil or to the *square of the diameter* of the pupil. The pupil of the human eye can become as small as approximately 1.5 mm. and as large as 8 mm. in diameter. Therefore, the quantity of light entering the eye may vary approximately 30 times as a result of changes in pupillary aperture.

Depth of Focus of the Lens System of the Eye. Figure 18–11 illustrates two separate eyes that are exactly alike except for the diameters of the pupillary apertures. In the upper eye the pupillary aperture is small, and in the lower eye the aperture is large. In front of each of these two eyes are two small point sources of light, and light from each passes through the pupillary aperture and focuses on the retina. Consequently, in both eyes the retina sees two spots of light in perfect focus. It is evident from the diagrams, however, that if the retina is moved forward or backward to an out-of-focus position, the size of each spot will not change much in the upper eye, but in the lower eye the size of each spot will increase greatly, becoming a "blur circle." In other words, the upper lens system has far greater *depth of focus* than the bottom lens system. When a lens system has great depth of focus, the retina can be considerably displaced from the focal plane and still the image remains in sharp focus; whereas, when a lens system has a shallow depth of focus, moving the retina only slightly away from the focal plane causes extreme blurring.

The greatest possible depth of focus occurs when the pupil is extremely small. The reason for

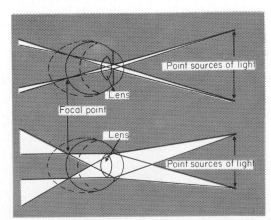

Figure 18–11. Effect of small and large pupillary apertures on the depth of focus.

this is that with a very small aperture the eye acts more or less as a pinhole camera. It will be recalled from the study of physics that light rays coming from an object and passing through a pinhole are in focus on any surface at all distances beyond the pinhole. In other words, the depth of focus of a pinhole camera is infinite.

"NORMAL" ABERRATIONS OF VISION

Spherical Aberration. The crystalline lens of the eye is not nearly so regularly formed as lenses made by good opticians. Indeed, the light rays passing through the peripheral edges of the eye lens are not brought to really sharp focus with the other light rays, as illustrated in Figure 18–12. This effect is known as "spherical aberration," and the lens system of the human eye is quite subject to such an error. Therefore, increasing the aperture of the pupil progressively decreases the sharpness of focus. This partially explains why visual acuity is decreased at low illumination levels, which cause the pupil to dilate.

Chromatic Aberration. The lens of the eye is also subject to "chromatic aberration," which is illustrated in Figure 18–13. This means that the refractive power of the lens is different for the different colors, so that different colors focus at different distances behind the lens. Furthermore, the greater the aperture of the lens, the greater are the errors of chromatic aberration, for those light rays passing near the center of the lens are proportionately less affected than are the rays passing through the periphery of the lens.

Diffractive Errors of the Eye. Still another error in the optical system of all eyes is "diffraction" of light rays. Diffraction means bending of light rays as they pass over sharp edges; this obviously occurs as the rays pass over the edges of the pupil. Diffractive errors become especially important when the pupil becomes very small, because "interference" patterns then appear on the retina. A thorough consideration of diffraction at this point is impossible, and this phenomenon is noted simply to explain that as the pupil becomes 1.5 mm. in size the sharpness of vision becomes less than when the pupil is approximately 2.5 mm. in size, despite the fact that the depth of focus is better the smaller the pupillary diameter.

Cataracts. Cataracts are an especially common eye abnormality that occurs in older people. A cataract is a cloudy or opaque area in the lens. In the early stage of cataract formation the proteins in the lens fibers immediately beneath the capsule become denatured. Later, these same proteins coagulate to form opaque areas in place of the normal transparent protein fibers of the

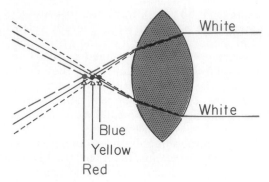

Figure 18–13. Chromatic aberration.

lens. Finally, in still later stages, calcium is often deposited in the coagulated proteins, thus further increasing the opacity.

When a cataract has obscured light transmission so greatly that it seriously impairs vision, the condition can be corrected by surgical removal of the entire lens. When this is done, however, the eye loses a large portion of its refractive power, which must be replaced by a powerful convex lens (about +15 diopters) in front of the eye, as will be explained in the following sections.

ERRORS OF REFRACTION

Emmetropia. As shown in Figure 18–14, the eye is considered to be normal or "emmetropic" if, when the ciliary muscle is completely relaxed, parallel light rays from distant objects are in sharp focus on the retina. This means that the emmetropic eye can, with its ciliary muscle completely relaxed, see all distant objects clearly, but to focus objects at close range it must contract its

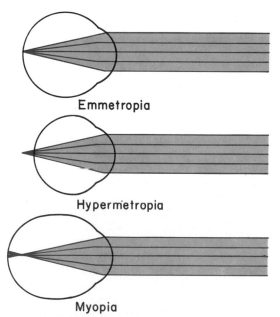

Emmetropia

Hypermetropia

Myopia

Figure 18–14. Parallel light rays focus on the retina in emmetropia, behind the retina in hypermetropia, and in front of the retina in myopia.

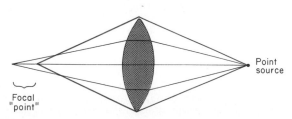

Point source

Focal "point"

Figure 18–12. Spherical aberration.

ciliary muscle and thereby provide various degrees of accommodation.

Hypermetropia (Hyperopia). Hypermetropia, which is also known as "far-sightedness," is usually due either to an eyeball that is too short or occasionally to a lens system that is too weak when the ciliary muscle is completely relaxed. In this condition, parallel light rays are not bent sufficiently by the lens system to come to a focus by the time they reach the retina. In order to overcome this abnormality, the ciliary muscle may contract to increase the strength of the lens. Therefore, the far-sighted person is capable, by using the mechanism of accommodation, of focusing distant objects on the retina. If he has used only a small amount of strength in his ciliary muscle to accommodate for the distant objects, then he still has much accommodative power left, and objects closer and closer to the eye can also be focused sharply until the ciliary muscle has contracted to its limit. The distance of the object away from the eye at this point is known as the "near point" of vision.

In old age, when the lens becomes presbyopic, the far-sighted person often is not able to accommodate his lens sufficiently to focus even distant objects, much less to focus near objects.

Myopia. In myopia, or "near-sightedness," when the ciliary muscle is completely relaxed, the light rays coming from distant objects are focused in front of the retina. This is usually due to too long an eyeball but it can occasionally result from too much power of the lens system of the eye.

No mechanism exists by which the eye can decrease the strength of its lens to less than that which exists when the ciliary muscle is completely relaxed. Therefore, the myopic person has no mechanism by which he can ever focus distant objects sharply on his retina. However, as an object comes nearer to his eye it finally comes near enough that its image will focus on the retina. Then, when the object comes still closer to the eye, the person can use his mechanism of accommodation to keep the image focused clearly. Therefore, a myopic person has a definite limiting "far point" for clear vision as well as a "near point"; when an object comes inside the "far point," he can use his mechanism of accommodation to keep the object in focus until the object reaches the "near point."

Correction of Myopia and Hypermetropia by Use of Lenses. It will be recalled that light rays passing through a concave lens diverge. Therefore, if the refractive surfaces of the eye have too much refractive power, as in myopia, some of this excessive refractive power can be neutralized by placing in front of the eye a concave spherical lens, which will diverge rays. On the other hand, in a person who has hypermetropia — that is, someone who has too weak a lens for the distance of the retina from the lens — the abnormal vision can be corrected by adding refractive power with a convex lens in front of the eye. These corrections are illustrated in Figure 18–15. One usually determines the strength of the concave or convex lens needed for clear vision by "trial and error" — that is, by trying first a strong lens and then a stronger or weaker lens until the one that gives the best visual acuity is found.

Astigmatism. Astigmatism is a refractive error of the lens system of the eye caused usually by an oblong shape of the cornea or, rarely, by an oblong shape of the

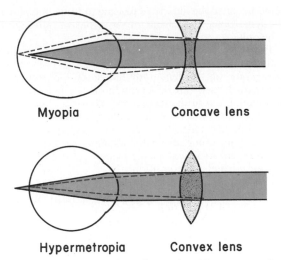

Figure 18–15. Correction of myopia with a concave lens, and correction of hypermetropia with a convex lens.

lens. A lens surface like the side of an egg lying edgewise to the incoming light would be an example of an astigmatic lens. The degree of curvature in a plane through the long axis of the egg is not nearly so great as the degree of curvature in a plane through the short axis. The same is true of an astigmatic lens. Because the curvature of the astigmatic lens along one plane is less than the curvature along the other plane, light rays striking the peripheral portions of the lens in one plane are not bent nearly so much as are rays striking the peripheral portions of the other plane.

This is illustrated in Figure 18–16, which shows what happens to rays of light emanating from a point source and passing through an oblong astigmatic lens. The light rays in the vertical plane, which is indicated by plane BD, are refracted greatly by the astigmatic lens because of the greater curvature in the vertical direction than in the horizontal direction. However, the light rays in the horizontal plane, indicated by plane AC, are bent not nearly so much as the light rays in the vertical plane. It is obvious, therefore, that the light rays passing through an astigmatic lens do not all come to a common focal

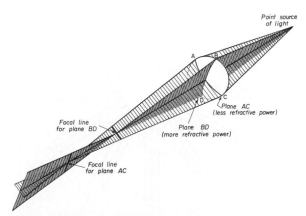

Figure 18–16. Astigmatism, illustrating that light rays focus at one focal distance in one focal plane and at another focal distance in the plane at right angles.

point because the light rays passing through one plane of the lens focus far in front of those passing through the other plane.

Placing an appropriate *spherical* lens in front of an astigmatic eye can bring the light rays that pass through *one plane* of the lens into focus on the retina, but spherical lenses can never bring *all* the light rays into complete focus at the same time. This is the reason why astigmatism is a very undesirable refractive error of the eyes. Furthermore, the accommodative powers of the eyes cannot compensate for astigmatism for the same reasons that spherical lenses placed in front of the eyes cannot correct the condition.

Correction of Astigmatism with a Cylindrical Lens. In correcting astigmatism with lenses it must always be remembered that two cylindrical lenses of equal strength may be crossed at right angles to give the same refractive effects as those of a spherical lens of the same strength. However, if one of the crossed cylindrical lenses has a different strength from that of the second lens, the light rays in one plane may not be brought to a common focal point with the light rays in the opposite plane. This is the situation that one usually finds in the astigmatic eye. In other words, one may consider an astigmatic eye as having a lens system made up of two cylindrical lenses of slightly different strengths. Another way of looking at the astigmatic lens system of the eye is that this system is a spherical lens with a superimposed cylindrical lens.

To correct the focusing of an astigmatic lens system, it is necessary to determine both the *strength* of the cylindrical lens needed to neutralize the excess cylindrical power of the eye lens and the *axis* of this abnormal cylindrical lens.

There are several methods for determining the axis of the abnormal cylindrical component of the lens system of an eye. One of these methods is based on the use of parallel black bars as shown in Figure 18–17. Some of these parallel bars are vertical, some horizontal, and some at various angles to the vertical and horizontal axes. After placing, by trial and error, various spherical

Figure 18–17. Chart composed of parallel black bars for determining the axis (meridian) of astigmatism.

lenses in front of the astigmatic eye, a strength of lens will usually be found that will cause sharp focus on one set of these parallel bars on the retina of the astigmatic eye. If there is no accompanying myopia or hypermetropia, the spherical lens may not be necessary.

It can be shown from the physical principles of optics discussed earlier in this chapter that the axis of the *out-of-focus* cylindrical component of the optical system is parallel to the black bars that are fuzzy in appearance. Once this axis is found, the examiner tries progressively stronger and weaker positive or negative cylindrical lenses, the axes of which are placed parallel to the out-of-focus bars, until the patient sees all the crossed bars with equal clarity. When this has been accomplished, the examiner directs the optician to grind a special lens having both the spherical correction plus the cylindrical correction at the appropriate axis.

Correction of Optical Abnormalities by Use of Contact Lenses. In recent years, either glass or plastic contact lenses have been fitted snugly against the anterior surface of the cornea. These lenses are held in place by a thin layer of tears that fill the space between the contact lens and the anterior eye surface.

A special feature of the contact lens is that it nullifies almost entirely the refraction that normally occurs at the anterior surface of the cornea. The reason for this is that the tears between the contact lens and the cornea have a refractive index almost equal to that of the cornea so that no longer does the anterior surface of the cornea play a significant role in the eye's optical system. Instead, the anterior surface of the contact lens now plays the major role and its posterior surface a minor role. Thus, the refraction of this lens now substitutes for the cornea's usual refraction. This is especially important in persons whose eye refractive errors are caused by an abnormally shaped cornea, such as persons who have an odd-shaped, bulging cornea — a condition called *keratoconus.* Without the contact lens the bulging cornea causes such severe abnormality of vision that almost no glasses can correct the vision satisfactorily; when a contact lens is used, however, the corneal refraction is neutralized, and normal refraction by the contact lens is substituted in its place.

The contact lens has several other advantages as well, including (1) the lens turns with the eye and gives a broader field of clear vision than do usual glasses, and (2) the contact lens has little effect on the size of the object that the person sees through the lens; on the other hand, lenses placed several centimeters in front of the eye do affect the size of the image even though they correct the focus.

SIZE OF THE IMAGE ON THE RETINA AND VISUAL ACUITY

If the distance from an object to the eye lens is 17 meters and the distance from the center of the lens to the image is 17 millimeters, the ratio of the object size to image size is 1000 to 1. Therefore, an object 17 meters in front of the eye and 1 meter in size produces an image on the retina 1 millimeter in size.

Theoretically, a point of light from a distant

point source, when focused on the retina, should be infinitely small. However, since the lens system of the eye is not perfect, such a retinal spot ordinarily has a total diameter of about 11 microns even with maximal resolution of the optical system. However, it is brightest in its very center and shades off gradually toward the edges, as illustrated by the two point images in Figure 18–18.

The average diameter of cones *in the fovea* of the retina, the central part of the retina where vision is most highly developed, is approximately 1.5 microns, which is one-seventh the diameter of the spot of light. Nevertheless, since the spot of light has a bright center point and shaded edges, a person can distinguish two separate points if their centers lie approximately 2 microns apart on the retina, which is slightly greater than the width of a foveal cone. This discrimination between points is illustrated in Figure 18–18.

The maximum visual acuity of the human eye for discriminating between point sources of light is 26 seconds. That is, when light rays from two separate points strike the eye with an angle of at least 26 seconds between them, they can usually be recognized as two points instead of one. This means that a person with maximal acuity looking at two bright pinpoint spots of light 10 meters away can barely distinguish the spots as separate entities when they are 1 millimeter apart.

The fovea is less than a millimeter in diameter, which means that maximum visual acuity occurs in only 3 degrees of the visual field. Outside this foveal area the visual acuity is reduced 5- to 10-fold, and it becomes progressively poorer as the periphery is approached. This is caused by the connection of many rods and cones to the same nerve fiber, as discussed in Chapter 20.

Clinical Method for Stating Visual Acuity. Usually the test chart for testing eyes is placed 20 feet away from the tested person, and ·if the person can see the letters of the size that he should be able to see at 20 feet, he is said to have 20/20 vision: that is, normal vision. If he can see

only letters that he should be able to see at 200 feet, he is said to have 20/200 vision. On the other hand, if he can see at 20 feet letters that he should be able to see only at 15 feet, he is said to have 20/15 vision. In other words, the clinical method for expressing visual acuity is to use a mathematical fraction that expresses the ratio of two distances, which is also the ratio of one's visual acuity to that of the normal person.

DETERMINATION OF DISTANCE OF AN OBJECT FROM THE EYE – DEPTH PERCEPTION

There are three major means by which the visual apparatus normally perceives distance, a phenomenon that is known as depth perception. These are (1) relative sizes of objects, (2) moving parallax, and (3) stereopsis.

Determination of Distance by Relative Sizes. If a person knows that a man is six feet tall and then he sees this man even with only one eye, he can determine how far away the man is simply by the size of the man's image on his retina. He does not consciously think about the size of this image, but his brain has learned to determine automatically from image sizes the distances of objects from the eye when the dimensions of these objects are already known.

Determination of Distance by Moving Parallax. Another important means by which the eyes determine distance is that of moving parallax. If a person looks off into the distance with his eyes completely still, he perceives no moving parallax, but, when he moves his head to one side or the other, the images of objects close to him move rapidly across his retinae while the images of distant objects remain rather stationary. For instance, if he moves his head 1 inch and an object is only 1 inch in front of his eye, the image moves almost all the way across his retinae, whereas the image of an object 200 feet away from his eyes does not move perceptibly. Thus, by this mechanism of moving parallax, one can tell the *relative distances* of different objects even though only one eye is used.

Determination of Distance by Stereopsis. Another method by which one perceives parallax is that of binocular vision. Because one eye is a little more than 2 inches to one side of the other eye, the images on the two retinae are different one from the other — that is, an object that is 1 inch in front of the bridge of the nose forms an image on the temporal portion of the retina of each eye, while a small object 20 feet in front of the nose has its image at closely corresponding points in the middle of each retina. This type of parallax is illustrated in Figure 18–19, which shows the images of a black spot and a square actually reversed on the

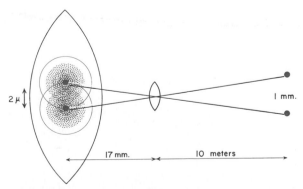

Figure 18–18. Maximum visual acuity for two point sources of light.

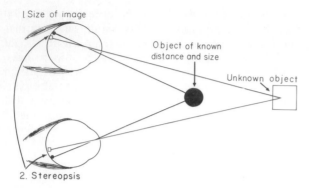

Figure 18–19. Perception of distance (1) by the size of the image on the retina, and (2) as a result of stereopsis.

retinae because they are at different distances in front of the eyes. This gives a type of parallax that is present all the time when both eyes are being used. It is almost entirely this binocular parallax (or stereopsis) that gives a person with two eyes far greater ability to judge relative distances *when objects are nearby* than a person who has only one eye. However, stereopsis is virtually useless for depth perception at distances beyond 200 feet.

OPTICAL INSTRUMENTS

THE OPHTHALMOSCOPE

The ophthalmoscope is an instrument designed so that an observer can look through it into another person's eye and see the retina with clarity. Though the ophthalmoscope appears to be a relatively complicated instrument, its principles are simple. The basic components are illustrated in Figure 18–20 and may be explained as follows.

If a bright spot of light is on the retina of an emmetropic eye, light rays from the spot diverge toward the lens system of the eye, and, after they pass through the lens system, they are parallel with each other because the retina is located in the focal plane of the lens. When these parallel rays pass into an emmetropic eye of another person, they focus to a point on the retina of the second person because his retina is in the focal plane of his lens. Therefore, any spot of light on the

retina of the observed eye comes to a focal spot on the retina of the observing eye. Likewise, when the bright spot of light is moved to different points on the observed retina, the focal spot on the retina of the observer also moves an equal amount. Thus, if the retina of one person is made to emit light, the image of his retina will be focused on the retina of the observer provided the two eyes are simply looking into each other. These principles, of course, apply only to completely emmetropic eyes.

To make an ophthalmoscope, one need only devise a means for illuminating the retina to be examined. Then, the reflected light from that retina can be seen by the observer simply by putting the two eyes close to each other. To illuminate the retina of the observed eye, an angulated mirror or a segment of a prism is placed in front of the observed eye in such a manner that light from a bulb is reflected into the observed eye. Thus, the retina is illuminated through the pupil, and the observer sees into the subject's pupil by looking over the edge of the mirror or prism, or preferably *through* an appropriately designed prism so that the light will not have to enter the pupil at an angle.

It was noted above that these principles apply only to persons with completely emmetropic eyes. If the refractive power of either eye is abnormal, it is necessary to correct this refractive power in order for the observer to see a sharp image of the observed retina. Therefore, the usual ophthalmoscope has a series of about 20 lenses mounted on a turret so that the turret can be rotated from one lens to another, and the correction for abnormal refractive power of either or both eyes can be made at the same time by selecting a single lens of appropriate strength. In normal young adults, when the two eyes come close together, a natural accommodative reflex occurs that causes approximately +2 diopters increase in the strength of the lens of each eye. To correct for this, it is necessary that the lens turret be rotated to approximately −4 diopters correction.

THE RETINOSCOPE

The retinoscope, illustrated in Figure 18–21, is an instrument that can be used to determine the refractive power of an eye even though the subject cannot converse with the observer. Such a procedure is valuable for fitting glasses to an infant.

To use the retinoscope, one places a bright spot of light behind and to one side of the observed eye, and stands 1 meter away, looking through a hole in the

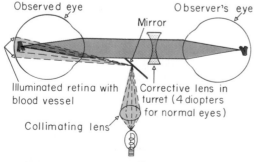

Figure 18–20. The optical system of the ophthalmoscope.

Figure 18–21. The retinoscope.

middle of a mirror. The observer then rotates this mirror from side to side, making a reflected beam of light travel across the pupil of the observed eye while the subject keeps his gaze intently on the observer's eye. If the observed eye is normal, when the edge of this beam of light first enters the pupil, the entire pupil suddenly glows red. If the eye has abnormal refractive power, the red glow appears either on the side of the pupil into which the light edge first shines or on the opposite side of the pupil — one or the other. *In hypermetropia the first glow appears on the side of the pupil from which the light beam is being moved. In myopia the first glow appears on the opposite side of the pupil.* The cause of this difference is that the lens of the hyperopic eye is too weak and that of the myopic eye too strong to focus the light from the edge of the pupil on the retina exactly in line with the observer's eye. For a fuller understanding of this effect, however, the student is referred to texts on physiologic optics.

One can fit glasses to a patient by placing selected lenses in front of the observed eye one at a time until the glow suddenly covers the pupil over its entire extent rather than spreading from one side of the pupil to the other. However, it should be noted that in retinoscopy one tests an eye that is focused on the observer's eye at 1 meter's distance. This must be taken into consideration in prescribing glasses; 1 diopter strength must be subtracted for far vision.

REFERENCES

Allen, E. W.: Essentials of Ophthalmic Optics. New York, Oxford University Press, 1979.

Campbell, C. J., *et al.*: Physiological Optics. Hagerstown, Md., Harper & Row, 1974.

Collins, R., and Van der Werff, T. J.: Mathematical Models of the Dynamics of the Human Eye. New York, Springer-Verlag, 1980.

Davson, H.: The Physiology of the Eye, 3rd Ed. New York. Academic Press, 1972.

Davson, H., and Graham, L. T., Jr.: The Eye. Vols. 1–6. New York, Academic Press, 1969–1974.

Dick, G. L.: Studies in Ocular Anatomy and Physiology. Kensington, N. S. W., New South Wales University Press, 1976.

Hartstein, J.: Basics of Contact Lenses, 3rd Ed. San Francisco, American Academy of Ophthalmology, 1979.

Kavner, R. S., and Dusky, L.: Total Vision. New York, A & W Publishers, 1980.

Kolder, H. E. J. W. (ed.): Cataracts. Boston, Little, Brown, 1978.

Lerman, S.: Radiant Energy and the Eye. New York, The Macmillan Co., 1979.

Miller, D.: Ophthalmology; The Essentials. Boston, Houghton Mifflin, 1979.

Morgan, M. W.: The Optics of Ophthalmic Lenses. Chicago, Professional Press, 1978.

Polyak, S.: The Vertebrate Visual System. Chicago, University of Chicago Press, 1957.

Records, R. E.: Physiology of the Human Eye and Visual System. Hagerstown, Md., Harper & Row, 1979.

Regan, D., *et al.*: The visual perception of motion in depth. *Sci. Am., 241*(1):136, 1979.

Roth, H. W., and Roth-Wittig, M.: Contact Lenses. Hagerstown, Md., Harper & Row, 1980.

Ruben, M.: Understanding Contact Lenses (and the Correction of the Abnormal Eye). London, Heinemann Health Books, 1975.

Safir, A. (ed.): Refraction and Clinical Optics. Hagerstown, Md., Harper & Row, 1980.

Sloane, A. E. (ed.): Manual of Refraction. Boston, Little, Brown, 1979.

Soft Contact Lenses. New York, Elsevier/North-Holland, 1977.

Toates, F. M.: Accommodation function of the human eye. *Physiol. Rev., 52*:828, 1972.

Van Heyningen, R.: What happens to the human lens in cataract. *Sci. Am., 233*(6):70, 1975.

Whitnall, S. E.: The Anatomy of the Human Orbit and Accessory Organs of Vision. Huntington, N.Y., R. E. Krieger Publishing Co., 1979.

Whitteridge, D.: Binocular vision and cortical function. *Proc. R. Soc. Med., 65*:947, 1972.

Witkovsky, P.: Peripheral mechanisms of vision. *Annu. Rev. Physiol., 33*:257, 1971.

19

The Eye: II. Receptor Functions of the Retina

The retina is the light-sensitive portion of the eye, containing the cones which are responsible for color vision, and the rods, which are mainly responsible for vision in the dark. When the rods and cones are excited, signals are transmitted through successive neurons in the retina itself and finally into the optic nerve fibers and cerebral cortex. The purpose of the present chapter is to explain specifically the mechanisms by which the rods and cones detect both white and colored light.

ANATOMY AND FUNCTION OF THE STRUCTURAL ELEMENTS OF THE RETINA

The Layers of the Retina. Figure 19–1 shows the functional components of the retina arranged in layers from the outside to the inside as follows: (1) pigment layer, (2) layer of rods and cones projecting into the pigment, (3) outer lining membrane, (4) outer nuclear layer, (5) outer plexiform layer, (6) inner nuclear layer, (7) inner plexiform layer, (8) ganglionic layer, (9) layer of optic nerve fibers, and (10) inner limiting membrane.

After light passes through the lens system of the eye and then through the vitreous humor, it enters the retina from the bottom (see Figure 19–1); that is, it passes through the ganglion cells, the plexiform layer, the nuclear layer, and the limiting membranes before it finally reaches the layer of rods and cones located all the way on the opposite side of the retina. This distance is a thickness of several hundred microns; visual acuity is obviously decreased by this passage through such non-homogeneous tissue. However, in the central region of the retina, as will be discussed below, the initial layers are pulled aside to prevent this loss of acuity.

The Foveal Region of the Retina and Its Importance in Acute Vision. A minute area in the center of the retina, illustrated in Figure 19–2, called the *macula* and occupying a total area of less than 1 square millimeter, is especially capable of acute and detailed vision. This area is composed entirely of cones, but the cones are very much elongated and have a diameter of only 1.5 microns in contradistinction to the very large cones located farther peripherally in the retina. The central portion of the macula, only 0.4 mm. in diameter, is called the *fovea;* in this region the blood vessels, the ganglion cells, the inner nuclear layer of cells, and the plexiform layers are all displaced to one side rather than resting directly on top of the cones. This allows light to pass unimpeded to the cones rather than through several layers of retina, which aids immensely in the acuity of visual perception by this region of the retina.

The Rods and Cones. Figure 19–3 is a diagrammatic representation of a photoreceptor, either a rod or a cone, though the cones are distinguished by having a conical upper end (the outer segment), as shown in Figure 19–4. In general, the rods are narrower and longer than the cones, but this is not always the case. In the peripheral portions of the retina the rods are 2 to 5

Figure 19–1. Plan of the retinal neurons. (From Polyak: The Retina. University of Chicago Press.)

244

Figure 19–2. Photomicrograph of the macula and of the fovea in its center. Note that the inner layers of the retina are pulled to the side to decrease the interference with light transmission. (From Bloom and Fawcett: A Textbook of Histology, 10th Ed. Philadelphia, W. B. Saunders Company, 1975; courtesy of H. Mizoguchi.)

microns in diameter while the cones are 5 to 8 microns in diameter; in the central part of the retina, in the fovea, the cones have a diameter of only 1.5 microns.

To the right in Figure 19–3 are labeled the four major functional segments of either a rod or a cone: (1) the outer segment, (2) the inner segment, (3) the nucleus, and (4) the synaptic body. In the outer segment the light-sensitive photochemical is found. In the case of the rods, this is *rhodopsin,* and in the cones it is one of several photochemicals almost exactly the same as rhodopsin except for a difference in spectral sensitivity. The cross-marks in the outer segment represent discs,

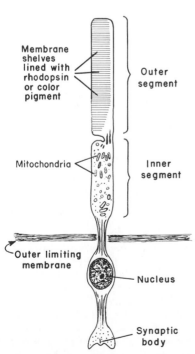

Figure 19–3. Schematic drawing of the functional parts of the rods and cones.

or "shelves," formed by infoldings of the cell membrane. The photosensitive pigments are incorporated into these membranes as part of their structures. They are concentrated at each surface of the membrane — both the inside and the outside surfaces. In this outer segment the concentration of the photosensitive pigment is approximately 40 per cent.

The inner segment contains the usual cytoplasm of the cell with the usual cytoplasmic organelles. Particularly important are the mitochondria, for we shall see later that the mitochondria in this segment play an important role in providing most of the energy for function of the photoreceptors.

The synaptic body is the portion of the rod and cone that connects with the subsequent neuronal cells, the horizontal and bipolar cells, that represent the next stages in the vision chain.

Figure 19–4 shows in more detail the photoreceptor discs in the outer segments of the rods and cones. Note especially their relationships to the cell membrane from which they originated.

Regeneration of Photoreceptors. The inner segments of the rods continually synthesize new rhodopsin. This in turn migrates to the base of the outer segment, where the cell membrane is continually forming new folds that become the discs of the rod and to which the rhodopsin attaches. Several new discs are formed each hour, and these migrate outward along the rod toward the tip, carrying the new rhodopsin with them. When the discs reach the top they degenerate and are dissoluted by the pigment epithelium. Thus, the light receptor portion of the rod is continually being replaced.

On the other hand, new disc formation does not seem to occur in the cones. However, new visual pigment does migrate throughout the outer segment, and local repair of the disc system does seem to occur.

These processes of disc generation and repair are probably necessary to provide continually viable photoreceptor chemical mechanisms in the photoreceptors.

The Pigment Layer of the Retina. The black pigment

Figure 19–4. Membranous structures of the outer segments of a rod (left) and a cone (right). (Courtesy of Dr. Richard Young.)

melanin in the pigment layer, and still more melanin in the choroid, prevent light reflection throughout the globe of the eyeball, and this is extremely important for clear vision. This pigment performs the same function in the eye as does the black paint inside the bellows of a camera. Without it, light rays would be reflected in all directions within the eyeball and would cause diffuse lighting of the retina rather than the contrast between dark and light spots required for formation of precise images.

The importance of melanin in the pigment layer and choroid is well illustrated by its absence in *albinos,* persons hereditarily lacking in melanin pigment in all parts of their bodies. When an albino enters a bright area, light that impinges on the retina is reflected in all directions by the white surface of the unpigmented choroid so that a single discrete spot of light that would normally excite only a few rods or cones is reflected everywhere and excites many of the receptors. Also, a large amount of diffuse light enters the eye through the unpigmented iris. Thus, the lack of melanin causes the visual acuity of albinos, even with the best of optical correction, to be rarely better than 20/100 to 20/200. The pigment layer also stores large quantities of *vitamin A.* This vitamin A is exchanged back and forth through the membranes of the outer segments of the rods and cones, which themselves are embedded in the pigment layer. We shall see later that vitamin A is an important precursor of the photosensitive pigments and that this interchange of vitamin A is very important for adjustment of the light sensitivity of the receptors.

The Blood Supply of the Retina — the Retinal Arterial System and the Choroid. The nutrient blood supply for the inner layers of the retina is derived from the central retinal artery, which enters the inside of the eye along with the optic nerve and then divides to supply the entire inner retinal surface. Thus, to a great extent, the retina has its own blood supply independent of the other structures of the eye.

However, the outer layer of the retina is adherent to the *choroid,* which is a highly vascular tissue between the retina and the sclera. The outer layers of the retina, including the outer segments of the rods and cones, depend mainly on diffusion from the choroid vessels for their nutrition, especially for their oxygen.

Retinal Detachment. The neural retina occasionally detaches from the pigment epithelium. In a few instances the cause of such detachment is injury to the eyeball that allows fluid or blood to collect between the retina and the pigment epithelium, but more often it is caused by contracture of fine collagenous fibrils in the vitreous humor, which pull the retina unevenly toward the interior of the globe.

Fortunately, partly because of diffusion across the detachment gap and partly because of the independent blood supply to the retina through the retinal artery, the retina can resist degeneration for a number of days and can become functional once again if surgically replaced in its normal relationship with the pigment epithelium. But, if not replaced soon, the retina finally degenerates and then is unable to function even after surgical repair.

PHOTOCHEMISTRY OF VISION

Both the rods and cones contain chemicals that decompose on exposure to light and, in the process, excite the nerve fibers leading from the eye. The chemical in the *rods* is called *rhodopsin*, and the light-sensitive chemicals in the *cones* have compositions only slightly different from that of rhodopsin.

In the present section we will discuss principally the photochemistry of rhodopsin, but we can apply almost exactly the same principles to the photochemistry of the color-sensitive substances of the cones.

THE RHODOPSIN-RETINAL VISUAL CYCLE, AND EXCITATION OF THE RODS

Rhodopsin and Its Decomposition by Light Energy. The outer segment of the rod that projects into the pigment layer of the retina has a concentration of about 40 per cent of the light-sensitive pigment called *rhodopsin* or *visual purple*. This substance is a combination of the protein *scotopsin* and the carotenoid pigment *retinal* (also called "retinene"). Furthermore, the retinal is a particular type called 11-*cis* retinal. This *cis* form of the retinal is important because only this form can combine with scotopsin to synthesize rhodopsin.

When light energy is absorbed by rhodopsin, the rhodopsin immediately begins to decompose, as shown in Figure 19–5. The cause of this is photoactivation of electrons in the retinal portion of

Figure 19–5. Photochemistry of the rhodopsin-retinal— vitamin A visual cycle.

the rhodopsin, which leads to an instantaneous change of the *cis* form of retinal into an all-*trans* form, which still has the same chemical structure as the *cis* form but has a different physical structure — a straight molecule rather than a curved molecule. Because the three-dimensional orientation of the reactive sites of the all-*trans* retinal no longer fits with that of the reactive sites on the protein scotopsin, it begins to pull away from the scotopsin. The immediate product is *bathorhodopsin* (also called "prelumirhodopsin"), which is a partially split combination of the all-*trans* retinal and scotopsin. However, bathorhodopsin is an extremely unstable compound and decays in nanoseconds to *lumirhodopsin*. This decays in microseconds to *metarhodopsin I,* then in about a millisecond to *metarhodopsin II,* and finally, much more slowly (in about a minute), to *pararhodopsin.* All of these are loose combinations of the all-*trans* retinal and scotopsin, but the pararhodopsin, too, is unstable, and it decomposes during the next few minutes into completely split products — scotopsin and all-*trans* retinal. During the first stages of splitting, the rods are excited, and signals are transmitted into the central nervous system.

Reformation of Rhodopsin. The first stage in reformation of rhodopsin, as shown in Figure 19–5, is to reconvert the all-*trans* retinal into 11-*cis* retinal. This process is catalyzed by the enzyme *retinal isomerase*. However, this process also requires metabolic energy from the rods and cones. Once the 11-*cis* retinal is formed, it automatically recombines with the scotopsin to reform rhodopsin, an exergonic process (which means that it gives off energy). The product, rhodopsin, is a stable compound until its decomposition is again triggered by absorption of light energy.

Excitation of the Rods When Rhodopsin Decomposes. Although the exact way in which rhodopsin decomposition excites the rod is still speculative, it is believed to occur in the following general way: The *retinal* portion of rhodopsin is a photosensitive compound that becomes activated in the presence of light. The initial effect of the light is to cause photoexcitation of electrons in the retinal molecule, raising these electrons to higher energy states. During this excited state, the internal physical structure (but not yet its chemical structure) begins to change, and the ultimate effect is conversion of the 11-*cis*-retinal into all-*trans*-retinal. All this occurs within nanoseconds or microseconds, and at the same time the retinal portion of the rhodopsin molecule undergoes a conformational change, from an angulated molecular structure of the *cis* form to a straight molecular structure of the *trans* form. Then, in rapid succession, the rhodopsin decomposes chemically through the several stages of decomposition products as described above.

But, how does this photoexcitation and decomposition of the rhodopsin molecule excite the rod? Rod stimulation is believed to occur at the very instant that the rhodopsin molecule becomes excited by the light. The instantaneous effect on the rod is a sudden *decrease* in electrical conductance of the rod membrane, which leads to a change in the membrane potential, as we shall discuss subsequently.

Because stimulation of the rod takes place at the very outset of rhodopsin decomposition, it is believed that the initial photoexcitation of the retinal portion of the rhodopsin molecule is the prime cause of the stimulation. This could occur in one of several ways: One of the suggestions has been that the excited electrons themselves in some way lead directly to a change in the membrane conductance. A second suggestion has been that the excited electrons cause a change in a second chemical substance that in turn affects membrane conductance. Still a third suggestion has been that the rhodopsin molecule itself undergoes an instantaneous conformational change that alters the actual physical structure of the membrane, in this way changing its conductance at the same time; this theory is based principally on the fact that the rhodopsin molecules are actually a physical part of the membrane structure itself.

The physical construction of the outer segment of the rod is compatible with all these concepts because the cell membrane folds inward to form tremendous numbers of shelf-like discs lying one on top of the other, each one lined on both the inside and outside of the membrane with aggregates of rhodopsin. This extensive relationship between rhodopsin and the cell membrane could explain why the rod is so exquisitely sensitive to light, being capable of detectable excitation following absorption of only one quantum of light energy.

Generation of the Receptor Potential.   Regardless of the precise mechanism by which the membrane of the outer segment becomes altered in the presence of decomposing rhodopsin, it is known that this excitation process *decreases* the conductance of this membrane for sodium ions. Based on this fact, the following theory for development of the receptor potential has been proposed:

Figure 19–6 illustrates movement of sodium ions in a complete electrical circuit through the inner and outer segments of the rod. The inner segment continually pumps sodium from inside the rod to the outside, thereby creating a negative potential on the inside of the entire cell. However, the membrane of the outer segment of the rod, in the unexcited condition, is very leaky to sodium. Therefore, sodium continually leaks back to the

Figure 19–6. Theoretical basis for the generation of a hyperpolarization receptor potential caused by rhodopsin decomposition.

inside of the rod and thereby neutralizes much of the negativity on the inside of the entire cell. Thus, under normal conditions, when the rod is not excited, there is a reduced amount of electronegativity inside the membrane of the rod.

When the rhodopsin in the outer segment of the rod is exposed to light and begins to decompose, however, this *decreases* the leakage of sodium to the interior of the rod even though sodium continues to be pumped out. Thus, a net loss of sodium from the rod creates increased negativity inside the membrane, and the greater the amount of light energy striking the rod, the greater the electronegativity. This process is called *hyperpolarization*. Furthermore, it is exactly opposite to the effect that occurs in almost all other sensory receptors in which the degree of negativity is generally reduced during stimulation rather than increased, producing a state of depolarization rather than hyperpolarization.

Characteristics of the Receptor Potential.   The receptor potential has two phases: an instantaneous, very low voltage phase, the electrical potential of which is directly proportional to the light energy; and a secondary phase of much greater voltage, the potential of which is proportional to the logarithm of the light energy. The first potential is believed to result from the immediate interaction of light with the rhodopsin. The second is believed to result from the sodium current mechanism described above.

This transduction of light energy into a logarithmic type of receptor potential seems to be an exceedingly important one for function of the eye, because it allows the eye to discriminate light intensities through a range many thousand times as great as would otherwise be possible.

Relationship Between Retinal and Vitamin A. The lower part of the scheme in Figure 19–5 illustrates that each of the two types of retinal can be converted into corresponding types of *retinol* and *retinyl ester,* both of which are forms of vitamin A. In turn, both of these can be reconverted into the two types of retinal. Thus, the two retinals are in dynamic equilibrium with vitamin A. Most of the vitamin A of the retina is stored in the pigment layer of the retina rather than in the rods themselves, but this vitamin A is readily available to the rods.

An important feature of the conversion of retinal into vitamin A, or the converse conversion of vitamin A into retinal, is that these processes require a longer time to approach equilibrium than it takes for conversion of retinal and scotopsin into rhodopsin, or for conversion (under the influence of strong light energy) of rhodopsin into retinal and scotopsin. Therefore, all the reactions of the upper part of Figure 19–5 can take place relatively rapidly in comparison with the slower interconversions between retinal and vitamin A.

Yet if the retina remains exposed to strong light for a long time, most of the stored rhodopsin will be converted eventually into vitamin A, thereby decreasing the concentration of all the photochemicals in the rods much more than would be true were it not for this subsequent conversion.

Conversely, during total darkness, essentially all the retinal already in the rods becomes converted into rhodopsin within a few minutes. This then allows much of the vitamin A to be converted into still additional retinal, which also becomes rhodopsin within another few minutes. Thus, when a person remains in complete darkness for a prolonged period of time, not only is almost all the retinal of his rods converted into rhodopsin but also much of the vitamin A stored in the pigment layer of the retina is absorbed by the rods and also converted into rhodopsin.

Night Blindness. Night blindness occurs in severe vitamin A deficiency. When the total quantity of vitamin A in the blood becomes greatly reduced, the quantities of vitamin A, retinal, and rhodopsin in the rods, as well as the color photosensitive chemicals in the cones, are all depressed, thus decreasing the sensitivities of the rods and cones. This condition is called night blindness because at night the amount of available light is far too little to permit adequate vision, though in daylight, sufficient light is available to excite the rods and cones despite their reduction in photochemical substances.

For night blindness to occur, a person often must remain on a vitamin A–deficient diet for months, because large quantities of vitamin A are normally stored in the liver and are made available to the rest of the body in times of need. However, once night blindness does develop it can sometimes be completely cured in a half hour or more by intravenous injection of vitamin A. This results from the ready conversion of vitamin A into retinal and thence into rhodopsin.

PHOTOCHEMISTRY OF COLOR VISION BY THE CONES

It was pointed out at the outset of this discussion that the photochemicals in the cones have almost exactly the same chemical composition as that of rhodopsin in the rods. The only difference is that the protein portions, the opsins, called *photopsins* in the cones, are different from the scotopsin of the rods. The retinal portions are exactly the same in the cones as in the rods. The color-sensitive pigments of the cones, therefore, are combinations of retinal and photopsins.

In the discussion of color vision later in the chapter, it will become evident that three different types of photochemicals are present in different cones, thus making these cones selectively sensitive to the different colors of blue, green, and red. These photochemicals are called respectively *blue-sensitive pigment, green-sensitive pigment,* and *red-sensitive pigment.* The absorption characteristics of the pigments in the three types of cones show peak absorbencies at light wavelengths, respectively, of 430, 535, and 575 millimicrons. These are also the wavelengths for peak light sensitivity for each type of cone, which begins to explain how the retina differentiates the colors. The approximate absorption curves for these three pigments are shown in Figure 19–7. The peak absorption for the rhodopsin of the rods, on the other hand, occurs at 505 millimicrons.

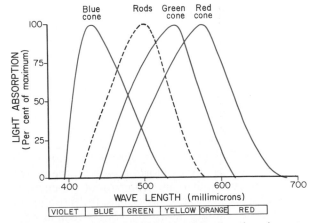

Figure 19–7. Light absorption by the respective pigments of the three color-receptive cones of the human retina. (Drawn from curves recorded by Marks, Dobelle, and MacNichol, Jr.: *Science, 143*:1181, 1964, and by Brown and Wald: *Science, 144*:45, 1964.)

Note that the peak absorption of the so-called "red" cone is actually in the orange color band. It is called the "red" cone because it responds to red more intensely than do any of the other cones.

AUTOMATIC REGULATION OF RETINAL SENSITIVITY — DARK AND LIGHT ADAPTATION

Relationship of Sensitivity to Pigment Concentration. The sensitivity of rods is approximately proportional to the antilogarithm of the rhodopsin concentration, and it is assumed that this relationship also holds true in the cones. Therefore, the sensitivity of the rods and cones can be altered up or down tremendously by only slight changes in concentrations of the photosensitive chemicals.

Light and Dark Adaptation. If a person has been in bright light for a long time, large proportions of the photochemicals in both the rods and cones have been reduced to retinal and opsins. Furthermore, most of the retinal of both the rods and cones has been converted into vitamin A. Because of these two effects, the concentrations of the photosensitive chemicals are considerably reduced, and the sensitivity of the eye to light is even more reduced. This is called *light adaptation*.

On the other hand, if the person remains in darkness for a long time, essentially all the retinal and opsins in the rods and cones become converted into light-sensitive pigments. Furthermore, large amounts of vitamin A are converted into retinal, which is then changed into additional light-sensitive pigments, the final limit being determined by the amount of opsins in the rods and cones. Because of these two effects, the visual receptors gradually become so sensitive that even the minutest amount of light causes excitation. This is called *dark adaptation*.

Figure 19–8 illustrates the course of dark adaptation when a person is exposed to total darkness after having been exposed to bright light for several hours. Note that sensitivity of the retina is very low when one first enters the darkness, but within 1 minute the sensitivity has increased 10-fold — that is, the retina can respond to light of one-tenth intensity. At the end of 20 minutes the sensitivity has increased about 6000-fold, and at the end of 40 minutes it has increased about 25,000-fold.

The resulting curve of Figure 59–8 is called the *dark adaptation curve*. Note, however, the inflection in the curve. The early portion of the curve is caused by adaptation of the cones, for these adapt much more rapidly than the rods because of a basic difference in the rate at which they resynthesize their photosensitive pigments. On the other hand, the cones do not achieve anywhere near the same degree of sensitivity as the rods. Therefore,

Figure 19–8. Dark adaptation, illustrating the relationship of cone adaptation to rod adaptation.

despite rapid adaptation by the cones, they cease adapting after only a few minutes, while the slowly adapting rods continue to adapt for many minutes or even hours, their sensitivity increasing tremendously. However, a large share of the greater sensitivity of the rods is also caused by convergence of as many as 100 rods onto a single ganglion cell in the retina; these rods summate to increase their sensitivity, as will be discussed in the following chapter.

Figure 19–9 illustrates several additional dark adaptation curves, but in this figure it is shown that the rate of dark adaptation differs depending on the previous degree of exposure of the retina to light. Curve number 1 shows the dark adaptation after a person had been in bright light for approximately 20 minutes, curve number 2 shows the rate after he had been in bright light for only a minute or so, and curve number 3 after he had been in bright light for many hours. Note that the eye exposed to bright light for a long time adapts slowly in comparison with the eye that has been in bright light for only a few minutes. The cause of this difference is probably the fact that long exposure to light converts most of the retinal into vitamin A that is then stored in the pigment

Figure 19–9. Dark and light adaptation. (The retina is considered to have a sensitivity of 1 when maximally lighted adapted.)

epithelium, and this is slow to return to the rods and cones.

To the right in Figure 19–9 is shown a *light adaptation curve,* illustrating that light adaptation occurs much more rapidly than dark adaptation. Also, the slow component caused by retinal–vitamin A interconversion does not play as prominent a role in light adaptation as in dark adaptation. Therefore, a person exposed to extremely bright light after having been in prolonged darkness becomes adjusted to the new light conditions in only a few minutes. This is in contrast to dark adaptation, which requires 10 to 20 minutes for moderate adaptation and 10 to 18 hours for maximal adaptation.

Other Mechanisms of Light and Dark Adaptation. In addition to adaptation caused by changes in concentrations of rhodopsin or color photochemicals, the eye has two other mechanisms for light and dark adaptation. The first of these is the *change in pupillary size,* which was discussed in the previous chapter. This can cause a degree of adaptation of approximately 30-fold because of changes in the amount of light allowed through the pupillary opening.

The other mechanism is *neural adaptation,* involving the neurons in the successive stages of the visual chain in the retina itself. That is, when the light intensity first increases, the intensities of the signals transmitted by the bipolar cells, the horizontal cells, the amacrine cells, and the ganglion cells are all very intense. However, the intensities of these signals all decrease rapidly. Although the degree of this adaptation is only a few-fold rather than the many thousand-fold that occurs during adaptation of the photochemical system, this neural adaptation occurs in a fraction of a second, in contrast to the many minutes required for full adaptation by the photochemicals.

Value of Light and Dark Adaptation in Vision. Between the limits of maximal dark adaptation and maximal light adaptation, the eye can change its sensitivity to light by as much as 500,000 to 1,000,000 times, the sensitivity automatically adjusting to changes in illumination.

Since the registration of images by the retina requires detection of both dark and light spots in the image, it is essential that the sensitivity of the retina always be adjusted so that the receptors respond to the lighter areas and not to the darker areas. An example of maladjustment of the retina occurs when a person leaves a movie theater and enters the bright sunlight, for even the dark spots in the images then seem exceedingly bright, and, as a consequence, the entire visual image is bleached, having little contrast between its different parts. Obviously, this is poor vision, and it remains poor until the retina has adapted sufficiently that the dark spots of the image no longer stimulate the receptors excessively.

Conversely, when a person enters darkness, the sensitivity of the retina is usually so slight that even the light spots in the image cannot excite the retina. But, after dark adaptation, the light spots begin to register. As an example of the extremes of

light and dark adaptation, the light intensity of the sun is approximately 30,000 times that of the moon; yet the eye can function well both in bright sunlight and in bright moonlight.

Negative After-Images. If one looks steadily at a scene for a while, the bright portions of the image cause light adaptation of the retina while the dark portions of the image cause dark adaptation. In other words, areas of the retina that are stimulated by light become less sensitive while areas that are exposed only to darkness gain in sensitivity. If the person then moves his eyes away from the scene and looks at a bright white surface, he sees exactly the same scene that he had been viewing, but the light areas of the scene now appear dark, and the dark areas appear light. This is known as the negative after-image, and it is a natural consequence of light and dark adaptation.

The negative after-image persists as long as any degree of light and dark adaptation remains in the respective portions of the retina. Referring back to Figure 19–9, one can see from the dark adaptation curves that a negative after-image could possibly persist as long as an hour under favorable conditions.

Photopic versus Scotopic Vision. *Photopic vision* means vision capable of discriminating color, while *scotopic vision* means vision capable of discriminating only between shades of black and white. In bright light one's vision is photopic, while below a critical light intensity, vision is scotopic. The reason for this difference is the following: In very dim light, only rods are capable of becoming dark-adapted to a sensitivity level required for light detection. Therefore, in dim light the retina is capable only of scotopic vision. On the other hand, in very bright light, the rods become light-adapted to the point that they either become inoperative or overshadowed by the signals from the cones; in contrast, the cones find bright light especially suitable for optimal function. Some physiologists believe that the cones in bright light inhibit rod function by transmitting inhibiting signals through the horizontal cells to the synaptic bodies of the rods. At any rate, in bright light, function of the retina appears to be based almost entirely on cone detection of the light signals.

FUSION OF FLICKERING LIGHTS BY THE RETINA

In a flickering light, the intensity alternately increases and decreases rapidly. An instantaneous flash of light excites the visual receptors for as long as $1/10$ to $1/5$ second, and because of the *persistence* of excitation, rapidly successive flashes of light become *fused* together to give the appearance of being continuous. This effect is well known when one observes motion pictures or television. The images on the motion picture screen are flashed at a rate of 24 frames per second, while those of the television screen are flashed at a rate of 60 frames per second. As a result, the images fuse together, and continuous motion is observed.

The frequency at which flicker fusion occurs,

Figure 19–10. Relationship of intensity of illumination to the critical frequency for fusion.

called the *critical frequency for fusion,* varies with the light intensity. Figure 19–10 illustrates the effect of intensity of illumination on the critical fusion frequency. At a low intensity, fusion results even when the rate of flicker is as low as 2 to 6 per second. However, in bright illumination, the critical frequency for fusion rises to as great as 60 flashes per second. This difference results at least partly from the fact that the cones, which operate mainly at high levels of illumination, can detect much more rapid alterations in illumination than can the rods, which are the important receptors in dim light.

COLOR VISION

From the preceding sections, we know that different cones are sensitive to different colors of light. The present section is a discussion of the mechanisms by which the retina detects the different gradations of color in the visual spectrum.

THE TRI-COLOR THEORY OF COLOR PERCEPTION

Many different theories have been proposed to explain the phenomenon of color vision, but they are all based on the well-known observation that the human eye can detect almost all gradations of colors when red, green, and blue monochromatic lights are appropriately mixed in different combinations.

The first important theory of color vision was that of Young, which was later expanded and given a more experimental basis by Helmholtz. Therefore, the theory is known as the *Young-Helmholtz theory.* According to this theory, there are three different types of cones, each of which responds maximally to a different color.

As time has gone by, the Young-Helmholtz theory has been expanded, and more details have been worked out. It now is generally accepted as the mechanism of color vision.

Spectral Sensitivities of the Three Types of Cones. On the basis of color vision tests, the spectral sensitivities of the three different types of cones in human beings are essentially the same as the light absorption curves for the three types of pigment found in the respective cones. These were illustrated in Figure 19–7 and are also shown in Figure 19–11. These curves can readily explain almost all the phenomena of color vision.

Interpretation of Color in the Nervous System. Referring to Figure 19–11, one can see that an orange monochromatic light with a wavelength of 580 millimicrons stimulates the red cones to a stimulus value of approximately 99 (99 per cent of the peak stimulation at optimum wavelength), while it stimulates the green cones to a stimulus value of approximately 42 and the blue cones not at all. Thus, the ratios of stimulation of the three different types of cones in this instance are 99:42:0. The nervous system interprets this set of ratios as the sensation of orange. On the other hand, a monochromatic blue light with a wavelength of 450 millimicrons stimulates the red cones to a stimulus value of 0, the green cones to a value of 0 and the blue cones to a value of 97. This set of ratios — 0:0:97 — is interpreted by the nervous system as blue. Likewise, ratios of 83:83:0 are interpreted as yellow and 31:67:36, as green.

This scheme also shows how it is possible for a person to perceive a sensation of yellow when a red light and a green light are shone into the eye at the same time, for this stimulates the red and green cones approximately equally, which gives a sensation of yellow even though no wavelength of light corresponding to yellow is present.

Perception of White Light. Approximately

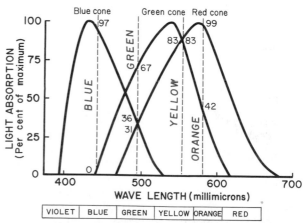

Figure 19–11. Demonstration of the degree of stimulation of the different color-sensitive cones by monochromatic lights of four separate colors: blue, green, yellow, and orange.

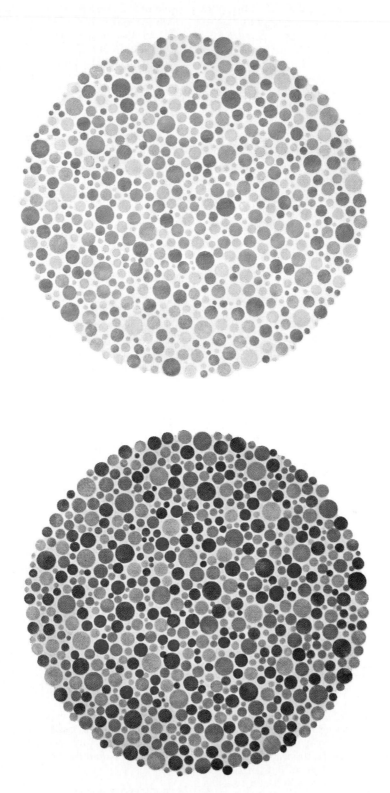

Figure 19–12. Two Ishihara charts. *Upper:* In this chart, the normal person reads "74," whereas the red-green color blind person reads "21." *Lower:* In this chart, the red-blind person (protanope) reads "2," while the green-blind person (deuteranope) reads "4." The normal person reads "42." (From Ishihara: Tests for Colour-Blindness. Tokyo, Kanehara and Co.)

equal stimulation of all the red, green, and blue cones gives one the sensation of seeing white. Yet there is no wavelength of light corresponding to white; instead, white is a combination of all the wavelengths of the spectrum. Furthermore, the sensation of white can be achieved by stimulating the retina with a proper combination of only three chosen colors that stimulate the respective types of cones approximately equally.

Integration of Color Sensations by the Retina and the Brain.   From psychological studies, we know that the interpretation of color is performed partly by the retina and partly by the brain. If a monochromatic green filter is placed in front of the left eye and a monochromatic red filter in front of the right eye, the visual object appears mainly yellow. This integration of color sensations obviously could not be occurring in the retina because one retina is allowed to respond only to green light and the other only to red light. However, sensations perceived in this way are not as clearly mixed as those perceived when the two monochromatic lights are mixed in the same retina. Therefore, at least some degree of the interpretation of color occurs in the retina itself even before the light information is transmitted into the brain. Some of the known features of color signal processing in the neuronal cells of the retina will be presented in the following chapter.

COLOR BLINDNESS

Red-Green Color Blindness.   When a single group of color receptive cones is missing from the eye, the person is unable to distinguish some colors from others. As can be observed by studying Figure 19–9 or 19–11, if the red cones are missing, light of 525 to 625 millimicrons' wavelength can stimulate only the green-sensitive cones, so that the *ratio* of stimulation of the different cones does not change as the color changes from green all the way through the red spectrum. Therefore, within this wavelength range, all colors appear to be the same to this "color blind" person.

On the other hand, if the green-sensitive cones are missing, the colors in the range from green to red can stimulate only the red-sensitive cones, and the person also perceives only one color within these limits. Therefore, when either the red or green types of cones are lacking, the person is said to be "red-green" color blind. However, when one or more types of cones are abnormal but still function partially, a person has "color weakness," instead of color blindness.

The person with loss of red cones is called a *protanope;* his overall visual spectrum is noticeably shortened at the long wavelength end because of lack of the red cones. The color blind person who lacks green cones is called a *deuteranope;* this person has a perfectly normal visual spectral width because the absent green cones operate in the middle of the spectrum where red or blue cones also operate.

Blue Weakness.   Occasionally, a person has "blue weakness," which results from diminished or absent blue receptors. If we observe Figure 19–11 once again, we can see that the blue cones are sensitive to a spectral range almost entirely different from that of both the red and green cones. Therefore, if the blue receptors are completely absent, the person has a greater preponderance of green, yellow, orange, and red in the visual spectrum than of blue, thus producing this rarely observed type of color weakness or blindness.

Tests for Color Blindness.   Tests for color blindness depend on the person's ability to distinguish various colors from each other and also on his ability to judge correctly the degree of contrast between colors. For instance, to determine whether or not a person is red-green color blind, he may be given many small tufts of wool whose colors encompass the entire visual spectrum. He is then asked to place those tufts that have the same colors in the same piles. If he is not color blind, he recognizes immediately that all the tufts have slightly different colors; however, if he is red-green color blind, he places the red, orange, yellow, and yellow-green colors all together as having essentially the same color.

Stilling and Ishihara Test Charts.   A rapid method for determining color blindness is based on the use of spot-charts such as those illustrated in Figure 19–12. These charts are arranged with a confusion of spots of several different colors. In the top chart, the normal person reads "74," while the red-green color blind person reads "21." In the bottom chart, the normal person reads "42," while the red blind protanope reads "2," and the green blind deuteranope reads "4."

If one will study these charts while at the same time observing the spectral sensitivity curves of the different cones in Figure 19–11, it can be readily understood how excessive emphasis can be placed on spots of certain colors by color blind persons in comparison with normal persons.

Genetics of Color Blindness.   Color blindness is sex-linked and results from absence of appropriate color genes in the X chromosomes. This lack of color genes is a recessive trait; therefore, color blindness will not appear as long as another X chromosome carries the genes necessary for development of the respective color-receptive cones.

Because the male human being has only one X chromosome, all three color genes must be present in this single chromosome if he is not to be color blind. In approximately 1 of every 50 times, the X chromosome lacks the red gene; in approximately 1 of every 16, it lacks the green gene; and, rarely, it lacks the blue gene. This means, therefore, that 2 per cent of all men are red color blind (protanopes) and 6 per cent are green color blind (deuteranopes), making a total of approximately 8 per cent who are red-green color blind. Because a female has two X chromosomes, red-green color blindness is a rare abnormality in the female.

REFERENCES

Benson, W. E.: Retinal Detachment: Diagnosis and Management. Philadelphia, Harper & Row, 1980.
Brindley, G. S.: Physiology of the Retina and Visual Pathway, 2nd Ed. Baltimore, Williams & Wilkins, 1970.

Callender, R., and Honig, B.: Resonance Raman studies of visual pigments. *Annu. Rev. Biophys. Bioeng., 6*:33, 1977.

Cervetto, L., and Fuortes, M. G. F.: Excitation and interactions in the retina. *Annu. Rev. Biophys. Bioeng., 7*:229, 1978.

Chignell, A. H.: Retinal Detachment Surgery. New York, Springer-Verlag, 1979.

Cunha-Vaz, J. G. (ed.): The Blood-Retinal Barriers. New York, Plenum Press, 1980.

Davson, H.: The Physiology of the Eye, 3rd Ed. New York, Academic Press, 1972.

Daw, N. W.: Neurophysiology of color vision. *Physiol. Rev., 53*:571, 1973.

Dick, G. L.: Studies in Ocular Anatomy and Physiology. Kensington, N. S. W., New South Wales University Press, 1976.

Fatt, I.: Physiology of the Eye: An Introduction to the Vegetative Function. Boston, Butterworths, 1978.

Favreau, O. E., and Corballis, M. C.: Negative aftereffects in visual perception. *Sci. Am., 235*(6):42, 1976.

Fine, B. S., and Yanoff, M.: Ocular Histology: A Text and Atlas. Hagerstown, Md., Harper & Row, 1979.

Freeman, R. D. (ed.): Developmental Neurobiology of Vision. New York, Plenum Press, 1979.

Friedlaender, M. H.: Allergy and Immunology of the Eye. Hagerstown, Md., Harper & Row, 1979.

Kaneko, A.: Physiology of the retina. *Annu. Rev. Neurosci., 2*:169, 1979.

Klein, R. M., and Katzin, H. M.: Cellular and Biochemical Aspects in Diabetic Retinopathy. Baltimore, Williams & Wilkins, 1978.

Kohner, E. M. (ed.): Diabetic Retinopathy. Boston, Little, Brown, 1978.

Land, E. H.: The retinex theory of color vision. *Sci. Am., 237*(6):108, 1977.

MacNichol, E. F., Jr.: Three-pigment color vision. *Sci. Am., 211*:48, 1964.

Marks, W. B., *et al.*: Visual pigments of single primate cones. *Science, 143*:1181, 1964.

Michael, C. R.: Color vision. *N. Engl. J. Med., 288*:724, 1973.

Michaelson, I. C.: Textbook of the Fundus of The Eye. New York, Churchill Livingstone, 1980.

Ming, A. L. S., and Constable, I. J.: Colour Atlas of Ophthalmology. Boston, Houghton Mifflin, 1979.

Padgham, C. A., and Saunders, J. E.: The Perception of Light and Color. New York, Academic Press, 1975.

Retina and Vitreous. Rochester, Minn., American Academy of Ophthalmology, 1978.

Rushton, W. A. H.: Visual pigments and color blindness. *Sci. Am., 232*(3):64, 1975.

Schepens, C. L.: Retinal Detachment and Allied Diseases. Philadelphia, W. B. Saunders Co., 1981.

Yannuzzi, L. A., *et al.* (eds.): The Macula: A Comprehensive Text and Atlas. Baltimore, Williams & Wilkins, 1978.

Young, R. W.: Proceedings: Biogenesis and renewal of visual cell outer segment membranes. *Exp. Eye Res., 18*:215, 1974.

Zinn, K. M., and Marmor, M. F. (eds.): The Retinal Pigment Epithelium. Cambridge, Mass., Harvard University Press, 1979.

20

The Eye:
III. Neurophysiology
of Vision

THE VISUAL PATHWAY

Figure 20–1 illustrates the visual pathway from the two retinae back to the *visual cortex*. After impulses leave the retinae they pass backward through the *optic nerves*. At the *optic chiasm* all the fibers from the nasal halves of the retinae cross to the opposite side where they join the fibers from the opposite temporal retinae to form the *optic tracts*. The fibers of each optic tract synapse in the *lateral geniculate body* and from here, the *geniculocalcarine fibers* pass through the *optic radiation*, or *geniculocalcarine tract*, to the *primary visual cortex* in the calcarine area of the occipital lobe.

In addition, visual fibers also pass to other areas of the brain: (1) from the optic tracts to the *suprachiasmatic nucleus of the hypothalamus,* presumably for controlling circadian rhythms; (2) from the optic tracts to the *brain stem motor nuclei,* for control of eye movements and head turning; (3) into the *pretectal nuclei,* for control of fixation of the eyes on objects of importance and also for activating the pupillary light reflex; (4) into the *superior colliculus,* for control of bilateral simultaneous movement of the two eyes; (5) into the *pulvinar* as a secondary visual pathway either directly from the optic tracts or indirectly from the superior colliculus — then from the pulvinar to the secondary visual areas, areas 18 and 19, of the occipital lobes; and (6) into other areas of the thalamus and brain stem, possibly partly for perception of light intensity.

NEURAL FUNCTION OF THE RETINA

NEURAL ORGANIZATION OF THE RETINA

The detailed anatomy of the retina was illustrated in Figure 19–1 of the preceding chapter, and Figure 20–2 illustrates the basic essentials of the retina's neural connections; to the left is the general organization of the neural elements in a peripheral retinal area and to the right the organization of the foveal area. Note that in the peripheral region both rods and cones converge on *bipolar cells* which in turn converge on *ganglion cells*. In the fovea, where only cones exist, there is little convergence; instead, the cones are represented by approximately equal numbers of bipolar and ganglion cells.

Not emphasized in the figure is the fact that in

Figure 20–1. The visual pathways from the eyes to the visual cortex. (Modified from Polyak: The Retina. University of Chicago Press.)

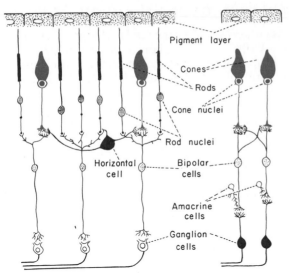

Figure 20–2. Neural organization of the retina: peripheral area to the left, foveal area to the right.

both the outer and inner plexiform layers (where the neurons synapse with each other) are many lateral connections between the different neural elements. Many of these lateral connections are collateral branches of the dendrites and axons of the bipolar and ganglion cells. But, in addition, two special types of cells are present in the inner nuclear layer that transmits signals laterally: (1) the *horizontal cells,* and (2) the *amacrine cells.*

Each retina contains about 125 million rods and 5.5 million cones; yet, as counted with the light microscope, only 900,000 optic nerve fibers lead from the retina to the brain. Thus, an average of 140 rods plus 6 cones converge on each optic nerve fiber. However, there are major differences between the peripheral retina and the central retina, for nearer the fovea fewer and fewer rods and cones converge on each optic fiber, and the rods and cones both become slenderer. These two effects progressively increase the acuity of vision toward the central retina. In the very central portion, in the *fovea,* there are no rods at all. Also, the number of optic nerve fibers leading from this part of the retina is almost equal to the number of cones, as shown to the right in Figure 20–2. This mainly explains the high degree of visual acuity in the central portion of the retina in comparison with the very poor acuity in the peripheral portions.

Another difference between the peripheral and central portions of the retina is the considerably greater sensitivity of the peripheral retina to weak light. This results partly from the fact that as many as 300 rods converge on the same optic nerve fiber in the most peripheral portions of the retina; the signals from the rods summate to give intense stimulation of the peripheral ganglion cells. But, in

addition, rods are more sensitive to weak light than are the cones because of intrinsic differences in the receptors themselves.

STIMULATION OF THE RODS AND CONES — THE RECEPTOR POTENTIAL

Stimulation of the rods and cones was discussed at length in the preceding chapter. Briefly, when light strikes either of these receptors, it decomposes a photochemical that in turn acts on the membrane of the *outer segment* of the receptor (the part that protrudes into the pigment layer) to cause a sustained *receptor potential* that lasts as long as the light continues. However, as pointed out in the previous chapter, this receptor potential is different from all other receptor potentials that have been recorded, for it is a *hyperpolarization* signal rather than a depolarization signal. Also, its intensity is proportional to the logarithm of light energy, in contrast to the more linear response of many other receptors. This logarithmic response is very important to vision, because it allows the eyes to detect contrasts in the image even when light intensities vary many thousand-fold, an effect that would not be possible if there were linear transduction of the signal.

Receptor potentials are transmitted unchanged through the bodies of the rods and cones. Neither the rods nor the cones generate action potentials. Instead, the receptor potentials themselves, acting at the synaptic bodies, induce signals in the successive neurons, the bipolar and horizontal cells.

STIMULATION OF THE BIPOLAR AND HORIZONTAL CELLS

The synaptic bodies of the rods and cones make intimate contact with the dendrites of both the bipolar and horizontal cells. For this reason, it has been believed that signals were transmitted from the rods and cones to the bipolar and horizontal cells by electrotonic conduction, that is, by flow of electrical current directly from the rods and cones into the bipolar and horizontal cells. However, it is now almost certain that the rods and cones secrete a transmitter substance that then induces the potential changes in the bipolar and horizontal cells. Unfortunately, the exact nature of the transmitter is yet unknown.

The transmitter from the rods and cones causes *depolarization of the horizontal cells* and *hyperpolarization of the bipolar cells.* Therefore, when the rods and cones are excited, the bipolar cells become excited, while the horizontal cells become inhibited.

Neither the bipolar cells nor the horizontal cells transmit action potentials. Instead, their signals, like those of the rods and cones, result from electrotonic depolarization or hyperpolarization of the entire neuronal membrane all at once.

Function of the Bipolar Cells. The bipolar cells are the main transmitting link for the visual signal from the rods and cones to the ganglion cells. They are entirely excitatory cells; that is, they can only excite the ganglion cells.

Function of the Horizontal Cells. The horizontal cells lie in the inner nuclear layer and spread widely in the retina, transmitting signals laterally as far as several hundred microns. They are inhibited by the synaptic bodies of the rods and cones and in turn transmit their inhibitory signals mainly to bipolar cells located in areas lateral to the excited rods and cones.

The horizontal cells, therefore, function as inhibitory pathways, in contrast to the bipolar cells, which are excitatory. Therefore, the signals transmitted by the horizontal cells from the excited rods and cones cause inhibition of the bipolar cells lateral to the excited point in the retina. That is, excited rods and cones transmit excitatory signals in a direct line through the bipolar cells in the area of excitation but transmit inhibitory signals through the surrounding bipolar cells.

The horizontal cells are of major importance for enhancing and helping to detect contrasts in the visual scene. They are also of importance in helping to differentiate colors. Both of these functions will be discussed in subsequent sections of this chapter.

Stimulation and Function of the Amacrine Cells. The amacrine cells, also located in the inner nuclear layer, are excited mainly by the bipolar cells but possibly also occasionally directly by the synaptic bodies of the rods and cones. These cells in turn synapse with the ganglion cells. However, their response is a *transient* one rather than the steady, continuous response of the bipolar and horizontal cells. That is, when the photoreceptors are first stimulated, the signal transmitted by the amacrine cells is very intense; this signal dies away to almost nothing in a fraction of a second.

Another difference between the amacrine cells and the bipolar and horizontal cells is that the amacrine cells often transmit action potentials (and can transmit signals by electrotonic conduction as well), but the significance of this difference is not known.

Bipolar cells, horizontal cells, and amacrine cells are all believed to secrete transmitter substances at their nerve terminations, but the types of transmitter substances are yet unknown. Some of the different transmitter substances that have been found in the retina include acetylcholine, dopamine, GABA, glutamate ions, and aspartate ions.

EXCITATION OF THE GANGLION CELLS

Spontaneous, Continuous Discharge of the Ganglion Cells. The ganglion cells transmit their signals through the optic nerve fibers to the brain in the form of action potentials. These cells, even when unstimulated, transmit continuous nerve impulses at an average rate of about 5 per second. The visual signal is superimposed onto this basic level of ganglion cell stimulation. It can be either an excitatory signal, with the number of impulses increasing to greater than 5 per second, or an inhibitory signal, with the number of nerve impulses decreasing to below 5 per second — often all the way to zero.

Summation at the Ganglion Cells of Signals from the Bipolar Cells, the Horizontal Cells, and the Amacrine Cells. The bipolar cells transmit the main direct *excitatory* information from the rods and the cones to the ganglion cells: the horizontal cells transmit *inhibitory* information from laterally displaced rods and cones to surrounding bipolar cells and then to the ganglion cells; the amacrine cells seem to transmit direct but short-lived transient signals that signal a *change* in the level of illumination of the retina. Thus, each of these three types of cells performs a separate function in stimulating the ganglion cells.

DIFFERENT TYPES OF SIGNALS TRANSMITTED BY THE GANGLION CELLS THROUGH THE OPTIC NERVE

Transmission of Luminosity Signals. The ganglion cells are of several different types, and they also have different patterns of stimulation by the bipolar, horizontal, and amacrine cells. A very few of the ganglion cells respond to the intensity *(luminosity)* of the light falling on the photoreceptors. The rate of impulses from these cells remains at a level greater than the natural rate of firing as long as the luminosity is high. It is the signals from these cells that are believed to apprise the brain of the overall level of light intensity of the observed scene. However, by far the greater number of ganglion cells are concerned with transmitting information concerning the form of the scene in terms of contrast borders, as will be discussed below.

Transmission of Signals Depicting Contrasts in the Visual Scene — The Process of Lateral Inhibition. Most of the ganglion cells do not respond to the actual level of illumination of the scene; instead they respond only to contrast borders in the scene. Since it seems that this is the major means by which the form of the scene is transmitted to the brain, let us explain how this process occurs.

When flat light is applied to the entire retina —

that is, when all the photoreceptors are stimulated equally by the incident light — the contrast type of ganglion cell is neither stimulated nor inhibited. The reason for this is that the signals transmitted *directly* from the photoreceptors through the bipolar cells are excitatory, whereas the signals transmitted *laterally* through the horizontal cells are inhibitory. These two effects neutralize each other. Now, let us examine what happens when a contrast border occurs in the visual scene. Figure 20–3 shows a spot of light shining on the retina and exciting the photoreceptors. The signal is transmitted directly through the bipolar cells and thence to the ganglion cells in the same area to cause excitation. At the same time these same excited photoreceptors transmit *lateral inhibitory* signals through the horizontal cells to the surrounding bipolar and ganglion cells. Thus, when there is a contrast border, with stimulated photoreceptors on one side of the border and unstimulated photoreceptors on the opposite side of the border, the mutual cancellation of the excitatory signals through the bipolar cells and the inhibitory signals through the horizontal cells no longer occurs. Consequently, the ganglion cells on either side of this border become either excited or inhibited — excited on the light side of the border and inhibited on the dark side.

A linear contrast border acts almost identically as does a spot of light; the ganglion cells on the light side of the border are stimulated and on the dark side are inhibited. On the other hand, all of the contrast type of ganglion cells that lie in the flatly illuminated portion of the scene still remain unstimulated.

This process of contrasting an excitatory signal with an inhibitory signal is essentially the same as the process of *lateral inhibition* that occurs in

Figure 20–4. Responses of ganglion cells to light in (1) an area excited by a spot of light and (2) an area immediately adjacent to the excited spot; the ganglion cells in this area are inhibited by the mechanism of lateral inhibition. (Modified from Granit: Receptors and Sensory Perception: A Discussion of Aims, Means, and Results of Electrophysiological Research into the Process of Reception. Yale University Press, 1955.)

most other types of sensory signal transmission. The process is a mechanism used by the nervous system for contrast detection and enhancement.

When impulses are recorded from ganglion cells, it is possible to observe the effects of contrast borders on the signals transmitted in optic nerve fibers. Figure 20–4 illustrates this effect. The upper recording is from a ganglion cell located in the area excited by a spot of light, whereas the lower recording is from a ganglion cell located a few hundred microns to the side of the spot. Note that when the spot of light is turned on, the ganglion cell in the center of the light becomes excited while the ganglion cell located laterally becomes inhibited.

Detection of Instantaneous Changes in Light Intensity — The On-Off Response. Many of the ganglion cells are especially excited by *change* in light intensity; this effect most often occurs in the same ganglion cells that transmit contrast border signals. For instance, the upper tracing of Figure 20–4 shows that when the light was first turned on the ganglion cell became strongly excited for a fraction of a second, and then the level of excitation diminished. The bottom tracing shows that a second ganglion cell located in the dark area lateral to the spot of light was markedly inhibited at the same time. Then when the light was turned off, exactly the opposite effects occurred. Thus, the responses of these two types of cells are called the "on-off" and the "off-on" responses.

This ability of the retina to detect and transmit signals related to *change* in light intensity is caused by a rapid phase of "adaptation" of some of the neurons in the visual chain. Since this effect is known to be extremely marked in the amacrine cells, it has been suggested that the amacrine cells are peculiarly adapted to detecting light intensity change.

This capability to detect change in light intensity is especially well developed in the peripheral retina. For instance, a minute gnat flying across the peripheral field of vision is instantaneously

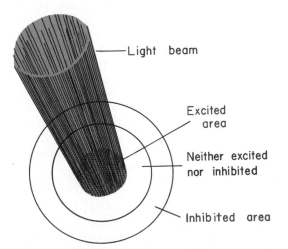

Figure 20–3. Excitation and inhibition of a retinal area caused by a small beam of light.

detected. On the other hand, the same gnat sitting quietly in the peripheral field of vision remains entirely below the threshold of visual detection.

Transmission of Color Signals by the Ganglion Cells. A single ganglion cell may be stimulated by a number of cones or by only a very few. When all three types of cones — the red, blue, and green types — all stimulate the same ganglion cell, the signal transmitted through the ganglion cell is the same for any color of the spectrum. Therefore, this signal plays no role in the detection of the different colors. Instead, it is a "luminosity" signal.

On the other hand, many of the ganglion cells are excited by only one color type of cone but inhibited by a second type. For instance, this frequently occurs for the red and green cones, red causing excitation and green causing inhibition — or, vice versa, that is, green causing excitation and red, inhibition. The same type of reciprocal effect also occurs between blue cones and red or green cones.

The mechanism of this opposing effect of colors is the following: One color type cone excites the ganglion cell by the direct excitatory route through a bipolar cell, while the other color type inhibits the ganglion cell by the indirect inhibitory route through a horizontal cell.

The importance of these color-contrast mechanisms is that they represent a mechanism by which the retina itself differentiates colors. Thus each color-contrast type of ganglion cell is excited by one color but inhibited by the "opponent." Therefore, the process of color analysis begins in the retina and is not entirely a function of the brain.

FUNCTION OF THE LATERAL GENICULATE BODY

ANATOMICAL ORGANIZATION OF THE LATERAL GENICULATE NUCLEI

Each lateral geniculate body is composed of six nuclear layers. Layers 2, 3, and 5 (from the inside outward) receive signals from the temporal portion of the ipsilateral retina, while layers 1, 4, and 6 receive signals from the nasal retina of the opposite eye.

All layers of the lateral geniculate body relay visual information to the *visual cortex* through the *geniculocalcarine tract*.

Though it has not been proved, the pairing of layers from the two eyes probably plays a role in *fusion of vision* from the two eyes, because corresponding retinal fields in the two eyes connect with respective neurons that are approximately superimposed over each other in the successive layers. Also, with a little imagination, one can postulate that interaction between the successive layers could be part of the mechanism by which *stereoscopic visual depth perception* occurs, because this depends on comparing the visual images of the two eyes and determining their slight differences, as was discussed in Chapter 18. However, both fusion of vision and stereopsis also require the visual cortex, as we shall discuss in more detail later in the chapter.

Characteristics of the Visual Signals in the Lateral Geniculate Body

The signals recorded in the relay neurons of the lateral geniculate body are similar to those recorded in the ganglion cells of the retina. A few of the neurons transmit luminosity signals, while the majority transmit signals depicting only contrast borders or opponent colors in the visual image; also, many of the neurons are particularly responsive to movement of objects across the visual scene. However, the signals of the geniculate neurons are different from those in the ganglion cells in that a greater number of the complex interactions are found. That is, a much higher percentage of the neurons respond to contrast in the visual scene or to movement. These more complex reactions presumably result from convergence of excitatory and inhibitory signals from two or more ganglion cells on the relay neurons of the lateral geniculate body.

Color Signals in the Lateral Geniculate Body. Signals related to black and white vision are mainly found in layers 1 and 2 of the lateral geniculate body, while color signals occur mainly in layers 3 through 6. A few of the neurons in these last four layers respond to all colors and therefore transmit "white light" information. However, about three-quarters of the neurons respond to "opponent colors;" that is, a given cell may be excited by red but be inhibited by green. Another cell will operate exactly oppositely. These are called the "red-green" cells. Still other lateral geniculate body cells respond to the opponent colors blue and yellow, with one of these exciting the cell and the other inhibiting it. The mechanism of this effect is the same as in the retina; that is, it is caused by convergence of signals from red and green cones onto the same neuron, one of these signals causing inhibition while the other causes excitation.

By various interactions of this type, the color information in the visual scene is gradually dissected, and the information is then transmitted to other areas of the brain as signals that express the *ratios* of different colors in the different areas of the visual scene.

FUNCTION OF THE PRIMARY VISUAL CORTEX

The ability of the visual system to detect spatial organization of the visual scene — that is, to detect the forms of objects, brightness of the individual parts of the objects, shading, and so forth — depends on function of the *primary visual cortex,* the anatomy of which is illustrated in Figure 20–5. This area lies mainly in the calcarine fissure located bilaterally on the medial aspect of each occipital cortex. Specific points of the retina connect with specific points of the visual cortex, the right halves of the two respective retinae connecting with the right visual cortex and the left halves connecting with the left visual cortex. The macula is represented at the occipital pole of the visual cortex and the peripheral regions of the retina are represented in concentric circles farther and farther forward from the occipital pole. The upper portion of the retina is represented superiorly in the visual cortex, and the lower portion, inferiorly. Note the large area of cortex receiving signals from the macular region of the retina. It is in this region that the fovea is represented, which gives the highest degree of visual acuity. Based on area, the fovea has 35 times as much representation in the primary visual cortex as do the peripheral portions of the retina.

DETECTION OF LINES AND BORDERS BY THE PRIMARY VISUAL CORTEX

If a person looks at a blank wall, only a few neurons of the primary visual cortex will be stimulated, whether the illumination of the wall is bright or weak. Therefore, the question must be asked: What does the visual cortex do? To answer this question, let us now place on the wall a large solid cross such as that illustrated to the left in Figure 20–6. To the right is illustrated the spatial pattern of the greater majority of the excited neurons that one finds in the visual cortex. *Note that the areas*

Retinal Image   Cortical Stimulation

Figure 20–6. Pattern of excitation occurring in the visual cortex in response to a retinal image of a dark cross.

of excitation occur along the sharp borders of the visual pattern. Thus, by the time the visual signal is recorded in the primary visual cortex, it is concerned mainly with the *contrasts* in the visual scene rather than with the flat areas. At each point in the visual scene where there is a change from dark to light or light to dark, the corresponding area of the primary visual cortex becomes stimulated. The intensity of stimulation is determined by the *gradient of contrast.* That is, the greater the sharpness in the contrast border and the greater the difference in intensities between the light and dark areas, the greater is the degree of stimulation.

Thus, the *pattern of contrasts* in the visual scene is impressed upon the neurons of the visual cortex, and this pattern has a spatial orientation roughly the same as that of the retinal image.

Detection of Orientation of Lines and Borders — Neuronal Columns. Not only does the visual cortex detect the *existence* of lines and borders in the different areas of the retinal image, but it also detects the *orientation* of each line or border — that is, whether it is a vertical or horizontal line or border, or lies at some degree of inclination. The mechanism of this effect is the following:

In each small area of the visual cortex the neurons are arranged in columns, each column containing about 100,000 neurons and having a diameter of about 1 mm., extending downward from the surface of the cortex through its six layers. The signals arriving in the cortex from the lateral geniculate body terminate in layer 4, and from here secondary signals spread upward or downward in the column. The neurons in the deeper portions of layer 4 respond in almost exactly the same way as the ganglion cells of the retina and the cells of the lateral geniculate body — that is, they respond to spots of light, borders, or lines. However, as the signal travels outward toward the surface of the cortex (into the outer portion of layer 4 and then into layers 3 and 2) or inward (into layers 5 and 6), the neurons

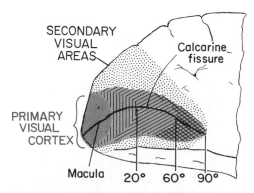

SECONDARY VISUAL AREAS

Calcarine fissure

PRIMARY VISUAL CORTEX

Macula   20°   60°   90°

Figure 20–5. The visual cortex.

respond no longer to just any spot, line, or border but instead only to lines or borders oriented in certain directions. Some respond to vertical lines or borders, others to lines or borders slightly angulated, still others to lines or borders more angulated, and so forth. This process of selective stimulation is presumably caused by convergence of signals from a number of layer 4 neurons. The effect is similar to that which occurs in the retina, some of the signals causing inhibition and others, excitation.

If the orientation of the border between the dark area and the light area in the visual scene corresponds with the orientation of the neural connections of inhibitory and excitatory input fibers to a given neuron of the visual cortex, the neuron would be excited. By having many different cortical neurons with slightly different synaptic connections, such interactions could lead to selective stimulation of one neuron for one orientation of a border, another neuron for another orientation, and so forth. This represents another stage in the mechanism for deciphering information in the visual scene.

Detection of Line Orientation Even When the Line Is Displaced Laterally.   Still other neurons in the columns are capable of detecting lines oriented in one direction even when the lines are moved to slightly different areas on the retina. These neurons presumably are excited by signals from many separate line-oriented cells in adjacent columns. The cells that detect line orientation when the line is not displaced are called *simple cells*, while those neurons that detect line orientation when the line is displaced are called *complex cells*.

Detection of Length of Lines.   Still a higher order for deciphering information from the visual scene is the ability of yet other neuronal cells to be stimulated by lines or borders of specific lengths. This type of detection presumably results from convergence of signals within the neuronal columns and between adjacent columns. The neurons that detect lines or borders of specific length are called *hypercomplex cells*.

Analysis of Color by the Visual Cortex.   One finds in the primary visual cortex specific cells that are stimulated by color intensity or by contrasts of the opponent colors, the red-green opponent colors and the blue-yellow opponent colors. These effects are almost identical to those found in the lateral geniculate body. However, the proportion of cells excited by the opponent color contrasts is vastly reduced from the proportion found in the lateral geniculate body. Since neuronal excitation by color contrasts is a means of deciphering color, it is believed that the primary visual cortex is concerned with an even higher order of detection of color than simply the deciphering of color itself.

Full appreciation of color, however, does not seem to be achieved in the primary visual cortex, for it has recently been found in a number of human beings that lesions of the ventral surface of the occipital lobe can cause loss of color perception. It is suggested, therefore, that this area might be the final region for color signal processing.

Interaction of Visual Signals from the Two Different Eyes in the Primary Visual Cortex.   From our earlier description of the lateral geniculate body, it will be recalled that the visual signals from the two separate eyes are relayed through separate lateral geniculate body neuronal layers. These signals from the two eyes are still separated from each other when they arrive in the primary visual cortex. The cortex is interlaced with zebra-like stripes of neurons, each stripe about 0.5 mm. wide; the signals from one eye enter every other stripe, and the signals from the other eye the opposite set of stripes. Each neuronal column of cells lies approximately one half in one of the stripes and the other half in the next stripe from the opposite eye. The signals also remain separated from each other when they excite the layer 4 neurons; this is also true for excitation of almost all the simple cells that detect simple line orientation. However, by the time the complex, and especially the hypercomplex, cells are excited, many of the signals from the two separate eyes have by then begun to converge. As we shall see later in the chapter, when these signals are not "in register" — that is, not both excited or inhibited together — *interference patterns* develop and excite still other cells. It is presumed that these patterns are the basis for controlling fusion of the visual images from the two eyes, and they are likely also the basis of stereopsis.

PERCEPTION OF LUMINOSITY

Although most of the neurons in the visual cortex are mainly responsive to contrasts caused by lines, borders, moving objects, or opponent colors in the visual scene, a few are directly responsive to the levels of luminosity in the different areas of the visual scene. Presumably, it is these cells that detect flat areas in the scene and also the overall level of luminosity. It is likely, too, that some of the visual signals entering the brain stem and thalamus help to determine luminosity.

EFFECT OF REMOVING THE PRIMARY VISUAL CORTEX

Removal of the primary visual cortex in the human being always causes loss of conscious vision. However, psychological studies have demonstrated that such persons can still react subconsciously to many aspects of vision, especially to changes in light intensity, and to crude aspects of form as well. The reactions include turning the eyes, turning the head, avoidance, and so on. In some low-level mammals a large share of the vision is still preserved even when the primary visual cortex is completely removed. This vision is believed to be subserved by neuronal pathways from the optic tracts to the superior colliculi and thence to the pulvinar and secondary visual cortical areas, areas 18 and 19 of the occipital lobe.

TRANSMISSION OF VISUAL INFORMATION INTO OTHER REGIONS OF THE CEREBRAL CORTEX

The primary visual cortex is located in the *calcarine fissure area,* mainly on the medial aspect of each hemisphere but also spreading slightly over the occipital pole. It is known as *Brodmann area 17* of the cortex, and it is also called the *striate area* because of its striated appearance to the naked eye.

Signals from the striate area project laterally in the occipital cortex into area 18 and then into area 19, as illustrated in Figure 20–7. These areas are called the *secondary visual cortex,* and they are also known as *visual association areas.* In reality, they are simply the loci for additional processing of visual information.

The visual projection images in areas 18 and 19 are organized into columns of cells in the same manner as described earlier for the primary visual cortex. There are also topographic representations of the visual field as found in the primary visual cortex. However, the neuronal cells respond to more complex patterns than do those in the primary visual cortex. For instance, some cells are stimulated by simple geometric patterns, such as curving borders, angles, and so forth. Presumably, these progressively more complex interpretations eventually decode the visual information, giving the overall impression of the visual scene that the person is observing.

Projection of Visual Information into the Temporal Cortex. From areas 18 and 19, visual signals next proceed to the posterior portion of the temporal lobes, Brodmann areas 20 and 21. In these areas simple visual patterns such as lines, borders, angles, and so forth fail to cause excitation of specific neurons. The degree of integration of visual information at this level, such

as interpretation of letters or words, is presumably much higher.

Effects of Destruction of the Secondary Visual Cortex. Human beings who have destructive lesions of any of the visual association areas, areas 18 and 19 in the occipital cortex or areas 20 and 21 in the temporal cortex, have difficulty with certain types of visual perception and visual learning. For instance, destruction in areas 18 and 19 generally makes it difficult to perceive form, such as shapes of objects, their sizes, and their meanings. It is believed that this type of lesion in the dominant hemisphere can cause the abnormality known as *dyslexia* or *word blindness,* which means that the person has difficulty understanding the meanings of words that are seen.

Destruction of the temporal projections of the visual system makes it especially difficult for animals, and presumably for human beings as well, to learn tasks that are based upon visual perceptions. For instance, a person might be able to see a plate of food perfectly well but be unable to utilize this visual information to direct a fork toward the food. Yet, when the person feels the plate with the other hand, the fork can be directed accurately by stereotactic information from the somesthetic cortex.

Effects of Electrical Stimulation of the Visual Areas. Electrical stimulation in the primary visual cortex or in the parietal association areas, areas 18 and 19, causes a person to have simple optic auras — that is, flashes of light, simple colors, or simple forms such as lines, stars, or so forth — but complicated forms are not seen.

Stimulation of the visual association areas of the temporal cortex, areas 20 and 21, occasionally elicits complicated visual perceptions, sometimes causing the person to see a scene that had been known many years before. This is in keeping with the interpretative function of this area for visual function.

THE FIELDS OF VISION; PERIMETRY

The *field of vision* is the area seen by an eye at a given instant. The area seen to the nasal side is called the *nasal field of vision*, and the area seen to the lateral side is called the *temporal field of vision.*

To diagnose blindness in specific portions of the retinae, one charts the field of vision for each eye by a process known as *perimetry*. This is done by having the subject look with one eye toward a central spot directly in front of the eye. Then a small dot of light or a small object is moved back and forth in all areas of the field of vision, both laterally and nasally and upward and downward, and the person indicates when the spot of light or object can be seen and when it cannot. At the same time, a chart (Fig. 20–8) is made for the eye, showing the areas in which the subject can and cannot see the spot. Thus, the field of vision is plotted.

In all perimetry charts, a blind spot caused by lack of rods and cones in the retina over the optic disc is found approximately 15 degrees lateral to the central point of vision, as illustrated in the figure.

Abnormalities in the Fields of Vision. Occasionally

Figure 20–7. The visual association fields and the cortical areas for control of eye movements.

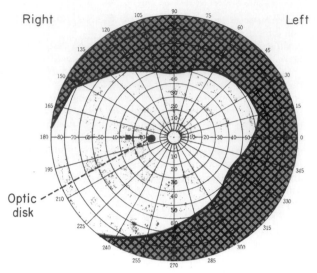

Figure 20–8. A perimetry chart, showing the field of vision for the left eye.

blind spots are found in other portions of the field of vision besides the optic disc area. Such blind spots are called *scotomata;* they frequently result from allergic reactions in the retina or from toxic conditions, such as lead poisoning or even excessive use of tobacco.

Still another condition that can be diagnosed by perimetry is *retinitis pigmentosa.* In this disease, portions of the retina degenerate and excessive melanin pigment deposits in the degenerated areas. Retinitis pigmentosa generally causes blindness in the peripheral field of vision first and then gradually encroaches on the central areas.

Effect of Lesions in the Optic Pathway on the Fields of Vision. One of the most important uses of perimetry is for localization of lesions in the visual nervous pathway. Lesions in the optic nerve, in the optic chiasm, in the optic tract, and in the geniculocalcarine tract all cause blind areas in the visual fields, and the "patterns" of these blind areas indicate the location of the lesion.

Destruction of an entire *optic nerve* obviously causes blindness of the respective eye. Destruction of the *optic chiasm,* as shown by the longitudinal line across the chiasm in Figure 20–1, prevents the passage of impulses from the nasal halves of the two retinae to the opposite optic tracts. Therefore, the nasal halves are both blinded, which means that the person is blind in both temporal fields of vision; this condition is called *bitemporal hemianopsia.* Such lesions frequently result from tumors of the adenohypophysis pressing upward on the optic chiasm.

Interruption of an *optic tract,* which is also shown by a line in Figure 20–1, denervates the corresponding half of each retina on the same side as the lesion, and, as a result, neither eye can see objects to the opposite side. This condition is known as *homonymous hemianopsia.* Destruction of the *optic radiation* or the *visual cortex* of one side also causes homonymous hemianopsia. A common condition that destroys the visual cortex is thrombosis of the posterior cerebral artery, which infarcts the occipital cortex except for the foveal area, thus often sparing central vision.

One can differentiate a lesion in the optic tract from a lesion in the geniculocalcarine tract or visual cortex by determining whether impulses can still be transmitted into the pretectal nuclei to initiate a pupillary light reflex. To do this, light is shown onto the blinded half of one of the retinae, and, if a pupillary light reflex can still occur, it is known that the lesion is at or beyond the lateral geniculate body, that is, in the geniculocalcarine tract or visual cortex. However, if the light reflex is also lost, then the lesion is in the optic tract itself.

EYE MOVEMENTS AND THEIR CONTROL

To make use of the abilities of the eye, almost equally as important as the system for interpretation of the visual signals from the eyes is the cerebral control system for directing the eyes toward the object to be viewed.

Muscular Control of Eye Movements. The eye movements are controlled by three separate pairs of muscles, shown in Figure 20–9: (1) the *medial* and *lateral recti,* (2) the *superior* and *inferior recti,* and (3) the *superior* and *inferior obliques.* The medial and lateral recti contract reciprocally to move the eyes from side to side. The superior and inferior recti contract reciprocally to move the eyes upward or downward. And the oblique muscles function mainly to rotate the eyeballs to keep the visual fields in the upright position.

Neural Pathways for Control of Eye Movements. Figure 20–9 also illustrates the nuclei of the third, fourth, and sixth cranial nerves and their innervation of the ocular muscles. Shown, too, are the interconnections among these three nuclei through the *medial longitudinal fasciculus.* Either by way of this fasciculus or by way of other closely associated pathways, each of the three sets of muscles to each eye is *reciprocally* innervated so that one muscle of the pair relaxes while the other contracts.

Figure 20–9. The extraocular muscles of the eye and their innervation.

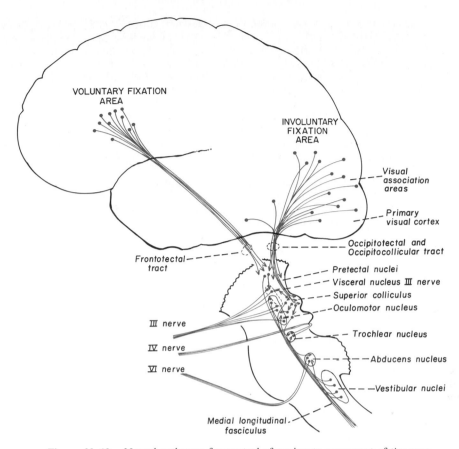

Figure 20–10. Neural pathways for control of conjugate movement of the eyes.

Figure 20–10 illustrates cortical control of the oculomotor apparatus, showing spread of signals from the occipital visual areas through occipitotectal and occipitocollicular tracts into the pretectal and superior colliculus areas of the brain stem. In addition, a frontotectal tract passes from the frontal cortex into the pretectal area. From both the pretectal and the superior colliculus areas, the oculomotor control signals then pass to the nuclei of the oculomotor nerves. Strong signals are also transmitted into the oculomotor system from the vestibular nuclei by way of the medial longitudinal fasciculus.

CONJUGATE MOVEMENT OF THE EYES

Simultaneous movement of both eyes in the same direction is called *conjugate movement* of the eyes. The signals to cause these movements probably originate in the reticular nuclei of the mesencephalon and pons in close association with the oculomotor nuclei. However, the movements are under strong control of the cerebral cortex, which transmits signals into the reticular nuclei by way of the pretectal nuclei and the superior colliculi. Signals from the vestibular nuclei also elicit conjugate movement of the eyes, mainly by sending signals through the medial longitudinal fasciculi.

FIXATION MOVEMENTS OF THE EYES

Perhaps the most important movements of the eyes are those that cause the eyes to "fix" on a discrete portion of the field of vision.

Fixation movements are controlled by two different neuronal mechanisms. The first of these allows the person to move his eyes voluntarily to find the object upon which he wishes to fix his vision; this is called the *voluntary fixation mechanism*. The second is an involuntary mechanism that holds the eyes firmly on the object once it has been found; this is called the *involuntary fixation mechanism*.

The voluntary fixation movements are controlled by a small cortical field located bilaterally in the premotor cortical regions of the frontal lobes, as illustrated in Figure 20–10. Bilateral dysfunction or destruction of these areas makes it difficult or almost impossible for the person to "unlock" his eyes from one point of fixation and then move them to another point. It is usually necessary for him to blink his eyes or put his hand over his eyes for a short time, which then allows him to move the eyes.

On the other hand, the fixation mechanism that causes the eyes to "lock" on the object of attention once it is found is controlled by the *secondary visual area of the occipital cortex* — mainly area 19 — which is also illustrated in Figure 20–10. When this area is destroyed bilaterally, the person has difficulty or becomes completely unable to keep his eyes directed toward a given fixation point.

To summarize, the posterior eye fields automatically "lock" the eyes on a given spot of the visual field and thereby prevent movement of the image across the retina. To unlock this visual fixation, voluntary impulses must be transmitted from the "voluntary" eye fields located in the frontal areas.

Mechanism of Fixation. Visual fixation results from a negative feedback mechanism that prevents the object of attention from leaving the foveal portion of the retina. The eyes even normally have three types of continuous but almost imperceptible movements: (1) a *continuous tremor* at a rate of 30 to 80 cycles per second caused by successive contractions of the motor units in the ocular muscles, (2) a *slow drift* of the eyeballs in one direction or another, and (3) sudden *flicking movements* which are controlled by the involuntary fixation mechanism. When a spot of light has become fixed on the foveal region of the retina, the tremorous movements cause the spot to move back and forth at a rapid rate across the cones, and the drifting movements cause it to drift slowly across the cones. However, each time the spot of light drifts as far as the edge of the fovea, a sudden reflex reaction occurs, producing a flicking movement that moves the spot away from this edge back toward the center. Thus, whenever the image drifts away from the point of fixation, an automatic response moves the image back toward the central portion of the fovea. These drifting and flicking motions are illustrated in Figure 20–11, which shows by the dashed lines the slow drifting across the retina and by the solid lines the flicks that keep the image from leaving the foveal region.

Fixation of the Eyes on Important Visual Highlights — Role of the Superior Colliculi. The eyes have an automatic capability for instantaneously *fixing* on an important highlight in the visual field. However, this capability is mostly lost when the superior colliculi are destroyed even though most other conjugate movements of eyes occur normally in the absence of the superior colliculi. The signals for fixation originate in the visual areas of the occipital cortex, primarily in the secondary visual areas, then pass to the superior colliculi, from there to reticular areas around the oculomotor nuclei, and thence into the motor nuclei themselves.

The superior colliculi are also important in causing sudden turning of the eyes to the side when a flash of light or some other sudden visual disturbance occurs on that side. In addition, signals are transmitted through the superior colliculi into the medial longitudinal fasciculus and other areas of the brain stem to cause turning of the whole head and perhaps even of the whole body toward the direction of the light. Other types of disturbances besides visual disturbances, such as strong sounds or even stroking the side of the body, will cause similar turning of the eyes, head, and body if the superior colliculi are intact. This effect, however, is absent or severely disturbed when the superior colliculi are destroyed. Therefore, it is frequently said that the superior colliculi play an important role in orienting the eyes, the head, and the body with respect to external signals — visual signals, auditory signals, somatic signals, and perhaps even others.

Saccadic Movement of the Eyes. When the visual scene is moving continually before the eyes, such as when a person is riding in a car or turning around, the eyes fix on one highlight after another in the visual field, jumping from one to the next at a rate of two to three jumps per second. The jumps are called *saccades*, and the movements are called *opticokinetic movements*. The saccades occur so rapidly that not more than 10 per cent of the total time is spent in moving the eyes, 90 per cent of the time being allocated to the fixation sites. Also, the brain suppresses the visual image during the saccades so that one is completely unconscious of the movements from point to point.

Saccadic Movements During Reading. During the process of reading, a person usually makes several saccadic movements of the eyes for each line. In this case the visual scene is not moving past the eyes, but the eyes are trained to scan across the visual scene to extract the important information. Similar saccades occur when a person observes a painting, except that the saccades occur in one direction after another from one highlight of the painting to another, then another, and so forth.

Fixation on Moving Objects — "Pursuit Movements." The eyes can also remain fixed on a moving object, which is called *pursuit movement*. A highly developed cortical mechanism automatically detects the course of movement of an object and then gradually develops a similar course of movement of the eyes. For instance, if an object is moving up and down in a wavelike form at a rate of several times per second, the eyes at first may be completely unable to fixate on it. However, after a second or so the eyes begin to jump coarsely in approximately the same pattern of movement as that of the object. Then after a few more seconds, the eyes develop progressively smoother and smoother movements and finally follow the course of movement almost exactly. This represents a high degree of automatic, subconscious computational ability by the cerebral cortex.

Vestibular Control of Eye Movements. Another type of eye movement is elicited by stimulation of the

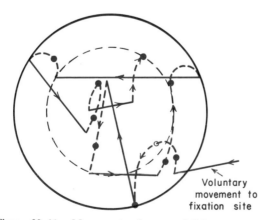

Voluntary movement to fixation site

Figure 20–11. Movements of a spot of light on the fovea, showing sudden "flicking" movements to move the spot back toward the center of the fovea whenever it drifts to the foveal edge. (The dashed lines represent slow drifting movements, and the solid lines represent sudden flicking movements.) (Modified from Whitteridge: Handbook of Physiology, Vol. 2, Sec. 1. Baltimore, The Williams & Wilkins Company, 1960, p. 1089.)

vestibular apparatus. The vestibular nuclei are connected directly with the brainstem nuclei that control ocular movements, and, whenever the head is accelerated in a vertical, longitudinal, lateral or angular direction, an immediate compensatory motion of the eyes occurs in the opposite direction. This allows the eyes to remain fixed on an object of attention despite rapid movements of the body or head.

Vestibular control of the eyes is especially valuable when a person is subjected to jerky motions of the body. For instance, when a person with bilateral destruction of the vestibular apparatuses rides over rough roads, fixing the eyes on the road or on any horizontal scene is extremely difficult. The opticokinetic type of movement is not capable of keeping the eyes fixed under such conditions because it has a latent period of about one-fifth second before the direction of movement of the visual scene can be detected and followed by the eyes. On the other hand, the vestibular type of eye movement has a short latent period, measured in thousandths of a second rather than one-fifth second.

Also when a person begins to rotate, the vestibular apparatuses cause a vestibular type of saccadic movements called *vestibular nystagmus*. That is, the eyes lag behind the rotating head, then jump forward, then lag behind again, jump again, and so forth. This type of nystagmus is discussed in Chapter 12 in relation to vestibular function.

Pathologic Types of Nystagmus. Occasionally, abnormalities occur in the control system for eye movements that cause continuous nystagmus (back and forth movements) despite the fact that neither the visual scene nor the body is moving. This is likely to occur when one of the vestibular apparatuses is damaged or when severe damage is sustained in the deep nuclei of the cerebellum. This is discussed further in Chapter 13.

Another pathologic type of eye movement that is sometimes called nystagmus occurs when the foveal regions of the two eyes have been destroyed or when the vision in these areas is greatly weakened. In such a condition the eyes attempt to fix the object of attention on the foveae but always overshoot the mark because of foveal insensitivity. Therefore, they oscillate back and forth but never achieve foveal fixation. Even though this condition is known clinically as a type of nystagmus, physiologically it is completely different from the nystagmus that keeps the eyes fixed on a moving scene.

FUSION OF THE VISUAL IMAGES

To make the visual perceptions more meaningful and also to aid in depth perception by the mechanism of stereopsis, which was discussed in Chapter 18, the visual images in the two eyes normally *fuse* with each other on "corresponding points" of the two retinae.

The visual cortex especially, and perhaps the lateral geniculate body as well, plays a very important role in fusion. It was pointed out earlier in the chapter that corresponding points of the two retinae transmit visual signals to different neuronal layers of the lateral geniculate body, and these signals in turn are relayed to parallel stripes of neurons in the visual cortex. Interactions occur between the stripes of cortical neurons; these cause *interference patterns of excitation* in still other neuronal cells when the two visual images are not precisely "in register" — that is, not precisely fused. This excitation presumably provides the signal that is transmitted to the oculomotor apparatus to cause convergence or divergence or rotation of the eyes so that fusion can be re-established. Once the corresponding points of the retinae are precisely in register with each other, the excitation of the specific cells in the visual cortex disappears.

The Neural Mechanism for Stereopsis. The visual images that appear on the retina during the process of stereopsis were discussed in Chapter 18. It was pointed out that because the two eyes are a little more than 2 inches apart the images on the two retinae are not exactly the same. The closer the object is to the eye the greater is the disparity between the two images. Consequently, it is impossible for all corresponding points in the visual image to be in complete register at the same time. Furthermore, the nearer the object is to the eye the less is the degree of register. Here again, specific cells in the primary visual cortex become excited in the areas of the visual field where highlights are out of register. Presumably, this excitation is the source of signals for detection of the distance of the object in front of the eyes; this mechanism is called *stereopsis*.

Strabismus. Strabismus, which is also called *squint* or *cross-eyedness*, means lack of fusion of the eyes in one or more of the coordinates described above. Three basic types of strabismus are illustrated in Figure 20–12: *horizontal strabismus, vertical strabismus,* and *torsional strabismus.* However, combinations of two or even of all three of the different types of strabismus often occur.

Strabismus is caused by an abnormal "set" of the fusion mechanism of the visual system. That is, in the early efforts of the child to fixate the two eyes on the same object, one of the eyes fixates satisfactorily while the other fails to fixate, or they both fixate satisfactorily but never simultaneously. Soon, the patterns of conjugate movements of the eyes become abnormally "set" so that the eyes never fuse.

Frequently, some abnormality of the eyes contributes to the failure of the two eyes to fixate on the same point. For instance, if at birth one eye has poor vision in comparison with the other, the good eye tends to fixate on the object of attention while the poor eye might never do so. Also, in hypermetropic infants, intense impulses must be transmitted to the ciliary muscles to focus the eyes, and some of these impulses overflow into the oculomotor nuclei to cause simultaneous convergence of the eyes, as will be discussed below. As a result, the child's fusion mechanism becomes "set" for continual inward deviation of the eyes.

Suppression of Visual Image from a Repressed Eye. In

Horizontal   Torsional   Vertical
strabismus   strabismus   strabismus

Figure 20–12. The three basic types of strabismus.

many patients with strabismus the eyes alternate in fixing on the object of attention. However, in other patients, one eye alone is used all the time while the other eye becomes repressed and is never used for vision. The vision in the repressed eye develops only slightly, usually remaining 20/400 or less. If the dominant eye then becomes blinded, vision in the repressed eye can develop only to a slight extent in the adult but far more in young children. This illustrates that visual acuity is highly dependent on proper development of the central synaptic connections from the eyes.

AUTONOMIC CONTROL OF ACCOMMODATION AND PUPILLARY APERTURE

The Autonomic Nerves to the Eyes. The eye is innervated by both parasympathetic and sympathetic fibers, as illustrated in Figure 20–13. The parasympathetic preganglionic fibers arise in the *Edinger-Westphal nucleus* (the visceral nucleus of the third nerve) and then pass in the *third nerve* to the *ciliary ganglion,* which lies about 1 cm. behind the eye. Here the preganglionic fibers synapse with postganglionic parasympathetic neurons that, in turn, send fibers through the *ciliary nerves* into the eyeball. These nerves excite the ciliary muscle and the sphincter of the iris.

The sympathetic innervation of the eye originates in the *intermediolateral horn cells* of the first thoracic segment of the spinal cord. From here, sympathetic fibers enter the sympathetic chain and pass upward to the *superior cervical ganglion* where they synapse with postganglionic neurons. Fibers from these spread along the carotid artery and successively smaller arteries until they reach the eye. There the sympathetic fibers innervate the radial fibers of the iris as well as several extraocular structures around the eye, which are discussed shortly in relation to Horner's syndrome. Also, they supply very weak innervation to the ciliary muscle.

CONTROL OF ACCOMMODATION

The accommodation mechanism — that is, the mechanism which focuses the lens system of the eye — is essential for a high degree of visual acuity. Accommodation results from contraction or relaxation of the ciliary muscle, contraction causing increased strength of the lens system, as explained in Chapter 18, and relaxation causing decreased strength. The question that must be answered now is: How does a person adjust accommodation to keep the eyes in focus all the time?

Accommodation of the lens is regulated by a negative feedback mechanism that automatically adjusts the focal power of the lens for the highest degree of visual acuity. When the eyes have been fixed on some far object and then suddenly fix on a near object, the lens accommodates for maximum acuity of vision usually within one second.

Though the precise control mechanism that causes this rapid and accurate focusing of the eye is still unclear, some of the known features of the mechanism are the following:

First, when the eyes suddenly change the distance of the fixation point, the lens always changes its strength in the proper direction to achieve a new state of focus. In other words, the lens *does not hunt* back and forth on the two sides of focus in an attempt to find the focus.

Second, different types of clues that can help the lens change its strength in the proper direction include the following: (1) *Chromatic aberration* appears to be important. That is, the red light rays focus slightly posteriorly to the blue light rays. The eyes appear to be able to detect which of these two types of rays is in better focus, and this clue relays information to the accommodation mechanism whether to make the lens stronger or weaker. (2) When the eyes fixate on a near object they also converge toward each other. *The neural mechanisms for convergence cause a simultaneous signal to strengthen the lens of the eye.* (3) *Since the fovea is a depressed area, the clarity of focus in the depth of the fovea versus the clarity of focus on the edges will be different.* It has been suggested that this also gives clues as to which way the strength of the lens needs to be changed. (4) It has been found that *the degree of accommodation of the lens oscillates slightly* all of the time, at a frequency up to 2 times per second. It has been suggested that the visual image becomes clearer when the oscillation of the lens strength is in the appropriate direction and poorer when the lens strength is in the wrong direction. This could give a rapid cue as to which way the strength of the lens needs to change to provide appropriate focus.

It is presumed that the cortical areas that control accommodation closely parallel those that control fixation movements of the eyes, with final integration of the visual signals in areas 18 and 19 and transmission of motor signals to the ciliary muscle through the pretectal area and Edinger-Westphal nucleus.

CONTROL OF THE PUPILLARY APERTURE

Stimulation of the parasympathetic nerves excites the pupillary sphincter, thereby decreasing the pupillary aperture; this is called *miosis.* On the other hand, stimulation of the sympathetic nerves excites the radial fibers of the iris and causes pupillary dilatation, which is called *mydriasis.*

The Pupillary Light Reflex. When light is shone into the eyes the pupils constrict, a reaction that is called the pupillary light reflex. The neuronal pathway for this reflex is illustrated in Figure

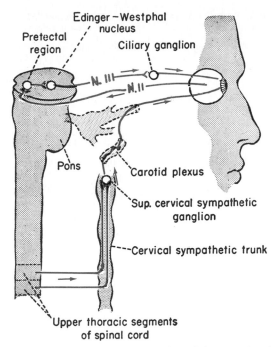

Figure 20–13. Autonomic innervation of the eye, showing also the reflex arc of the light reflex. (Modified from Ranson and Clark: Anatomy of the Nervous System. Philadelphia, W. B. Saunders Company, 1959.)

20–13. When light impinges on the retina, the resulting impulses pass through the optic nerves and optic tracts to the pretectal nuclei. From here, impulses pass to the *Edinger-Westphal nucleus* and finally back through the *parasympathetic nerves* to constrict the sphincter of the iris. In darkness, the reflex becomes inhibited, which results in dilatation of the pupil.

The function of the light reflex is to help the eye adapt extremely rapidly to changing light conditions, the importance of which was explained in relation to retinal adaptation in the previous chapter. The limits of pupillary diameter are about 1.5 mm. on the small side and 8 mm. on the large side. Therefore, the range of light adaptation that can be effected by the pupillary reflex is about 30 to 1.

Pupillary Reflexes in Central Nervous System Disease. Certain central nervous system diseases block the transmission of visual signals from the retinae to the Edinger-Westphal nucleus. Such blocks frequently occur as a result of *central nervous system syphilis, alcoholism, encephalitis,* or so forth. The block usually occurs in the pretectal region of the brain stem, though it can also result from destruction of the small afferent fibers in the optic nerves.

The light signals to the Edinger-Westphal nucleus are of the inhibitory type. Therefore, when they are blocked, the nucleus becomes chronically active, causing the pupils thereafter to remain partially constricted in addition to their failure to respond to light.

When the light reflex is lost, the pupils can still constrict an additional amount if the Edinger-Westphal

nucleus is stimulated through some other pathways. For instance, when the eyes fixate on a near object, the signals that cause accommodation of the lens (and also those that cause convergence of the two eyes) cause a mild degree of pupillary constriction at the same time. This is called the *accommodation reflex.* Such a pupil that fails to respond to light but does respond to accommodation and also is very small (an *Argyll Robertson pupil*) is an important diagnostic sign of central nervous system disease — very often syphilis.

Horner's Syndrome. The sympathetic nerves to the eye are occasionally interrupted, and this interruption frequently occurs in the cervical sympathetic chain. This results in *Horner's syndrome*, which consists of the following effects: First, because of interruption of fibers to the pupillary dilator muscle, the pupil remains persistently constricted to a smaller diameter than that of the pupil of the opposite eye. Second, the superior eyelid droops because this eyelid is normally maintained in an open position during the waking hours partly by contraction of a smooth muscle, the *superior palpebral muscle,* which is innervated by the sympathetics. Therefore, destruction of the sympathetics makes it impossible to open the superior eyelid nearly as widely as normally. Third, the blood vessels on the corresponding side of the face and head become persistently dilated. And, fourth, sweating cannot occur on the side of the face and head affected by Horner's syndrome.

REFERENCES

Armington, J. C.: The Electroretinogram. New York, Academic Press, 1974.

Bizzi, E.: The coordination of eye-head movements. *Sci. Am.,* 231(4):100, 1974.

Critchley, M., and Critchley, E. A.: Dyslexia Defined. Springfield, Ill., Charles C Thomas, 1978.

Dunn-Rankin, P.: The visual characteristics of words. *Sci. Am.,* 238(1):122, 1978.

Ewert, J. P.: The neural basis of visually guided behavior. *Sci. Am.,* 230(3):34, 1974.

Fatt, I.: Physiology of the Eye: An Introduction to the Vegetative Function. Boston, Butterworths, 1978.

Fraser, S. E., and Hunt, R. K.: Retinotectal specificity: Models and experiments in search of a mapping function. *Annu. Rev. Neurosci.,* 3:319, 1980.

Goldchrist, A. L.: The perception of surface blacks and whites. *Sci. Am.,* 240(3):112, 1979.

Glickstein, M., and Gibson, A. R.: Visual cells in the pons of the brain. *Sci. Am.,* 235(5):90, 1976.

Gogel, W. C.: The adjacency principle in visual perception. *Sci. Am.,* 238(5):126, 1978.

Guyton, J. S., and Kirkman, N.: Ocular movement: I. Mechanics, pathogenesis, and surgical treatment of alternating hypertropia (dissociated vertical divergence, double hypertropia) and some related phenomena. *Am. J. Ophthalmol.,* 41:438, 1956.

Hess, E. H.: The role of pupil size in communication. *Sci. Am.,* 235(5):110, 1975.

Hubbell, W. L., and Bownds, M. D.: Visual transduction in vertebrate photoreceptors. *Annu. Rev. Neurosci.,* 2:17, 1979.

Hubel, D. H.: Eleventh Bowditch Lecture. Effects of distortion of sensory input on the visual system of kittens. *Physiologist, 10:17,* 1967.

Hubel, D. H., and Wiesel, T. N.: Receptive fields of cells in striate cortex of very young, visually inexperienced kittens. *J. Neurophysiol., 26:994,* 1963.

Hubel, D. H., and Wiesel, T. N.: Cortical and callosal connections concerned with vertical meridian of visual fields in the cat. *J. Neurophysiol., 30:1561,* 1967.

Hubel, D. H., and Wiesel, T. N.: Brain mechanisms of vision. *Sci. Am.,* 241(3):150, 1979.

Kuffler, S. W.: The single-cell approach in the visual system and the study of receptive fields. *Invest. Ophthalmol., 12:794,* 1973.

Johansson, G.: Visual motion perception. *Sci. Am., 232*(6):1975.

Julesz, B.: Experiments in the visual perception of texture. *Sci. Am., 232*(4):34, 1975.

Kool, K. A., and Marshall, R. E.: Visual Evoked Potentials in Central Disorders of the Visual System. New York, Harper & Row, 1979.

McIlwain, J. T.: Large receptive fields and spatial transformations in the visual system. *Int. Rev. Physiol., 10*:223, 1976.

Neuroanatomy and Neuro-Ophthalmology, May–June 1978. Rochester, Minn., American Academy of Ophthalmology, 1978.

Ordy, J. M., and Brizzee, K. R. (eds.): Sensory Systems and Communication in the Elderly. New York, Raven Press, 1979.

Polyak, S.: The Retina. Chicago, University of Chicago Press, 1941.

Raphan, T., and Cohen, B.: Brainstem mechanisms for rapid and slow eye movements. *Annu. Rev. Physiol., 40*:527, 1978.

Regan, D., *et al.*: The visual perception of motion in depth. *Sci. Am. 241*(1):136, 1979.

Reinecke, R. D. (ed.): Strabismus. New York, Grune & Stratton, 1978.

Rodieck, R. W.: Visual pathways. *Annu. Rev. Neurosci., 2*:193, 1979.

Sekuler, R., and Levinson, E.: The perception of moving targets. *Sci. Am., 236*(1):60, 1977.

Singer, W.: Control of thalamic transmission by corticofugal and ascending reticular pathways in the visual system. *Physiol. Rev., 57*:386, 1977.

Smith, J. L.: Neuro-Ophthalmology, Focus 1980. New York, Masson Publishing USA, 1979.

Toates, F. M.: Accommodation function in the human eye. *Physiol. Rev., 52*:828, 1972.

Van Essen, D. C.: Visual areas of the mammalian cerebral cortex. *Annu. Rev. Neurosci., 2*:227, 1979.

Walsh, T. J.: Neuro-Ophthalmology: Clinical Signs and Symptoms. Philadelphia, Lea & Febiger, 1978.

Wurtz, R. H., and Albano, J. E.: Visual-motor function of the primate superior colliculus. *Annu. Rev. Neurosci., 3*:189, 1980.

Yannuzzi, L. A., *et al.* (eds.): The Macula: A Comprehensive Text and Atlas. Baltimore, Williams & Wilkins, 1978.

21

The Sense of Hearing

Hearing, like many somatic senses, is a mechanoreceptive sense, for the ear responds to mechanical vibration of the sound waves in the air. The purpose of the present chapter is to describe and explain the mechanism by which the ear receives sound waves, discriminates their frequencies, and finally transmits auditory information into the central nervous system.

THE TYMPANIC MEMBRANE AND THE OSSICULAR SYSTEM

TRANSMISSION OF SOUND FROM THE TYMPANIC MEMBRANE TO THE COCHLEA

Figure 21–1 illustrates the *tympanic membrane* (commonly called the *eardrum*) and the *ossicular system,* which transmits sound through the middle ear. The tympanic membrane is cone-shaped, with its concavity facing downward and outward toward the auditory canal. Attached to the very center of the tympanic membrane is the *handle* of the *malleus*. At its other end the malleus is tightly bound to the *incus* by ligaments so that whenever the malleus moves the incus moves with it. The opposite end of the incus in turn articulates with the stem of the *stapes,* and the *faceplate* of the stapes lies against the membranous labyrinth in the opening of the oval window where sound waves are transmitted into the inner ear, the *cochlea*.

The ossicles of the middle ear are suspended by ligaments in such a way that the combined malleus and incus act as a single lever having its fulcrum approximately at the border of the tympanic membrane. The large *head* of the malleus, which is on the opposite side of the fulcrum from the handle, almost exactly balances the other end of the lever so that changes in position of the body will not increase or decrease the tension on the tympanic membrane.

The articulation of the incus with the stapes causes the stapes to push forward on the cochlear fluid every time the handle of the malleus moves inward and to pull backward on the fluid every time the malleus moves outward, which promotes inward and outward motion of the faceplate at the oval window.

The handle of the malleus is constantly pulled inward by ligaments and by the tensor tympani muscle, which keeps the tympanic membrane tensed. This allows sound vibrations on *any* portion of the tympanic membrane to be transmitted to the malleus, which would not be true if the membrane were lax.

Impedance Matching by the Ossicular System. The amplitude of movement of the stapes faceplate with each sound vibration is only three-fourths as much as the amplitude of the handle of the malleus. Therefore, the ossicular lever system does not amplify the movement distance of the stapes, as is commonly believed. Instead, the system actually reduces the amplitude but increases the *force* of movement about 1.3 times. However, the surface area of the tympanic membrane is approximately 55 sq. mm., while the surface area of the stapes averages 3.2 sq. mm. This 17-fold difference times the 1.3-fold ratio of the lever system allows all the energy of a sound wave impinging on the tympanic membrane to be

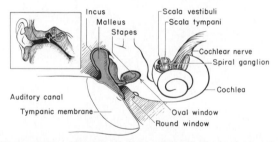

Figure 21–1. The tympanic membrane, the ossicular system of the middle ear, and the inner ear.

applied to the small faceplate of the stapes, causing approximately 22 times as much *pressure* on the fluid of the cochlea as is exerted by the sound wave against the tympanic membrane. Since fluid has far greater inertia than air, it is easily understood that increased amounts of pressure are needed to cause vibration in the fluid. Therefore, the tympanic membrane and ossicular system provide *impedance matching* between the sound waves in air and the sound vibrations in the fluid of the cochlea. Indeed, the impedance matching is about 50 to 75 per cent of perfect for sound frequencies between 300 to 3000 cycles per second, which allows almost full utilization of the energy in the incoming sound waves.

In the absence of the ossicular system and tympanum, sound waves can travel directly through the air of the middle ear and can enter the cochlea at the oval window. However, the sensitivity for hearing is then 30 decibels less than for ossicular transmission — equivalent to a decrease from a very loud voice to a barely audible voice level.

Attenuation of Sound by Contraction of the Stapedius and Tensor Tympani Muscles. When loud sounds are transmitted through the ossicular system into the central nervous system, a reflex occurs after a latent period of 40 to 80 milliseconds to cause contraction of both the stapedius and tensor tympani muscles. The tensor tympani muscle pulls the handle of the malleus inward while the stapedius muscle pulls the stapes outward. These two forces oppose each other and thereby cause the entire ossicular system to develop a high degree of rigidity, thus greatly reducing the ossicular transmission of low frequency sound, mainly frequencies below 1000 cycles per second.

This *attenuation reflex* can reduce the intensity of sound transmission by as much as 30 to 40 decibels, which is about the same difference as that between a whisper and the sound emitted by a loud voice. The function of this mechanism is probably two-fold:

1. To *protect* the cochlea from damaging vibrations caused by excessively loud sound. It is mainly low frequency sounds (the ones that are attenuated) that are frequently loud enough to damage the basilar membrane of the cochlea. Unfortunately, because of the 40 or more millisecond latency for reaction of the reflex, the sudden, loud, thunderous sounds that result from explosions can still cause extensive cochlear damage.

2. To *mask* low frequency sounds in loud environments. This usually removes a major share of the background noise and allows a person to concentrate on sounds above 1000 cycles per second frequency. It is in this upper frequency range that most of the pertinent information in voice communication is transmitted.

Another function of the tensor tympani and stapedius muscles is to decrease a person's hearing sensitivity to his or her own speech. This effect is activated by collateral signals transmitted to these muscles at the same time that the brain activates the voice mechanism.

TRANSMISSION OF SOUND THROUGH BONE

Because the inner ear, the *cochlea,* is embedded in a bony cavity in the temporal bone called the bony labyrinth, vibrations of the entire skull can cause fluid vibrations in the cochlea itself. Therefore, under appropriate conditions, a tuning fork or an electronic vibrator placed on any bony protuberance of the skull causes the person to hear the sound if it is intense enough. Unfortunately, the energy available even in very loud sound in the air is not sufficient to cause hearing through the bone except when a special electromechanical sound-transmitting device is applied directly to the bone, usually to the mastoid process.

THE COCHLEA

FUNCTIONAL ANATOMY OF THE COCHLEA

The cochlea is a system of coiled tubes, shown in Figure 21–1, and in cross-section in Figures 21–2 and 21–3, with three different tubes coiled side by side: the *scala vestibuli,* the *scala media*, and the *scala tympani.* The scala vestibuli and scala media are separated from each other by *Reissner's membrane* (also called the *vestibular membrane*), and

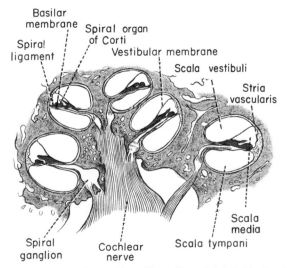

Figure 21–2. The cochlea. (From Goss C. M. (ed.): Gray's Anatomy of the Human Body. Lea & Febiger.)

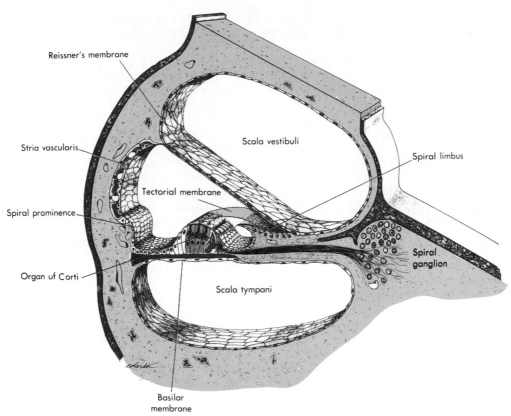

Figure 21–3. A section through one of the turns of the cochlea. (Drawn by Sylvia Colard Keene. From Bloom and Fawcett: A Textbook of Histology. Philadelphia, W. B. Saunders Company, 1975.)

the scala tympani and scala media are separated from each other by the *basilar membrane*. On the surface of the basilar membrane lies a structure, the *organ of Corti*, which contains a series of mechanically sensitive cells, the *hair cells*. These are the receptive end-organs that generate nerve impulses in response to sound vibrations.

Figure 21–4 diagrams the functional parts of the uncoiled cochlea for transmission of sound vibrations. First, note that Reissner's membrane is missing from this figure. This membrane is so thin and so easily moved that it does not obstruct the passage of sound vibrations from the scala vestibuli into the scala media at all. Therefore, so far

Figure 21–4. Movement of fluid in the cochlea following forward thrust of the stapes.

as the transmission of sound is concerned, the scala vestibuli and scala media are considered to be a single chamber. The importance of Reissner's membrane is to maintain a special fluid in the scala media that is required for normal function of the sound receptive hair cells, as discussed later in the chapter.

Sound vibrations enter the scala vestibuli from the faceplate of the stapes at the oval window. The faceplate covers this window and is connected with the window's edges by a relatively loose annular ligament so that it can move inward and outward with the sound vibrations. Inward movement causes the fluid to move into the scala vestibuli and scala media, which immediately increases the pressure in the entire cochlea and causes the round window to bulge outward.

Note in Figure 21–4 that the distal ends of the scala vestibuli and scala tympani are continuous with each other through an opening at the end, the *helicotrema*. If the stapes moves inward *very slowly*, fluid from the scala vestibuli is pushed through the helicotrema into the scala tympani, and this causes the round window to bulge outward. However, if the stapes vibrates inward and outward rapidly, the fluid simply does not have time to pass all the way to the helicotrema, then to the round window, and back again to the oval window between each two successive vibrations. Instead, the fluid wave takes a shortcut through the basilar membrane, causing it to bulge back and forth with each sound vibration. We shall see later that each frequency of sound causes a different "pattern" of vibration in the basilar membrane and that this is one of the important means by which the sound frequencies are discriminated from each other.

The Basilar Membrane and Resonance in the Cochlea.   The basilar membrane contains 20,000 to 30,000 *basilar fibers* that project from the bony center of the cochlea, the *modiolus*, toward the outer wall. These fibers are stiff, elastic, reedlike structures that are fixed at their basal ends but not at their distal ends except that the distal ends are embedded in the loose basilar membrane. Because the fibers are stiff and also free at one end, they can vibrate like reeds of a harmonica.

The lengths of the basilar fibers increase progressively as one goes from the oval and round windows toward the helicotrema, from a length of approximately 0.04 mm. near the windows to 0.5 mm. at the helicotrema, a 12-fold increase in length.

The diameters of the fibers, on the other hand, decrease from the base to the helicotrema, so that their overall stiffness decreases more than 100-fold. As a result, the stiff, short fibers near the base of the cochlea have a tendency to vibrate at a high frequency, while the long, limber fibers near the helicotrema have a tendency to vibrate at a low frequency.

In addition to the differences in stiffness of the basilar fibers, they are also differently "loaded" by the fluid mass of the cochlea. That is, when a fiber vibrates back and forth, all the fluid between the vibrating fiber and the oval and round windows must also move back and forth at the same time. For a fiber vibrating near the base of the cochlea (near the two windows), the total mass of moving fluid is slight in comparison with that for a fiber vibrating near the helicotrema. This difference, too, favors high frequency vibration near the windows and low frequency vibration near the tip of the cochlea.

Thus, high frequency resonance of the basilar membrane occurs near the base, and low frequency resonance occurs near the apex because of (1) difference in stiffness of the fibers and (2) difference in "loading."

TRANSMISSION OF SOUND WAVES IN THE COCHLEA— THE "TRAVELING WAVE"

If the foot of the stapes moves inward instantaneously, the round window must also bulge outward instantaneously because the cochlea is bounded on all sides by bony walls. Since the fluid wave will not have time to move all the way from the oval window to the helicotrema and back to the round window, the initial effect is to cause the basilar membrane at the very base of the cochlea to bulge in the direction of the round window. However, the elastic tension that is built up in the basilar fibers as they bend toward the round window initiates a wave that "travels" along the basilar membrane toward the helicotrema, as illustrated in Figure 21–5. Figure 21–5A shows movement of a high frequency wave down the basilar membrane; Figure 21–5B, a medium frequency wave; and Figure 21–5C, a very low frequency wave. Movement of the wave along the basilar membrane is comparable to the movement of a pressure wave along the arterial walls, a widely known phenomenon, or it is also comparable to the wave that travels along the surface of a pond.

Pattern of Vibration of the Basilar Membrane for Different Sound Frequencies.   Note in Figure 21–5 the different patterns of transmission for sound waves of different frequencies. Each wave is relatively weak at the outset but becomes strong when it reaches that portion of the basilar membrane that has a natural resonant frequency equal to the respective sound frequency. At this point the basilar membrane can vibrate back and forth with such great ease that the energy in the wave is completely dissipated. Consequently, the wave ceases at this point and fails to travel the remaining distance along the basilar membrane. Thus, a high frequency sound wave travels only a short

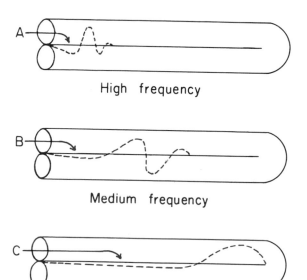

Figure 21–5.   "Traveling waves" along the basilar membrane for high, medium, and low frequency sounds.

Figure 21–6. (A) Amplitude pattern of vibration of the basilar membrane for a medium frequency sound. (B) Amplitude patterns for sounds of all frequencies between 50 and 8000 per second, showing the points of maximum amplitude (the resonance points) on the basilar membrane for the different frequencies.

distance along the basilar membrane before it reaches its resonant point and dies out; a medium frequency sound wave travels about halfway and then dies out; and, finally, a very low frequency sound wave travels the entire distance along the membrane.

Another feature of the traveling wave is that it travels fast along the initial portion of the basilar membrane but progressively more slowly as it goes farther and farther into the cochlea. The cause of this is the high coefficient of elasticity of the basilar fibers near the stapes but a progressively decreasing coefficient farther along the membrane. This rapid initial transmission of the wave allows the high frequency sounds to travel far enough into the cochlea to spread out and separate from each other on the basilar membrane. Without this spread, all the high frequency waves would be bunched together within the first millimeter or so of the basilar membrane, and their frequencies could not be discriminated one from the other.

Amplitude Pattern of Vibration of the Basilar Membrane. The dashed curves of Figure 21–6A show the position of a sound wave on the basilar membrane when the stapes (*a*) is all the way inward, (*b*) has moved back to the neutral point, (*c*) is all the way outward, and (*d*) has moved back again to the neutral point but is moving inward. The shaded area around these different waves shows the maximum extent of vibration of the basilar membrane during a complete vibratory cycle. This is the amplitude pattern of vibration of

the basilar membrane for this particular sound frequency.

Figure 21–6B shows the amplitude patterns of vibration for different frequencies, showing that the maximum amplitude for 8000 cycles occurs near the base of the cochlea, while that for frequencies less than 400 to 500 cycles per second is all the way at the tip of the basilar membrane near the helicotrema.

Note in Figure 21–6B that the basal end of the basilar membrane vibrates at least weakly for all frequencies. However, beyond the resonant area for each given frequency, the vibration of the basilar membrane cuts off sharply. The principal method by which sound frequencies, especially those above 400 to 500 cycles per second, are discriminated from each other is based on the "place" of maximum stimulation of the nerve fibers from the organ of Corti lying on the basilar membrane, as will be explained in the following section.

FUNCTION OF THE ORGAN OF CORTI

The organ of Corti, illustrated in Figures 21–2, 21–3, and 21–7, is the receptor organ that generates nerve impulses in response to vibration of the basilar membrane. Note that the organ of Corti lies on the surface of the basilar fibers and basilar membrane. The actual sensory receptors in the organ of Corti are two types of *hair cells,* a single row of *internal hair cells,* numbering about 3500 and measuring about 12 microns in diameter, and three to four rows of *external hair cells,* numbering about 20,000 and having diameters of only about 8 microns. The bases and sides of the hair cells synapse with a network of cochlear nerve endings. These lead to the *spiral ganglion of Corti,* which lies in the modiolus (the center) of the cochlea. The spiral ganglion in turn sends axons into the *cochlear nerve* and thence into the central nervous system at the level of the upper medulla. The relationship of the organ of Corti to the spiral ganglion and to the cochlear nerve is illustrated in Figure 21–2.

Excitation of the Hair Cells. Note in Figure 21–7 that minute hairs, or cilia, project upward from the hair cells and either touch or are embedded in the surface gel coating of the *tectorial membrane* which lies above the cilia in the scala media. These hair cells are similar to the hair cells found in the macula and cristae ampullaris of the vestibular apparatus, which were discussed in Chapter 12. Bending of the hairs in one direction depolarizes the hair cells, and this in turn excites the nerve fibers synapsing with their bases.

Figure 21–8 illustrates the mechanism by which vibration of the basilar membrane excites the hair endings. This shows that the upper ends of the hair

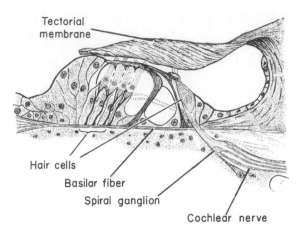

Figure 21–7. The organ of Corti, showing especially the hair cells and the tectorial membrane against the projecting hairs.

cells are fixed tightly in a structure called the *reticular lamina*. Furthermore, the reticular lamina is very rigid and is continuous with a rigid triangular structure called the *rods of Corti* that rests on the basilar fibers. Therefore, the basilar fiber, the rods of Corti, and the reticular lamina all move as a unit.

Upward movement of the basilar fiber rocks the reticular lamina upward and *inward*. Then, when the basilar membrane moves downward, the reticular lamina rocks downward and *outward*. The inward and outward motion causes the hairs to shear back and forth against the tectorial membrane, thus exciting the cochlear nerve fibers whenever the basilar membrane vibrates.

Mechanism by Which the Hair Cells Excite the Nerve Fibers — Receptor Potentials. Back-and-forth bending of the hairs causes alternate changes in the electrical potential across the hair cell membrane. This alternating potential is the *receptor potential* of the hair cell, and it in turn stimulates the cochlear nerve endings that terminate on the hair cells. Most physiologists believe that the receptor potential stimulates the endings by direct electrical excitation.

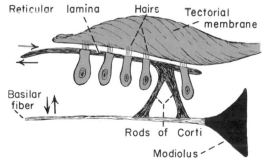

Figure 21–8. Stimulation of the hair cells by the to-and-fro movement of the hairs in the tectorial membrane.

When the basilar fiber bends toward the scala vestibuli (in the upward direction in Figure 21–8), the hair cell becomes depolarized, and it is this depolarization that excites an increased number of action potentials in the nerve fiber. When the basilar fiber moves in the opposite direction, the hair cell becomes hyperpolarized, and the number of action potentials decreases.

The Endocochlear Potential. To explain even more fully the electrical potentials generated by the hair cells, we need to explain still another electrical phenomenon called the endocochlear potential: The scala media is filled with a fluid called *endolymph* in contradistinction to the *perilymph* present in the scala vestibuli and scala tympani. The scala vestibuli and scala tympani in most young children and in some adults communicate directly with the subarachnoid space around the brain, so that the perilymph is almost identical with cerebrospinal fluid. On the other hand, the endolymph that fills the scala media is an entirely different fluid probably secreted by the *stria vascularis,* a highly vascular area on the outer wall of the scala media. Endolymph contains a very high concentration of potassium and a very low concentration of sodium, which is exactly opposite to the perilymph.

An electrical potential of approximately 80 mv. exists all the time between the endolymph and the perilymph, with positivity inside the scala media and negativity outside. This is called the *endocochlear potential,* and it is believed to be generated by continual secretion of positive potassium ions into the scala media by the stria vascularis.

The importance of the endocochlear potential is that the tops of the hair cells project through the reticular lamina into the endolymph of the scala media while perilymph bathes the lower bodies of the hair cells. Furthermore, the hair cells have a negative intracellular potential of −70 millivolts with respect to the perilymph, but −150 millivolts with respect to the endolymph at their upper surfaces where the hairs project into the endolymph. It is believed that this high electrical potential at the hair border of the cell greatly sensitizes the cell, thereby increasing its ability to respond to slight movement of the hairs.

DETERMINATION OF PITCH – THE "PLACE" PRINCIPLE

In the minds of most persons, sound pitch and sound frequency are the same thing. However, the two are slightly different in the following way: Pitch is the conscious perception of the sound frequency and may not be the same as the true sound frequency. The pitch is especially likely to deviate from the true sound frequency at both very high and very low frequency; also, the pitch usually changes slightly as the intensity of the sound changes even though the frequency remains constant. Yet, from the point of view of the following discussion, we can still consider the two to be essentially the same.

From earlier discussions in this chapter it is already apparent that low pitch (or low frequency) sounds cause maximal activation of the basilar membrane near the apex of the cochlea, sounds of high pitch (or high frequency) activate the basilar membrane near the base of the cochlea, and intermediate frequencies activate the membrane at intermediate distances between these two extremes. Furthermore, there is spatial organization of the cochlear nerve fibers from the cochlea to the cochlear nuclei in the brain stem, the fibers from each respective area of the basilar membrane terminating in a corresponding area in the cochlear nuclei. We shall see later that this spatial organization continues all the way up the brain stem to the cerebral cortex. The recording of signals from the auditory tracts in the brain stem and from the auditory receptive fields in the cerebral cortex shows that specific neurons are activated by specific pitches. Therefore, the major method used by the nervous system to detect different pitches is to determine the position along the basilar membrane that is most stimulated. This is called the *place principle* for determination of pitch.

Yet, referring again to Figure 21–6, one can see that the distal end of the basilar membrane at the helicotrema is stimulated by all sound frequencies below 400 to 500 cycles per second. Therefore, it has been difficult to understand from the place principle how one can differentiate between very low sound frequencies. It is postulated that these low frequencies are discriminated mainly by the so-called *frequency principle*. That is, the low frequency sounds cause volleys of impulses at the same low frequencies to be transmitted by the cochlear nerve into the cochlear nuclei. And it is believed that the cochlear nuclei then distinguish the different frequencies. In fact, destruction of the entire apical half of the cochlea, which destroys the basilar membrane where all of the lower frequency sounds are normally detected, still does not completely eliminate the discrimination of low frequency sounds.

DETERMINATION OF LOUDNESS

Loudness is determined by the auditory system in at least three different ways: First, as the sound becomes louder, the amplitude of vibration of the basilar membrane and hair cells also increases so that the hair cells excite the nerve endings at more rapid rates. Second, as the amplitude of vibration increases, it causes more and more of the hair cells on the fringes of the vibrating portion of the basilar membrane to become stimulated, thus causing *spatial summation* of impulses — that is, transmission through many nerve fibers, rather than through a few. Third, certain hair cells do not become stimulated until the vibration of the basilar membrane reaches a relatively high intensity, and it is believed that stimulation of these cells in some way apprises the nervous system that the sound is then very loud.

Detection of Changes in Loudness — The Power Law. It was pointed out in Chapter 8 that a person interprets changes in intensity of sensory stimuli approximately in proportion to a power function of the actual intensity. In the case of sound, the interpreted sensation changes approximately in proportion to the cube root of the actual sound intensity. To express this another way, the ear can discriminate differences in sound intensity from the softest whisper to the loudest possible noise, representing an *approximate one trillion times* increase in sound energy. Yet the ear interprets this much difference in sound level as approximately a 10,000-fold change. Thus, the scale of intensity is greatly "compressed" by the sound perception mechanisms of the auditory system. This obviously allows a person to interpret differences in sound intensities over an extremely wide range, a far broader range than would be possible were it not for compression of the scale.

The Decibel Unit. Because of the extreme changes in sound intensities that the ear can detect and discriminate, sound intensities are usually expressed in terms of the logarithm of their actual intensities. A 10-fold increase in sound energy (or a $\sqrt{10}$-fold increase in sound pressure, because energy is proportional to the square of pressure) is called 1 *bel*, and one-tenth bel is called 1 *decibel*. One decibel represents an actual increase in intensity of 1.26 times.

Another reason for using the decibel system in expressing changes in loudness is that, in the usual sound intensity range for communication, the ears can detect approximately a 1 decibel change in sound intensity.

The "Zero" Decibel Reference Level. The usual method for expressing the intensity of sound is to state the pressure difference between the peak of the sound compression wave and the trough of the wave. A pressure of *0.0002 dyne per square centimeter* is considered by audiologists to be unit intensity, and this is expressed as *zero decibels* when converted to the decibel scale because the logarithm of unity is zero. This sound level is also approximately the minimum that can be detected by the normal ear at the optimal frequency of 2000 cycles per second. (On the other hand, sound engineers frequently consider a sound pressure of 1 dyne per square centimeter to be zero decibels.)

Threshold for Hearing Sound at Different Frequencies. Figure 21–9 shows the energy threshold at which sounds of different frequencies can barely be heard by the ear. This figure illustrates that a 2000 cycle per second sound can be heard even when its intensity is as low as 70 decibels below 1 dyne/cm.^{2} sound pressure level, which is one ten-millionth microwatt/cm.^{2}. On the other hand, a 100 cycle per second sound can be detected only if its intensity is 10,000 times as great as this.

Frequency Range of Hearing. The frequencies of sound that a young person can hear, before aging has occurred in the ears, is generally stated to be between 30 and 20,000 cycles per second. However, referring again to Figure 21–9, we see that the sound range depends to a great extent on intensity. If the intensity is 60 decibels

Figure 21–9. Relationship of the threshold of hearing and the threshold of somesthetic perception to the sound energy level at each sound frequency. (Modified from Stevens and Davis: Hearing. John Wiley & Sons.)

below the 1 dyne/cm.² sound pressure level, the sound range is 500 to 5000 cycles per second, and only with intense sounds can the complete range of 30 to 20,000 cycles be achieved. In old age, the frequency range falls to 50 to 8,000 cycles per second or less, as is discussed later in the chapter.

CENTRAL AUDITORY MECHANISMS

THE AUDITORY PATHWAY

Figure 21–10 illustrates the major auditory pathways. It shows that nerve fibers from the *spiral ganglion of the organ of Corti* enter the *cochlear nuclei* located in the

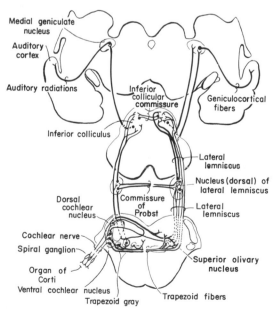

Figure 21–10. The auditory pathway. (Modified from Crosby, Humphrey, and Lauer: Correlative Anatomy of the Nervous System. The Macmillan Co.)

upper part of the medulla. At this point, all the fibers synapse, and second order neurons pass mainly to the opposite side of the brain stem through the *trapezoid body* to the *superior olivary nucleus*. However, some of the second order fibers pass ipsilaterally to the superior olivary nucleus on the same side. Most of the fibers entering the superior olivary nucleus on either side terminate here, but some pass on through this nucleus. From the superior olivary nucleus the auditory pathway then passes upward through the *lateral lemniscus,* and many of the fibers terminate in the *nucleus of the lateral lemniscus,* but many also bypass this nucleus and pass on to the inferior colliculus where most terminate; a few pass on without terminating to higher levels. A few fibers cross from the nucleus of the lateral lemniscus through the *commissure of Probst* to the contralateral nucleus, and still other fibers cross through the *inferior collicular commissure* from one inferior colliculus to the other. From the inferior colliculus, the pathway passes through the *peduncle of the inferior colliculus* to the *medial geniculate nucleus,* where all the fibers synapse. From here, the auditory tract spreads by way of the *auditory radiation* to the *auditory cortex* located mainly in the superior temporal gyrus.

Several points of importance in relation to the auditory pathway should be noted. First, impulses from either ear are transmitted through the auditory pathways of both sides of the brain stem with only slight preponderance of transmission in the contralateral pathway. In at least three different places in the brain stem crossing-over occurs between the two pathways: (a) in the trapezoid body, (b) in the commissure of Probst, and (c) in the commissure connecting the two inferior colliculi.

Second, many collateral fibers from the auditory tracts pass directly into the reticular activating system of the brain stem. This system projects diffusely upward into the cerebral cortex and downward into the spinal cord.

Third, the pathway for transmission of sound impulses from the cochlea to the cortex consists of at least four neurons and sometimes as many as six. Neurons *may* or *may not* synapse in the superior olivary nuclei, in the nuclei of the lateral lemniscus, and in the inferior colliculi. Therefore, some of the tracts are more direct than others, which means that some impulses arrive at the cortex well ahead of others even though they might have originated at exactly the same time.

Fourth, several important pathways also exist from the auditory system into the cerebellum: (a) directly from the cochlear nuclei, (b) from the inferior colliculi, (c) from the reticular substance of the brain stem, and (d) from the cerebral auditory areas. These activate the *cerebellar vermis* instantaneously in the event of a sudden noise.

Fifth, a high degree of spatial orientation is maintained in the fiber tracts from the cochlea all the way to the cortex. In fact, there are three different spatial representations of sound frequencies in the cochlear nuclei, two representations in the inferior colliculi, one precise representation for discrete sound frequencies in the auditory cortex, and several less precise representations in the auditory association areas.

Firing Rates at Different Levels of the Auditory Tract. Single nerve fibers entering the cochlear nuclei from the eighth nerve can fire at rates up to 1000 per second, the rate being determined mainly by the loudness of the sound. At low sound frequencies, the nerve impulses are usually synchronized with the sound waves but they do not necessarily occur with every wave.

In the auditory tracts of the brain stem, the firing is usually no longer synchronized with the sound frequency except at sound frequencies below 200 cycles per second. And above the level of the inferior colliculi, even this synchronization is mainly lost. These findings demonstrate that the sound signals are not transmitted unchanged directly from the ear to the higher levels of the brain; instead, information from the sound signals begins to be dissected from the impulse traffic at levels as low as the cochlear nuclei. We will have more to say about this later, especially in relation to perception of direction from which sound comes.

Another significant feature of the auditory pathways is that low rates of impulse firing continue even in the absence of sound all the way from the cochlear nerve fibers to the auditory cortex. When the basilar membrane moves toward the scala vestibuli, the impulse traffic increases; and when the basilar membrane moves toward the scala tympani, the impulse traffic decreases. Thus, the presence of this background signal allows information to be transmitted from the basilar membrane when the membrane moves in either direction: positive information in one direction and negative information in the opposite direction. Were it not for the background signal, only the positive half of the information could be transmitted. This type of so-called "carrier wave" method for transmitting information is utilized in many parts of the brain, as has been discussed in several of the preceding chapters.

Function of the Auditory Relay Nuclei. Very little is known about the function of the different nuclei in the auditory pathway. However, cats and even monkeys can still detect very low intensity sound when the cerebral cortex is removed bilaterally, which indicates that the nuclei in the brain stem and thalamus can perform many auditory functions even without the cerebral cortex. However, discrimination of tonal patterns and sound sequences is considerably impaired. In human beings, *bilateral* destruction of the cortical auditory centers may give a different picture: it is said to cause severe hearing loss; but, unfortunately, this has not been studied adequately.

FUNCTION OF THE CEREBRAL CORTEX IN HEARING

The projection of the auditory pathway to the cerebral cortex is illustrated in Figure 21–11, which shows that the auditory cortex lies princi-

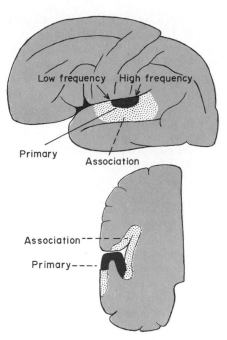

Figure 21–11. The auditory cortex.

pally on the *supratemporal plane of the superior temporal gyrus* but also extends over the *lateral border of the temporal lobe,* over much of the *insular cortex,* and even into the most lateral portion of the *parietal operculum.*

Two separate areas are shown in Figure 21–11: the *primary auditory cortex* and the *auditory association cortex* (also called the *secondary auditory cortex*). The primary auditory cortex is directly excited by projections from the medial geniculate body, while the auditory association areas are usually excited secondarily by impulses from the primary auditory cortex and by projections from thalamic association areas adjacent to the medial geniculate body.

Locus of Sound Frequency Perception in the Primary Auditory Cortex. Certain parts of the primary auditory cortex are known to respond to high frequencies and other parts to low frequencies. In monkeys, the posteromedial part of the supratemporal plane responds to high frequencies, while the anterolateral part responds to low frequencies. Presumably, the same frequency localization occurs in the human cortex, but this is yet unproven.

The frequency range to which each individual neuron in the auditory cortex responds is much narrower than that in the cochlear and brain stem relay nuclei. Referring back to Figure 21–6B, we note that the basilar membrane near the base of the cochlea is stimulated by all frequency sounds, and in the cochlear nuclei this same breadth of sound representation is found. Yet by the time the excitation has reached the cerebral cortex, each sound-responsive neuron responds to only a narrow range of frequencies rather than to a broad range. Therefore, somewhere along the pathway, processing mechanisms in some way "sharpen" the frequency response. It is believed that this sharpening effect is caused mainly by the phenomenon of lateral inhibition, which was discussed in Chapter 7 in relation to mechanisms for transmitting information in nerves. That is, stimulation of the cochlea at one frequency causes inhibition of signals caused by sound frequencies on either side of the stimulated frequency, this effect resulting from collateral fibers angling off the primary signal pathway and exerting inhibitory influences on adjacent pathways. The same effect has also been demonstrated to be important in sharpening patterns of somesthetic images, visual images, and other types of sensations.

A large share of the neurons in the auditory cortex, especially in the auditory association cortex, do not respond to specific sound frequencies in the ear. It is believed that these neurons "associate" different sound frequencies with each other or associate sound information with information from other sensory areas of the cortex. Indeed, the parietal portion of the auditory association cortex partly overlaps somatic sensory area II, which could provide easy opportunity for association of auditory information with somatic sensory information.

Discrimination of Sound "Patterns" by the Auditory Cortex. Complete bilateral removal of the auditory cortex does not prevent an animal from detecting sounds or reacting in a crude manner to the sounds. However, it does greatly reduce or sometimes even abolish its ability to discriminate different sound pitches and especially *patterns of sound*. For instance, an animal that has been trained to recognize a combination or sequence of tones, one following the other in a particular pattern, loses this ability when the auditory cortex is destroyed, and, furthermore, it cannot relearn this type of response. Therefore, the auditory cortex is important in the discrimination of *tonal* and *sequential sound patterns*.

In the human being, lesions affecting the auditory association areas but not affecting the primary auditory cortex will allow the person full capability to hear and differentiate sound tones as well as to interpret at least a few simple patterns of sound. However, he will often be unable to interpret the *meaning* of the sound that he hears. For instance, lesions in the posterior portion of the superior temporal gyrus often make it impossible for the person to interpret the meanings of words even though he hears them perfectly well and can even repeat them. These functions of the auditory association areas and their relationship to the overall intellectual functions of the brain were discussed in detail in Chapter 15.

DISCRIMINATION OF DIRECTION FROM WHICH SOUND EMANATES

A person determines the direction from which sound emanates by two principal mechanisms: (1) by the time lag between the entry of sound into one ear and into the opposite ear and (2) by the difference between the intensities of the sounds in the two ears. The first mechanism functions best for frequencies below 3000 cycles per second, and the intensity mechanism operates best at higher frequencies because the head acts as a sound barrier at these frequencies. The time lag mechanism discriminates direction much more exactly than the intensity mechanism, for the time lag mechanism does not depend on extraneous factors but only on an exact interval of time between two acoustical signals. If a person is looking straight toward the sound, the sound reaches both ears at exactly the same instant, while, if the right ear is closer to the sound than the left ear, the sound signals from the right ear are perceived ahead of those from the left ear.

If a sound emanates from the right side 45 degrees from the frontal direction and if still a second sound emanates also from the right but 45 degrees from behind, the difference in time of arrival of the two sounds at the two ears will be exactly the same. For this reason, it is difficult to distinguish whether the sound is originating from the frontal or the posterior quadrant. The principal method by which a person determines this is to rotate his head quickly. If he turns his head toward the right when the sound is coming from the frontal quadrant, the time lag between the two ears becomes smaller. If the sound is originating from the posterior quadrant, the time lag becomes greater. A sudden sound that occurs so rapidly that the person does not have time to move his head often cannot be properly localized to the frontal or posterior quadrant.

Neural Mechanisms for Detecting Sound Direction. Destruction of the auditory cortex on both sides of the brain, in either human beings or lower mammals, causes loss of almost all ability to detect the direction from which sound comes. Yet, the mechanism for this detection process begins in the superior olivary nuclei, even though it requires the neural pathways all the way from these nuclei to the cortex for interpretation of the signals. The mechanism is believed to be the following:

Some neurons in the superior olivary nucleus are inhibited by signals from one ear but excited by signals from the other ear. Therefore, if the signals from both ears reach these cells at the same time, they cancel each other and no subsequent signal is transmitted to the auditory cortex. However, if the sound reaches one ear before the other, then the two signals do not cancel each other, and the time interval between the sounds in the two ears determines the degree of cancellation, thus providing the clue required to discriminate the direction of the sound.

Let us add still another feature to the mechanism: Because of multiple neuronal relays between the cochlear nuclei and the superior olivary nuclei, the signals reaching some of the olivary neurons arrive later than others. Therefore, the signals for some of these neurons are cancelled when the time interval between the sounds in the two ears is very short while for other neurons the signals are cancelled when the time interval is very long. Thus, a spatial pattern of neuronal stimulation develops, with sound from directly in front of the head stimulating one set of olivary neurons maximally and sounds from different side angles stimulating other sets of neurons maximally. This spatial orientation of signals is then transmitted all the way to the auditory cortex where sound direction is determined by the locus in the cortex that is stimulated maximally. It is believed that the signals for determining sound direction are transmitted through a slightly different pathway and that this pathway terminates in the cerebral cortex in a slightly different locus from the transmission pathway and the termination locus of the tonal patterns of sound.

This mechanism for detection of sound direction indicates again how information in sensory signals is dissected out as the signals pass through different levels of neuronal activity. In this case, the "quality" of sound direction is separated from the "quality" of sound tones at the level of the superior olivary nuclei.

CENTRIFUGAL CONDUCTION OF IMPULSES FROM THE CENTRAL NERVOUS SYSTEM

Retrograde pathways have been demonstrated at each level of the central nervous system all the way from the auditory cortex to the cochlea. The final pathway is mainly from the superior olivary nucleus to the organ of Corti.

These retrograde fibers are inhibitory. Indeed, direct stimulation of discrete points in the olivary nucleus have been shown to inhibit specific areas of the organ of Corti, reducing their sound sensitivities as much as 15 to 20 decibels. One can readily understand how this could allow a person to direct attention to sounds of particular qualities while rejecting sounds of other qualities. This is readily demonstrated when one listens to a single instrument in a symphony orchestra.

HEARING ABNORMALITIES

TYPES OF DEAFNESS

Deafness is usually divided into two types; first, that caused by impairment of the cochlea or auditory nerve, which is usually classed under the heading "nerve deafness," and, second, that caused by impairment of the middle ear mechanisms for transmitting sound into the cochlea, which is usually called "conduction deafness." Obviously, if either the cochlea or the auditory nerve is completely destroyed the person is permanently deaf. However, if the cochlea and nerve are still intact but the ossicular system has been destroyed or ankylosed ("frozen" in place by fibrosis or calcification), sound waves can still be conducted into the cochlea by means of bone conduction.

Tuning Fork Test for Differentiation Between Nerve Deafness and Conduction Deafness. To test an ear for bone conduction with a tuning fork, one places a vibrating fork in front of the ear, and the subject listens to the tone of the fork until he can no longer hear it. Then the butt of the still weakly vibrating fork is immediately placed against the mastoid process. If his bone conduction is better than his air conduction, he will again hear the sound of the tuning fork. If this occurs, his deafness may be considered to be conduction deafness. However, if on placing the butt of the fork against the mastoid process he cannot hear the sound of the tuning fork, his bone conduction is probably decreased as much as his air conduction, and the deafness is presumably due to damage in the cochlea or in the nervous system rather than in the ossicular system — that is, it is nerve deafness.

The Audiometer. To determine the nature of hearing disabilities more exactly than can be accomplished by the above method, the audiometer is used. This is simply an earphone connected to an electronic oscillator capable of emitting pure tones ranging from low frequencies to high frequencies. Based on previous studies of normal persons, the instrument is calibrated so that the zero intensity level of sound at each frequency is the loudness that can barely be heard by the normal person. However, a calibrated volume control can increase or decrease the loudness of each tone above or below the zero level. If the loudness of a tone must be increased to 30 decibels above normal before it can be heard, the subject is said to have a *hearing loss* of 30 decibels for that particular tone.

In performing a hearing test using an audiometer, one tests approximately 8 to 10 frequencies covering the auditory spectrum, one at a time, and the hearing loss is determined for each of these frequencies. Then the

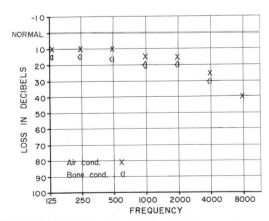

Figure 21–12. Audiogram of the old-age type of nerve deafness.

Figure 21–13. Audiogram of deafness resulting from middle ear sclerosis.

so-called "audiogram" is plotted as shown in Figures 21–12 and 21–13, depicting the hearing loss for each of the frequencies in the auditory spectrum.

The audiometer, in addition to being equipped with an earphone for testing air conduction by the ear, is also equipped with an electronic vibrator for testing bone conduction from the mastoid process into the cochlea.

The Audiogram in Nerve Deafness. In nerve deafness — this term including damage to the cochlea, to the auditory nerve, or to the central nervous system circuits from the ear — the person has lost the ability to hear sound as tested by both the air conduction apparatus and the bone conduction apparatus. An audiogram depicting nerve deafness is illustrated in Figure 21–12. In this figure the deafness is mainly for high frequency sound. Such deafness could be caused by damage to the base of the cochlea. This type of deafness occurs to some extent in almost all older persons.

Other patterns of nerve deafness frequently occur as follows: (1) deafness usually for low frequency sounds caused by excessive and prolonged exposure to very loud sounds (the rock band or the jet airplane engine) because low frequency sounds are usually louder and more damaging to the organ of Corti, and (2) deafness for all frequencies caused by drug sensitivity of the organ of Corti, especially sensitivity to some antibiotics such as streptomycin, kanamycin, and chloramphenicol.

The Audiogram in Conduction Deafness. A second and frequent type of deafness is that caused by fibrosis of the middle ear following repeated infection in the middle ear or in the hereditary disease called *otosclerosis*. In this instance the sound waves cannot be transmitted easily to the oval window. Figure 21–13 illustrates an audiogram from a person with "middle ear deafness" of this type. In this case the bone conduction is essentially normal, but air conduction is greatly depressed at all frequencies, more so at the low frequencies. In this

type of deafness, the faceplate of the stapes frequently becomes "ankylosed" by bony overgrowth to the edges of the oval window. In this case, the person becomes totally deaf for air conduction, but can be made to hear again almost normally by removing the stapes and replacing it with a minute Teflon or metal prosthesis that transmits the sound from the incus to the oval window.

REFERENCES

Aitkin, L. M.: Tonotopic organization at higher levels of the auditory pathway. *Int. Rev. Physiol., 10*:249, 1976.

Beagley, H. A. (ed.): Auditory Investigation: The Scientific and Technological Basis. New York, Oxford University Press, 1979.

Bench, J., and Bamford, J. (eds.): Speech-Hearing Tests and the Spoken Language of Hearing-Impaired Children. New York, Academic Press, 1979.

Brugge, J. F., and Geisler, C. D.: Auditory mechanisms of the lower brainstem. *Annu. Rev. Neurosci., 1*:363, 1978.

Busnel, R., and Fish, J. F. (eds.): Animal Sonar Systems. New York, Plenum Press, 1979.

Carterette, E. C., and Friedman, M. P.: Hearing. New York, Academic Press, 1978.

Dallos, P.: The Auditory Periphery. New York, Academic Press, 1973.

Davis, H.: Biophysics and physiology of the inner ear. *Physiol. Rev., 37*:1, 1957.

Egerton, B. J., and Danhauer, J. L.: Clinical Implications of Speech Discrimination Testing Using Nonsense Stimuli. Baltimore, University Park Press, 1979.

Evans, E. F., and Wilson, J. P. (eds.): Psychophysics and Physiology of Hearing. New York, Academic Press, 1977.

Gerber, S. E.: Introductory Hearing Science, Philadelphia, W. B. Saunders Co., 1974.

Harris, J. D.: The Electrophysiology and Layout of the Auditory Nervous System. Indianapolis, The Bobbs-Merrill Co., 1974.

Heasley, B. E.: Auditory Processing Disorders and Remediation, 2nd Ed. Springfield, Ill., Charles C Thomas, 1980.

Jarvis, J. F.: An Introduction to the Anatomy and Physiology of Speech and Hearing. Cape Town, South Africa, Juta & Co., 1978.

Lipscomb, D. M. (ed.): Noise and Audiology. Baltimore, University Park Press, 1978.

Naunton, R. F., and Fernandez, C. (eds.): Evoked Electrical Activity in the Auditory Nervous System. New York, Academic Press, 1978.

Rintelmann, W. F. (ed.): Hearing Assessment. Baltimore, University Park Press, 1979.

Rosenblum, E. H.: Fundamentals of Hearing for Health Professionals. Boston, Little, Brown, 1979.

Sataloff, J., *et al.*: Hearing Loss, 2nd Ed. Philadelphia, J. B. Lippincott Co., 1980.

Scheich, O. C. H., and Schreiner, C. (eds.): Hearing Mechanisms and Speech. New York, Springer-Verlag, 1979.

Singh, R. P.: Anatomy of Hearing and Speech. New York, Oxford University Press, 1980.

Skinner, P. H., and Shelton, R. L.: Speech, Language, and Hearing: Normal Processes and Disorders. Reading, Mass., Addison-Wesley Publishing Co., 1978.

Starr, A.: Neurophysiological mechanisms of sound localization. *Fed. Proc., 33*:1911, 1974.

Tobias, J. V. (ed.): Foundations of Modern Auditory Theory. Vols. 1 and 2. New York, Academic Press, 1970.

Van Hattum, R. J.: Communication Disorders. New York, The Macmillan Co., 1980.

Wever, E. G., and Lawrence, M.: Physiological Acoustics. Princeton, Princeton University Press, 1954.

Yanick, P., Jr., and Freifeld, S. (eds.): The Application of Signal Processing Concepts of Hearing Aids. New York, Grune & Stratton, 1978.

22

The Chemical Senses — Taste and Smell

THE SENSE OF TASTE

Taste is mainly a function of the *taste buds* in the mouth, but it is also common experience that one's sense of smell also contributes strongly to taste perception. In addition, the texture of food, as detected by tactual senses of the mouth, and the presence of such elements in the food as pepper, which stimulate pain endings, greatly condition the taste experience. The importance of taste lies in the fact it allows a person to select food in accord with desires and perhaps also in accord with the needs of the tissues for specific nutritive substances.

On the basis of psychological studies, there are generally believed to be four *primary* sensations of taste: *sour, salty, sweet, and bitter.* Yet we know that a person can perceive literally hundreds of different tastes. These are all supposed to be combinations of the four primary sensations in the same manner that all the colors of the spectrum are combinations of three primary color sensations, as described in Chapter 19. There might be other, less conspicuous classes or subclasses of primary sensations; nevertheless, the following discussion is based on the usual classification of only four primary tastes.

THE PRIMARY SENSATIONS OF TASTE

The Sour Taste. The sour taste is caused by acids, and the intensity of the taste sensation is approximately proportional to the logarithm of the *hydrogen ion concentration.* That is, the more acidic the acid, the stronger becomes the sensation.

The Salty Taste. The salty taste is elicited by ionized salts. The quality of the taste varies somewhat from one salt to another because the salts also elicit other taste sensations besides saltiness. The cations of the salts are mainly responsible for the salty taste, but the anions also contribute at least to some extent.

The Sweet Taste. The sweet taste is not caused by any single class of chemicals. A list of some of the types of chemicals that cause this taste includes: sugars, glycols, alcohols, aldehydes, ketones, amides, esters, amino acids, sulfonic acids, halogenated acids, and inorganic salts of lead and beryllium. Note specifically that most of the substances that cause a sweet taste are organic chemicals. It is especially interesting that very slight changes in the chemical structure, such as addition of a simple radical, can often change the substance from sweet to bitter.

The third column of Table 22–1 shows the relative intensities of taste of certain substances that cause the sweet taste. *Sucrose,* which is common table sugar, is considered to have an index of 1. Note that one of the substances has a sweet index 5000 times as great as that of sucrose. However, this extremely sweet substance, known as *P-4000,* is unfortunately extremely toxic and therefore cannot be used as a sweetening agent. *Saccharin,* on the other hand, is also more than 600 times as sweet as common table sugar, and since it is not toxic (except that it might be mildly carcinogenic), it can be used with impunity as a sweetening agent.

The Bitter Taste. The bitter taste, like the sweet taste, is not caused by any single type of chemical agent, but, here again, the substances that give the bitter taste are almost entirely organic substances. Two particular classes of substances are especially likely to cause bitter taste sensations: (1) long chain organic substances and (2) alkaloids. The alkaloids include many of the drugs used in medicines such as quinine, caffeine, strychnine, and nicotine.

Some substances that at first taste sweet have a bitter after-taste. This is true of saccharin, which makes this substance objectionable to some people. Some substances have a sweet taste on the

TABLE 22-1 RELATIVE TASTE INDICES OF DIFFERENT SUBSTANCES

Sour Substances	Index	Bitter Substances	Index	Sweet Substances	Index	Salty Substances	Index
Hydrochloric acid	1.	Quinine	1	Sucrose	1	NaCl	1
Formic acid	1.1	Brucine	11	1-propoxy-2-amino-		NaF	2
Chloracetic acid	0.9	Strychnine	3.1	4-nitrobenzene	5000	CaCl$_2$	1
Acetyllactic acid	0.85	Nicotine	1.3	Saccharin	675	NaBr	0.4
Lactic acid	0.85	Phenylthiourea	0.9	Chloroform	40	NaI	0.35
Tartaric acid	0.7	Caffeine	0.4	Fructose	1.7	LiCl	0.4
Malic acid	0.6	Veratrine	0.2	Alanine	1.3	NH$_4$Cl	2.5
Potassium H tartrate	0.58	Pilocarpine	0.16	Glucose	0.8	KCl	0.6
Acetic acid	0.55	Atropine	0.13	Maltose	0.45		
Citric acid	0.46	Cocaine	0.02	Galactose	0.32		
Carbonic acid	0.06	Morphine	0.02	Lactose	0.3		

From Derma: *Proc. Oklahoma Acad. Sc.*, 27:9, 1947; and Pfaffman: Handbook of Physiology, Sec. I, Vol. I, p. 507, 1959. Baltimore, The Williams & Wilkins Co.

front of the tongue, where taste buds with special sensitivity to the sweet taste are principally located, and a bitter taste on the back of the tongue, where taste buds more sensitive to the bitter taste are located.

The bitter taste, when it occurs in high intensity, usually causes the person or animal to reject the food. This is undoubtedly an important purposive function of the bitter taste sensation because many of the deadly toxins found in poisonous plants are alkaloids, and these all cause intensely bitter taste.

Threshold for Taste

The threshold for stimulation of the sour taste by hydrochloric acid averages 0.0009 N; for stimulation of the salty taste by sodium chloride, 0.01 M; for the sweet taste by sucrose, 0.01 M; and for the bitter taste by quinine, 0.000008 M. Note especially how much more sensitive is the bitter taste sense to stimuli than all the others, which would be expected since this sensation provides an important protective function.

Table 22-1 gives the relative taste indices (the reciprocals of the taste thresholds) of different substances. In this table, the intensities of the four different primary sensations of taste are referred, respectively, to the intensities of taste of hydrochloric acid, quinine, sucrose, and sodium chloride, each of which is considered to have a taste index of 1.

Taste Blindness. Many persons are taste blind for certain substances, especially for different types of thiourea compounds. A substance used frequently by psychologists for demonstrating taste blindness is *phenylthiocarbamide*, for which approximately 15 to 30 per cent of all people exhibit taste blindness, the exact percentage depending on the method of testing and the concentration of the substance.

THE TASTE BUD AND ITS FUNCTION

Figure 22-1 illustrates a taste bud, which has a diameter of about $^1/_{30}$ millimeter and a length of about $^1/_{16}$ millimeter. The taste bud is composed of about 40 modified epithelial cells, some of which

are supporting cells and others are *taste cells*. The taste cells are continually being replaced by mitotic division from the surrounding epithelial cells so that some are young cells and others are mature cells that lie toward the center of the bud and soon dissolute. The life span of each taste cell is about ten days.

The outer tips of the taste cells are arranged around a minute *taste pore*, shown in Figure 22-1. From the tip of each cell, several *microvilli,* or *taste hairs,* about 2 to 3 microns in length and 0.1 to 0.2 micron in width, protrude outward through the taste pore to approach the cavity of the mouth. These microvilli are believed to provide the receptor surface for taste.

Interwoven among the taste cells is a branching terminal network of several *taste nerve fibers* that are stimulated by the taste cells. These fibers invaginate into folds of the taste cell membranes, so that there is extremely intimate contact between the taste cells and the nerves. Several taste buds can be innervated by the same taste fiber.

An interesting feature of the taste buds is that they completely degenerate when the taste nerve fibers are destroyed. Then, if the taste fibers regrow to the epithelial surface of the mouth, the local epithelial cells regroup themselves to form

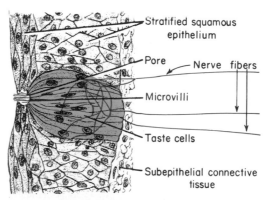

Figure 22-1. The taste bud.

new taste buds. This illustrates the important principle of "trophic" function of nerve fibers in certain parts of the body. The cause of the tropism is unknown, but it has been postulated to be a protein trophic factor secreted by the nerve endings.

Location of the Taste Buds. The taste buds are found on three of four different types of papillae of the tongue, as follows: (1) A large number of taste buds are on the walls of the troughs that surround the circumvallate papillae, which form a V line toward the posterior of the tongue. (2) Moderate numbers of taste buds are on the fungiform papillae over the front surface of the tongue. (3) Moderate numbers are on the foliate papillae located in the folds along the lateral surfaces of the tongue. Additional taste buds are located on the palate and a few on the tonsillar pillars and at other points around the nasopharynx. Adults have approximately 10,000 taste buds, and children a few more. Beyond the age of 45 many taste buds rapidly degenerate, causing the taste sensation to become progressively less critical.

Especially important in relation to taste is the tendency for taste buds subserving particular primary sensations of taste to be localized in special areas. The sweet taste is localized *principally* on the anterior surface and tip of the tongue, the salty and sour tastes on the two lateral sides of the tongue, and the bitter taste on the circumvallate papillae on the posterior of the tongue.

Specificity of Taste Buds for the Primary Taste Stimuli. Psychological tests using different types of taste stimuli carefully applied to individual taste buds, one at a time, have suggested that we have four distinctly different varieties of taste buds, each sensitive for only one type of taste. Yet, microelectrode studies from single taste buds while they are stimulated successively by the four different primary taste stimuli have shown that most of them can be excited by two, three, or even four of the primary taste stimuli, though usually with one or two of these predominating. Thus, at present, there are conflicting beliefs about the degree of specificity of taste buds, some physiologists believing them always to be highly specific for only one primary taste stimulus and other physiologists believing this to be true only in a statistical sense because of dominance of one taste perception over the others.

Regardless of which of the two theories is correct, one can well understand that the hundreds of different types of tastes that we experience result from different quantitative degrees of stimulation of the four primary sensations of taste, as well as simultaneous stimulation of smell in the nose and tactile and pain nerve endings in the mouth.

Mechanism of Stimulation of Taste Buds. *The Receptor Potential.* The membrane of the taste cell, like that of other sensory receptor cells, normally is negatively charged on the inside with respect to the outside. Application of a taste substance to the taste hairs causes partial loss of this negative potential. The decrease in potential, within a wide range, is approximately proportional to the logarithm of concentration of the stimulating substance. This change in potential in the taste cell is the *receptor potential* for taste.

The mechanism by which the stimulating substance reacts with the taste hairs to initiate the receptor potential is unknown. It is believed by some physiologists that the substance is simply adsorbed to receptors on the membrane surface of the taste hair and that this adsorption changes the physical characteristics of the hair membrane. This in turn makes the taste cell more permeable to sodium ions and thus depolarizes the cell. The substance is gradually washed away from the taste hair by the saliva, thus removing the taste stimulus. Supposedly, the type of receptor substance or substances in each taste hair determines the types of taste substances that will elicit responses.

Generation of Nerve Impulses by the Taste Bud. The taste nerve fiber endings are encased by folds of the taste cell membranes. In some way not understood the receptor potentials of the taste cells generate impulses in the taste fibers. On first application of the taste stimulus, the rate of discharge of the nerve fibers rises to a peak in a small fraction of a second, but then it adapts within the next 2 seconds back to a much lower steady level. Thus, a strong immediate signal is transmitted by the taste nerve, and a much weaker continuous signal is transmitted as long as the taste bud is exposed to the taste stimulus.

TRANSMISSION OF TASTE SIGNALS INTO THE CENTRAL NERVOUS SYSTEM

Figure 22–2 illustrates the neuronal pathways for transmission of taste signals from the tongue and pharyngeal region into the central nervous system. Taste impulses from the anterior two thirds of the tongue pass first into the *fifth nerve*

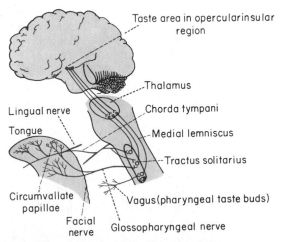

Figure 22–2. Transmission of taste impulses into the central nervous system.

and then through the *chorda tympani* into the *seventh nerve*, thence into the *tractus solitarius* in the brain stem. Taste sensations from the circumvallate papillae on the back of the tongue and from other posterior regions of the mouth are transmitted through the *ninth nerve* also into the *tractus solitarius* but at a slightly lower level. Finally, a few taste impulses are transmitted into the *tractus solitarius* from the base of the tongue and other parts of the pharyngeal region by way of the *vagus nerve*.

All taste fibers synapse in the *nuclei of the tractus solitarius* and send second order neurons to a small area of the *thalamus* located slightly medial to the thalamic terminations of the facial regions of the dorsal column–medial lemniscal system. From the thalamus, third order neurons are transmitted to the *lower tip of the postcentral gyrus in the parietal cortex* where it curls deep into the sylvian fissure. This lies in close association with, or even superimposed on, the tongue area of somatic area I. Third order neurons also project to the nearby *opercular-insular area,* located deep in the sylvian fissure as well.

From this description of the taste pathways, it immediately becomes evident that they parallel closely the somatic pathways from the tongue.

Taste Reflexes. From the tractus solitarius a large number of impulses are transmitted directly into the *superior* and *inferior salivatory nuclei,* and these in turn transmit impulses to the submaxillary and parotid glands to help control the secretion of saliva during the ingestion of food.

Adaptation of Taste. Everyone is familiar with the fact that taste sensations adapt rapidly, often with almost complete adaptation within 1 to 5 minutes of continuous stimulation. Yet, from electrophysiological studies of taste nerve fibers, it seems that the taste buds themselves do not adapt enough to account for all or even most of the taste adaptation. They have a rapid period of adaptation during the first 2 to 3 seconds after contact with the taste stimulus. The first burst of impulses from the taste bud allows one to detect extremely minute concentrations of taste substances, but normal concentrations of taste substances cause prolonged discharge of the taste fibers. Therefore, the progressive adaptation that occurs in the sensation of taste has been postulated to occur in the central nervous system itself, though the mechanism and site of this is not known. If this is true, it is a mechanism that is different from that of other sensory systems, which adapt almost entirely in the receptors.

SPECIAL ATTRIBUTES OF THE TASTE SENSE

Affective Nature of Taste. *Pleasantness* and *unpleasantness* are called the ''affective'' attributes of a sensa-

Figure 22–3. The affective nature of the different primary sensations of taste at progressively increasing degrees of taste stimulus. (From Engel in Woodworth and Schlosberg: Experimental Psychology. Holt, Rinehart & Winston, Inc.)

tion. Figure 22–3 illustrates the affective effects of different types of taste at different concentrations of the stimulating substances, showing, strangely enough, that the sweet taste is likely to be unpleasant at a very low concentration but very pleasant at high concentrations. The other types of taste, on the other hand, are likely to be pleasant at low concentrations but exceedingly unpleasant at high concentrations. This is particularly true of the bitter taste.

Importance of the Sense of Smell in Taste. Persons with severe colds frequently state that they have lost their sense of taste. However, on testing, the taste sensations are found to be completely normal. This illustrates that much of what we call taste is actually smell. Odors from the food can pass upward into the nasopharynx, often stimulating the olfactory system thousands of times as strongly as the taste system. For instance, if the olfactory system is intact, alcohol can be ''tasted'' in 1/25,000 the concentration required when the olfactory system is not intact.

Taste Preference and Control of the Diet. Taste preferences mean simply that an animal will choose certain types of food in preference to others, and it automatically uses this to help control the type of diet it eats. Furthermore, its taste preferences often change in accord with the needs of the body for certain specific substances. The following experimental studies illustrate this ability of an animal to choose food in accord with the need of its body: First, adrenalectomized animals automatically select drinking water with a high concentration of sodium chloride in preference to pure water, and this in many instances is sufficient to supply the needs of the body and prevent death as a result of salt depletion. Second, an animal injected with excessive amounts of insulin develops a depleted blood sugar, and it automatically chooses the sweetest food from among many samples. Third, parathyroidectomized animals automatically choose drinking water with a high concentration of calcium chloride.

These same phenomena are also observed in many instances of everyday life. For instance, the salt licks of the desert region are known to attract animals from far and wide, and even the human being rejects any food that has an unpleasant affective sensation, which certainly in many instances protects our bodies from undesirable substances.

The phenomenon of taste preference almost certainly results from some mechanism located in the central nervous system and not from a mechanism in the taste buds themselves, because many experiments have demonstrated that taste preference can occur in animals even in the absence of changes in stimulus threshold of the taste buds for the substances involved. Another reason for believing this to be a central phenomenon is that previous experience with unpleasant or pleasant tastes plays a major role in determining one's different taste preferences. For instance, if a person becomes sick immediately after eating a particular type of food, the person generally develops a negative taste preference, or taste aversion, for that particular food thereafter; the same effect can be demonstrated in animals.

THE SENSE OF SMELL

Smell is the least understood sense. This results partly from the location of the olfactory membrane high in the nose where it is difficult to study and partly from the fact that the sense of smell is a subjective phenomenon that cannot be studied with ease in lower animals. Still another complicating problem is the fact that the sense of smell is almost rudimentary in the human being in comparison with that of some lower animals.

THE OLFACTORY MEMBRANE

The olfactory membrane lies in the superior part of each nostril, as illustrated in Figure 22–5. Medially it folds downward over the surface of the septum, and laterally it folds over the superior turbinate and even over a small portion of the upper surface of the middle turbinate. In each nostril the olfactory membrane has a surface area of approximately 2.4 square centimeters.

The Olfactory Cells. The receptor cells for the smell sensation are the *olfactory cells,* which are actually bipolar nerve cells derived originally from the central nervous system itself. There are about 100 million of these cells in the olfactory epithelium interspersed among *sustentacular cells,* as shown in Figure 22–4. The mucosal end of the olfactory cell forms a knob called the *olfactory rod* from which 6 to 12 *olfactory hairs,* or *cilia,* 0.3 micron in diameter and several microns in length, project into the mucus that coats the inner surface of the nasal cavity. These projecting olfactory hairs are believed to react to odors in the air and then to stimulate the olfactory cells, as discussed below. Spaced among the olfactory cells in the olfactory membrane are many small *glands of Bowman* that secrete mucus onto the surface of the olfactory membrane.

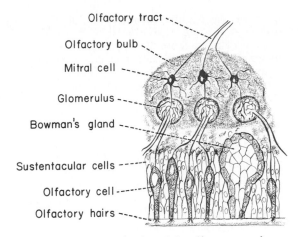

Figure 22–4. Organization of the olfactory membrane.

STIMULATION OF THE OLFACTORY CELLS

The Necessary Stimulus for Smell. We do not know what it takes chemically to stimulate the olfactory cells. Yet we do know the physical characteristics of the substances that cause olfactory stimulation: First, the substance must be volatile so that it can be sniffed into the nostrils. Second, it must be at least slightly water-soluble so that it can pass through the mucus to the olfactory cells. And, third, it must also be lipid-soluble, presumably because the olfactory cilia and outer tips of the olfactory cells are composed principally of lipid materials.

Regardless of the basic mechanism by which the olfactory cells are stimulated, it is known that they become stimulated only when air blasts upward into the superior region of the nose. Therefore, smell occurs in cycles along with the inspirations, which indicates that the olfactory receptors respond in milliseconds to the volatile agents. Because smell intensity is exacerbated by blasting air through the upper reaches of the nose, the sensitivity of smell can be greatly increased by the well-known sniffing technique.

Receptor Potentials in Olfactory Cells. The olfactory cells are believed to react to olfactory stimuli in the same manner that most other sensory receptors react to their specific stimuli; that is, by generating a receptor potential, which in turn initiates nerve impulses in the olfactory nerve fibers. An experiment that probably demonstrates this property of the olfactory receptors is the following: An electrode is placed on the surface of the olfactory membrane, and its electrical potential with respect to the remainder of the body is recorded. When an odorous substance is blown into the nostril, the potential becomes negative and remains negative as long as the odorous air continues to pass through the nostril. This electrical recording is called the *electro-olfactogram,* and it is believed to result from summation of receptor potentials developed in the receptor olfactory cells and perhaps also in the sustentacular cells that seem to be electrically connected to the olfactory cells.

Over a wide range, both the amplitude of the electro-olfactogram and the rate of olfactory nerve impulses are approximately proportional to the logarithm of the stimulus strength, which illustrates that the olfactory receptors tend to obey principles of transduction similar to those of other sensory receptors.

Adaptation.   The olfactory receptors adapt approximately 50 per cent in the first second or so after stimulation. Thereafter, they adapt further very slowly. Yet we all know from our own experience that smell sensations adapt almost to extinction within a minute or so after one enters a strongly odorous atmosphere. Since the psychological adaptation is far more rapid than the adaptation of the receptors, it has been suggested that most of this adaptation occurs in the central nervous system, as has also been postulated for adaptation of taste sensations.

Search for the Primary Sensations of Smell.   Most physiologists are convinced that the many smell sensations are subserved by a few rather discrete primary sensations, in the same way that taste is subserved by sour, sweet, bitter, and salty sensations. But, thus far, only minor success has been achieved in classifying the primary sensations of smell. Yet, on the basis of psychological tests and action potential studies from various points in the olfactory nerve pathways, it has been postulated that about seven different primary classes of olfactory stimulants preferentially excite separate olfactory cells. These classes of olfactory stimulants may be characterized as follows.

1. Camphoraceous
2. Musky
3. Floral
4. Pepperminty
5. Ethereal
6. Pungent
7. Putrid

However, it is unlikely that this list actually represents the true primary sensations of smell, even though it does illustrate the results of one of the many attempts to classify them. Indeed, several clues in recent years have indicated that there may be as many as *50* or more primary sensations of smell — a marked contrast to only *three* primary sensations of color detected by the eyes and only *four* primary sensations of taste detected by the tongue. For instance, persons have been found who have *odor blindness* for single substances; and such discrete odor blindness has been identified for more than 50 different substances. Since it is presumed that odor blindness for each substance represents a lack of the appropriate receptor cell for that substance, it is postulated that the sense of smell might be subserved by 50 or more primary smell sensations.

Two basic theories have been postulated to explain the abilities of different receptors to respond selectively to different types of olfactory stimulants: the *chemical theory* and the *physical theory*. The chemical theory assumes that *receptor chemicals* in the membranes of the olfactory cilia react specifically with the different types of olfactory stimulants. The type of receptor chemical determines the type of stimulant that will elicit a response in the olfactory cell. The reaction between the stimulant and the receptor substance supposedly increases the permeability of the olfactory ciliary membrane, and this in turn creates the receptor potential in the olfactory cell that generates impulses in the olfactory nerve fibers.

The physical theory assumes that differences in *physical receptor sites* on the olfactory ciliary membranes of separate olfactory cells allow specific olfactory stimulants to adsorb to the membranes of different olfactory cells. A fact supporting this theory is that some substances with very different chemical properties, but with almost identical molecular shapes, have the same odor. Yet, this principle does not hold for most odoriferous substances so that the physical theory is probably of historical rather than factual importance.

Affective Nature of Smell.   Smell, equally as much as taste, has the affective qualities of either pleasantness or unpleasantness. Because of this, smell is as important as, if not more important than, taste in the selection of food. Indeed, a person who has previously eaten food that has disagreed with him is often nauseated by the smell of that same type of food on a second occasion. Other types of odors that have proved to be unpleasant in the past may also provoke a disagreeable feeling; on the other hand, perfume of the right quality can wreak havoc with masculine emotions. In addition, in some lower animals odors are the primary excitant of sexual drive.

Threshold for Smell.   One of the principal characteristics of smell is the minute quantity of the stimulating agent in the air often required to effect a smell sensation. For instance, the substance *methyl mercaptan* can be smelled when only 1/25,000,000,000 milligram is present in each milliliter of air. Because of this low threshold, this substance is mixed with natural gas to give it an odor that can be detected when it leaks from a gas pipe.

Measurement of Smell Threshold.   One of the problems in studying smell has been difficulty in obtaining accurate measurements of the threshold stimulus required to induce smell. The simplest technique is simply to allow a person to sniff different substances in the usual manner of smelling. Indeed, some investigators feel that this is as satisfactory as almost any other procedure. However, to eliminate variations from person to person, more objective methods have been developed: One of these has been to place a box containing the volatilized agent over the subject's head. Appropriate precautions are taken to exclude odors from the person's own body. The person is allowed to breathe naturally, but the volatilized agent is distributed evenly in the air that is breathed.

Gradations of Smell Intensities. Though the threshold concentrations of substances that evoke smell are extremely slight, concentrations only 10 to 50 times above the threshold values evoke maximum intensity of smell. This is in contrast to most other sensory systems of the body, in which the ranges of detection are tremendous — for instance, 500,000 to 1 in the case of the eyes and 1,000,000,000,000 to 1 in the case of the ears. This perhaps can be explained by the fact that smell is concerned more with detecting the presence or absence of odors than with quantitative detection of their intensities.

TRANSMISSION OF SMELL 'SIGNALS INTO THE CENTRAL NERVOUS SYSTEM

The function of the central nervous system in olfaction is almost as vague as the function of the peripheral receptors. However, Figures 22–4 and 22–5 illustrate the general plan for transmission of olfactory signals into the central nervous system. Figure 22–4 shows a number of separate *olfactory cells* sending axons into the *olfactory bulb* to end on *dendrites from mitral cells* in a structure called the *glomerulus*. Approximately 25,000 axons enter each glomerulus and synapse with about 25 mitral cells that in turn send signals into the brain. Also in the glomerulus are smaller cells, the *tufted cells*, that send signals to the brain as well — perhaps to the older portions of the olfactory nervous system.

Figure 22–5 shows the major pathways for transmission of olfactory signals from the mitral and tufted cells into the brain. The fibers from the cells travel through the olfactory tract and terminate either primarily or after relay neurons in two principal areas of the brain called the *medial*

olfactory area and the *lateral olfactory area,* respectively. The medial olfactory area is composed of a large group of nuclei located in the midportion of the brain superiorly and anteriorly to the hypothalamus. This group includes the *olfactory trigone,* the *medial part of the anterior perforated substance,* the *paraolfactory area,* and the *nucleus of the stria terminalis.*

The lateral olfactory area is composed of the *prepyriform area,* the *lateral part of the anterior perforated substance,* and part of the *amygdaloid nuclei.*

Secondary olfactory tracts pass from the nuclei of both the medial olfactory area and the lateral olfactory area into the *hypothalamus, septum, thalamus, hippocampus, gyrus subcallosus,* and *brain stem nuclei.* These secondary areas control the automatic responses of the body to olfactory stimuli, including automatic feeding activities and also emotional responses, such as fear, excitement, and pleasure and sexual drives.

Secondary olfactory tracts also spread from the lateral olfactory area into the *uncus,* the lateroposterior orbitofrontal cortex, and the prefrontal cortex. It is probably in this lateral olfactory area, especially in the amygdala, its associated cortical regions in the temporal cortex, and the lateroposterior orbitofrontal cortex, that the more complex aspects of olfaction are integrated, such as association of olfactory sensations with somatic, visual, tactile, and other types of sensation. However, complete removal of the lateral olfactory area hardly affects the primitive responses to olfaction, such as licking the lips, salivation, and other feeding responses caused by the smell of food or such as the various emotions associated with smell. On the other hand, its removal does abolish the more complicated conditioned reflexes depending on olfactory stimuli. Therefore, cortical portions of this region are often considered to be the *primary olfactory cortex* for smell. In human beings, tumors in the region of the uncus, amygdala, or lateroposterior orbitofrontal cortex frequently cause the person to perceive abnormal smells.

Centrifugal Control of the Olfactory Bulb by the Central Nervous System. The central nervous system also transmits impulses in a backward direction to the olfactory bulb. These originate mainly from undetermined areas in the brain stem and olfactory portion of the cerebrum and terminate on small *granule* cells in the center of the bulb, which in turn send axons to the mitral and tufted cells to inhibit these.

Mechanism of Function of the Olfactory Tracts. Electrophysiological studies of the olfactory system show that the mitral and tufted cells are continually active, and superimposed on this background are increases or decreases in impulse traffic caused by different odors. Thus, the olfactory stimuli presumably *modulate* the frequency of impulses in the olfactory system and in this way transmit the olfactory information.

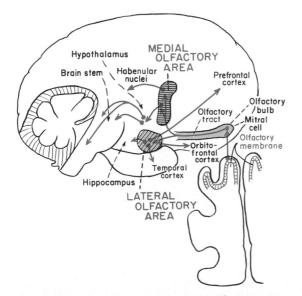

Figure 22–5. Neural connections of the olfactory system.

REFERENCES

Alberts, J. R.: Producing and interpreting experimental olfactory deficits. *Physiol. Behav., 12*:657, 1974.

Bradley, R. M., and Mistretta, C. M.: Investigations of taste function and swallowing in fetal sheep. *Symp. Oral Sens. Percept., 4*:185, 1973.

Dastoli, F. R.: Taste receptor proteins. *Life Sci., 14*:1417, 1974.

Denton, D. A.: Salt appetite. *In* Code, C. F., and Heidel, W. (eds.): Handbook of Physiology. Sec. 6, Vol. 1. Baltimore, Williams & Wilkins, 1967, p. 433.

Douek, E.: The Sense of Smell and Its Abnormalities. New York, Churchill Livingstone, 1974.

Forss, D. A.: Odor and flavor compounds from lipids. *Prog. Chem. Fats Other Lipids, 13*:177, 1972.

Hodgson, E. S.: Taste receptors. *Sci. Am., 204*:135, 1961.

Kare, M. R., and Maller, O.: The Chemical Sense and Nutrition. Baltimore, The Johns Hopkins Press, 1967.

Lat, J.: Self-selection of dietary components. *In* Code, C. F., and Heidel, W. (eds.): Handbook of Physiology. Sec. 6, Vol. 1. Baltimore, Williams & Wilkins, 1967, p. 367.

Moulton, D. G.: Spatial patterning of response to odors in the peripheral olfactory system. *Physiol. Rev., 56*:578, 1976.

Moulton, D. G., and Beidler, L. M.: Structure and function in the peripheral olfactory system. *Physiol. Rev., 47*:1, 1967.

Norsiek, F. W.: The sweet tooth. *Am. Sci., 60*:41, 1972.

Oakley, B., and Benjamin, R. M.: Neural mechanisms of taste. *Physiol. Rev., 46*:173, 1966.

Ohloff, G., and Thomas, A. F. (eds.): Gustation and Olfaction. New York, Academic Press, 1971.

Schultz, E. F., and Tapp, J. T.: Olfactory control of behavior in rodents. *Psychol. Bull., 79*:21, 1973.

Shepherd, G. M.: Synaptic organization of the mammalian olfactory bulb. *Physiol. Rev., 52*:864, 1972.

Shepherd, G. M.: The olfactory bulb: A simple system in the mammalian brain. *In* Brookhart, J. M., and Mountcastle, V. B. (eds.): Handbook of Physiology. Sec. 1, Vol. 1. Baltimore, Williams & Wilkins, 1977, p. 945.

Todd, J. H.: The chemical languages of fishes. *Sci. Am., 224*:98, 1971.

Weiffenbach, J. M. (ed.): Taste and Development: The Genesis of Sweet Preference. Washington, D.C., U.S. Government Printing Office, 1977.

Wenzel, B. M., and Sieck, M. H.: Olfaction. *Annu. Rev. Physiol., 28*:381, 1966.

Zotterman, Y.: Olfaction and Taste. New York, The Macmillan Co., 1963.

Part IV

NERVOUS CONTROL OF BODY FUNCTIONS

23

Nervous Regulation of the Circulation and of Respiration

Because the nervous system is the major overall controller of our bodily activities, it is equally as important to understand the ways in which the nervous system interfaces with the peripheral parts of the body as to understand the nervous system itself. Therefore, the remaining chapters of this text will help to explain some of the more important ways in which the nervous system controls what we call the *vegetative functions* of the body, meaning the life processes of the body, such as the control of arterial pressure, respiration, gastrointestinal function, body temperature, and even sexual functions.

The present chapter will address the control of the circulation and respiration.

NERVOUS REGULATION OF THE CIRCULATION

The circulation is regulated partly by non-nervous mechanisms that are intrinsic to the circulation itself and partly by extrinsic mechanisms, especially by the nervous system. The intrinsic mechanisms consist of such functions as intrinsic control of rhythmicity within the heart muscle itself and local control of blood flow by each tissue of the body when the tissue needs more or less nutrients.

Nervous control of the circulation has two very important features: First, nervous regulation can function extremely rapidly, some of the nervous effects beginning to occur within 1 second and reaching full development within 5 to 30 seconds. Second, the nervous system provides a means for controlling large parts of the circulation simultaneously, often in spite of the effect that this has on the blood flow to individual tissues. For instance, when it is important to raise the arterial pressure temporarily, the nervous system can arbitrarily

cut off, or at least greatly decrease, blood flow to major segments of the circulation despite the fact that the local blood flow regulatory mechanisms oppose this.

AUTONOMIC CONTROL OF THE CIRCULATION

The autonomic nervous system was discussed in detail in Chapter 17. However, it is so important to the regulation of the circulation that its specific anatomical and functional characteristics relating to the circulation deserve special attention here.

By far the most important part of the autonomic nervous system for regulation of the circulation is the *sympathetic nervous system*. The *parasympathetic nervous system* is important only for its regulation of heart function, as we shall see later in the chapter.

The Sympathetic Nervous System. Figure 23–1 illustrates the anatomy of sympathetic nervous control of the circulation. Sympathetic vasomotor nerve fibers leave the spinal cord through all the thoracic and the first one to two lumbar spinal nerves. These pass into the sympathetic chain and thence by two routes to the blood vessels throughout the body: (1) through the *peripheral sympathetic nerves* and (2) through the *spinal nerves*. The precise pathways of these fibers in the spinal cord and in the sympathetic chains were discussed in Chapter 17. It suffices to say here that, with rare exceptions, all vascular areas of the body are supplied with sympathetic nerve fibers.

Distribution of Sympathetic Nerve Fibers to the Peripheral Vasculature. Figure 23–2 illustrates the distribution of sympathetic nerve fibers to the peripheral blood vessels and shows that all the vessels, except the capillaries, sphincters, and most of the metarterioles, are innervated.

The innervation of the small arteries and arterioles allows sympathetic stimulation to increase

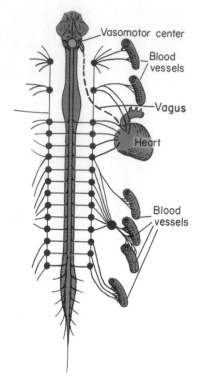

Figure 23–1. The vasomotor center and its control of the circulatory system through the sympathetic and vagus nerves.

the *resistance* and thereby to change the rate of blood flow through the tissues. The innervation of large vessels, particularly of the veins, makes it possible for sympathetic stimulation to change the volume of these vessels and thereby to alter the volume of the peripheral circulatory system, which plays a major role in the regulation of cardiovascular function, as we shall see later in this chapter and subsequent chapters.

Sympathetic Nerve Fibers to the Heart. In addition to sympathetic nerve fibers supplying the blood vessels, these fibers also go to the heart. This innervation was discussed in Chapter 5. It will be recalled that sympathetic stimulation mark-

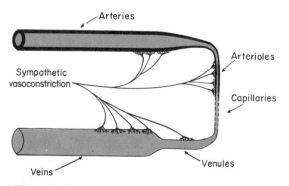

Figure 23–2. Innervation of the systemic circulation.

edly increases the activity of the heart, increasing the heart rate and enhancing its strength of pumping.

Parasympathetic Control of Heart Function, Especially Heart Rate. Though the parasympathetic nervous system is exceedingly important for many other autonomic functions of the body, it plays only a minor role in regulation of the circulation. Its only really important effect is its control of heart rate. It also has a slight effect on control of cardiac contractility; however, this effect is far overshadowed by the sympathetic nervous system control of contractility. Parasympathetic nerves pass to the heart in the vagus nerve, as illustrated in Figure 23–1.

The effects of parasympathetic stimulation on heart function were discussed in detail in Chapter 5. Principally, parasympathetic stimulation causes a marked *decrease* in heart rate and a slight decrease in contractility.

The Sympathetic Vasoconstrictor System and Its Control by the Central Nervous System

The sympathetic nerves carry both vasoconstrictor and vasodilator fibers, but by far the most important of these are the *sympathetic vasoconstrictor* fibers. Sympathetic vasoconstrictor fibers are distributed to essentially all segments of the circulation. However, this distribution is greater in some tissues than in others. It is less potent in both skeletal and cardiac muscle and in the brain, while it is powerful in the kidneys, the gut, the spleen, and the skin.

The Vasomotor Center and Its Control of the Vasoconstrictor System — Vasomotor Tone. Located bilaterally in the reticular substance of the lower third of the pons and upper two-thirds of the medulla, as illustrated in Figure 23–3, is an area called the *vasomotor center*. This center transmits impulses downward through the cord and thence through the vasoconstrictor fibers to all the blood vessels of the body.

The upper and lateral portions of the vasomotor center are *tonically active*. That is, they have an inherent tendency to transmit nerve impulses all the time, thereby maintaining even normally a slow rate of firing in essentially all vasoconstrictor nerve fibers of the body at a rate of about one-half to two impulses per second. This continual firing is called *sympathetic vasoconstrictor tone*. These impulses maintain a partial state of contraction in the blood vessels, a state called *vasomotor tone*.

The brain stem can be severed above the lower third of the pons without significantly changing the normal activity of the vasomotor center. This center remains tonically active and continues to transmit approximately normal numbers of im-

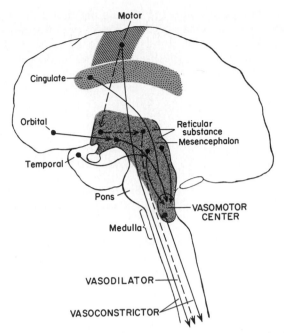

Figure 23–3. Areas of the brain that play important roles in the nervous regulation of the circulation.

pulses to the sympathetic vasoconstrictor fibers throughout the body.

Figure 23–4 demonstrates the significance of vasoconstrictor tone. In the experiment of this figure, total spinal anesthesia was administered to an animal, which completely blocked all transmission of nerve impulses from the central nervous system to the periphery. As a result, the arterial pressure fell from 100 to 50 mm. Hg, illustrating the effect of loss of vasoconstrictor tone through-

out the body. A few minutes later a small amount of the hormone norepinephrine was injected — norepinephrine is the substance secreted at the endings of sympathetic nerve fibers throughout the body. As this hormone was transported in the blood to all the blood vessels, the vessels once again became constricted, and the arterial pressure rose to a level even greater than normal for a minute or two until the norepinephrine was destroyed.

The Inhibitory Area of the Vasomotor Center. The medial and lower portion of the vasomotor center does not participate in excitation of the vasoconstrictor fibers. Instead, stimulation of this area transmits *inhibitory* impulses into the upper lateral parts of the vasomotor center, thereby *decreasing the degree of sympathetic vasoconstrictor tone* and consequently allowing dilatation of the blood vessels. Thus, the vasomotor center is composed of two parts, a bilateral *excitatory part* that can excite the vasoconstrictor fibers and cause vascular constriction and a medial *inhibitory part* that can inhibit vasoconstriction, thus allowing vasodilatation.

Control of Heart Activity by the Vasomotor Center. At the same time that the vasomotor center is controlling the degree of vascular constriction, it also controls heart activity. The lateral portions of the vasomotor center transmit excitatory impulses through the sympathetic nerve fibers to the heart to increase heart rate and contractility, while the medial portion of the vasomotor center, which lies in immediate apposition to the *dorsal motor nucleus of the vagus nerve,* transmits impulses through the vagus nerve to the heart to decrease heart rate. Therefore, the

Figure 23–4. Effect of total spinal anesthesia on the arterial pressure, showing a marked fall in pressure resulting from loss of vasomotor tone.

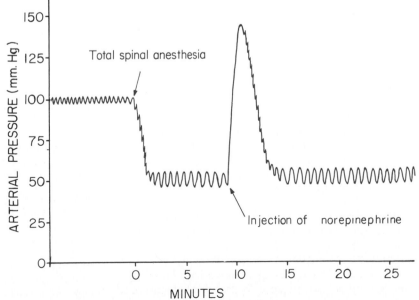

vasomotor center can either increase or decrease heart activity, this ordinarily increasing at the same time that vasoconstriction occurs throughout the body and ordinarily decreasing at the same time that vasoconstriction is inhibited. However, these interrelationships are not invariable, because some signals that pass down the vagus nerves to the heart can by-pass the vasomotor center.

Control of the Vasomotor Center by Higher Nervous Centers. Large numbers of areas throughout the *reticular substance* of the *pons, mesencephalon,* and *diencephalon* can either excite or inhibit the vasomotor center. This reticular substance is illustrated in Figure 23–3 by the diffuse shaded area. In general, the more lateral and superior portions of the reticular substance cause excitation, while the more medial and inferior portions cause inhibition.

The *hypothalamus* plays a special role in the control of the vasoconstrictor system, for it can exert powerful excitatory or inhibitory effects on the vasomotor center. The *posterolateral portions* of the hypothalamus cause mainly excitation, while the *anterior part* can cause mild excitation or inhibition, depending on the precise part of the anterior hypothalamus stimulated.

Many different parts of the *cerebral cortex* can also excite or inhibit the vasomotor center. Stimulation of the *motor cortex,* for instance, excites the vasomotor center because of impulses transmitted downward into the hypothalamus and thence to the vasomotor center. Also, stimulation of the *anterior temporal lobe,* the *orbital areas of the frontal cortex,* the *anterior part of the cingulate gyrus,* the *amygdala,* the *septum,* and the *hippocampus* can all either excite or inhibit the vasomotor center, depending on the precise portion of these areas that is stimulated and upon the intensity of the stimulus.

Thus, widespread areas of the brain can have profound effects on the vasomotor center and in turn on the sympathetic vasoconstrictor system of the body, either further enhancing the degree of vasoconstriction or inhibiting the vasoconstrictor tone and thereby causing vasodilatation.

Norepinephrine — The Sympathetic Vasoconstrictor Transmitter Substance. The substance secreted at the endings of the vasoconstrictor nerves is norepinephrine. Norepinephrine acts directly on the smooth muscle of the vessels to cause vasoconstriction, as was discussed in Chapter 12.

The Adrenal Medullae and Their Relationship to the Sympathetic Vasoconstrictor System. Sympathetic impulses are transmitted to the adrenal medullae at the same time that they are transmitted to all the blood vessels. These impulses cause the medullae to secrete both epinephrine and norepinephrine into the circulating blood, as was described in Chapter 16. These two hormones are carried in the bloodstream to all parts of the body, where they act directly on the blood vessels usually to cause vasoconstriction, but sometimes the epinephrine causes vasodilatation, as will be discussed later in the chapter.

The Sympathetic Vasodilator System and Its Control by the Central Nervous System

The sympathetic nerves to skeletal muscles carry sympathetic vasodilator fibers as well as constrictor fibers. In lower animals, such as the cat, these fibers release *acetylcholine* at their endings, though in primates the vasodilator substance might be epinephrine. The vasodilator acts on the smooth muscle of the blood vessels to cause vasodilatation in contrast to the vasoconstrictor effect of norepinephrine.

The pathways for central nervous system control of the vasodilator system are illustrated by the dashed lines in Figure 23–3. The principal area of the brain controlling this system is the *anterior hypothalamus,* which transmits impulses to a relay station in the *subcollicular region* of the mesencephalon. From here impulses are transmitted down the cord to the *sympathetic preganglionic neurons* in the lateral horns of the cord. These then transmit vasodilator impulses to the blood vessels of the muscles.

Note also in Figure 23–3 that stimulation of the *motor cortex* excites the *sympathetic vasodilator system* by transmitting impulses downward into the hypothalamus.

Importance of the Sympathetic Vasodilator System. It is doubtful that the sympathetic vasodilator system plays a very important role in the control of the circulation, because complete block of the sympathetic nerves to the muscles hardly affects the ability of the muscles to control their own blood flow in response to their needs. Yet, it is possible, if not probable, that at the onset of exercise the sympathetic vasodilator system causes initial vasodilation in the skeletal muscles to allow an *anticipatory increase in blood flow* even before the muscles require increased nutrients.

"PATTERNS" OF CIRCULATORY RESPONSES ELICITED BY DIFFERENT CENTRAL NERVOUS SYSTEM CENTERS

Stimulation of the Vasomotor Center — The Mass Action Effect. Stimulation of the lateral portions of the vasomotor center causes widespread activation of the vasoconstrictor fibers throughout the body, while stimulation of the medial portions of the vasomotor center causes widespread *inhibition of vasoconstriction.* In many conditions the entire vasomotor center acts as a unit, stimulating all vasoconstrictors throughout the body and also the heart, as well as stimulating the adrenal medullae to secrete epinephrine and norepinephrine that circulate in the blood to excite the circulation still further. The results of this "mass action" are three-fold: First, the peripheral resistance increases in most parts of the circulation, thereby elevating the arterial pressure. Second, the capacity vessels, particularly the veins, are excited at the same time, greatly decreasing their capacity; this forces increased quantities of blood into the heart, thereby increasing the cardiac output. Third, the heart is simultaneously stimulated so that it can handle the increased cardiac output.

Thus, the overall effect of this "mass action" is to prepare the circulation for increased delivery of blood flow to the body.

Stimulation of the Hypothalamus — The "Alarm" Pattern. Under normal conditions, the hypothalamus probably does not transmit large numbers of impulses into the sympathetic vascular control system. However, on occasion the hypothalamus becomes strongly stimulated and can then activate both the vasoconstrictor and vasodilator systems or either of them separately.

Diffuse stimulation of the hypothalamus (or of closely allied areas such as the septum) activates the vasodilator system to the muscles, thereby increasing the blood flow through the muscles; at the same time it causes intense vasoconstriction throughout the remainder of the body and an intense increase in heart activity. The arterial pressure rises, the cardiac output increases, the heart rate increases, and the circulation is ready to supply nutrients to the muscles if there be need. Also, impulses are transmitted simultaneously throughout the central nervous system to cause a state of generalized excitement and attentiveness, these often increasing to such a pitch that the overall pattern of the reaction is that of *alarm*.

Thus, the "alarm" pattern contains all the ingredients of the "mass action" pattern as well as the elements of muscle vasodilation and extreme psychic excitement. This pattern seems to have the purposeful effect of preparing the animal or person to perform on a second's notice whatever activity is required.

The "Motor" Pattern of Circulatory Stimulation. When the motor cortex transmits signals to the skeletal muscle to cause motor activities, it also sends signals to the circulatory system to cause the following effects: First, it excites the alarm system just described, and this generally activates the heart and increases arterial pressure, making the circulatory system ready to supply increased blood flow to the muscles. This effect also causes vasoconstriction in most nonmuscular parts of the body, such as the kidneys, the skin, and the gut, thereby forcing a larger share of the blood flow through the active muscles. Second, impulses pass directly from the motor cortex to the sympathetic neurons of the spinal cord. These enhance the vasoconstriction in the nonmuscular parts of the body, thereby raising the arterial pressure still more and helping to increase muscle blood flow. They possibly also inhibit the vasoconstrictor nerves to the excited muscles.

The motor pattern of circulatory responses can also be elicited by stimulation of several areas of the reticular substance in the brain stem. Stimulation of one of these areas, the *fields of Forel*, elicits a response almost precisely the same as that caused by direct activation of the motor cortex. Therefore, it is possible, if not likely, that this area of the reticular substance plays a major role in control of the circulatory system in exercise.

Emotional Fainting — Vasovagal Syncope. A particularly interesting circulatory reaction occurs in persons who faint because of intense emotional experiences. In this condition, the muscle vasodilator system becomes powerfully activated so that blood flow through the muscles increases several-fold. Intense vagal stimulation of the heart also occurs, causing the heart rate to slow markedly. This overall effect is called *vasovagal syncope*. The arterial pressure falls instantly, which in turn reduces the blood flow to the brain and causes the person to lose consciousness. It is probable, therefore, that emotional fainting results from powerful stimulation of the anterior hypothalamic vasodilator center.

REFLEX CONTROL OF ARTERIAL PRESSURE

The Arterial Baroreceptor Control System — Baroreceptor Reflexes

By far the best known of the mechanisms for arterial pressure control is the *baroreceptor reflex*. Basically, this reflex is initiated by stretch receptors, called either *baroreceptors* or *pressoreceptors,* located in the walls of the large systemic arteries. A rise in pressure stretches the baroreceptors and causes them to transmit signals into the central nervous system, and other signals are in turn sent to the circulation to reduce arterial pressure back toward the normal level.

Physiologic Anatomy of the Baroreceptors. Baroreceptors are spray-type nerve endings lying in the walls of the arteries; they are stimulated when stretched. A few baroreceptors are located in the wall of almost every large artery of the thoracic and neck regions; but, as illustrated in Figure 23–5, baroreceptors are extremely abundant, in (1) the walls of the internal carotid arteries slightly above the carotid bifurcations, areas

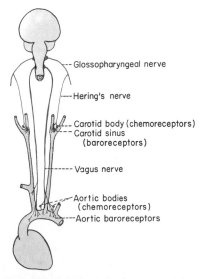

Figure 23–5. The baroreceptor system.

known as the *carotid sinuses,* and (2) the walls of the aortic arch.

Figure 23–5 also shows that impulses are transmitted from each carotid sinus through the very small *Hering's nerve* to the glossopharyngeal nerve and thence to the medullary area of the brain stem. Impulses from the arch of the aorta are transmitted through the vagus nerves also to the medulla. Hering's nerve is especially important in physiologic experiments because baroreceptor impulses can be recorded from it with ease.

Response of the Baroreceptors to Pressure. Figure 23–6 illustrates the effect of different arterial pressures on the rate of impulse transmission in a Hering's nerve. Note that the carotid sinus baroreceptors are not stimulated at all by pressures between 0 and 60 mm. Hg, but above 60 mm. Hg they respond progressively more and more rapidly and reach a maximum at about 180 mm. Hg. The responses of the aortic baroreceptors are similar to those of the carotid receptors, except that they respond, in general, at pressure levels about 30 mm. Hg higher.

Note especially that the increase in number of impulses for each unit change in arterial pressure, expressed as $\Delta I/\Delta P$ in the figure, is greatest at a pressure level near the normal mean arterial pressure. This means that the increase in baroreceptor control of arterial pressure occurs just at the level where the response needs to be most marked. That is, in the normal operating range of arterial pressure, even a slight change in pressure causes strong sympathetic reflexes to readjust the arterial pressure back toward normal.

The baroreceptors respond extremely rapidly to changes in arterial pressure; the number of impulses even increases during systole and decreases again during diastole. Furthermore, the baroreceptors *respond much more to a rapidly changing pressure* than to a stationary pressure. That is, if the mean arterial pressure is 150 mm. Hg but at that moment is rising rapidly, the rate of impulse transmission may be as much as twice that when the pressure is stationary at 150 mm. Hg. On the other hand, if the pressure is falling, the rate might be as little as one-quarter that for a stationary pressure.

The Reflex Initiated by the Baroreceptors. The baroreceptor impulses *inhibit the vasoconstrictor center* of the medulla and *excite* the vagal center. The net effects are (1) *vasodilatation* throughout the peripheral circulatory system and (2) *decreased heart rate* and *strength of contraction.* Therefore, excitation of the baroreceptors by pressure in the arteries reflexly *causes the arterial pressure to decrease.* Conversely, low pressure has opposite effects, reflexly causing the pressure to rise back toward normal.

Figure 23–7 illustrates a typical reflex change in arterial pressure caused by clamping the common carotids. This procedure reduces the carotid sinus pressure; as a result, the baroreceptors become inactive and lose their inhibitory effect on the vasomotor center. The vasomotor center then becomes much more active than usual, causing the arterial pressure to rise and to remain elevated during the ten minutes that the carotids are clamped. Removal of the clamps allows the pressure to fall immediately to slightly below normal as a momentary overcompensation and then to return to normal in another minute or so.

Function of the Baroreceptors During Changes in Body Posture. The ability of the baroreceptors to maintain relatively constant arterial pressure is extremely important when a person sits or stands after having been lying down. Immediately upon standing, the arterial pressure in the head and upper part of the body obviously tends to fall, and marked reduction of this pressure can cause loss of

Figure 23–6. Response of the baroreceptors at different levels of arterial pressure.

Figure 23–7. Typical carotid sinus reflex effect on arterial pressure caused by clamping both common carotids.

consciousness. Fortunately, however, the falling pressure at the baroreceptors elicits an immediate reflex, resulting in strong sympathetic discharge throughout the body, and this minimizes the decrease in pressure in the head and upper body.

The "Buffer" Function of the Baroreceptor Control System. Because the baroreceptor system opposes increases and decreases in arterial pressure, it is often called a *pressure buffer system,* and the nerves from the baroreceptors are called *buffer nerves.*

Figure 23–8 illustrates the importance of this buffer function of the baroreceptors. The upper record in this figure shows an arterial pressure recording for 2 hours from a normal dog and the lower record from a dog whose baroreceptor nerves from both the carotid sinuses and the aorta had previously been removed. Note the extreme variability of pressure in the denervated dog caused by simple events of the day such as lying down, standing, excitement, eating, defecation, noises, and so forth.

In summary, we can state that the primary purpose of the arterial baroreceptor system is to reduce the daily variation in arterial pressure to about one-half to one-third that which would occur were the baroreceptor system not present. But note in Figure 23–8 that the average arterial pressure over any prolonged period is almost exactly the same whether the baroreceptors are present or not, illustrating the unimportance of the baroreceptor system for long-term regulation of arterial pressure even though it is extremely potent in preventing the rapid changes of arterial pressure that occur moment-by-moment or hour-by-hour.

Unimportance of the Baroreceptor System for Long-Term Regulation of Arterial Pressure — Adaptation of the Baroreceptors. The baroreceptor control system is probably of no importance whatsoever in long-term regulation of arterial pressure for a very simple reason: The baroreceptors themselves adapt in one to three days to whatever pressure level they are exposed to. That is, if the pressure rises from the normal value of 100 mm. Hg up to 200 mm. Hg, extreme numbers of baroreceptor impulses are at first transmitted. During the next few seconds, the rate of firing diminishes considerably; then it diminishes very slowly during the next one to two days, at the end of which time the rate will have returned essentially to the normal level despite the fact that the arterial pressure remains 200 mm. Hg. Conversely, when the arterial pressure falls to a very low value, the baroreceptors at first transmit no impulses at all, but gradually over a period of several days the rate of baroreceptor firing returns again to the original control level.

This adaptation of the baroreceptors obviously prevents the baroreceptors reflex from functioning

Figure 23–8. Two hour records of arterial pressure in a normal dog (above) and in the same dog (below) several weeks after the baroreceptors had been denervated. (Courtesy of Dr. Allen W. Cowley, Jr.)

as a control system to buffer arterial pressure changes that last longer than a few days at a time. Therefore, prolonged regulation of arterial pressure requires other control systems, principally the renal–body fluid–pressure control system (along with its associated hormonal mechanisms).

Control of Arterial Pressure by the Vasomotor Center in Response to Diminished Brain Blood Flow — The CNS Ischemic Response

Normally, most nervous control of blood pressure is achieved by reflexes originating in the baroreceptors, the chemoreceptors, and the low pressure receptors, all of which are located in the peripheral circulation outside the brain. However, when blood flow to the vasomotor center in the lower brain stem becomes decreased enough to cause nutritional deficiency, a condition called *ischemia,* the neurons in the vasomotor center itself respond directly to the ischemia and become strongly excited. When this occurs, the systemic arterial pressure often rises to a level as high as the heart can possibly pump. This effect is believed to be caused by failure of the slowly flowing blood to carry carbon dioxide away from the vasomotor center; the local concentration of carbon dioxide increases greatly and has an extremely potent effect in stimulating the sympathetic nervous system. It is possible that other factors, such as the buildup of lactic acid and other acidic substances, also contribute to the marked stimulation of the vasomotor center and to the elevation in pressure. This arterial pressure elevation in response to cerebral ischemia is known as the *central nervous system ischemic response* or simply *CNS ischemic response*.

The magnitude of the ischemic effect on vasomotor activity is tremendous; it can elevate the mean arterial pressure for as long as ten minutes sometimes to as high as 270 mm. Hg. *The degree of sympathetic vasoconstriction caused by intense cerebral ischemia is often so great that some of the peripheral vessels become totally or almost totally occluded.* The kidneys, for instance, will entirely cease their production of urine because of arteriolar constriction in response to the sympathetic discharge. Therefore, *the CNS ischemic response is one of the most powerful of all the activators of the sympathetic vasoconstrictor system.*

Importance of the CNS Ischemic Response as a Regulator of Arterial Pressure. Despite the extremely powerful nature of the CNS ischemic response, it does not become very active until the arterial pressure falls far below normal, down to *levels below 50 mm. Hg* and below, reaching its greatest degree of stimulation at a pressure of 15 to 20 mm. Hg. Therefore, it is not one of the mechanisms for regulating normal arterial pressure. Instead it operates principally as an *emergency arterial pressure control system that acts rapidly and extremely powerfully to prevent further decrease in arterial pressure whenever blood flow to the brain decreases dangerously close to the lethal level.* It is sometimes called the "last ditch stand" pressure control mechanism.

REGULATION OF RESPIRATION

The nervous system adjusts the rate of alveolar ventilation almost exactly to the demands of the body so that the blood oxygen pressure (Po_2) and carbon dioxide pressure (Pco_2) are hardly altered even during strenuous exercise or other types of respiratory stress.

The following discussion describes the operation of this nervous system for regulation of respiration.

THE RESPIRATORY CENTER

The so-called "respiratory center" is a widely dispersed group of neurons located bilaterally in the reticular substance of the medulla oblongata and pons, as illustrated in Figure 23–9. It is divided into three major areas: (1) a dorsal medullary group of neurons, which is mainly an *inspiratory area,* (2) a ventral respiratory group of neurons, which is mainly an *expiratory area,* and (3) an area in the pons that helps to control the respiratory rate, called the *pneumotaxic area.* It is the inspiratory area that plays the fundamental role in the control of respiration. Therefore, let us discuss its function first.

The Inspiratory Area

The inspiratory area lies bilaterally in the dorsal portion of the medulla, extending approximately the entire length of the medulla. Its neurons are very near to and interconnect closely with the tractus solitarius, which is the sensory termination of both the vagal and glossopharyngeal nerves; each of these nerves in turn transmits sensory signals from the peripheral chemoreceptors, in this way helping to control pulmonary ventilation. In addition, the vagi also transmit sensory signals from the lungs that help to control lung inflation and respiratory rate, as we shall discuss in a subsequent section of this chapter.

Rhythmical Oscillation in the Inspiratory Area. The basic rhythm of respiration is generated in the inspiratory area. Even when all incoming nerve fiber connections to this area have been sectioned or blocked, the area still emits repetitive bursts of action potentials that cause rhythmical inspiratory cycles.

During expiration the inspiratory center becomes dormant, but after a few seconds the inspiratory center suddenly and automatically turns on again. This seems to result from an inherent,

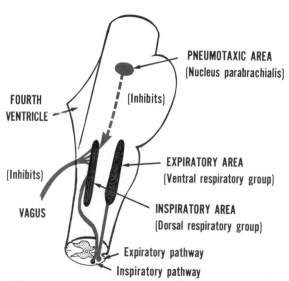

Figure 23–9. Organization of the respiratory center.

intrinsic excitability of the inspiratory neurons themselves that causes reverberatory oscillation to occur from neuron to neuron within the dorsal respiratory group; this neuronal activity initiates the inspiratory nervous signals to the diaphragm and other inspiratory muscles. During the next few seconds the intensity of the inspiratory signal increases rapidly, causing the diaphragm and other inspiratory muscles to contract more and more forcefully. In normal respiration this ''ramp'' increase in inspiratory signal lasts for about two seconds, at the end of which time it suddenly comes to a halt. Then the inspiratory neurons remain dormant again for approximately the next three seconds in normal respiration before the entire cycle repeats itself once more, this repetition continuing on and on throughout the life of the person.

Function of the Pneumotaxic Center to Limit the Duration of Inspiration and to Increase Respiratory Rate. The pneumotaxic center, located in the pons, transmits impulses continuously to the inspiratory area. The primary effect of these is to help turn off the inspiratory signal before the lungs become too full of air. When the pneumotaxic signals are strong, inspiration might last for as short as one-half second. When the pneumotaxic signal is extremely weak the inspiratory ramp signal will continue to ascend the crescendo of strength for perhaps as long as five to seven seconds, thus filling the lungs with a great excess of air.

Thus, the function of the pneumotaxic center is primarily to limit inspiration. However, this has a secondary effect on the rate of breathing because limitation of inspiration shortens the entire period of respiration. Therefore, a new cycle of inspiration begins again at a much earlier time. Thus, a strong pneumotaxic signal can increase the rate of breathing up to 30 to 40 breaths per minute while a weak pneumotaxic signal may reduce the rate of respiration to only a few breaths per minute.

Limitation of Inspiration by Vagal Lung Inflation Signals — The Hering-Breuer Reflex. Located in the walls of the bronchi and bronchioles throughout the lungs are *stretch receptors* that transmit signals through the vagi into the inspiratory center when overstretched. These signals affect inspiration in almost exactly the same way as signals from the pneumotaxic center; that is, they limit the duration of inspiration. Therefore, when the lungs become overly inflated, the stretch receptors activate an appropriate feedback response to limit further inspiration. This is called the *Hering-Breuer reflex*. This reflex also has the same effect as the pneumotaxic signals in increasing the rate of respiration because of the reduced period of inspiration.

Though in the past it was believed that the Hering-Breuer reflex plays an important role in controlling even normal lung inflation, recent experimental studies have shown that the reflex is not activated until the tidal volume increases to greater than approximately 1.5 liters. Therefore, the reflex appears to be mainly a protective mechanism for preventing excess lung inflation rather than an important ingredient in the normal control of ventilation.

The Expiratory Area

Located bilaterally in the medulla, and also extending the entire length of the medulla, is a ventral respiratory group of neurons which when stimulated excites the expiratory muscles. This expiratory area remains dormant during most normal quiet respiration, because quiet respiration is achieved by contraction only of the inspiratory muscles while expiration results from passive recoil of the elastic structures of the lung and surrounding chest cage. Furthermore, no evidence has been found that the expiratory area participates in the basic rhythmical oscillation that controls respiration.

On the other hand, when the respiratory drive for increased pulmonary ventilation becomes greater than normal, signals then spill over into the expiratory area from the basic oscillating mechanism in the inspiratory area. As a consequence, the expiratory muscles then contribute their powerful contractile forces to the pulmonary ventilatory process. Unfortunately, the neurophysiological basis for this interaction between the inspiratory and expiratory centers is not yet known.

Control of Respiratory Center Activity

Pulmonary ventilation must change vastly under different conditions, especially when the body's metabolic rate is increased so that oxygen utilization and carbon dioxide formation are increased as much as 20-fold. These vast changes in pulmonary ventilation are achieved in two different ways: (1) by feedback control of respiratory center activity in response to changes in the chemical composition of the blood, especially its concentrations of carbon dioxide, hydrogen ions, and oxygen, and (2) by control from other parts of the nervous system, especially during exercise. The main purpose of the remainder of this chapter is to discuss this control of ventilation in response to the needs of the body.

CHEMICAL CONTROL OF RESPIRATION

The ultimate goal of respiration is to maintain proper concentrations of oxygen, carbon dioxide, and hydrogen ions in the body fluid. It is fortunate, therefore, that respiratory activity is highly responsive to changes in any one of these.

Excess carbon dioxide or hydrogen ions affect respiration mainly by direct excitatory effects on the respiratory center itself, causing greatly increased strength of both the inspiratory and expiratory signals to the respiratory muscles. The resulting increase in ventilation increases the elimination of carbon dioxide from the blood; this also removes hydrogen ions from the blood because of decreased blood carbonic acid.

Oxygen, on the other hand, does not seem to have a significant direct effect on the respiratory center of the brain in controlling respiration. Instead, it probably acts entirely on peripheral chemoreceptors located in the carotid and aortic bodies, and these in turn transmit appropriate neuronal signals to the respiratory center for control of respiration.

Let us discuss first the direct stimulation of the respiratory center itself by carbon dioxide and hydrogen ions.

Figure 23–10. Stimulation of the inspiratory area by the *chemosensitive area* located bilaterally in the medulla, lying only a few microns beneath the ventral medullary surface. Note also that hydrogen ions stimulate the chemosensitive area, while mainly carbon dioxide in the fluid gives rise to the hydrogen ions.

DIRECT CHEMICAL CONTROL OF RESPIRATORY CENTER ACTIVITY BY CARBON DIOXIDE AND HYDROGEN IONS

The Chemosensitive Area of the Respiratory Center. Thus far, we have discussed mainly three different areas of the respiratory center: the inspiratory area, the expiratory area, and the pneumotaxic area. However, it is believed that none of these is affected directly by changes in blood carbon dioxide concentration or hydrogen ion concentration. Instead, a very sensitive *chemosensitive* area, illustrated in Figure 23–10, is located bilaterally and ventrally in the substance of the medulla, lying only a few microns beneath the surface anterior to the entry of the glossopharyngeal and vagal nerves into the medulla. This area is highly sensitive to changes in either blood CO_2 or hydrogen ion concentration, and it in turn excites the other portions of the respiratory center. It has especially potent effects on increasing the degree of activity of the inspiratory center, increasing both the rate of rise of the inspiratory ramp signal and also the intensity of the signal. This in turn has an automatic secondary effect of increasing the frequency of the respiratory rhythm.

Response of the Chemosensitive Neurons to Hydrogen Ions — The Primary Stimulus

The sensor neurons in the chemosensitive area are especially excited by hydrogen ions; in fact, it

is believed that hydrogen ions are perhaps the only important direct stimulus for these neurons. Unfortunately, though, hydrogen ions do not easily cross either the blood-brain barrier or the blood–cerebrospinal fluid barrier. For this reason, changes in hydrogen ion concentration in the blood actually have considerably less effect in stimulating the chemosensitive neurons than do changes in carbon dioxide, even though carbon dioxide stimulates these neurons indirectly, as will be explained below.

Effect of Blood Carbon Dioxide on Stimulating the Chemosensitive Area

Though carbon dioxide has very little direct effect on stimulating the neurons in the chemosensitive area, it does have a very potent indirect effect. It does this by reacting with the water of the tissues to form carbonic acid. This in turn dissociates into hydrogen and bicarbonate ions; the hydrogen ions then have a potent direct stimulatory effect. These effects are illustrated in Figure 23–10.

But, why is it that blood CO_2 has a much more potent effect on stimulating the chemosensitive neurons than do blood hydrogen ions? The answer is that hydrogen ions, as noted above, pass through both the blood-brain barrier and the blood–cerebrospinal fluid barrier only very poorly while carbon dioxide passes through both these barriers almost as if they did not exist. Consequently, whenever the blood carbon dioxide concentration increases, so also does the P_{CO_2}

increase in both the interstitial fluid of the medulla and also in the cerebrospinal fluid. And, in both of these fluids the carbon dioxide immediately reacts with the water to form hydrogen ions. Thus, paradoxically, more hydrogen ions are released into the respiratory chemosensitive sensory area when the blood carbon dioxide concentration increases than when the blood hydrogen ion concentration increases. For this reason, respiratory center activity is affected considerably more by changes in blood carbon dioxide than by changes in blood hydrogen ions, a fact that we will subsequently discuss quantitatively.

Stimulation of the Chemosensitive Area by Carbon Dioxide in the Cerebrospinal Fluid

On first thought, one would suspect that most stimulation of respiratory center activity would result from changes in carbon dioxide and hydrogen ion concentrations in the interstitial fluid of the respiratory center itself. However, most respiratory physiologists now believe that an increase in carbon dioxide concentration in the cerebrospinal fluid has more effect on stimulating the chemosensitive area than does a change in carbon dioxide in the interstitial fluid. This concept is still controversial but if it is true, the reason is probably a difference in the degree of acid-base buffering of the two fluids. The cerebrospinal fluid has very little protein buffer, while the interstitial fluid is lined on all sides by cells containing high concentrations of acid-base buffers. Therefore, a given change in carbon dioxide concentration in the cerebrospinal fluid will cause far more change in hydrogen ion concentration than in the interstitial fluid. And, since the chemosensitive neurons are located immediately beneath the surface of the medulla, diffusion of hydrogen ions into these neurons from the cerebrospinal fluid seems to be the major factor in the control of respiration.

One of the advantages of this cerebrospinal fluid system for control of respiration is the rapidity with which it can function. The cerebrospinal fluid is in intimate contact with the very rich blood supply of the arachnoid plexus. Therefore, within seconds after the blood P_{CO_2} changes, so also do the P_{CO_2} and hydrogen ion concentration of the cerebrospinal fluid change. On the other hand, a minute or more is required for full change of the P_{CO_2} in the brain interstitial fluid.

Quantitative Effects of Blood P_{CO_2} and Hydrogen Ion Concentration on Alveolar Ventilation

Figure 23–11 illustrates quantitatively the approximate effects of blood P_{CO_2} and blood pH

(which is an inverse measure of hydrogen ion concentration) on alveolar ventilation. Note the marked increase in ventilation caused by *acute* increase in P_{CO_2}. But note also the much smaller effect of increased hydrogen ion concentration (that is, decreased pH).

Finally, note that this *difference* in stimulation of ventilation is especially great in the normal P_{CO_2} and pH ranges: P_{CO_2}s between 40 and 45 mm. Hg and pHs between 7.45 and 7.35. Therefore, from a practical point, changes in blood carbon dioxide play by far the greatest role in the normal minute-by-minute control of pulmonary ventilation.

Value of Carbon Dioxide as a Regulator of Alveolar Ventilation. Since carbon dioxide is one of the end-products of metabolism, its concentration in the body fluids greatly affects the chemical reactions of the cells and also affects the tissue pH. For these reasons, the tissue fluid P_{CO_2} must be regulated exactly. In the preceding chapter, it was pointed out that blood and interstitial fluid P_{CO_2} are determined to a great extent by the rate of alveolar ventilation. Therefore, stimulation of the respiratory center by carbon dioxide provides an important feedback mechanism for regulation of the concentration of carbon dioxide throughout the body. That is, (1) an increase in P_{CO_2} stimulates the respiratory center; (2) this increases alveolar ventilation and reduces the alveolar carbon dioxide; (3) as a result, the tissue P_{CO_2} returns

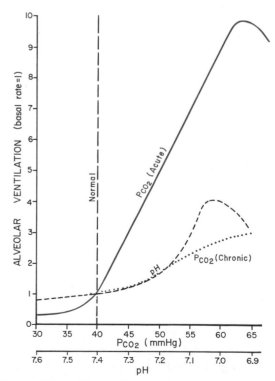

Figure 23–11. Effects of increased arterial P_{CO_2} (both acute and chronic) and decreased arterial pH on the rate of alveolar ventilation.

most of the way back toward normal. In this way, the respiratory center maintains the P_{CO_2} of the tissue fluids at a relatively constant level and, therefore, might well be called a "carbon dioxide pressostat."

THE PERIPHERAL CHEMORECEPTOR SYSTEM FOR CONTROL OF RESPIRATORY ACTIVITY— ROLE OF OXYGEN IN RESPIRATORY CONTROL

Aside from the direct sensitivity of the respiratory center itself to CO_2 and hydrogen ions, special chemical receptors called *chemoreceptors,* located outside the central nervous system, are also responsive to changes in oxygen, carbon dioxide, and hydrogen ion concentrations. These transmit signals to the respiratory center to help regulate respiratory activity. These chemoreceptors are located in the *carotid* and *aortic bodies,* which are illustrated in Figure 23–12 along with their afferent nerve connections to the respiratory center. The *carotid bodies* are located bilaterally in the bifurcations of the common carotid arteries, and their afferent nerve fibers pass through Hering's nerves to the glossopharyngeal nerves and thence to the medulla. The *aortic bodies* are located along the arch of the aorta; their afferent nerve fibers pass to the medulla through the vagi. Each of these chemoreceptor bodies receives a special blood supply through a minute artery directly from the adjacent arterial trunk.

Stimulation of the Chemoreceptors by Decreased Arterial Oxygen. Changes in arterial oxygen concentration have *no* direct stimulatory effect on the

Figure 23–13. Effect of arterial P_{O_2} on impulse rate from the carotid body of a cat. (Curve drawn from data from several sources, but primarily from Von Euler.)

respiratory center itself, but when the oxygen concentration in the arterial blood falls below normal, the chemoreceptors become strongly stimulated. This effect is illustrated in Figure 23–13, which shows the relationship between *arterial* P_{O_2} and rate of nerve impulse transmission from a carotid body. Note that the impulse rate is particularly sensitive to changes in arterial P_{O_2} in the range between 60 and 30 mm. Hg, which is the range in which the arterial hemoglobin saturation with oxygen decreases rapidly.

Quantitative Effect of Low Blood P_{O_2} on Alveolar Ventilation

Low blood P_{O_2} normally will not increase alveolar ventilation significantly until the alveolar P_{O_2} falls almost to one-half normal. This is illustrated in Figure 23–14. The lowermost curve of this figure shows that changing the alveolar arterial P_{O_2} from slightly more than 100 mm. Hg down to about 60 mm. Hg has an imperceptible effect on ventilation. But, then, as the P_{O_2} falls still further, down to 40 and then to 30 mm. Hg, alveolar ventilation increases 1.5- to 1.7-fold. However, contrast this rather feeble increase in alveolar

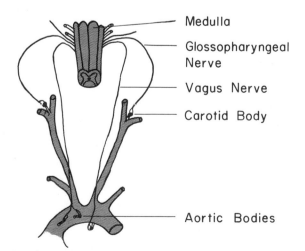

Figure 23–12. Respiratory control by the carotid and aortic bodies.

Figure 23–14. Effect of arterial P_{O_2} on alveolar ventilation and on the subsequent decrease in arterial P_{CO_2}. (From Gray: Pulmonary Ventilation and Its Physiological Regulation. Charles C Thomas.)

ventilation to the four-fold increase caused by decreasing blood pH to 7.0 or the ten-fold increase caused by increasing the P_{CO_2} only 50 per cent. Thus, it is clear that the normal effect of changes in blood P_{O_2} on respiratory activity is very slight, especially when compared with the effect of P_{CO_2}.

Cause of the Poor Acute Effect of Low P_{O_2} on Respiration — The "Braking" Effect of the P_{CO_2} and pH Regulatory Mechanisms. The cause of the poor effect of P_{O_2} changes on respiratory control is a "braking" effect caused by *both* the carbon dioxide and the hydrogen ion control mechanisms. This phenomenon can be explained by referring again to Figure 23–14, which shows the slight increase in ventilation as the alveolar P_{O_2} is decreased. The increase in ventilation that does occur blows off carbon dioxide from the blood and therefore decreases the P_{CO_2}, which is also illustrated in the figure; at the same time it also decreases the hydrogen ion concentration. Therefore, two powerful respiratory inhibitory effects are caused by (a) diminished carbon dioxide and (b) diminished hydrogen ions. These two exert an inhibitory "braking" effect that opposes the excitatory effect of the diminished oxygen. As a result, they keep the decreased oxygen from causing a marked increase in ventilation until the P_{O_2} falls to 20 to 40 mm. Hg, a range that is incompatible with life for more than a few minutes. Therefore, the maximum effect of decreased alveolar oxygen on alveolar ventilation, in the range compatible with life, is normally only a 66 per cent increase.

Thus, one can see that for the control of the usual normal respiration the P_{CO_2} and pH feedback control mechanisms are extremely powerful in relation to the P_{O_2} feedback control of respiration. Indeed, under normal conditions the P_{O_2} mechanism is of almost no significance in the control of respiration.

Yet, under some abnormal conditions the P_{CO_2} and hydrogen ion concentrations *increase at the same time that the arterial P_{O_2} decreases*. Under these conditions, all three of the feedback mechanisms support each other, and the P_{O_2} mechanism then exerts its full share of respiratory stimulation, sometimes becoming even more potent as a controller of respiration than are the P_{CO_2} and hydrogen ion mechanisms.

Effects of the Oxygen Lack Mechanism at High Altitudes. When a person first ascends to high altitudes or in any other way is exposed to a rarefied atmosphere, the diminished oxygen in the air stimulates the oxygen lack control system of respiration. The respiration at first increases to a maximum of about two-thirds above normal, which is a comparatively slight increase. Once again, the cause of this slight increase is the tremendous "braking" effect of the carbon diox-

ide and hydrogen ion control mechanisms on the oxygen lack mechanism.

However, over about a week, the respiratory center gradually becomes "adapted" to the diminished carbon dioxide, so that this now depresses the respiratory center very little. Thus, the "braking" effect on the oxygen control is gradually lost, and alveolar ventilation then rises to as high as 5 to 7 times normal. This is part of the acclimatization that occurs as a person slowly ascends a mountain, thus allowing the person to adjust respiration gradually to a level fitted for the higher altitude.

Why Oxygen Regulation of Respiration Is Not Normally Needed. On first thought, it seems strange that oxygen should play so small a role in the normal regulation of respiration, particularly since one of the primary functions of the respiratory center is to provide adequate intake of oxygen. However, oxygen control of respiration is not needed under most normal circumstances for the following reason:

The respiratory system ordinarily maintains an alveolar P_{O_2} actually *higher* than the level needed to saturate almost completely the hemoglobin of the arterial blood. It does not matter whether alveolar ventilation is normal or 10 times normal, the blood will still be essentially fully saturated. Also, alveolar ventilation can decrease to as low as one-half normal, and the blood still remains within 10 per cent of complete saturation. Therefore, one can see that alveolar ventilation can change tremendously without significantly affecting oxygen transport to the tissues.

On the other hand, changes in alveolar ventilation do have a tremendous effect on tissue carbon dioxide concentration, as was explained earlier in the chapter and illustrated in Figure 23–14. Therefore, it is exceedingly important that carbon dioxide — not oxygen — be the major controller of respiration under normal conditions.

REGULATION OF RESPIRATION DURING EXERCISE

In strenuous exercise, oxygen utilization and carbon dioxide formation can increase as much as 20-fold (Fig. 23–15). Yet, except in very heavy exercise, alveolar ventilation ordinarily increases almost the same amount so that the blood P_{O_2}, P_{CO_2}, and pH all remain *almost exactly normal*.

In trying to analyze the factors that cause increased ventilation during exercise, one is tempted immediately to ascribe this to the chemical alterations in the body fluids during exercise, including increase of carbon dioxide, increase of hydrogen ions, and decrease of oxygen. However, this is not valid, for measurements of arterial P_{CO_2}, pH, and P_{O_2} show that none of these usually

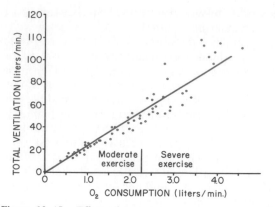

Figure 23–15. Effect of exercise on oxygen consumption and ventilatory rate. (From Gray: Pulmonary Ventilation and Its Physiological Regulation. Charles C Thomas.)

changes significantly and certainly not enough to account for the increase in ventilation. Indeed, even if a very high P_{CO_2} should develop during exercise, this still would be sufficient to account for only two thirds of the increased ventilation of heavy muscular exercise, for, as shown in Figure 23–16, the minute respiratory volume in exercise is about 50 per cent greater than that which can be effected by maximal carbon dioxide stimulation.

Therefore, the question must be asked: What is it during exercise that causes the intense respiration? This question has not been answered, but at least two different effects seem to be predominantly concerned:

1. The cerebral cortex, on transmitting impulses to the contracting muscles, is believed to transmit collateral impulses into the reticular substance of the brain stem to excite the respiratory center. This is analogous to the stimulatory effect that causes the arterial pressure to rise during exercise when similar collateral impulses pass to the vasomotor center.

2. During exercise, the body movements, especially of the limbs, are believed to increase pulmonary ventilation by exciting joint proprioceptors that then transmit excitatory impulses to the respiratory center. The reason for believing this is that even passive movements of the limbs often increase pulmonary ventilation several-fold.

It is possible that still other factors are also important in regulating respiration during exercise. For instance, some experiments even suggest that hypoxia developing in the muscles during exercise elicits afferent nerve signals to the respiratory center to excite respiration. However, since the increase in ventilation begins immediately upon the initiation of exercise, most of the increase in respiration probably results from the two neurogenic factors noted above, namely *stimulatory impulses from the higher centers of the brain* and *proprioceptive stimulatory reflexes*.

Interrelationship Between Chemical Factors and Nervous Factors in the Control of Respiration During Exercise. Figure 23–17 illustrates the different factors that operate in the control of respiration during exercise, showing two neurogenic factors: (1) direct stimulation of the respiratory center by the cerebral cortex and (2) indirect stimulation by proprioceptors. It shows also the

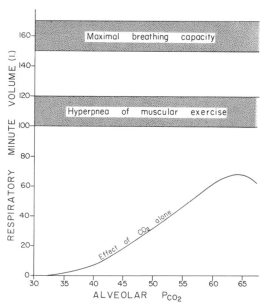

Figure 23–16. Relationship of hyperpnea caused by muscular exercise to that caused by increased alveolar P_{CO_2}. (Modified from Comroe: The Lung: Clinical Physiology and Pulmonary Function Tests. Chicago, Year Book Medical Publishers.)

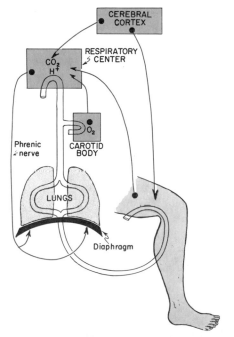

Figure 23–17. The different factors that enter into regulation of respiration during exercise.

three humoral factors of carbon dioxide, hydrogen ions, and oxygen.

When a person exercises, usually the nervous factors stimulate the respiratory center almost exactly the proper amount to supply the extra oxygen requirements for the exercise and to blow off the extra carbon dioxide. But, occasionally, the nervous signals are either too strong or too weak in their stimulation of the respiratory center. Then, the chemical factors play a very significant role in bringing about the final adjustment in respiration required to keep the carbon dioxide and hydrogen ion concentrations of the body fluids as nearly normal as possible. This effect is illustrated in Figure 23–18, which shows changes in alveolar ventilation and in arterial P_{CO_2} during a one-minute period of exercise and then for another minute after the exercise is over. Note that the alveolar ventilation increases without an initial increase in arterial P_{CO_2}; this increase is caused by a stimulus that originates in the brain at the same time that the brain excites the muscles. Often, the increase in alveolar ventilation is so great that it actually *decreases* arterial P_{CO_2} below normal, as shown in the figure, even though the exercising muscles are beginning to form large amounts of carbon dioxide. The reason for this is that the ventilation forges ahead of the increase in carbon dioxide formation. Thus, the brain provides an "anticipatory" stimulation of respiration at the onset of exercise, causing excessive alveolar ventilation even before this is needed.

Note also in the figure that after a short delay the decrease in arterial P_{CO_2} finally acts on the respiratory center to reduce the alveolar ventilation back toward normal for a fraction of a minute; soon thereafter, the large amount of carbon dioxide formed by the muscles gradually increases the P_{CO_2} up toward the normal level, and the alveolar ventilation increases once again.

The anticipatory signal from the brain thus initiates the increase in alveolar ventilation during exercise; then the chemical feedback factors (mainly arterial P_{CO_2}) make additional adjustments, either upward or downward, to balance the rate of alveolar ventilation with the rate of metabolism in the body. Because of the direct brain stimulus, the final level of P_{CO_2}, hydrogen ion concentration, and P_{O_2} in the arterial blood is almost exactly normal during exercise — sometimes slightly above normal and sometimes slightly below normal.

Finally, note in Figure 23–18 that exactly the opposite effects occur when exercise is over. The shutting-off of the brain stimulus returns the alveolar ventilation toward normal instantaneously, but this gets ahead of the decrease in carbon dioxide formation by the muscles so that a sequence of chemical-directed feedback readjustments is necessary before the alveolar ventilation finally becomes stabilized.

Now for a final comment regarding the brain factor for stimulation of respiration during exercise: Many experiments indicate that this brain factor is partly if not entirely a learned response. That is, with repeated periods of exercise of the same degree of strenuousness, the brain seems to become progressively more able to establish the proper amount of brain signal to maintain the chemical factors at their normal levels during exercise. Therefore, there is much reason to believe that some of the higher centers of learning in the brain are important in this brain factor — probably even the cerebral cortex.

Figure 23–18. Changes in alveolar ventilation and arterial P_{CO_2} during a 1-minute period of exercise and also following termination of the exercise. (Extrapolated to the human being from data in dogs; from Bainton: *J. Appl. Physiol., 33*:778, 1972.)

REFERENCES

Bainton, C. R.: Effect of speed versus grade and shivering on ventilation in dogs during active exercise. *J. Appl. Physiol., 33*:778, 1972.

Biscoe, T. J.: Carotid body: Structure and function. *Physiol. Rev., 51*: 527, 1971.

Brown, A. M.: Cardiac reflexes. *In* Berne, R. M., *et al.* (eds.): Handbook of Physiology. Sec. 2, Vol. I. Baltimore, Williams & Wilkins, 1979, p. 677.

Coleridge, J. C. G., and Coleridge, H. M.: Chemoreflex regulation of the heart. *In* Berne, R. M., *et al.* (eds.): Handbook of Physiology. Sec. 2, Vol. I, Baltimore, Williams & Wilkins, 1979, p. 653.

Cunningham, D. J. C.: Integrative aspects of the regulation of breathing: A personal view. *In* MTP International Review of Science: Physiology. Vol. 2. Baltimore, University Park Press, 1974, p. 303.

Cushing, H.: Concerning a definite regulatory mechanism of the vasomotor center which controls blood pressure during cerebral compression. *Bull. Johns Hopkins Hosp., 12*:290, 1901.

Downing, S. E.: Baroreceptor regulation of the heart. *In* Berne, R. M., *et al.* (eds.): Handbook of Physiology. Sec. 2, Vol. I. Baltimore, Williams & Wilkins, 1979, p. 621.

Guyton, A. C.: Arterial Pressure and Hypertension. Philadelphia, W. B. Saunders Co., 1980.

Guz, A.: Regulation of respiration in man. *Annu. Rev. Physiol., 37*:303, 1975.

Kirchheim, H. R.: Systemic arterial baroreceptor reflexes. *Physiol. Rev., 56*:100, 1976.

Loeschcke, H. H.: Respiratory chemosensitivity in the medulla oblongata. *Acta Neurobiol. Exp., 33*:97, 1973.

Mancia, G., *et al.:* Reflex control of circulation by heart and lungs. *Int. Rev. Physiol., 9*:111, 1976.

Mitchell, R. A., and Berger, A. J.: Neural regulation of respiration. *Am. Rev. Resp. Dis., 111*:206, 1975.

Rosell, S.: Nervous control of microcirculation. *In* Kaley, G., and Altura, B. M. (eds.): Microcirculation. Vol. II. Baltimore, University Park Press, 1977.

Sagawa, K., *et al.:* Nervous control of the circulation. *In* MTP International Review of Science: Physiology. Baltimore, University Park Press, 1974. Vol. 1, p. 197.

Smith, O. A.: Reflex and central mechanisms involved in the control of the heart and circulation. *Annu. Rev. Physiol., 36*:93, 1974.

Von Euler, C., and Lagercrantz, H. (eds.): Central Nervous Control Mechanisms in Breathing. New York, Pergamon Press, 1980.

24

Regulation of the Gastrointestinal Tract, Food Intake, and Body Temperature

THE INTRINSIC NERVES OF THE GASTROINTESTINAL TRACT

The gastrointestinal tract has an *intrinsic nervous system* of its own that begins in the esophagus and extends all the way to the anus. This system controls most gastrointestinal functions, especially gastrointestinal movements and secretion. On the other hand, both parasympathetic and sympathetic nervous signals to the gastrointestinal tract from the brain can strongly alter the degree of activity of this intrinsic nervous system, parasympathetic activity in general increasing its activity and sympathetic stimulation decreasing the activity.

The intrinsic nervous system is composed principally of two layers of neurons and appropriate connecting fibers: the outer layer, called the *myenteric plexus* or *Auerbach's plexus*, lies between the longitudinal and circular muscular layers; the inner layer, called the *submucosal plexus* or *Meissner's plexus*, lies in the submucosa. The myenteric plexus controls mainly the *gastrointestinal movements*, while the submucosal plexus is important in controlling *secretion* and also subserves many *sensory functions*, receiving signals principally from the gut epithelium and from stretch receptors in the gut wall.

In general, stimulation of the myenteric plexus increases the activity of the gut, causing four principal effects: (1) increased tonic contraction, or "tone," of the gut wall, (2) increased intensity of the rhythmic contractions, (3) increased rate of rhythmic contraction, and (4) increased velocity of conduction of excitatory waves along the gut wall. On the other hand, some myenteric plexus fibers are inhibitory rather than excitatory; these fibers are believed to be *purinergic* — that is, they secrete ATP or some similar purine-based transmitter substance. The excitatory fibers are mainly *cholinergic* — that is, they secrete acetylcholine, though some probably secrete one or more other excitatory transmitters as well.

The intrinsic nervous system, including both the submucosal sensory plexus and the myenteric motor plexus, is especially responsible for many neurogenic reflexes that occur locally in the gut, such as reflexes from the mucosal epithelium to increase the activity of the gut muscle or to cause localized secretion of digestive juices by the submucosal glands.

Autonomic Control of the Gastrointestinal Tract. The gastrointestinal tract receives extensive parasympathetic and sympathetic innervation that is capable of altering the overall activity of the entire gut or of specific parts of it, particularly of its upper end down to the stomach and its distal end from the mid-colon region to the anus.

Parasympathetic Innervation. The parasympathetic supply to the gut is divided into *cranial* and *sacral divisions*, which were discussed in Chapter 17. Except for a few parasympathetic fibers to the mouth and pharyngeal regions of the alimentary tract, the cranial parasympathetics are transmitted almost entirely in the *vagus nerves*. These fibers provide extensive innervation to the esophagus, stomach, pancreas, and first half of the large intestine (but rather little innervation to the small intestine). The sacral parasympathetics originate in the second, third, and fourth sacral segments of the spinal cord and pass through the *nervi erigentes* to the distal half of the large intestine. The sigmoidal, rectal, and anal regions of the large intestine are considerably better supplied with parasympathetic fibers than are the other portions. These fibers function especially in the defecation reflexes, which are discussed later in the chapter.

The postganglionic neurons of the parasympathetic system are probably part of the myenteric plexus, so that stimulation of the parasympathetic nerves causes a general increase in activity of this plexus. This in turn excites the gut wall and facilitates most of the intrinsic excitatory nervous reflexes of the gastrointestinal tract.

Sympathetic Innervation. The sympathetic fibers to the gastrointestinal tract originate in the spinal cord between the segments T-8 and L-3. The preganglionic fibers, after leaving the cord, enter the sympathetic chains and pass through the chains to outlying ganglia, such as the *celiac ganglion* and various *mesenteric ganglia*. Here, the postganglionic neuron bodies are located, and postganglionic fibers spread from them along with the blood vessels to all parts of the gut. The sympathetics innervate essentially all portions of the gastrointestinal tract rather than being more extensively supplied to the most orad and most analward portions as is true of the parasympathetics. The sympathetic nerve endings secrete *norepinephrine*.

In general, stimulation of the sympathetic nervous system inhibits activity in the gastrointestinal tract, causing effects essentially opposite to those of the parasympathetic system. It exerts its effects in two different ways: (1) by direct effect of the norepinephrine on the smooth muscle to inhibit this, and (2) by an inhibitory effect of the norepinephrine on the neurons of the intrinsic nervous system. Thus, strong stimulation of the sympathetic system can totally block movement of food through the gastrointestinal tract.

Afferent Nerve Fibers from the Gut. Many afferent nerve fibers arise in the gut. Some of these have their cell bodies in the submucosal plexus and terminate mainly in the myenteric plexus. These nerves can be stimulated by (a) irritation of the gut mucosa, (b) excessive distension of the gut, or (c) the presence of specific chemical substances in the gut. Signals transmitted through these fibers can cause excitation or, under some conditions, inhibition of intestinal movements or intestinal secretion.

In addition to the afferent fibers that terminate in the intramural plexus, other afferent fibers whose cell bodies lie in the dorsal root ganglia of the spinal cord or in the cranial nerve ganglia transmit signals all the way to the central nervous system, traveling along the sympathetic or parasympathetic nerves. For example, pain nerve fibers, except those from the esophagus, course along the sympathetic nerves to the spinal cord. Also, about 80 per cent of the nerve fibers in the vagus nerves are afferent rather than efferent. These fibers transmit signals into the medulla to help initiate vagal signals that in turn control several important functions of the gastrointestinal tract, as described in this chapter.

Function of the Myenteric Plexus in Peristalsis. Even though peristalsis is a basic characteristic of all tubular smooth muscle structures, it occurs only weakly in portions of the gastrointestinal tract that have congenital absence of the myenteric plexus. Also, it is greatly depressed or completely blocked in the entire gut when the person is treated with atropine to paralyze the cholinergic nerve endings of the myenteric plexus. Furthermore, since the myenteric plexus is strongly affected in most parts of the gastrointestinal tract, except in the small intestine, by the parasympathetic nerves, the intensity of peristalsis in these areas and its velocity of conduction can be altered by parasympathetic stimulation.

Therefore, *even though the basic phenomenon of peristalsis is not dependent on the myenteric nerve plexus, effectual* peristalsis does require an active myenteric plexus.

Analward Peristaltic Movements. Peristalsis, theoretically, can occur in either direction from a stimulated point, but it normally dies out rapidly in the orad direction while continuing for a considerable distance analward. The cause of this directional transmission of peristalsis has never been ascertained, though several suggestions have been offered, as follows:

Receptive Relaxation and the "Law of the Gut." Some physiologists believe the directional movement of peristalsis to be caused by a special organization of the myenteric plexus, which allows preferential transmission of analward signals. One reason for believing this is the effect of electrical stimulation on the gut: An electrical stimulus causes a contractile ring to appear near the point of the stimulus but at the same time sometimes causes relaxation, called "receptive relaxation," several centimeters down the gut toward the anus. It is believed that this relaxation could occur only as a result of conduction in the myenteric plexus. Obviously, a leading wave of receptive relaxation could allow food to be propelled more easily analward than in the orad direction.

This response to electrical stimulation is also called the "law of the gut" or sometimes simply the "myenteric reflex." It can be particularly well demonstrated in the esophagus and in the pyloric region of the stomach.

INGESTION OF FOOD

The amount of food that a person ingests is determined principally by the intrinsic desire for food called *hunger*. The type of food that a person preferentially seeks is determined by *appetite*. These mechanisms in themselves are extremely important automatic regulatory systems for maintaining an adequate nutritional supply for the body, and they will be discussed later in the chapter. The present discussion is confined to the actual mechanical aspects of food ingestion, including especially *mastication* and *swallowing*.

Mastication (Chewing)

The teeth are admirably designed for chewing, the anterior teeth (incisors) providing a strong cutting action and the posterior teeth (molars) a grinding action. All the jaw muscles working together can close the teeth with a force as great as 55 pounds on the incisors and 200 pounds on the molars. When this is applied to a small object, such as a small seed between the molars, the actual force *per square inch* may be several thousand pounds.

Most of the muscles of chewing are innervated by the motor branch of the 5th cranial nerve, and the chewing process is controlled by nuclei in the hindbrain. Stimulation of the reticular formation near the hindbrain centers for taste can cause continual rhythmic chewing movements. Also, stimulation of areas in the hypothalamus, amygdaloid nuclei, and even in the cerebral cortex near the sensory areas for taste and smell can cause chewing.

Much of the chewing process is caused by the *chewing reflex,* which may be explained as follows: The presence of a bolus of food in the mouth causes reflex inhibition of the muscles of mastication, which allows the lower jaw to drop. The drop in turn initiates a stretch reflex of the jaw muscles that leads to *rebound* contraction. This automatically raises the jaw to cause closure of the teeth, but it also compresses the bolus again against the linings of the mouth, which inhibits the jaw muscles once again, allowing the jaw to drop and rebound another time, and this is repeated again and again.

Chewing of the food is important for digestion of all foods, but it is especially important for most fruits and raw vegetables, because these have undigestible cellulose membranes around their nutrient portions which must be broken before the food can be utilized. Chewing aids in the digestion of food for the following simple reason: Since the *digestive enzymes act only on the surfaces of food particles,* the rate of digestion is highly dependent on the total surface area exposed to the intestinal secretions. Also, grinding the food to a very fine particulate consistency prevents excoriation of the gastrointestinal tract and increases the ease with which food is emptied from the stomach into the small intestine and thence into all succeeding segments of the gut.

Swallowing (Deglutition)

Swallowing is a complicated mechanism, principally because the pharynx most of the time subserves several other functions besides swallowing and is converted for only a few seconds at a time into a tract for propulsion of food. Especially is it important that respiration not be seriously compromised during swallowing.

In general, swallowing can be divided into: (1) the *voluntary stage,* which initiates the swallowing process, (2) the *pharyngeal stage,* which is involuntary and constitutes the passage of food through the pharynx into the esophagus, and (3) the *esophageal stage,* another involuntary phase which promotes passage of food from the pharynx to the stomach.

Voluntary Stage of Swallowing.   When the food is ready for swallowing, it is "voluntarily" squeezed or rolled posteriorly in the mouth by pressure of the tongue upward and backward against the palate, as shown in Figure 24–1. Thus, the tongue forces the bolus of food into the pharynx. From here on, the process of swallowing becomes entirely, or almost entirely, automatic and ordinarily cannot be stopped.

Pharyngeal Stage of Swallowing.   When the bolus of food is pushed backward in the mouth, it stimulates *swallowing receptor areas* all around the opening of the pharynx, especially on the tonsillar pillars, and impulses from these pass to the brain stem to initiate a series of automatic pharyngeal muscular contractions as follows:

1.   The soft palate is pulled upward to close the posterior nares, in this way preventing reflux of food into the nasal cavities.

2.   The palatopharyngeal folds on either side of the pharynx are pulled medialward to approximate each other. In this way these folds form a sagittal slit through which the food must pass into the posterior pharynx. This slit performs a selective action, allowing food that has been masticated properly to pass with ease while impeding the passage of large objects. Since this stage of swal-

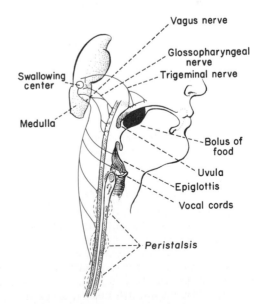

Figure 24–1.   The swallowing mechanism.

lowing lasts only 1 second, any large object is usually impeded too much to pass through the pharynx into the esophagus.

3. The vocal cords of the larynx are strongly approximated, and the epiglottis swings backward over the superior opening of the larynx. Both of these effects prevent passage of food into the trachea. Especially important is the approximation of the vocal cords, but the epiglottis helps to prevent food from ever getting as far as the vocal cords. Destruction of the vocal cords or of the muscles that approximate them can cause strangulation. On the other hand, removal of the epiglottis usually does not cause serious debility in swallowing.

4. The entire larynx is pulled upward and forward by muscles attached to the hyoid bone; this movement of the larynx stretches the opening of the esophagus. At the same time, the upper 3 to 4 centimeters of the esophagus, an area called the *upper esophageal sphincter* or the *pharyngoesophageal sphincter,* relaxes, thus allowing food to move easily and freely from the posterior pharynx into the upper esophagus. This sphincter, between swallows, remains tonically and strongly contracted, thereby preventing air from going into the esophagus during respiration. The upward movement of the larynx also lifts the glottis out of the main stream of food flow so that the food usually passes on either side of the epiglottis rather than over its surface; this adds still another protection against passage of food into the trachea.

5. At the same time that the larynx is raised and the pharyngoesophageal sphincter is relaxed, the superior constrictor muscle of the pharynx contracts, giving rise to a rapid peristaltic wave passing downward over the pharyngeal muscles and into the esophagus, which also propels the food into the esophagus.

To summarize the mechanics of the pharyngeal stage of swallowing — the trachea is closed, the esophagus is opened, and a fast peristaltic wave originating in the pharynx then forces the bolus of food into the upper esophagus, the entire process occurring in 1 to 2 seconds.

Nervous Control of the Pharyngeal Stage of Swallowing. The most sensitive tactile areas of the pharynx for initiation of the pharyngeal stage of swallowing lie in a ring around the pharyngeal opening, with greatest sensitivity in the tonsillar pillars. Impulses are transmitted from these areas through the sensory portions of the trigeminal and glossopharyngeal nerves into a region of the medulla oblongata closely associated with the *tractus solitarius* which receives essentially all sensory impulses from the mouth.

The successive stages of the swallowing process are then automatically controlled in orderly sequence by neuronal areas distributed throughout the reticular substance of the medulla and lower portion of the pons. The sequence of the swallowing reflex remains the same from one swallow to the next, and the timing of the entire cycle also remains constant from one swallow to the next. The areas in the medulla and lower pons that control swallowing are collectively called the *deglutition* or *swallowing center*.

The motor impulses from the swallowing center to the pharynx and upper esophagus that cause swallowing are transmitted by the 5th, 9th, 10th, and 12th cranial nerves and even a few of the superior cervical nerves.

In summary, the pharyngeal stage of swallowing is principally a reflex act. It is almost never initiated by direct stimuli to the swallowing center from higher regions of the central nervous system. Instead, it is almost always initiated by voluntary movement of food into the back of the mouth, which, in turn, elicits the swallowing reflex.

Effect of the Pharyngeal Stage of Swallowing on Respiration. The entire pharyngeal stage of swallowing occurs in less than 1 to 2 seconds, thereby interrupting respiration for only a fraction of a usual respiratory cycle. The swallowing center specifically inhibits the respiratory center of the medulla during this time, halting respiration at any point in its cycle to allow swallowing to proceed. Yet, even while a person is talking, swallowing interrupts respiration for such a short time that it is hardly noticeable.

Esophageal Stage of Swallowing. The esophagus functions primarily to conduct food from the pharynx to the stomach, and its movements are organized specifically for this function.

Normally the esophagus exhibits two types of peristaltic movements — *primary peristalsis* and *secondary peristalsis*. Primary peristalsis is simply a continuation of the peristaltic wave that begins in the pharynx and spreads into the esophagus during the pharyngeal stage of swallowing. This wave passes all the way from the pharynx to the stomach in approximately 5 to 10 seconds. However, food swallowed by a person who is in the upright position is usually transmitted to the lower end of the esophagus even more rapidly than the peristaltic wave itself, in about 4 to 8 seconds, because of the additional effect of gravity pulling the food downward. If the primary peristaltic wave fails to move all the food that has entered the esophagus into the stomach, secondary peristaltic waves result from distension of the esophagus by the retained food. These waves are essentially the same as the primary peristaltic waves, except that they originate in the esophagus itself rather than in the pharynx. Secondary peristaltic waves continue to be initiated until all the food has emptied into the stomach.

The peristaltic waves of the esophagus are controlled almost entirely by vagal reflexes that are part of the overall swallowing mechanism. These reflexes are transmitted through *vagal afferent fibers* from the esophagus to the medulla and then back again to the esophagus through *vagal efferent fibers*.

The musculature of the pharynx and the upper quarter of the esophagus is skeletal muscle, and, therefore, the peristaltic waves in these regions are controlled only by skeletal nerve impulses. In the lower two thirds of the esophagus, the musculature is smooth, but even this portion of the esophagus is normally under the control of the vagus nerve. However, when the vagus nerves to the esophagus are sectioned, the myenteric nerve plexus of the esophagus becomes excitable enough after several days to cause secondary peristaltic waves even without support from the vagal reflexes. Therefore, following paralysis of the swallowing reflex, food forced into the upper esophagus and then pulled by gravity to the lower esophagus still passes readily into the stomach.

Receptive Relaxation of the Stomach. As the esophageal peristaltic wave passes toward the stomach, a wave of relaxation precedes the constriction. Furthermore, the entire stomach and, to a lesser extent, even the duodenum become relaxed as this wave reaches the lower end of the esophagus. Especially important, also, is relaxation of the gastroesophageal sphincter at the juncture between the esophagus and the stomach. In other words, the constrictor and the stomach are prepared well ahead of time to receive food being propelled down the esophagus during the swallowing act.

NERVOUS CONTROL OF FOOD MOVEMENT THROUGH THE STOMACH, SMALL INTESTINE, AND COLON

Movement of food through the stomach, small intestine, and colon is caused by various forms of peristaltic propulsive movements. Most of these movements are controlled by the intrinsic nervous system of the gastrointestinal wall. That is, when a segment of bowel becomes overfilled, the stretch of the nerve endings elicits a local peristaltic reflex, as explained earlier in the chapter, causing propulsion of the food forward.

In general, parasympathetic stimulation by way of the vagi and sacral nerves increases the rate of peristalsis, and sympathetic stimulation normally inhibits it.

Intrinsic GI Reflexes That Inhibit Rate of Food Movement. At several points in the gastrointestinal tract special reflex mechanisms prevent too rapid movement of food along the gastrointestinal tract. For instance, when the stomach empties too

much food into the upper portions of the small intestine, stretch of the intestinal walls transmits signals backwards along the myenteric plexus to the stomach to inhibit its peristaltic movements. This obviously allows the small intestine to receive food at a rate slow enough for it to process the food appropriately. Another reflex occurs from the colon to the lower end of the small intestine; when the colon becomes overfilled, myenteric reflex signals inhibit peristalsis in the small intestine and thereby prevent movement of the intestinal contents into the colon at a rate more rapid than these can be processed.

DEFECATION

Most of the time, the rectum is empty of feces. This results partly from the fact that a weak functional sphincter exists approximately 20 cm. from the anus at the juncture between the sigmoid and the rectum. However, when a mass movement forces feces into the rectum the desire for defecation is normally initiated, including reflex contraction of the rectum and relaxation of the anal sphincters.

Continual dribble of fecal matter through the anus is prevented by tonic constriction of (1) the *internal anal sphincter,* a circular mass of smooth muscle that lies immediately inside the anus, and (2) the *external anal sphincter,* composed of striated voluntary muscle that both surrounds the internal sphincter and also extends distal to it; the external sphincter is controlled by the somatic nervous system and therefore is under voluntary control.

The Defecation Reflexes. Ordinarily, defecation results from the *defecation reflexes* which can be described as follows: When the feces enter the rectum, distension of the rectal wall initiates afferent signals that spread through the *myenteric plexus* to initiate peristaltic waves in the descending colon, sigmoid, and rectum, forcing feces toward the anus. As the peristaltic wave approaches the anus, the internal anal sphincter is inhibited by the usual phenomenon of *receptive relaxation,* and if the external anal sphincter is relaxed, defecation will occur. This overall effect is the *intrinsic defecation reflex* of the colon itself.

However, the intrinsic defecation reflex itself is usually weak, and to be effective in causing defecation it must be fortified by another type of defecation reflex, a *parasympathetic defecation reflex* that involves the sacral segments of the spinal cord, as illustrated in Figure 24–2. When the afferent fibers in the rectum are stimulated, signals are transmitted into the spinal cord and thence, reflexly, back to the descending colon, sigmoid, rectum, and anus by way of parasym-

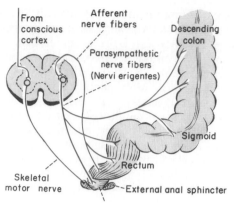

Figure 24–2. The afferent and efferent pathways of the

pathetic nerve fibers in the *nervi erigentes*. These parasympathetic signals greatly intensify the peristaltic waves and convert the intrinsic defecation reflex from an ineffectual weak movement into a powerful process of defecation that is sometimes effective in emptying the large bowel in one movement all the way from the splenic flexure to the anus. Also, the afferent signals entering the spinal cord initiate other effects, such as taking a deep breath, closure of the glottis, and contraction of the abdominal muscles to force downward on the fecal contents of the colon while at the same time causing the pelvic floor to pull outward and upward on the anus to evaginate the feces downward.

However, despite the defecation reflexes other effects are also necessary before actual defecation occurs because relaxation of the internal sphincter and forward movement of feces toward the anus normally initiates an instantaneous contraction of the external sphincter, which still temporarily prevents defecation. Except in babies and mentally inept persons, the conscious mind then takes over voluntary control of the external sphincter and either inhibits it to allow defecation to occur or further contracts it if the moment is not socially acceptable for defecation. When the contraction is maintained, the defecation reflexes die out after a few minutes and usually will not return until an additional amount of feces enters the rectum, which may not occur until several hours thereafter.

When it becomes convenient for the person to defecate, the defecation reflexes can sometimes be excited by taking a deep breath to move the diaphragm downward and then contracting the abdominal muscles to increase the pressure in the abdomen, thus forcing fecal contents into the rectum to elicit new reflexes. Unfortunately, reflexes initiated in this way are never as effective as those that arise naturally, for which reason people who too often inhibit their natural reflexes become severely constipated.

In the newborn baby and in some persons with transected spinal cords, the defecation reflexes cause automatic emptying of the lower bowel without the normal control exercised through contraction of the external anal sphincter.

AUTONOMIC CONTROL OF GASTROINTESTINAL SECRETION

The nervous system of the gastrointestinal tract not only controls peristaltic movement of food but also controls secretion by many of the gastrointestinal glands, especially salivary secretion in the mouth, gastric juice secretion in the stomach, and mucus secretion in the distal colon and in the sigmoid.

Nervous Regulation of Salivary Secretion

Figure 24–3 illustrates the nervous pathways for regulation of salivation, showing that the salivary glands are controlled by *parasympathetic nervous signals* from the *salivatory nuclei*. The salivatory nuclei are located approximately at the junction of the medulla and pons and are excited by both taste and tactile stimuli from the tongue and other areas of the mouth. Many taste stimuli, especially the sour taste, elicit copious secretion of saliva — often as much as 5 to 10 ml. per minute or 8 to 20 times the basal rate of secretion. Also, certain tactile stimuli, such as the presence of smooth objects in the mouth (a pebble, for instance), cause marked salivation, while rough objects cause less salivation and occasionally even inhibit salivation.

Salivation can also be stimulated or inhibited by

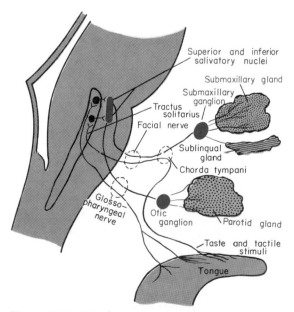

Figure 24–3. Nervous regulation of salivary secretion.

impulses arriving in the salivatory nuclei from higher centers of the central nervous system. For instance, when a person smells or eats favorite foods, salivation is far greater than when disliked food is smelled or eaten. The *appetite area* of the brain that partially regulates these effects is located in close proximity to the parasympathetic centers of the anterior hypothalamus, and it functions to a great extent in response to signals from the taste and smell areas of the cerebral cortex or amygdala.

Finally, salivation also occurs in response to reflexes originating in the stomach and upper intestines — particularly when very irritating foods are swallowed or when a person is nauseated because of some gastrointestinal abnormality. The swallowed saliva presumably helps to remove the irritating factor in the gastrointestinal tract by diluting or neutralizing the irritant substances.

Regulation of Gastric Secretion by Nervous and Hormonal Mechanisms

Gastric secretion is regulated by both nervous and hormonal mechanisms, nervous regulation being effected through the parasympathetic fibers of the vagus nerves as well as through local intrinsic nerve plexus reflexes, and hormonal regulation taking place by means of the hormone *gastrin*. Thus, regulation of gastric secretion is different from the regulation of salivary secretion, which is effected entirely by nervous mechanisms.

Vagal Stimulation of Gastric Secretion

Nervous signals to cause gastric secretion originate in the dorsal motor nuclei of the vagi and pass via the vagus nerves to the intrinsic nerve plexus of the stomach and thence to the oxyntic glands. In response, these glands secrete vast quantities of both pepsin and acid, but with a higher proportion of pepsin than in gastric juice elicited in other ways. Also, vagal signals to all the mucus-secreting glands and epithelial lining cells cause increased mucus secretion as well.

Still another effect of vagal stimulation is to cause the antral part of the stomach mucosa to secrete the hormone *gastrin*. As will be explained in the following paragraphs, this hormone then acts on the gastric glands to cause additional flow of highly acidic gastric juice. Thus, vagal stimulation excites stomach secretion both directly by stimulation of the gastric glands and indirectly through the gastrin mechanism.

Stimulation of Gastric Secretion by Gastrin

When food enters the stomach, it causes the antral portion of the stomach mucosa to secrete the hormone gastrin. This hormone is secreted by *gastrin cells*, also called *G cells*, in the pyloric glands and to a lesser extent in the proximal glands of the duodenum. Gastrin is a large peptide secreted in two forms, a large form called *G-34*, containing 34 amino acids, and a smaller form, *G-17*, containing 17 amino acids. Though both of these are important, the smaller form is more abundant.

The food causes release of this hormone in two ways: (1) The actual bulk of the food distends the stomach, and this causes the hormone gastrin to be released from the antral mucosa. (2) Certain substances called secretagogues — such as food extractives, partially digested proteins, alcohol (in low concentration), caffeine, and so forth — also cause gastrin to be liberated from the antral mucosa.

Both of these stimuli — the distension and the chemical action of the secretagogues — elicit gastrin release by means of a local nerve reflex. That is, they stimulate sensory nerve fibers in the stomach epithelium which in turn synapse with the intrinsic nerve plexus. This then transmits efferent signals to the gastrin cells, causing them to secrete the gastrin. Therefore, any factor that blocks this reflex will also block the formation of gastrin. For instance, anesthetization of the gastric mucosa to block the sensory stimuli will prevent gastrin release; administration of atropine, which blocks the action on the gastrin cells of the acetylcholine released by the intrinsic nerves and also by the vagus nerves, will also prevent gastrin release.

Gastrin is absorbed into the blood and carried to the gastric glands where it stimulates mainly the oxyntic cells and to much less extent the peptic cells, also. The oxyntic cells increase their rate of hydrochloric acid secretion as much as eight-fold, and the chief cells increase their rate of pepsin secretion two- to four-fold.

The rate of secretion in response to gastrin is somewhat less than to vagal stimulation, 200 ml. per hour in contrast to about 500 ml. per hour, indicating that the gastrin mechanism is a less potent mechanism for stimulation of stomach secretion than is vagal stimulation. However, the gastrin mechanism usually continues for several hours in contrast to a much shorter period of time for vagal stimulation. Therefore, as a whole, it is likely that the gastrin mechanism is equally as important as, if not more important than, the vagal mechanism for control of gastric secretion. Yet, when both of these work together, the total secretion is much greater than the sum of the individual secretions caused by each of the two mechanisms. In other words, *the two mechanisms multiply each other rather than simply add to each other*.

Feedback Inhibition of Gastric Acid Secretion. When the acidity of the gastric juices increases to a pH of 2.0, the gastrin mechanism for stimulating gastric secretion becomes totally blocked. This effect probably results from two different factors. First, greatly enhanced acidity depresses or blocks the extraction of gastrin itself from the antral mucosa. Second, the acid seems to extract an inhibitory hormone from the gastric mucosa or to cause an inhibitory reflex that inhibits gastric acid secretion.

Obviously, this feedback inhibition of the gastric glands plays an important role in protecting the stomach against excessively acid secretions, which would readily cause peptic ulceration. However, in addition to this protective effect, the feedback mechanism is also important in maintaining optimal pH for function of the peptic enzymes in the digestive process because whenever the pH rises gastrin begins to be secreted again.

REGULATION OF FOOD INTAKE

Hunger.   The term hunger means a craving for food, and it is associated with a number of objective sensations. For instance, in a person who has not had food for many hours, the stomach undergoes intense rhythmic contractions called *hunger contractions*. These cause a tight or gnawing feeling in the pit of the stomach and sometimes actually cause pain called *hunger pangs*. In addition to the hunger pangs, the hungry person also becomes more tense and restless than usual.

Some physiologists actually define hunger as the tonic contractions of the stomach. However, even after the stomach is completely removed, the psychic sensations of hunger still occur, and craving for food still makes the person search for an adequate food supply.

Appetite.   The term appetite is often used in the same sense as hunger except that it usually implies desire for specific types of food instead of food in general. Therefore, appetite helps a person choose the quality of food to eat.

Satiety.   Satiety is the opposite of hunger. It means a feeling of fulfillment in the quest for food. Satiety usually results from a filling meal, particularly when the person's nutritional storage depots, the adipose tissue and the glycogen stores, are already filled.

NEURAL CENTERS FOR REGULATION OF FOOD INTAKE

Hunger and Satiety Centers.   Stimulation of the *lateral hypothalamus* causes an animal to eat voraciously, while stimulation of the *ventromedial nuclei of the hypothalamus* causes complete satiety, and, even in the presence of highly appetizing food, the animal will still refuse to eat. Conversely, destructive lesions of the two respective areas cause results exactly opposite to those caused by stimulation. That is, ventromedial le-

sions cause voracious and continued eating until the animal becomes extremely obese, sometimes as large as 4 times normal in size. And lesions of the lateral hypothalamic nuclei cause complete lack of desire for food and progressive inanition of the animal. Therefore, we can label the lateral nuclei of the hypothalamus as the *hunger center* or *feeding center*, while we can label the ventromedial nuclei of the hypothalamus as a *satiety center*.

The feeding center operates by directly exciting the emotional drive to search for food (while also stimulating other emotional drives as well — see Chapters 16 and 17). On the other hand, it is believed that the satiety center operates primarily by inhibiting the feeding center.

Other Neural Centers That Enter into Feeding.   If the brain is sectioned between the hypothalamus and the mesencephalon, the animal can still perform the basic mechanical features of the feeding process. It can salivate, lick its lips, chew food, and swallow. Therefore, the actual mechanics of feeding are all controlled by centers in the brain stem. The function of the hypothalamus in feeding, then, is to control the quantity of food intake and to excite the lower centers to activity.

Higher centers than the hypothalamus also play important roles in the control of feeding, particularly in the control of appetite. These centers include especially the amygdala and the cortical areas of the limbic system, all of which are closely coupled with the hypothalamus. It will be recalled from the discussion of the sense of smell that the amygdala is one of the major parts of the olfactory nervous system. Destructive lesions in the amygdala have demonstrated that some of its areas greatly increase feeding, while others inhibit feeding. In addition, stimulation of some areas of the amygdala elicits the mechanical act of feeding. However, the most important effect of destruction of the amygdala on both sides of the brain is a "psychic blindness" in the choice of foods. In other words, the animal (and presumably the human being as well) loses or at least partially loses the mechanism of appetite control of type and quality of food that it eats.

The cortical regions of the limbic system, including the infraorbital regions, the hippocampal gyrus, and the cingulate gyrus, all have areas that when stimulated can either increase or decrease feeding activities. These areas seem especially to play a role in the animal's drive to search for food when it is hungry. It is presumed that these centers are also responsible, probably operating in association with the amygdala and hypothalamus, for determining the quality of food that is eaten. For instance, a previous unpleasant experience with almost any type of food often destroys a person's appetite for that food thenceforth.

FACTORS THAT REGULATE FOOD INTAKE

We can divide the regulation of food into (1) *nutritional regulation,* which is concerned primarily with maintenance of normal quantities of nutrient stores in the body, and (2) *alimentary regulation,* which is concerned primarily with the immediate effects of feeding on the alimentary tract and is sometimes called *peripheral regulation* or *short-term regulation.*

Nutritional Regulation. An animal that has been starved for a long time and is then presented with unlimited food eats a far greater quantity than does an animal that has been on a regular diet. Conversely, an animal that has been force-fed for several weeks eats little when allowed to eat according to its own desires. Thus, the feeding center in the hypothalamus is geared to the nutritional status of the body. Some of the nutritional factors that control the degree of activity of the feeding center are the following:

Availability of Glucose to the Body Cells – The Glucostatic Theory of Hunger and of Feeding Regulation. It has long been known that a decrease in blood glucose concentration is associated with development of hunger, which has led to the so-called glucostatic theory of hunger and of feeding regulation: When the blood glucose level falls too low, this automatically causes the animal to increase his feeding, which eventually returns the glucose concentration back toward normal. Two other observations also support the glucostatic theory: (1) An increase in blood glucose level increases the measured electrical activity in the satiety center in the ventromedial nuclei of the hypothalamus and simultaneously decreases the electrical activity in the feeding center of the lateral nuclei. (2) Chemical studies show that the ventromedial nuclei (the satiety center) concentrate glucose while other areas of the hypothalamus fail to concentrate glucose; therefore, it is assumed that glucose acts by increasing the degree of satiety.

Effect of Blood Amino Acid Concentration on Feeding. An increase in amino acid concentration in the blood also reduces feeding, and a decrease enhances feeding. In general, though, this effect is not as powerful as the glucostatic mechanism.

Effect of Fat Metabolites on Feeding — Long-Term Regulation. The overall degree of feeding varies almost inversely with the amount of adipose tissue in the body. That is, as the quantity of adipose tissue increases, the rate of feeding decreases. Therefore, many physiologists believe that *long-term regulation* of feeding is controlled mainly by fat metabolites of undiscovered nature. This is called the "lipostatic" theory of feeding regulation. In support of this is the fact that the long-term average concentration of free fatty acids in the blood is directly proportional to the quantity of adipose tissue in the body. Therefore, it is likely that the free fatty acids or some other similar fat metabolites act in the same manner as glucose and amino acids to cause a negative feedback regulatory effect on feeding. It is also possible, if not probable, that this is the most important long-term regulator of feeding.

Interrelationshp Between Body Temperature and Food Intake. When an animal is exposed to cold, it tends to overeat; when exposed to heat, it tends to undereat. This is caused by interaction within the hypothalamus between the temperature-regulating system (see p. 317) and the food intake–regulating system. It is important because increased food intake in the cold animal (a) increases its metabolic rate and (b) provides increased fat for insulation, both of which tend to correct the cold state.

Summary of Long-Term Regulation. Even though our information on the different feedback factors in long-term feeding regulation is imprecise, we can make the following general statement: When the nutrient stores of the body fall below normal, the feeding center of the hypothalamus becomes highly active, and the person exhibits increased hunger; on the other hand, when the nutrient stores are abundant, the person loses the hunger and develops a state of satiety.

Alimentary Regulation (Short-Term, Nonmetabolic Regulation). The degree of hunger or satiety at different times of the day depends to a great extent on habit. For instance, normally people have the habit of eating three meals a day, and, if they miss one, they are likely to develop a state of hunger at mealtime despite completely adequate nutritional stores in their tissues. But, in addition to habit, several other short-term physiological stimuli — mainly related to the alimentary tract — can alter one's desire for food for several hours at a time, as follows:

Gastrointestinal Filling. When the gastrointestinal tract becomes distended, especially the stomach or the duodenum, inhibitory signals temporarily suppress the feeding center, thereby reducing the desire for food. This effect probably depends mainly on sensory signals transmitted through the vagi, but part of the effect still persists after the vagi and the sympathetic nerves from the upper gastrointestinal tract have been severed. Therefore, somatic sensory signals from the stretched abdomen might also play a role. And, recently it has been found that hormonal feedback also suppresses feeding, for *cholecystokinin* that is released in response mainly to fat entering the duodenum has a strong effect on inhibition of further eating.

Obviously, these mechanisms are of particular importance in bringing one's feeding to a halt during a heavy meal.

Metering of Food by Head Receptors. When a

person with an esophageal fistula is fed large quantities of food, even though this food is immediately lost again to the exterior the degree of hunger is decreased after a reasonable quantity of food has passed through the mouth. This effect occurs despite the fact that the gastrointestinal tract does not become the least bit filled. Therefore, it is postulated that various "head factors" relating to feeding, such as chewing, salivation, swallowing, and tasting, "meter" the food as it passes through the mouth, and after a certain amount has passed through, the hypothalamic feeding center becomes inhibited. However, the inhibition caused by this metering mechanism is considerably less intense and less lasting, usually lasting only 20 to 40 minutes, than is the inhibition caused by gastrointestinal filling.

Importance of Having Both Long- and Short-term Regulatory Systems for Feeding. The long-term regulatory system, especially the lipostatic feedback mechanism, obviously helps an animal to maintain constant stores of nutrients in its tissues, preventing these from becoming too low or too high. On the other hand, the short-term regulatory stimuli make the animal feed only when the gastrointestinal tract is receptive to food. Thus, food passes through its gastrointestinal tract fairly continuously so that its digestive, absorptive, and storage mechanisms can all work at a steady pace rather than only when the animal needs food for energy. Indeed, the digestive, absorptive, and storage mechanisms can increase their rates of activity above normal only four- to five-fold, while the rate of usage of stored nutrients for energy sometimes increases to 20 times normal.

It is important, then, that feeding occur rather continuously (but at a rate that the gastrointestinal tract can accommodate), regulated principally by the short-term regulatory mechanisms. However, it is also important that the intensity of the daily rhythmic feeding habits be modulated up or down by the long-term regulatory system, based principally on the level of nutrient stores in the body.

OBESITY

Energy Input Versus Energy Output. When greater quantities of energy (in the form of food) enter the body than are expended, the body weight increases. Therefore, obesity is obviously caused by excess energy input over energy output. For each 9.3 Calories of excess energy entering the body, 1 gram of fat is stored.

Excess energy input occurs *only during the developing phase of obesity*, and once a person has become obese, all that is required to remain obese is that the energy input equal the energy output. For the person to reduce, the input must be *less* than the output. Indeed, studies of obese persons have shown that their intake of

food in the static stage of obesity (after the obesity has already been attained) is approximately the same as that for normal persons.

Effect of Muscular Activity on Energy Output. About one-third the energy used each day by the normal person goes into muscular activity, and in the laborer as much as two-thirds or occasionally three-fourths is used in this way. Since muscular activity is by far the most important means by which energy is expended in the body, it is frequently said that obesity results from *too high a ratio of food intake to daily exercise*.

Abnormal Feeding Regulation as a Pathological Cause of Obesity

The preceding discussion of the mechanisms that regulate feeding emphasized that the rate of feeding is normally regulated in proportion to the nutrient stores in the body. When these stores begin to approach an optimal level in a normal person, feeding is automatically reduced to prevent overstorage. However, in many obese persons this is not true, for feeding does not slacken until body weight is far above normal. Therefore, in effect, obesity is often caused by an abnormality of the feeding regulatory mechanism. This can result from either psychogenic factors that affect the regulation or actual abnormalities of the hypothalamus itself.

Psychogenic Obesity. Studies of obese patients show that a large proportion of obesity results from psychogenic factors. Perhaps the most common psychogenic factor contributing to obesity is the prevalent idea that healthy eating habits require three meals a day and that each meal must be filling. Many children are forced into this habit by overly solicitous parents, and the children continue to practice it throughout life. In addition, persons are known often to gain large amounts of weight during or following stressful situations, such as the death of a parent, a severe illness, or even mental depression. It seems that eating is often a means of release from tension.

Hypothalamic Abnormalities as a Cause of Obesity. In the preceding discussion of feeding regulation, it was pointed out that lesions in the ventromedial nuclei of the hypothalamus cause an animal to eat excessively and become obese. It has also been discovered that these lesions are associated with excess insulin production, which in turn increases fat depositon. Also, many persons with hypophysial tumors that encroach on the hypothalamus develop progressive obesity, illustrating that obesity in the human being, too, can definitely result from damage to the hypothalamus. Though in the normal obese person hypothalamic damage is almost never found, it is possible that the functional organization of the feeding center is different in the obese person from that of the nonobese person. For instance, an obese person who has reduced to normal weight usually develops hunger that is demonstrably far greater than that of the normal person. This indicates that the "setting" of the obese person's feeding center is at a much higher level of nutrient storage than is that of the normal person.

REGULATION OF BODY TEMPERATURE — THE "HYPOTHALAMIC THERMOSTAT"

Figure 24–4 illustrates approximately what happens to the temperature of the nude body after a few hours' exposure to dry air ranging from 30° to 170° F. Obviously, the precise dimensions of this curve vary, depending on the movement of air, the amount of moisture in the air, and even the nature of the surroundings. However, in general, between approximately 60° and 130° F. in dry air, the nude body is capable of maintaining indefinitely a normal body core temperature somewhere between 98° and 100° F.

The temperature of the body is regulated almost entirely by nervous feedback mechanisms, and almost all of these operate through *temperature regulating centers* located in the *hypothalamus.* However, for these feedback mechanisms to operate, there must also exist temperature detectors, discussed next, to determine when the body temperature becomes either too hot or too cold.

Thermostatic Detection of Excess Body Temperature — Role of the Preoptic Area of the Hypothalamus

In recent years, experiments have been performed in which minute areas in the brain have been either heated or cooled by use of a so-called *thermode.* This small, needle-like device is heated by electrical means or by passing hot water through it, or it is cooled by cold water. The principal area in the brain in which heat from a thermode affects body temperature control is the preoptic area of the hypothalamus, and to a lesser extent the adjacent regions of the anterior hypothalamus.

Using the thermode, the preoptic area of the hypothalamus has been found to contain large numbers of heat-sensitive neurons that seem to function as temperature sensors for controlling body temperature. These neurons increase their firing rate as the temperature rises, the rate sometimes increasing as much as 10-fold with an increase in body temperature of 10° C.

In addition to the heat-sensitive neurons, a few cold-sensitive neurons have also been found in other parts of the hypothalamus, in the septum, and in the reticular substance of the mid-brain, all of which increase their rate of firing when exposed to cold. However, the number of these are few, and it is likely that they play a much smaller, if any, role in regulating body temperature.

When the preoptic area is heated, the body immediately breaks out into a profuse sweat while at the same time the skin blood vessels over the entire body become greatly vasodilated. Thus, there is the immediate reaction to cause the body to lose heat, thereby helping to return the body temperature toward the normal level. In addition, excess body heat production is inhibited. Therefore, it is clear that the preoptic area of the hypothalamus has the capability of serving as a thermostatic body temperature control center.

Detection of Cold — Role of Skin and Spinal Cord Receptors

One of the ways in which the body detects cold is by reduced rates of discharge of the heat-sensitive neurons in the preoptic area. However, by the time the internal body temperature has fallen a few tenths of a degree below normal, these neurons have generally become completely inactive so that their signal level cannot be decreased any further. Therefore, detection of cold temperature in the body relies on other temperature receptors; mainly the cold receptors of the skin but to some extent cold receptors also in the spinal cord, abdomen, and possibly other internal structures of the body.

It will be recalled from the discussion of the temperature receptors in Chapter 9 that the skin is endowed with both *cold* and *warmth* receptors. However, there are far more cold receptors than warmth receptors; in fact, 10 times as many in some parts of the body. Therefore, peripheral detection of temperature mainly concerns detecting cool and cold instead of warm temperatures.

When the skin is chilled over the entire body, immediate reflex effects are invoked to increase the temperature of the body in several ways: (1) by

Figure 24–4. Effect of high and low atmospheric temperatures for several hours' duration on the internal body temperature, showing that the internal body temperature remains stable despite wide changes in atmospheric temperature.

providing a strong stimulus to cause shivering, with resultant increase in the rate of body heat production, (2) by inhibiting the process of sweating if this should be occurring, and (3) by promoting skin vasoconstriction to diminish the transfer of body heat to the skin.

Thus, it is clear that the heat center in the preoptic area of the hypothalamus plays a major role in preventing overheating of the body, while the cold receptors in many areas of the body — especially the skin — play very important roles in preventing low body temperatures.

Integration of the Heat and Cold Temperature Signals in the Posterior Hypothalamus

Even though a large share of the signals for cold detection arise in peripheral receptors, these signals help to control body temperature mainly through the hypothalamus. However, the area of the hypothalamus that they stimulate is not the preoptic area but instead an area located bilaterally in the posterior hypothalamus approximately at the level of the mammary bodies. The thermostatic signals from the preoptic area are also transmitted into this posterior hypothalamus area. It is here that the signals from the preoptic area and the signals from the body periphery are combined to provide the heat-producing or heat-losing reactions of the body.

The overall heat-controlling mechanism of the hypothalamus is called the *hypothalamic thermostat.*

NEURONAL EFFECTOR MECHANISMS TO INCREASE OR DECREASE BODY TEMPERATURE

When the hypothalamic thermostat detects that the body temperature is either too hot or too cold, it institutes appropriate heat-decreasing or heat-increasing procedures. The student is familiar with most of these from personal experience, but special features are the following:

Mechanisms for Reducing Body Temperature

The thermostatic system employs three important mechanisms to reduce body heat when the temperature becomes too great:

1. In almost all areas of the body *the skin blood vessels are intensely dilated.* This is caused by *inhibition of the sympathetic centers in the posterior hypothalamus that cause vasoconstriction.* Full vasodilatation can increase the rate of heat transfer to the skin as much as 8-fold.

Figure 24–5. Effect of hypothalamic temperature on: (1) evaporative heat loss from the body and (2) heat production caused primarily by muscular activity and shivering. This figure demonstrates the extremely critical temperature level at which increased heat loss begins and increased heat production stops. (Drawn from data in Benzinger, Kitzinger, and Pratt, in Hardy (ed.): Temperature, Part 3, p. 637. Reinhold Publishing Corp.)

2. *Sweating is strongly stimulated.* This effect is illustrated by the solid curve in Figure 24–5, which shows a sharp increase in the rate of evaporative heat loss resulting from sweating when the body core temperature rises above the critical temperature level of 37° C. (98.6° F.). An additional 1° C. increase in body temperature causes enough sweating to remove 10 times the basal rate of body heat production.

3. Heat production by such mechanisms as shivering and chemical thermogenesis is strongly inhibited.

Mechanisms for Increasing Body Heat When the Temperature Is Too Low

In the cold state, the thermostatic mechanism institutes exactly opposite procedures. These are:

1. *Skin vasoconstriction throughout the body* caused by stimulation of the posterior hypothalamic sympathetic centers.

2. *Pilo-erection* — that is, hairs "standing on end." Obviously, this effect is not important in the human being, but in lower animals the upright projection of the hairs entraps a thick layer of insulator air next to the skin so that the transfer of heat to the surroundings is greatly depressed.

3. *Increase in heat production* by causing (a) shivering, (b) sympathetic excitation of heat pro-

duction, and (c) thyroxine secretion. These require additional explanation, as follows:

Hypothalamic Stimulation of Shivering. Located in the dorsomedial portion of the posterior hypothalamus near the wall of the third ventricle is an area called the *primary motor center for shivering.* This area is normally inhibited by heat signals from the preoptic heat thermostatic area but is driven by cold signals from the skin and spinal cord. Therefore, as illustrated by the dashed curve in Figure 24–5, in response to cold, this center becomes activated and transmits impulses through bilateral tracts down the brain stem, into the lateral columns of the spinal cord, and, finally, to the anterior motoneurons. These impulses are nonrhythmic and do not cause the actual muscle shaking. Instead, they increase the tone of the skeletal muscles throughout the body. When the tone rises above a certain critical level, shivering begins. This probably results from feedback oscillation of the muscle spindle stretch reflex mechanism. During maximum shivering, body heat production can rise to as high as 4 to 5 times normal.

Sympathetic "Chemical" Excitation of Heat Production. Either sympathetic stimulation or circulating norepinephrine and epinephrine in the blood can cause an immediate increase in the rate of cellular metabolism; this effect is called *chemical thermogenesis,* and it is believed to result at least partially from the ability of norepinephrine and epinephrine to uncouple oxidative phosphorylation, as a result of which more oxidation of foodstuffs must occur to produce the energy required for normal function of the body. Therefore, the rate of cellular metabolism increases.

The degree of chemical thermogenesis that occurs in an animal is almost directly proportional to the amount of *brown* fat that exists in the animal's tissues. This is a type of fat that contains large numbers of mitochondria in its cells, and these cells are supplied by a strong sympathetic innervation. Upon sympathetic stimulation, the oxidative metabolism of the mitochondria is greatly stimulated, but this probably occurs in an uncoupled manner so that only small amounts of ATP are formed. Regardless of the chemical mechanism, the energy release caused by the oxidative metabolism provides a very important source of heat to the body.

The process of acclimatization greatly affects the intensity of chemical thermogenesis; some animals that have been exposed for several weeks to a very cold environment exhibit as much as a 100 to 500 per cent increase in metabolism when acutely exposed to cold, in contrast to the unacclimatized animal, which responds with an increase in metabolism of perhaps one-third as much.

In adult human beings, who have almost no brown fat, it is rare that chemical thermogenesis increases the rate of heat production more than 10 to 15 per cent. However, in infants, who *do* have a small amount of brown fat in the interscapular space, chemical thermogenesis can increase the rate of heat production as much as 100 per cent, which is probably a very important factor in maintaining normal body temperature in the neonate.

Increased Thyroxine Output as a Cause of Increased Heat Production. Cooling the preoptic area of the hypothalamus also increases the production of the neurosecretory hormone *thyrotropin-releasing hormone* by the hypothalamus. This hormone is carried by way of the hypothalamic portal veins to the adenohypophysis where it stimulates the secretion of thyroid-stimulating hormone. Thyroid-stimulating hormone, in turn, stimulates increased output of thyroxine by the thyroid gland, as will be explained in Chapter 25. The increased thyroxine increases the rate of cellular metabolism throughout the body. However, this increase in metabolism does not occur immediately but requires several weeks for the thyroid gland to hypertrophy before it reaches its new level of thyroxine secretion.

Exposure of animals to extreme cold for several weeks can cause their thyroid gland to increase in size as much as 20 to 40 per cent. However, human beings rarely allow themselves to be exposed to the same degree of cold as that to which animals have been subjected. Therefore, we still do not know, quantitatively, how important the thyroid method of adaptation to cold is in the human being. Yet, isolated measurements have shown that military personnel residing for several months in the Arctic develop increased metabolic rates; Eskimos also have abnormally high basal metabolic rates. Also, the continuous stimulatory effect of cold on the thyroid gland can probably explain the much higher incidence of toxic thyroid goiters in persons living in colder climates than in those living in warmer climates.

THE FEEDBACK GAIN FOR BODY TEMPERATURE CONTROL

Feedback gain is a measure of the effectiveness of a control system. In the case of body temperature control, it is important for the internal body temperature to change as little as possible despite marked changes in the environmental temperature, and the gain is approximately equal to the ratio of change in environmental temperature to change in body temperature. Experiments have shown that the body temperature changes about 1° C. for each 25° to 30° C. change in environmental temperature. Therefore, the feedback gain of the hypothalamic thermostat mechanism for control of body temperature averages about 27, which is an extremely high gain for a biological control system (the baroreceptor arterial pressure control system, for instance, has a gain less than 2).

BEHAVIORAL CONTROL OF BODY TEMPERATURE

Aside from the thermostatic mechanism for body temperature control, the body has still another temperature-controlling mechanism that is even more potent than all the above mechanisms together. This is behavioral control of temperature, which can be explained as follows: Whenever the internal body temperature becomes too high, signals from the thermostatic brain areas give the person a psychic sensation of being overheated. Conversely, whenever the body becomes too cold, signals from the skin and probably also from other receptors elicit the feeling of cold discomfort. Therefore, the person makes appropriate environmental adjustments to re-establish comfort. This is a much more powerful system of body temperature control than most physiologists have recognized in the past. Indeed, for people, this is the only really effective mechanism for body heat control in severely cold environs.

The obvious types of behavioral adjustments include selecting appropriate clothing, moving the body to a different environmental setting, increasing the delivery of heat or cold from appropriate heaters or air conditioners, and so forth.

It is important to note that many other of our body's control systems utilize similar behavior mechanisms to achieve highly refined degrees of control. For instance, even respiration is probably controlled to a great extent in this way — that is, when a person perceives that he is being subjected to air hunger, he consciously breathes more to make up the deficit. Therefore, it is not valid to think of the body's homeostatic control systems as operating only in the subconscious portions of the brain.

FEVER

Fever, which means a body temperature above the usual range of normal, may be caused by abnormalities in the brain itself or by toxic substances that affect the temperature regulating centers. Some causes of fever are presented in Figure 24–6. These include bacterial diseases, brain tumors, and environmental conditions that may terminate in heat stroke.

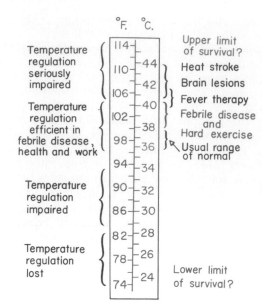

Figure 24–6. Body temperatures under different conditions. (From DuBois: Fever. Charles C Thomas.)

Resetting the Hypothalamic Thermostat in Febrile Diseases — Effect of Pyrogens

Many proteins, breakdown products of proteins, and certain other substances, such as lipopolysaccharide toxins secreted by bacteria, can cause the set-point of the hypothalamic thermostat to rise. Substances that cause this effect are called *pyrogens*. It is pyrogens secreted by toxic bacteria or pyrogens released from degenerating tissues of the body that cause fever during disease conditions. When the set-point of the hypothalamic thermostat becomes increased to a higher level than normal, all the mechanisms for raising the body temperature are brought into play, including heat conservation and increased heat production. Within a few hours after the thermostat has been set to a higher level, the body temperature also approaches this level.

Mechanism of Action of Pyrogens in Causing Fever — Role of "Endogeneous Pyrogen." Some physiologists believe that exogenous pyrogenic substances such as bacterial toxins act directly on the hypothalamic thermostat to increase its setting. However, there is reason to believe that most pyrogens affect the hypothalamic thermostat indirectly in the following manner:

When bacterial or other pyrogens are injected into a person they usually do not affect the hypothalamic thermostat immediately; instead, the effect is delayed for many minutes to several hours. This delay is believed to result from the fact that the pyrogens must first react with the polymorphonuclear leukocytes, monocytes, and certain of the reticuloendothelial cells to form still another substance called *endogenous pyrogen*. The endogenous pyrogen is then transmitted in the blood to the hypothalamus and has an extremely powerful direct effect on the preoptic heat-sensitive neurons in increasing the set-point of the hypothalamic thermostat to febrile levels.

To give one an idea of the extremely powerful effect of pyrogens in resetting the hypothalamic thermostat, only a few *nanograms* of purified endogenous pyrogen injected into an animal can cause severe fever.

Effect of Dehydration on the Hypothalamic Thermostat. Dehydration is another factor that can cause the body temperature to rise considerably. Part of this elevation of temperature probably results from lack of available fluid for sweating, but dehydration can also cause temperature elevation even in a cold environment. Consequently, dehydration almost certainly affects the hypothalamic centers directly to set the hypothalamic thermostat to febrile levels.

Characteristics of Febrile Conditions

Chills. When the setting of the thermostat is suddenly changed from the normal level to a higher-than-normal value as a result of tissue destruction, pyrogenic substances, or dehydration, the body temperature usually takes several hours to reach the new temperature setting. For instance, the temperature setting of the hypothalamic thermostat, as illustrated in Figure 24–7, might suddenly rise to 103° F. Because the blood temperature is less than the temperature setting of the hypothalamic thermostat, the usual responses to cause elevation of body temperature occur. During this period the person experiences chills and feels extremely cold, even though body temperature may already be above normal. Also, the skin is cold because of vasoconstriction, and the person shakes all over because of shivering. Chills continue until the body temperature rises to the hypothalamic setting of 103° F. Then, when the temperature of the body reaches this value, the person no longer experiences chills but instead feels neither cold nor hot. As long as the factor that is causing the hypothalamic thermostat to be set at this high value continues its effect, the body temperature is regulated more or less in the normal manner but at the high temperature level.

The Crisis of "Flush." If the factor that is causing the high temperature is suddenly removed, the hypothalamic thermostat is suddenly set at a lower value — perhaps even back to the normal level, as illustrated in Figure 24–7. In this instance, the body temperature is still 103° F., but the hypothalamus is attempting to regulate the temperature to 98.6° F. This situation is analogous to excessive heating of the preoptic area, which causes intense sweating and sudden development of a hot skin because of vasodilatation everywhere. This sudden change of events in a febrile disease is known as the "crisis" or, more appropriately, the "flush." In olden days, before the advent of antibiotics, the crisis was always awaited, for once this occurred the doctor knew immediately that the patient's temperature would soon be falling.

REFERENCES

Alfin-Slater, R. B., and Kirtchevsky, D. (eds.): Nutrition and the Adult: Macronutrients. New York, Plenum Press, 1979.
Atanassova, E., and Papasova, M.: Gastrointestinal motility. *Int. Rev. Physiol.*, 12:35, 1977.
Baile, C. A., and Forbes, J. M.: Control of feed intake and regulation of energy balance in ruminants. *Physiol. Rev.*, 54:160, 1974.
Barry, R. J., and Eggenton, J.: Electrical activity of the intestine. *Biomembranes*, 4B:917, 1974.
Benzinger, T. H.: Heat regulation: Homeostasis of central temperature in man. *Physiol. Rev.*, 49:671, 1969.
Bray, G. A., and Campfield, L. A.: Metabolic factors in the control of energy stores. *Metabolism*, 24:99, 1975.
Brooks, F. P., and Evers, P. W. (eds.): Nerves and the Gut. Thorofare, N.J., C. B. Slack, 1977.
Davenport, H. W.: A Digest of Digestion, 2nd Ed. Chicago, Year Book Medical Publishers, 1978.
Elizondo, R.: Temperature regulation in primates. *Int. Rev. Physiol*, 15:71, 1977.
Garrow, J. S.: Energy Balance and Obesity in Man. New York, Elsevier/North-Holland, 1978.
Grossman, M. I.: Neural and hormonal regulation of gastrointestinal function: An overview. *Annu. Rev. Physiol.*, 41:27, 1979.
Hardy, R. N.: Temperature and Animal Life. Baltimore, University Park Press, 1979.
Heller, H. C., *et al.*: The thermostat of vertebrate animals. *Sci. Am.*, 239(2):102, 1978.
Hensel, H.: Neural processes in thermoregulation. *Physiol. Rev.*, 53: 948, 1973.
Hensel, H.: Thermoreceptors. *Annu. Rev. Physiol.*, 36:233, 1974.
Hunt, S. M., *et al.*: Nutrition: Principles and Clinical Practice. New York, John Wiley & Sons, 1980.
Kluger, M. J.: Temperature regulation, fever, and siease. *In* Robertshaw, D. (ed.): International Review of Physiology: Environmental Physiology III. Vol. 20. Baltimore, University Park Press, 1979, p. 209.
Panksepp, J.: Hypothalamic regulation of energy balance and feeding behavior. *Fed. Proc.*, 33:1150, 1974.
Robertshaw, D.: Role of the adrenal medulla in thermoregulation. *Int. Rev. Physiol.*, 15:189, 1977.
Sernka, T. J., and Jacobson, E. D.: Gastrointestinal Physiology: The Essentials. Baltimore, Williams & Wilkins, 1979.
Sloan, A. W.: Man in Extreme Environments. Springfield, Ill, Charles C Thomas, 1979.
Thompson, C. I.: Controls of Eating. New York, Spectrum Publications, 1979.

Figure 24–7. Effects of changing the setting of the "hypothalamic thermostat."

25

Hypothalamic and Pituitary Control of Hormones and of Reproduction

One of the means by which the nervous system controls bodily activity is by increasing or decreasing the secretion of many of the body's hormones. In previous chapters we have already discussed part of this function, such as control of the secretion of epinephrine and norepinephrine by the autonomic nervous system and control of different local hormones in the gastrointestinal tract.

In this chapter we will discuss a much more global means by which the nervous system controls the secretion of hormones by most of the body's endocrine glands. These hormones in turn control many if not most of the body's metabolic function, as well as reproduction.

The nervous system's central control area for this global system is the *hypothalamus,* which controls the secretions of at least eight important hormones by the pituitary gland. These pituitary hormones in turn control the secretion of still other hormones by the thyroid gland, the adrenal glands, and the ovaries or testes. The function of the hypothalamus, and therefore its control effects on this pyramidal hormonal system, is itself controlled by nerve signals from almost all other parts of the brain, especially signals elicited by such subconscious nervous effects as the emotions, sex drives, body temperature, hunger, thirst, and even the crying of a baby.

It will not be possible to describe in the limited pages of this text this entire system and its multiple effects on the body. Yet, in this chapter we will discuss the most important features of the system, (1) the relationship of the hypothalamus to the pituitary gland and (2) the neurohormonal factors that promote the onset of reproduction.

THE PITUITARY GLAND AND ITS RELATIONSHIP TO THE HYPOTHALAMUS

The *pituitary gland* (Fig. 25–1), also called the *hypophysis,* is a small gland—about 1 cm. in diameter and 0.5 to 1 gram in weight—that lies in the *sella turcica* at the base of the brain and is connected with the hypothalamus by the *pituitary* (or *hypophysial*) *stalk.* Physiologically, the pituitary gland is divisible into two distinct portions: the *anterior pituitary,* also known as the *adenohypophysis,* and the *posterior pituitary,* also known as the *neurohypophysis.* Between these is a

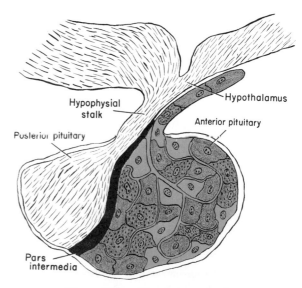

Figure 25–1. The pituitary gland.

small, relatively avascular zone called the *pars intermedia,* which is almost absent in the human being while much larger and much more functional in some lower animals.

Embryologically, the two portions of the pituitary originate from different sources, the anterior pituitary from *Rathke's pouch*, which is an embryonic invagination of the pharyngeal epithelium, and the posterior pituitary from an outgrowth of the hypothalamus. The origin of the anterior pituitary from the pharyngeal epithelium explains the epithelioid nature of its cells, while the origin of the posterior pituitary from neural tissue explains the presence of large numbers of glial-type cells in this gland.

Six very important hormones plus several less important ones are secreted by the *anterior* pituitary, and two important hormones are secreted by the *posterior* pituitary. The hormones of the anterior pituitary play major roles in the control of metabolic functions throughout the body, as shown in Figure 25-2. (1) *Growth hormone* promotes growth of the animal by affecting many metabolic functions throughout the body, especially protein formation. (2) *Adrenocorticotropin* controls the secretion of some of the adrenocortical hormones, which in turn affect the metabolism of glucose, proteins, and fats. (3) *Thyroid-stimulating hormone* controls the rate of secretion of thyroxine by the thyroid gland, and thyroxine in turn controls the rates of most chemical reactions of the entire body. (4) *Prolactin* promotes mammary gland development and milk production. And two separate gonadotropic hormones, (5) *follicle-stimulating hormone* and (6) *luteinizing*

hormone, control growth of the gonads as well as their reproductive activities.

The two hormones secreted by the posterior pituitary play other roles. (1) *Antidiuretic hormone* (also called *vasopressin*) controls the rate of water excretion into the urine and in this way helps to control the concentration of water in the body fluids. (2) *Oxytocin* (a) helps to deliver milk from the glands of the breast to the nipples during suckling, and (b) probably helps in the delivery of the baby at the end of gestation.

CONTROL OF PITUITARY SECRETION BY THE HYPOTHALAMUS

Almost all secretion by the pituitary is controlled by either hormonal or nervous signals from the hypothalamus. Indeed, when the pituitary gland is removed from its normal position beneath the hypothalamus and transplanted to some other part of the body, its rates of secretion of the different hormones (except for prolactin) fall to low levels — in the case of some of the hormones, almost to zero.

Secretion from the posterior pituitary is controlled by nerve fibers originating in the hypothalamus and terminating in the posterior pituitary. In contrast, secretion by the anterior pituitary is controlled by hormones called *hypothalamic releasing* and *inhibitory hormones* (or *factors*) secreted within the hypothalamus itself and then conducted to the anterior pituitary through minute blood vessels called *hypothalamic-hypophysial portal vessels.* In the anterior pituitary these releasing and inhibitory hormones act on the glandular cells to control their secretion. This system of control will be discussed in detail later in the chapter.

The hypothalamus receives signals from almost all possible sources in the nervous system. Thus, when a person is exposed to pain, a portion of the pain signal is transmitted into the hypothalamus. Likewise, when a person experiences some powerful depressing or exciting thought, a portion of the signal is transmitted into the hypothalamus. Olfactory stimuli denoting pleasant or unpleasant smells transmit strong signal components directly and through the amygdaloid nuclei into the hypothalamus. *Even the concentrations of nutrients, electrolytes, water, and various hormones* in the blood excite or inhibit various portions of the hypothalamus. Thus, the hypothalamus is a collecting center for information concerned with the well-being of the body, and in turn much of this information is used to control secretions of the many globally important pituitary hormones.

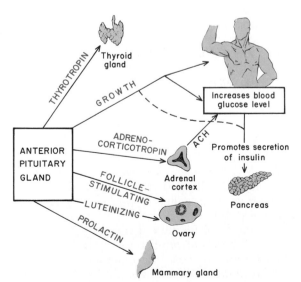

Figure 25–2. Metabolic functions of the anterior pituitary hormones.

THE ANTERIOR PITUITARY GLAND AND ITS REGULATION BY HYPOTHALAMIC RELEASING FACTORS

CELL TYPES OF THE ANTERIOR PITUITARY

The anterior pituitary gland is composed of several different types of cells. In general, there is one type of cell for each type of hormone that is formed in this gland; with special staining techniques these various cell types can be differentiated from one another. The only major exception to this is that the same cell type seems to secrete both luteinizing hormone and follicle-stimulating hormone.

However, through the use of usual acid-base histological stains, the cell types can be separated into only three types, commonly known as (1) *acidophils,* which stain strongly with acidic dyes; (2) *basophils,* which stain strongly with basic dyes; and (3) *chromophobes,* which do not stain with either. The *acidophils* produce *growth hormone* and *prolactin;* the *basophils* produce *luteinizing hormone, follicle-stimulating hormone, adrenocorticotropin,* and *thyroid-stimulating hormone;* and the *chromophobes* are believed to be cells mainly in nonsecreting stages of development.

THE HYPOTHALAMIC-HYPOPHYSIAL PORTAL SYSTEM

The anterior pituitary is a highly vascular gland with extensive capillary sinuses among the glandular cells. Almost all the blood that enters these sinuses passes first through a capillary bed in the tissue of the lower tip of the hypothalamus and then through small *hypothalamic-hypophysial portal vessels* into the anterior pituitary sinuses. Thus, Figure 25–3 illustrates a small artery supplying the lowermost portion of the hypothalamus called the *median eminence.* Small vascular tufts project into the substance of the median eminence and then return to its surface, coalescing to form the hypothalamic-hypophysial portal vessels.

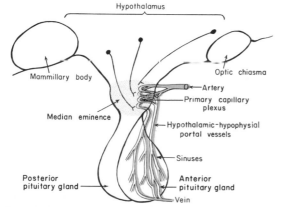

Figure 25–3. The hypothalamic-hypophysial portal system.

These in turn pass downward along the pituitary stalk to supply the anterior pituitary sinuses.

Secretion of Hypothalamic Releasing and Inhibitory Hormones into the Median Eminence. Special neurons in the hypothalamus synthesize and secrete hormones called *hypothalamic releasing* and *inhibitory hormones* (or *releasing* and *inhibitory factors*) that control the secretion of the anterior pituitary hormones. These neurons originate in various parts of the hypothalamus and send their nerve fibers into the median eminence and the tuber cinereum, the hypothalamic tissue that extends into the pituitary stalk. The endings of these fibers are different from most endings in the central nervous system in that their function is not to transmit signals from one neuron to another but merely to secrete the hypothalamic releasing and inhibitory hormones (factors) into the tissue fluids. These hormones are immediately absorbed into the capillaries of the hypothalamic-hypophysial portal system and carried directly to the sinuses of the anterior pituitary gland.

Function of the Releasing and Inhibitory Hormones. The function of the releasing and inhibitory hormones is to control the secretion of the anterior pituitary hormones. For each type of anterior pituitary hormone there is a corresponding hypothalamic releasing hormone; for some of the anterior pituitary hormones there is also a corresponding hypothalamic inhibitory factor. For most of the anterior pituitary hormones it is the releasing hormone that is important; but, for prolactin, an inhibitory hormone probably exerts most control. The hypothalamic releasing and inhibitory hormones that are of major importance are:

1. *Thyroid-stimulating hormone releasing hormone* (TRH), which causes release of thyroid-stimulating hormone

2. *Corticotropin releasing hormone* (CRH), which causes release of adrenocorticotropin

3. *Growth hormone releasing hormone* (GHRH), which causes release of growth hormone, and *growth hormone inhibitory hormone* (GHIH), which is the same as the hormone *somatostatin* and which inhibits the release of growth hormone

4. *Luteinizing hormone releasing hormone* (LRH), which causes release of both luteinizing hormone and follicle-stimulating hormone — this hormone is also called *gonadotropin releasing hormone* (GHRH)

5. *Prolactin inhibitory hormone* (PIH), which causes inhibition of prolactin secretion

In addition to these more important hypothalamic hormones, still another excites the secretion of prolactin and several hypothalamic inhibitory hormones inhibit some of the other anterior pituitary hormones. Each of the more important hypothalamic hormones will be discussed in detail at the time that the specific hormonal system controlled by it is presented in this chapter.

Specific Areas in the Hypothalamus That Control Secretion of Specific Hypothalamic Releasing and Inhibitory Factors. It is believed that all or most of the hypothalamic hormones are secreted at nerve endings in the median eminence before being transported to the anterior pituitary gland. Electrical stimulation of this region excites these nerve endings and therefore causes release of essentially all the hypothalamic factors. However, the neuronal cell bodies that give rise to these median eminence nerve endings are located in other discrete areas of the hypothalamus or in closely related areas of the basal brain. Unfortunately, the specific loci of the neurons that secrete the different hypothalamic hormones are so incompletely known that it would be misleading to attempt a delineation here.

PHYSIOLOGICAL FUNCTIONS OF THE ANTERIOR PITUITARY HORMONES

All the major pituitary hormones besides growth hormone exert their effects by stimulating target glands such as the thyroid gland, the adrenal cortex, the ovaries, the testicles, and the mammary glands. First, we will discuss briefly the functions of four of the pituitary hormones, *growth hormone, thyroid-stimulating hormone, adrenocorticotropin,* and *prolactin.* The functions of the two gonadotropic hormones, *luteinizing hormone* and *follicle-stimulating hormone,* will be discussed later in the chapter.

GROWTH HORMONE

Growth hormone is secreted by the anterior pituitary gland throughout the entire life of a person. Its rate of secretion is controlled by *growth hormone–releasing hormone,* which is formed in the hypothalamus and transmitted to the anterior pituitary gland through the hypothalamic-hypophysial portal system.

Growth hormone has two major functions: The first of these is to promote growth of the infant into the child and then of the child into the adult. One of the growth promoting effects is to cause growth of the bones, thus making the skeleton grow progressively longer and longer. However, the body stops increasing in height at adolescence because the long bones of the body then lose their capability for growth, not because of cessation of production of growth hormone. In addition to causing the bones to grow, this hormone promotes growth of essentially all other tissues of the body.

The second function of growth hormone is to control several of the metabolic functions of the body. Though these have not been defined in great detail, it is clear that growth hormone is essential for protein formation and for its maintenance in essentially all cells of the body. This, presumably, is the principal cause of growth. Growth hormone also enhances fat utilization but at the same time decreases carbohydrate use by the cells.

When growth hormone is not secreted by the anterior pituitary gland of a child, growth fails to occur, and the result is a so-called *pituitary dwarf* who retains childish features and often attains a height no greater than two to three feet. On the other hand, excess production of growth hormone by the anterior pituitary gland, caused usually by a tumor of the pituitary's growth hormone–producing cells, will cause the person to become a *giant.*

THYROID-STIMULATING HORMONE AND ITS CONTROL OF THYROID GLAND SECRETION

The thyroid gland secretes two hormones, *thyroxin* and *diiodothyronine,* that are very important in controlling the overall rate of metabolism of almost all tissues of the body — that is in controlling how rapidly the chemical reactions occur in all the tissues. When the rate of metabolism is great, a large amount of heat is also formed in the body, so that these thyroid hormones also play an important role in controlling body temperature.

Control of thyroid hormone secretion is vested in the hypothalamus and anterior pituitary gland. The hypothalamus secretes *thyroid-stimulating hormone–releasing hormone.* This then passes by way of the hypothalamic-hypophysial portal system to the anterior pituitary gland where it causes the release of *thyroid-stimulating hormone;* the thyroid-stimulating hormone, in turn, is the controller of the secretion of the thyroid hormones. Therefore, damage to either the hypothalamus or the anterior pituitary gland, especially the latter, can greatly reduce the rate of production of the thyroid hormones.

In the absence of the thyroid hormones, the person develops hypothyroidism, in which all the bodily activities become very sluggish, and often also becomes obese. On the other hand, overactivity of the hypothalamus or anterior pituitary gland can cause *hyperthyroidism,* in which the bodily functions become greatly overactive. Many of the body's tissues can actually be seriously damaged because of this overactivity. The person also is very excitable and nervous. Hyperthyroidism is often caused by psychic stress that elicits excessive signals through the hypothalamus.

Fortunately, in the normal person there is a feedback mechanism for control of thyroid secretion. That is, when thyroid secretion becomes too great, the hypothalamic-pituitary control system itself becomes inhibited, thus returning the body to normal thyroid secretion.

ADRENOCORTICOTROPIN AND ITS CONTROL OF THE ADRENOCORTICAL HORMONES

Each person has two adrenal glands, lying respectively adjacent to the superior poles of the two kidneys. The cortical portions of these glands secrete several different steroid hormones, the two most important of which are *cortisol* and *aldosterone*. The rate of secretion of aldosterone is controlled mainly by such factors as plasma potassium ion concentration and by the hormone angiotensin. On the other hand, the secretion of cortisol by the adrenal cortex is controlled almost entirely by the rate of secretion of adrenocorticotropin by the anterior pituitary. And the rate of secretion of adrenocorticotropin is itself controlled by *corticotropin-releasing hormone,* which is formed in the hypothalamus and transported to the pituitary gland through the hypothalamic-hypophysial portal system.

Cortisol has powerful controlling effects on many metabolic functions of the body, including protein metabolism, carbohydrate metabolism, and fat metabolism. For instance, it has an opposite effect on protein metabolism to that of growth hormone — that is, it reduces the amount of protein in most of the tissues. In doing so, it releases amino acids into the circulating blood that can be used elsewhere in the body when they are required to repair damaged tissues. For this reason as well as others, cortisol is a very valuable hormone to help the body resist tissue destruction during stress. Cortisol also enhances the conversion of amino acids into carbohydrates, which in turn are used for energy. It increases the utilization of fats for energy as well.

The hypothalamic control of cortisol secretion is especially important. Within minutes after a person experiences serious physical stress, such as a broken bone, excessive heat, hemorrhage, or almost any other life-threatening occurrence, the level of cortisol circulating in the body fluids increases many times, sometimes 20-fold or more. And the cortisol in turn plays a very significant role in helping the cells resist the destructive effects of the stress.

PROLACTIN AND ITS CONTROL OF MILK SECRETION

Under normal conditions, the rate of prolactin secretion is relatively slight. However, during pregnancy its secretion increases progressively until it becomes about ten times normal by the time the baby is born. The prolactin helps to promote growth of protein tissues in the fetus. But its most important function is its ability to cause development of the breasts during pregnancy and to cause milk secretion after birth of the baby.

Even though prolactin stimulates development of the breasts during pregnancy, the large quantities of estrogens and progesterone that are secreted by the placenta during pregnancy inhibit milk production until the baby is born. But after birth, when the placenta is no longer available to secrete the estrogens and progesterone, the prolactin then causes rapid secretion of milk by the breasts. Furthermore, everytime the baby suckles a breast, nerve signals pass from the breast, up the spinal cord, and into the hypothalamus to cause an increase in prolactin secretion and therefore production of more milk.

The hypothalamus controls prolactin secretion somewhat differently from the way that it controls the secretion of other anterior pituitary hormones. It does so by an inhibitory hormone, *prolactin inhibitory hormone,* rather than by a releasing hormone. That is, the hypothalamus normally secretes an excess of prolactin inhibitory hormone, which keeps the rate of secretion of prolactin at a relatively low level. However, during pregnancy and during periods of milk production, the hypothalamus *decreases* its rate of formation of prolactin inhibitory hormone, in this way allowing increased production of prolactin.

Because of the essential role of the hypothalamus in milk secretion, strong psychic stimuli, particularly emotional states of anguish, can actually cause the mother's milk-secreting apparatus to dry up.

CONTROL OF MALE SEXUAL FUNCTIONS BY THE GONADOTROPIC HORMONES — FSH AND LH

The anterior pituitary gland secretes two major gonadotropic hormones: (1) *follicle-stimulating hormone* (FSH); and (2) *luteinizing hormone* (LH). These are glycoprotein hormones that play major roles in the control of both male and female sexual function.

Regulation of Testosterone Production by LH. Testosterone is produced by the interstitial cells of Leydig only when the testes are stimulated by LH from the pituitary gland, and the quantity of testosterone secreted varies approximately in proportion to the amount of LH available.

Injection of purified LH into a child causes fibroblasts in the interstitial areas of the testes to develop into interstitial cells of Leydig, though mature Leydig cells are not normally found in the child's testes until after the age of approximately 10. Also, simultaneous administration of *prolactin* (another pituitary hormone that is closely associated with the gonadotropic hormones) greatly potentiates the effect of LH in promoting testosterone production.

Stimulation of Spermatogenesis by Follicle-Stimulating Hormone (FSH) and Testosterone. The conversion of primary spermatocytes into secondary spermatocytes in the seminiferous tubules is stimulated by FSH from the anterior pituitary gland. However, FSH cannot by itself cause complete formation of spermatozoa. For spermatogenesis to proceed to completion, testosterone must be secreted simultaneously by the interstitial cells. Thus, FSH seems to initiate the proliferative process of spermatogenesis, and testosterone diffusing from the interstitial cells into the seminiferous tubules apparently is necessary for final maturation of the spermatozoa. Indeed, once spermatogenesis has begun, testosterone alone can maintain this process for many weeks to months without additional FSH. Because testosterone is secreted by the interstitial cells under the influence of LH, both FSH and LH must be secreted by the anterior pituitary gland if spermatogenesis is to occur.

REGULATION OF PITUITARY SECRETION OF LH AND FSH BY THE HYPOTHALAMUS

The gonadotropins, like corticotropin and thyrotropin, are secreted by the anterior pituitary gland mainly in response to nervous activity in the hypothalamus. For instance, in the female rabbit, coitus with a male rabbit elicits nervous activity in the hypothalamus that in turn stimulates the anterior pituitary to secrete FSH and LH. These hormones then cause rapid ripening of follicles in the rabbit's ovaries, followed a few hours later by ovulation.

Many other types of nervous stimuli are also known to affect gonadotropin secretion. For instance, in sheep, goats, and deer, nervous stimuli in response to changes in weather and amount of light in the day increase the quantities of gonadotropins during one season of the year, the mating season, thus allowing birth of the young during an appropriate period for survival. Also, psychic stimuli can affect fertility of the male animal, as exemplified by the fact that transporting a bull under uncomfortable conditions can often cause almost complete temporary sterility. In the human being, it is known too that various psychogenic stimuli feeding into the hypothalamus can cause marked excitatory or inhibitory effects on gonadotropin secretion, in this way sometimes greatly altering the degree of fertility.

Luteinizing Hormone–Releasing Hormone (LHRH), the Hypothalamic Hormone That Stimulates Gonadotropin Secretion. In both the male and the female the hypothalamus controls gonadotropin secretion by way of the hypothalamic-hypophysial portal system, as was discussed earlier in the chapter. Although there are two different gonadotropic hormones, luteinizing hormone and follicle-stimulating hormone, only one hypothalamic-releasing hormone has been discovered; this is *luteinizing hormone–releasing hormone* (LHRH). Though this hormone has an especially strong effect on inducing luteinizing hormone secretion by the anterior pituitary gland, it has a potent effect in causing follicle stimulating hormone secretion as well.

Luteinizing hormone–releasing hormone plays a similar role in controlling gonadotropin secretion in the female, where the interrelationships are far more complex. Therefore, its nature and its functions will be discussed in more detail later in the chapter.

Reciprocal Inhibition of Hypothalamic–Anterior Pituitary Secretion of Gonadotropic Hormones by Testicular Hormones. *Feedback Control of Testosterone Secretion.* Injection of testosterone into either a male or a female animal strongly inhibits the secretion of luteinizing hormone but only slightly inhibits the secretion of the follicle-stimulating hormone. This inhibition depends on normal function of the hypothalamus; therefore, it is quite clear that the following negative feedback control system operates continuously to control very precisely the rate of testosterone secretion:

1. The hypothalamus secretes *luteinizing hormone–releasing hormone* which stimulates the anterior pituitary gland to secrete *luteinizing hormone*.

2. Luteinizing hormone in turn stimulates *hyperplasia of the Leydig cells* of the testes and also stimulates production of *testosterone* by these cells.

3. The testosterone in turn feeds back negatively to the hypothalamus, inhibiting production of luteinizing hormone–releasing hormone. This obviously limits the rate at which testosterone will be produced. On the other hand, when testosterone production is too low, lack of inhibition of the hypothalamus leads to subsequent return of testosterone secretion to the normal level.

Feedback Control of Spermatogenesis — Role of "Inhibin." It is known, too, that spermatogenesis by the testes inhibits the secretion of FSH. Conversely, failure of spermatogenesis causes markedly increased secretion of FSH; this is especially true when the seminiferous tubules are destroyed, including destruction of the Sertoli cells in addition to the germinal cells. Therefore, it is believed that the Sertoli cells secrete a hormone that has a direct inhibitory effect mainly on the anterior pituitary gland (but perhaps slightly on the hypothalamus as well) to inhibit the secretion of FSH. A hormone having a molecular weight between 25,000 and 100,000 and called *inhibin* has been discovered that probably is responsible for most of the feedback control of FSH secretion and of spermatogenesis. This feedback cycle is the following:

1. Follicle-stimulating hormone induces proliferation of the germinal epithelium of the seminiferous tubules and at the same time stimulates the Sertoli cells that provide nutrition for the developing spermatozoa.

2. The Sertoli cells (or less likely the germinal epithelial cells) release inhibin that in turn feeds back negatively to the anterior pituitary gland to inhibit the production of FSH. Thus, this feedback cycle maintains a rate of spermatogenesis that is required for male reproductive function.

PUBERTY AND REGULATION OF ITS ONSET

Initiation of the onset of puberty has long been a mystery. In the earliest history of humanity, the belief was simply that the testicles "ripened" at this time. With the discovery of the gonadotropins ripening of the anterior pituitary gland was considered responsible. Now it is known from experiments in which both testicular and pituitary tissues have been transplanted from infant animals into adult animals that both the testes and the anterior pituitary of the infant are capable of performing adult functions if appropriately stimulated. Therefore, it is now almost certain that *during childhood the hypothalamus, not the two glands, is responsible: that is, the hypothalamus simply does not secrete gonadotropin-releasing hormones.* Also, it is known that even the minutest amount of testosterone inhibits the production of gonadotropin-releasing hormones by the childhood hypothalamus. This leads to the theory that the childhood hypothalamus is so extremely sensitive to inhibition that the minutest amount of testosterone secreted by the testicles inhibits the entire system. For reasons yet unknown, the hypothalamus loses this inhibitory sensitivity at the time of puberty, which allows the secretory mechanisms to develop full activity. Thus, puberty is now believed to result from a maturing process of the hypothalamic sexual control centers.

REGULATION OF THE FEMALE MONTHLY RHYTHM — INTERPLAY BETWEEN THE OVARIAN AND HYPOTHALAMIC-PITUITARY HORMONES

Function of the Hypothalamus in the Regulation of Gonadotropin Secretion — Luteinizing Hormone–Releasing Hormone (LHRH). As was pointed out earlier in the chapter, secretion of most of the anterior pituitary hormones is controlled by releasing hormones formed in the hypothalamus and transported to the anterior pituitary gland by way of the hypothalamic-hypophysial portal system. In the case of the gonadotropins, at least one releasing factor, *luteinizing hormone–releasing hormone (LHRH)* is important. This has been purified and has been found to be a decapeptide having the following formula:

GLU-HIS-TRP-SER-TYR-GLY-LEU-ARG-PRO-GLY-NH$_2$

Though some research workers believe that another substance similar to this is follicle-stimulating hormone–releasing hormone (FSHRH), it has been found that the above purified LHRH causes release not only of luteinizing hormone but also of follicle-stimulating hormone. Therefore, since there is reason to believe that this decapeptide is in reality both LHRH and FSHRH combined in the same molecule, it is sometimes called simply *gonadotropin-releasing hormone* (GnRH).

Hypothalamic Centers for Stimulating Release of LHRH. Several different areas that profoundly influence the rate of secretion of the hypothalamic gonadotropin-releasing hormone LHRH have been found in the hypothalamus. In monkeys — and presumably in people — the midbasal region of the hypothalamus is the area most importantly involved. In lower animals, the area around the infundibulum causes a continuous tonic secretion of gonadotropin-releasing hormone, while two other areas modulate the rate of release. These areas are (1) a center in the preoptic area that causes cyclic variation in the secretory rate and (2) a center in the posterior hypothalamus that allows the psychic attitude of the animal to enhance or decrease the secretion of gonadotropin-releasing hormone.

Effect of Psychic Factors on the Female Sexual Cycle. It is well known that the young woman on first leaving home to go to college almost as often as not experiences disruption or irregularity of the female sexual cycle. Likewise, serious stresses of almost any type can interfere with the cycle. Finally, in many lower animals no ovulation occurs at all until after copulation; the sexual excitation attendant to the sexual act initiates a sequence of events that leads first to secretion in the hypothalamus of LHRH, then to secretion of the anterior pituitary gonadotropins, and finally to ovarian secretion of the female sex hormones and to ovulation. It is these effects that are believed to be mediated through the posterior hypothalamic center for modulating the output of LHRH.

Negative Feedback Effect of Estrogen and Progesterone on Secretion of Follicle-Stimulating Hormone

and Luteinizing Hormone. Estrogen in small amounts and progesterone in large amounts inhibit the production of FSH and LH. Both of these feedback effects seem to operate mainly by the actions of these hormones on the hypothalamus, though it is possible that they have very slight direct feedback actions on the anterior pituitary gland as well.

Positive Feedback Effect of Estrogen Before Ovulation — the Preovulatory Luteinizing Hormone Surge. For reasons not completely understood, the anterior pituitary gland secretes greatly increased amounts of LH on the day immediately before ovulation. This effect is illustrated in Figure 25–4, and the figure shows a much smaller preovulatory surge of FSH as well.

Experiments have shown that infusion of estrogen into a female for a period of two to three days during the first half of the ovarian cycle will cause rapidly accelerating growth of the follicles and also rapidly accelerating secretion of ovarian estrogens. During this period the secretion of both the follicle-stimulating hormone and luteinizing hormone by the anterior pituitary gland is at first suppressed slightly. Then abruptly the secretion of luteinizing hormone increases about eight-fold, and the secretion of follicle-stimulating hormone increases about two-fold. This abrupt increase in secretion of the gonadotropins seems to result from a *positive feedback effect* of the estrogen in place of the normal negative feedback that occurs during the remainder of the female sexual cycle. The precise cause of the positive feedback is not known, but nevertheless it is an absolutely necessary and integral part of the control mechanism. Without the normal preovulatory surge of luteinizing hormone, ovulation will never occur.

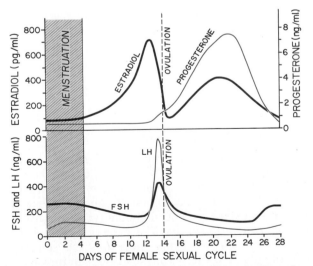

Figure 25–4. Plasma concentrations of the gonadotropins and ovarian hormones during the normal female sexual cycle.

FEEDBACK OSCILLATION OF THE HYPOTHALAMIC-PITUITARY-OVARIAN SYSTEM

Now, after discussing much of the known information about the interrelationships of the different components of the female hormonal system, we can digress from the area of proven fact into the realm of speculation and attempt to explain the feedback oscillation that controls the rhythm of the female sexual cycle. It seems to operate in approximately the following sequence of three successive events:

1. The Postovulatory Secretion of the Ovarian Hormones and Depression of Gonadotropins. The easiest part of the cycle to explain is the events that occur during the postovulatory phase — between ovulation and the beginning of menstruation. During this time the corpus luteum secretes very large quantities of both progesterone and estrogen. The combined effect of the estrogen and the progesterone on the hypothalamus is to inhibit the secretion of LHRH and therefore to cause strong negative feedback depression of secretion of the gonadotropins, both FSH and LH, during this period of time. These effects are illustrated in Figure 25–4.

2. The Follicular Growth Phase. A few days before menstruation, the corpus luteum involutes, and the secretion of both estrogen and progesterone decreases to a low ebb. This releases the hypothalamus from the feedback effect of the estrogen and progesterone so that LHRH increases again, followed in succession by a several hundred per cent increase also of FSH and LH. These hormones initiate new follicular growth and progressive increase in the secretion of estrogen, reaching a peak of estrogen secretion at about 12.5 to 13 days after the onset of menstruation. During the first 11 to 12 days of this follicular growth the rates of secretion of the gonadotropins FSH and LH decrease; then comes a sudden increase in secretion of both of these hormones, leading to the next stage of the cycle.

3. Preovulatory Surge of LH and FSH; Ovulation. At approximately 11.5 to 12 days after the onset of menstruation, the decline in secretion of FSH and LH comes to an abrupt halt. It is believed that the high level of estrogens at this time causes a positive feedback effect, as explained earlier, which leads to a terrific surge of secretion — especially of LH and to a lesser extent of FSH. This effect may be related to the fact that the follicular secretory cells are becoming exhausted so that their rate of secretion of estrogens had already begun to fall about one day prior to the LH surge. Whatever the cause of this preovulatory LH and FSH surge, the LH leads to both ovulation and formation of the corpus luteum. Thus, the hormonal system begins a new round of the female sexual cycle.

PUBERTY AND MENARCHE

Puberty means the onset of adult sexual life, and menarche means the onset of menstruation. As pointed out earlier in the chapter, the period of puberty is caused by a gradual increase in gonadotropic hormone secretion by the pituitary, beginning approximately the eighth year of life and usually culminating in the onset of menstruation between the ages of 11 and 16.

In the female, as in the male, the infantile pituitary gland and ovaries are capable of full function if appropriately stimulated. However, the hypothalamus is extremely sensitive to the inhibitory effects of estrogens, which keeps its stimulation of the pituitary almost completely suppressed throughout childhood. Then, at puberty, for reasons not understood, the hypothalamus matures; its excessive sensitivity to the negative feedback inhibition becomes greatly diminished, which allows enhanced production of gonadotropins and the onset of adult female sexual life.

Figure 25–5 illustrates (a) the increasing levels of estrogen secretion at puberty, (b) the cyclic variation during the monthly sexual cycles, (c) the further increase in estrogen secretion during the first few years of sexual life, (d) then progressive decrease in estrogen secretion toward the end of sexual life, and (e) finally almost no estrogen secretion beyond the menopause.

THE MENOPAUSE

At an average age of approximately 40 to 50 years the sexual cycles usually become irregular, and ovulation fails to occur during many of these cycles. After a few months to a few years, the cycles cease altogether, as illustrated in Figure 25–5. This period during which the cycles cease and the female sex hormones diminish rapidly to almost none at all is called the *menopause*.

The cause of the menopause is "burning out" of the ovaries. Throughout a woman's sexual life about 450 of the primordial follicles grow into vesicular follicles and ovulate, while literally thousands of the ova degenerate. At the age of about 45 only a few primordial follicles still remain to be stimulated by FSH and LH, and the production of estrogens by the ovary decreases as the number of primordial follicles approaches zero (also illustrated in Figure 25–5). When estrogen production falls below a critical value, the estrogens can no longer inhibit the production of FSH and LH; nor can they cause an ovulatory surge of LH and FSH to cause oscillatory cycles. Instead, FSH and LH (mainly FSH) are produced thereafter in large and

Figure 25–5.   Estrogen secretion throughout sexual life.

continuous quantities. Estrogens are produced in subcritical quantities for a short time after the menopause, but over a few years, as the final remaining primordial follicles become atretic, the production of estrogens by the ovaries falls almost to zero.

The Female Climacteric.   The term "female climacteric" means the entire time, lasting from several months to several years, during which the sexual cycles become irregular and gradually stop. In this period the woman must readjust her life from one that has been physiologically stimulated by estrogen and progesterone production to one devoid of these feminizing hormones. The secretion of estrogens decreases rapidly, and essentially no progesterone is secreted after the last ovulatory cycle. The loss of the estrogens often causes marked physiological changes in the function of the body, including (1) "hot flashes" characterized by extreme flushing of the skin, (2) psychic sensations of dyspnea, (3) irritability, (4) fatigue, (5) anxiety, and (6) occasionally, various psychotic states. These symptoms are of sufficient magnitude in approximately 15 per cent of women to warrant treatment. If psychotherapy fails, daily administration of an estrogen in small quantities will reverse the symptoms, and, by gradually decreasing the dose, the postmenopausal woman is likely to avoid severe symptoms; unfortunately, such treatment prolongs the symptoms.

THE MALE SEXUAL ACT

NEURONAL STIMULUS FOR PERFORMANCE OF THE MALE SEXUAL ACT

The most important source of impulses for initiating the male sexual act is the glans penis, for the glans contains a highly organized sensory end-organ system that transmits into the central nervous system a special modality of sensation called *sexual sensation*. The massaging action of intercourse on the glans stimulates the sensory end-organs, and the sexual sensations in turn pass through the pudendal nerve, thence through the sacral plexus into the sacral portion of the spinal cord, and finally up the cord to undefined areas of the cerebrum. Impulses may also enter the spinal cord from areas adjacent to the penis to aid in stimulating the sexual act. For instance, stimulation of the anal epithelium, the scrotum, and perineal structures in general can all send impulses into the cord which add to the sexual sensation. Sexual sensations can even originate in internal structures, such as irritated areas of the urethra, the bladder, the prostate, the seminal vesicles, the testes, and the vas deferens. Indeed, one of the causes of "sexual drive" is probably overfilling of the sexual organs with secretions. Infection and inflammation of these sexual organs sometimes cause almost continual sexual desire, and "aphrodisiac" drugs, such as cantharides, increase the sexual desire by irritating the bladder and urethral mucosa.

The Psychic Element of Male Sexual Stimulation. Appropriate psychic stimuli can greatly enhance the ability of a person to perform the sexual act. Simply thinking sexual thoughts or even dreaming that the act of intercourse is being performed can cause the male sexual act to occur and to culminate in ejaculation. Indeed, *nocturnal emissions* during dreams occur in many males during some stages of sexual life, especially during the teens.

Integration of the Male Sexual Act in the Spinal Cord. Though psychic factors usually play an important part in the male sexual act and can actually initiate or inhibit it, the cerebrum is probably not absolutely necessary for its performance, for appropriate genital stimulation can cause ejaculation in some animals and occasionally in a human being after their spinal cords have been cut above the lumbar region. Therefore, the male sexual act results from inherent reflex mechanisms integrated in the sacral and lumbar spinal cord, and these mechanisms can be initiated by either psychic stimulation or actual sexual stimulation.

STAGES OF THE MALE SEXUAL ACT

Erection. Erection is the first effect of male sexual stimulation, and the degree of erection is proportional to the degree of stimulation, whether this be psychic or physical.

Erection is caused by parasympathetic impulses that pass from the sacral portion of the spinal cord through the nervi erigentes to the penis. These parasympathetic impulses dilate the arteries of the penis and simultaneously constrict the veins, thus allowing arterial blood to build up under high pressure in the *erectile tissue* of the penis, illustrated in Figure 25–6. This erectile tissue is nothing more than large, cavernous, venous sinusoids, which are normally relatively empty but which become dilated tremendously when arterial blood

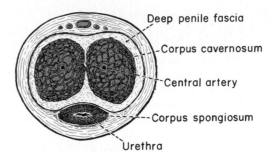

Figure 25–6. Erectile tissue of the penis.

flows into them under pressure, since the venous outflow is partially occluded. Also, the erectile bodies are surrounded by strong fibrous coats; therefore, high pressure within the sinusoids causes ballooning of the erectile tissue to such an extent that the penis becomes hard and elongated.

Lubrication. During sexual stimulation, the parasympathetic impulses, in addition to promoting erection, cause the glands of Littré and the bulbo-urethral glands to secrete mucus. Thus mucus flows through the urethra during intercourse to aid in the lubrication of coitus. However, most of the lubrication of coitus is provided by the female sexual organs rather than by the male. Without satisfactory lubrication, the male sexual act is rarely successful because unlubricated intercourse causes pain impulses which inhibit rather than excite sexual sensations.

Emission and Ejaculation. Emission and ejaculation are the culmination of the male sexual act. When the sexual stimulus becomes extremely intense, the reflex centers of the spinal cord begin to emit sympathetic impulses that leave the cord at L-1 and L-2 and pass to the genital organs through the hypogastric plexus to initiate emission, which is the forerunner of ejaculation.

Emission is believed to begin with contraction of the epididymis, the vas deferens, and the ampulla to cause expulsion of sperm into the internal urethra. Then, contractions of the muscular coat of the prostate gland followed lastly by contraction of the seminal vesicles expel prostatic fluid and seminal fluid, forcing the sperm forward. All these fluids mix with the mucus already secreted by the bulbo-urethral glands to form the semen. The process to this point is *emission*.

The filling of the internal urethra then elicits signals that are transmitted through the pudendal nerves to the sacral regions of the cord. In turn, rhythmic nerve impulses are sent from the cord to skeletal muscles, mainly the bulbocavernosus muscles, that encase the base of the erectile tissue, causing rhythmic, wavelike increases in pressure in this tissue, which "ejaculates" the semen from the urethra to the exterior. This is the process of *ejaculation*.

THE FEMALE SEXUAL ACT

Stimulation of the Female Sexual Act. As is true in the male sexual act, successful performance of the female sexual act depends on both psychic stimulation and local sexual stimulation.

The psychic factors that constitute "sex drive" in women are difficult to assess. The sex hormones, and the adrenocortical hormones as well, seem to exert a direct influence on the woman to create such a sex drive, but, on the other hand, the growing female child in modern society is often taught that sex is something to be hidden and that it is immoral. As a result of this training, much of the natural sex drive is inhibited, and whether the woman will have little or no sex drive ("frigidity") or will be more highly sexed probably depends partly on a balance between natural factors and previous training.

Local sexual stimulation in women occurs in more or less the same manner as in men, for massage, irritation, or other types of stimulation of the perineal region, sexual organs, and urinary tract create sexual sensations. The *clitoris* is especially sensitive for initiating sexual sensations. As in the male, the sexual sensory signals are mediated to the sacral segments of the spinal cord through the pudendal nerve and sacral plexus. Once these signals have entered the spinal cord, they are transmitted thence to the cerebrum. Also, local reflexes that are at least partly responsible for the female orgasm are integrated in the sacral and lumbar spinal cord.

Female Erection and Lubrication. Located around the introitus and extending into the clitoris is erectile tissue almost identical with the erectile tissue of the penis. This erectile tissue, like that of the penis, is controlled by the parasympathetic nerves that pass through the nervi erigentes from the sacral plexus to the external genitalia. In the early phases of sexual stimulation, the parasympathetics dilate the arteries and constrict the veins of the erectile tissues, and this allows rapid accumulation of blood in the erectile tissue so that the introitus tightens around the penis; this aids the male greatly in his attainment of sufficient sexual stimulation for ejaculation to occur.

Parasympathetic impulses also pass to the bilateral Bartholin's glands located beneath the labia minora to cause secretion of mucus immediately inside the introitus. This mucus is responsible for much of the lubrication during sexual intercourse, though much is also provided by other vaginal secretions as well and a small amount from the male urethral glands. The lubrication in turn is necessary for establishing during intercourse a satisfactory massaging sensation rather than an irritative sensation, which may be provoked by a dry vagina. A massaging sensation constitutes the optimal type of sensation for evoking the appropriate reflexes that culminate in both the male and female climaxes.

The Female Orgasm. When local sexual stimulation reaches maximum intensity, and especially when the local sensations are supported by appropriate psychic conditioning signals from the cerebrum, reflexes are initiated that cause the female orgasm, also called the *female climax*. The female orgasm is analogous to ejaculation in the male, and it perhaps helps promote fertilization of the ovum. Indeed, the human female is known to be somewhat more fertile when inseminated by normal sexual intercourse rather than by artificial methods, thus indicating an important function of the female orgasm. Possible effects that could result in this are:

First, during the orgasm the perineal muscles of the female contract rhythmically, which results from spinal cord reflexes similar to those that cause ejaculation in the male. It is possible, also, that these same reflexes increase uterine and fallopian tube motility during the orgasm, thus helping to transport the sperm toward the ovum, but the information on this subject is scanty.

Second, in many lower animals, copulation causes the posterior pituitary gland to secrete oxytocin; this effect is probably mediated through the amygdaloid nuclei and then through the hypothalamus to the pituitary. The oxytocin in turn causes increased contractility of the uterus, which also is believed to cause rapid transport of the sperm. Sperm have been shown to traverse the entire length of the fallopian tube in the cow in approximately five minutes, a rate at least 10 times as fast as that which the sperm themselves could achieve. Whether or not this occurs in the human female is unknown.

In addition to the possible effects of the orgasm on fertilization, the intense sexual sensations that develop during the orgasm also pass to the cerebrum and cause intense muscle tension throughout the body. But after culmination of the sexual act, this gives way during the succeeding minutes to a sense of satisfaction characterized by relaxed peacefulness, an effect called *resolution*.

REFERENCES

Arimura, A.: Hypothalamic gonadotropin-releasing hormone and reproduction. *Int. Rev. Physiol., 13*:1, 1977.

Austin, C. R., and Short, R. V. (eds.): Mechanisms of Hormone Action. New York, Cambridge University Press, 1979.

Bargmann, W., *et al.* (eds.): Neurosection and Neuroendocrine Activity; Evolution, Structure and Function. New York, Springer-Verlag, 1978.

Besser, G. M. (ed.): The Hypothalamus and Pituitary. Philadelphia, W. B. Saunders Co., 1977.

Bowers, C. Y., *et al.*: Hypothalamic peptide hormones; Chemistry and physiology. *In* DeGroot, L. J., *et al.* (eds.): Endocrinology. Vol. 1. New York, Grune & Stratton, 1979, p. 65.

Brodish, A., and Lymangrover, J. R.: The hypothalamic-pituitary adrenocortical system. *Int. Rev. Physiol., 16*:93, 1977.

Davis, J. C., and Hipkin, L. J.: Clinical Endocrine Pathology. Philadelphia, J. B. Lippincott Co., 1977.

DeGroot, L. J. (ed.): Endocrinology. New York, Grune & Stratton, 1979.

Dillon, R. S.: Handbook of Endocrinology: Diagnosis and Management of Endocrine and Metabolic Disorders, 2nd Ed. Philadelphia, Lea & Febiger, 1980.

Ezrin, C., *et al.* (eds.): Systematic Endocrinology, 2nd Ed. Hagerstown, Md., Harper & Row, 1979.

Ezrin, C., *et al.* (eds.): Pituitary Diseases. Boca Raton, Fla., CRC Press, 1980.

Fink, G., and Geffen, L. B.: The hypothalamo-hypophysial system: Model for central peptidergic and monoaminergic transmission. *In* Porter, R. (ed.): International Review of Physiology: Neurophysiology III. Vol. 17. Baltimore, University Park Press, 1978, p. 1.

Goss, R. F.: The Physiology of Growth. New York, Academic Press, 1977.

Guillemin, R., and Burgus, R.: The hormones of the hypothalamus. *Sci. Am., 227*:24, 1972.

Jeffcoate, S. L., and Hutchinson, J. S. M. (eds.): The Endocrine Hypothalamus. New York, Academic Press, 1978.

Jubiz, W.: Endocrinology. New York, McGraw-Hill, 1979.

Kastrup, K. W., and Neilsen, J. H. (eds.): Growth Factors: Cellular Growth Processes, Growth Factors, Hormonal Control of Growth. New York, Pergamon Press, 1978.

Kleeman, C. R., and Beri, T.: The neurohypophysial hormones: Vasopressin. *In* DeGroot, L. F., *et al.* (eds.): Endocrinology. Vol. 1, New York, Grune & Stratton, 1979, p. 253.

Kostyo, J. L., and Isaksson, O.: Growth hormone and the regulation of somatic growth. *Int. Rev. Physiol., 13*:255, 1977.

Krulick, L.: Central neurotransmitters and the secretion of prolactin, GH, LH, and TSH. *Annu. Rev. Physiol., 41*:603, 1979.

Krulick, L., and Fawcett, C. P.: The hypothalamic hypophysiotropic hormones. *Int. Rev. Physiol., 16*:35, 1977.

Li, C. H. (ed.): Hypothalamic Hormones. New York, Academic Press, 1979.

McCann, S. M., and Ojeda, S. R.: The role of brain monoamines, acetylcholine and prostaglandins in the control of anterior pituitary function. *In* DeGroot, L. J., *et al.* (eds.): Endocrinology. Vol. 1. New York, Grune & Stratton, 1979, p. 55.

Merimee, T. J.: Growth hormone: Secretion and action. *In* DeGroot, L. J., *et al.* (eds.): Endocrinology. Vol. 1. New York, Grune & Stratton, 1979, p. 123.

Nelson, D. H.: Regulatory mechanisms of the pituitary and pituitary-adrenal axis. *In* Frohlich, E. D. (ed.): Pathophysiology, 2nd Ed. Philadelphia, J. B. Lippincott Co., 1976, p. 327.

Ontjes, D. A., *et al.*: The anterior pituitary gland. *In* Bondy, P. K., and Rosenberg, L. E. (eds.): Metabolic Control and Disease, 8th Ed. Philadelphia, W. B. Saunders Co., 1980, p. 1165.

Polleri, A., and MacLeod, R. M. (eds.): Neuroendocrinology; Biological and Clinical Aspects. New York, Academic Press, 1979.

Ryan, W. G., *et al.* (eds.): Endocrine Disorders: A Pathophysiologic Approach, 2nd Ed. Chicago, Year Book Medical Publishers, 1980.

Sowers, J. R. (eds.): Hypothalamic Hormones. Stroudsburg, Pa., Dowden, Hutchinson & Ross, 1980.

Tepperman, J.: Metabolic and Endocrine Physiology: An Introductory Text. Chicago, Year Book Medical Publishers, 1980.

Tolis, G., *et al.* (eds.): Clinical Neuroendocrinology. New York, Raven Press, 1979.

Vale, W., *et al.*: Regulatory peptides of the hypothalamus. *Annu. Rev. Physiol., 39*:473, 1977.

Vorherr, H.: Oxytocin. *In* DeGroot, L. J., *et al.* (eds.): Endocrinology. Vol. 1. New York, Grune & Stratton, 1979, p. 277.

Weiner, R. L., and Ganong, W. F.: Role of brain monoamines and histamine in regulation of anterior pituitary secretion. *Physiol. Rev. 58*:905, 1978.

Williams, R. H.: Textook of Endocrinology, 5th Ed. Philadelphia, W. B. Saunders Co., 1975.

INDEX

Page numbers in *italics* indicate illustrations. Page numbers followed by t indicate tables.